FIFTH EDITION

Nutrition

FOR HEALTH, FITNESS & SPORT

Melvin H. Williams

Old Dominion University

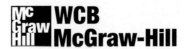
WCB
McGraw-Hill

Boston   Burr Ridge, IL   Dubuque, IA   Madison, WI   New York   San Francisco   St. Louis
Bangkok   Bogotá   Caracas   Lisbon   London   Madrid   Mexico City   Milan
New Delhi   Seoul   Singapore   Sydney   Taipei   Toronto

WCB/McGraw-Hill

A Division of The McGraw-Hill Companies

NUTRITION FOR HEALTH, FITNESS & SPORT, FIFTH EDITION

 This book is printed on recycled, acid-free paper containing 10% postconsumer waste.

1 2 3 4 5 6 7 8 9 0 QPD/QPD 9 0 9 8 7

ISBN 0–697–29510–9

Vice president, editorial director: *Kevin T. Kane*
Publisher: *Edward E. Bartell*
Executive editor: *Colin Wheatley*
Senior developmental editor: *Kassi Radomski*
Marketing manager: *Pamela S. Cooper*
Project manager: *Kay J. Brimeyer*
Production supervisor: *Mary E. Haas*
Coordinator of freelance design: *Michelle D. Whitaker*
Photo research coordinator: *Lori Hancock*
Compositor: *Shepherd, Inc.*
Typeface: *10.2/12.2 Goudy*
Printer: *Quebecor Printing Book Group/Dubuque, IA*

Freelance cover/interior design: *Diane Beasley*
Cover images: © *Index Stock Photography; Inset* © *Tony Stone Images/Chicago Inc.*

PHOTO CREDITS
Chapter 1: 1.4: © Bob Daemmrich/Stock Boston; 1.5: © Mark Antman/The Image Works; 1.7: © Comstock; **Chapter 2:** 2.2 (all), 2.7: © Bob Coyle; 2.8: © David Corona; **Chapter 3:** 3.3: © Melvin Williams; 34.: © David Corona; **Chapter 4:** 4.3: © David Corona; **Chapter 5:** 5.4: © David Corona; **Chapter 6:** 6.3: © David Corona; **Chapter 9:** 9.4: © David Corona; 9.9: © Michael DiSpezio; 9.12: AP/Wide World Photos; **Chapter 10:** 10.2: University of Michigan; 10.3: © Neil Michel/Life Measurement Instruments; **Chapter 11:** 11.3: © David Corona; 11.5: © Melvin Williams; **Chapter 12:** 12.2: © EKM; 12.12: © Melvin Williams.

Library of Congress Cataloging-in-Publication Data

Williams, Melvin H.
   Nutrition for health, fitness & sport / Melvin H. Williams. —
5th ed.
     Previous ed. has title: Nutrition for fitness and health.
     Includes bibliographical references and index.
     ISBN 0–697–29510–9
     1. Nutrition.   2. Physical fitness.   3. Sports—Physiological
aspects.   I. Williams, Melvin H. Nutrition for fitness and sport.
II. Title.
QP141.W514   1999   97–41026
613.2—dc21   CIP

www.mhhe.com

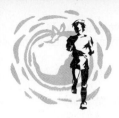

Contents

3

Human Energy   64

4

Carbohydrates: The Main Energy Food   94

5

Fat: An Important Energy Source During Exercise   137

6

Protein: The Tissue Builder   178

7

Vitamins: The Organic Regulators   208

8

Minerals: The Inorganic Regulators   241

9

Water, Electrolytes, and Temperature Regulation 274

10

Body Weight and Composition for Health and Sport 314

Appendixes   416

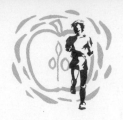

Preface

As we move toward the year 2000, our love affair with fitness and sports continues to grow. Americans and Canadians are no longer nations of spectators; more of us are becoming participants in physical activities such as aerobic dancing, bicycling, golf, running, swimming, tennis, weight lifting, and a host of other recreational activities and sports. Improvement in health and fitness is one of the major reasons that more and more people initiate an exercise program. But many also are finding the joy of athletic competition, such as participation in local 10-kilometer road races.

Research has shown that adults who become physically active also may become more interested in other aspects of their life-styles—particularly nutrition—that may affect their health in a positive way. Indeed, research findings continue to indicate that our diet is one of the most important determinants of our health status.

Moreover, individuals who compete athletically are always looking for a means to improve performance, be it a new piece of equipment or an improved training method. In this regard, proper nutrition may be an important factor in improving physical and athletic performance.

Nutrition is the study of foods and their effects upon health, development, and performance of the individual. The science of human nutrition has made a significant contribution to our knowledge of essential nutrient needs during the early part of this century. More recently, nutrition research has focused on the effects of foods, and their specific constituents, on health and performance. However, because most nutritional studies with humans cannot be controlled under exacting laboratory conditions, human nutrition science is not as precise as other scientific areas of study such as chemistry and physics. Given the basic physiological drives for food and fluid and the psychological overtones that surround our eating behaviors, certain individuals and commercial organizations have exploited this imprecise nature of human nutrition science for financial gains by distorting nutritional facts. Quackery represents fraudulent misrepresentation, and the area of nutrition is filled with numerous nutritional products and dietary supplements that may be classified as fraudulent and marketed to all segments of the population, from young children to the geriatric.

Because they are more likely to be interested in preserving their health, physically active individuals are major targets for those who market and sell nutritional supplements. A variety of media for active people, including the Internet and magazines, are filled with advertisements extolling the virtues of various supplements that are said to do everything from preventing aging to improving athletic performance. Some of these supplements include essential nutrients, such as calcium and vitamin E, whereas others contain compounds of dubious nutritional value, such as coenzyme Q_{10} and vitamin B_{15}, a nonvitamin. One purpose of this book is to help dispel the myths and misconceptions associated with nutrition for physically active individuals.

This book uses a question–answer approach, which is convenient when you have occasional short periods to study such as riding a bus or during a lunch break. In addition, the questions are arranged in a logical sequence, the answer to one question often leading into the question that follows. Where appropriate, cross-referencing within the text is used to expand the discussion. No deep scientific background is needed for the chemical aspects of nutrition and energy expenditure, as these have been simplified. Instructors who use this book as a course text may add details of biochemistry as they feel necessary.

Chapter 1 introduces you to the interrelationships between exercise and nutrition and their effects on health-related and sports-related fitness, while Chapter 2 provides a broad overview of sound guidelines relative to nutrition for optimal health and physical performance. Chapter 3 focuses upon energy and energy pathways in the body, the key to all physical activities.

Chapters 4 through 9 deal with the six basic nutrients—carbohydrate, fat, protein, vitamins, minerals, and water—with emphasis on the health and performance implications for the physically active individual. Chapters 10 through 12 review concepts of body composition and weight control, with suggestions on how to gain or lose body weight through diet and exercise, as well as the implications of such changes for health and athletic performance. Numerous appendixes complement the text, providing data on caloric expenditure during exercise, methods to determine body composition, how to use the

Internet to obtain sound information regarding nutrition and exercise, nutritional value of fast foods, and other information pertinent to physically active individuals.

Key concepts are presented at the beginning of each chapter, a kind of preliminary summary. These can be used for previewing the chapter and for reinforcement once the chapter has been completed. Key terms also are listed at the beginning of the chapter and highlighted, in most cases, when they are first defined in the text. Although some terms may appear in the text before they are defined, a thorough glossary includes the key terms as well as other terms warranting definition.

The bibliographic references are of three types. Books listed provide broad coverage of the major topics in the chapter. Review articles are detailed analyses of selected topics, usually involving a synthesis and analysis of specific research studies. The specific studies listed are primary research studies. The reference lists have been completely updated for this fifth edition and provide the scientific basis for the new concepts or additional support for those concepts previously developed. These references provide greater in-depth reading materials for the interested student. Although the content of this book is based on appropriate scientific studies, a reference-citation style is not used, that is, each statement is not referenced by a bibliographic source. However, names of authors may be used to highlight a reference source where deemed appropriate.

Your involvement in practical activities is encouraged. There are a number of opportunities for the reader to get actively involved: estimation of your percent body fat, estimation of the number of Calories to maintain body weight, designing a 1,200-Calorie diet, calculating the caloric expenditure for a given exercise, or initiating a sound exercise program based upon contemporary principles of exercise prescription.

This book is designed primarily to serve as a college text in professional preparation programs in health and physical education, exercise science, sports medicine, and sports nutrition. It is also directed to the physically active individual interested in the nutritional aspects of physical and athletic performance.

Those who may desire to initiate a physical training program may also find the nutritional information useful, as well as the guidelines for initiating a training program. This book may serve as a handy reference for coaches, trainers, and athletes. With the tremendous expansion of youth sports programs, parents may find the information valuable relative to the nutritional requirements of their active children.

In summary, the major purpose of this book is to help provide a sound knowledge base relative to the role that nutrition, complemented by exercise, may play in the enhancement of both health and sport performance. Hopefully, the information provided in this text will help not only the reader to develop a more healthful diet, but communicate this information to others. Bon appetit!

Supplementary Materials

For instructors

Instructor's Manual and Test Bank

The Instructor's Manual contains objectives, key terms, and outlines for each chapter, and the test bank section contains true-false and multiple-choice questions.

The fifth edition manual once again benefits from the expertise of Gayle A. Runke, M.S., who is presently an assistant professor in the Health, Physical Education, and Recreation department at Southwest Missouri State University. In addition to having co-authored the Instructor's Manual that accompanies the fourth edition of *Nutrition for Fitness & Sport*, she has also written two editions of the Instructor's Manuals that accompany *Lifetime Fitness and Wellness*, also by Melvin Williams.

MicroTest III Computerized Test Bank Instructors who adopt this text can receive the computerized test bank for Windows or Macintosh. This software allows the instructor to select, edit, delete, or add questions, and print tests and answer keys.

Transparencies Twenty-five two-color and black and white acetates feature key illustrations from the text.

Nutrition Videos and Videodiscs Available to qualified adopters. Please contact your local WCB/McGraw-Hill sales representative or Customer Service at 800-338-3987.

Nutri-News Upon request, adopters are given the password to this electronic newsletter (located on the WCB/McGraw-Hill nutrition web site at *http://www.mhhe.com/hper/nutrition/*) made up of nutrition-related articles.

For students

Workbook The Workbook is designed to help students review the concepts presented in the text, and put them to practical use. It contains a variety of exercises and activities including sample multiple-choice, matching, true-false, problems, and essay questions.

The Workbook was prepared by Charlene Harkins, M.Ed., R.D., L.D. Charlene is also certified with the American College of Sports Medicine (ACSM), and is a Fellow of the American Dietetics Association. She presently teaches health and nutrition classes at the University of Minnesota-Duluth.

Annual Editions: Nutrition Supplement any of your nutrition texts with this compilation of carefully selected nutrition-related articles from magazines, newspapers, and journals, which is updated annually.

NutriQuest™ Students will learn more about their own personal health habits with this new dietary analysis software program that allows users to track energy intake and expenditure, set weight goals, and more. This software is available on disk or CD-ROM for Macintosh and Windows.

Questions About These Supplements? If you have any questions about these supplements, please contact your WCB/McGraw-Hill sales representative, or call Customer Service at 800-338-3987.

Acknowledgements

The reviewers of each edition play an integral role in the changes that are made, and this edition is no exception. I wish to extend a special note of appreciation to those who reviewed the fourth edition text, and the fifth edition manuscript:

E. Wayne Askew, Ph.D.
Buffalo State College

Jack C. Benson, M.S.
Eastern Washington University

Jennifer A. Brown, Ed.D.
Auburn University at Montgomery

Laura deGhetaldi, M.S.
University of Colorado at Boulder

Christopher M. DeWitt, Ph.D.
University of South Carolina—Aiken

Pat McSwegin, Ph.D.
University of Missouri—Kansas City

T.C. Proctor, R.D.
Orange Coast College

Christine Rosenbloom, Ph.D.
Georgia State University

Gwyneth Short, M.S., ATC
University of Northern Colorado

Peter M. Tiidus, Ph.D.
Wilfrid Laurier University

Chester J. Zelasko, Ph.D.
Buffalo State College

I would like to acknowledge deep gratitude to Kassi Radomski, Senior Developmental Editor, Nutrition, for her very cooperative and helpful support during the developmental process of this book, and to Kay J. Brimeyer, Senior Project Manager, for her assistance during the production process. Many thanks also to Kris Queck for her meticulous review as a copyeditor. Finally, to the memory of Pat McSwegin for her friendship and input over the years to the development of this book.

Melvin H. Williams
Virginia Beach, Virginia

Introduction to Nutrition for Health, Fitness and Sports Performance

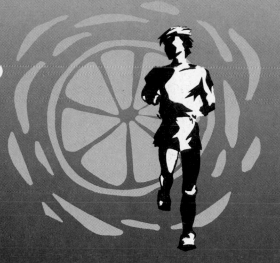

KEY CONCEPTS

- Six of the ten chronic diseases in the United States and Canada (heart diseases, cancer, stroke, lung diseases, diabetes, and liver diseases) may be prevented by appropriate life-style behaviors.

- The two primary determinants of health status are genetics and lifestyle.

- Two of the key health promotion objectives set by the Public Health Service in *Healthy People 2000* are increased levels of physical activity and exercise and improved dietary practices.

- Health-related fitness includes a healthy body weight, cardiovascular-respiratory fitness, adequate muscular strength and endurance, and sufficient flexibility.

- Physical inactivity may be dangerous to your health. As documented in the *Surgeon General's Report on Physical Activity and Health,* exercise, as a form of physical activity, is becoming increasingly important as a means to help prevent, and even treat, many chronic diseases.

- One of the key points of the Surgeon General's report is that physical activity need not be strenuous to achieve health benefits, but additional benefits may be gained through greater amounts of physical activity.

- The primary purpose of the food we eat is to provide us with nutrients essential for the numerous physiological and biochemical functions that support life.

- Poor eating habits span all ages. The Public Health Service in *Healthy People 2000* notes that poor nutrition is a major health problem in the United States.

- Basic guidelines for A Healthy North American Diet include maintenance of proper body weight and consumption of a wide variety of natural foods high in complex carbohydrates and low in fat.

- Although both proper exercise and sound nutrition habits may confer health benefits separately, health benefits may be maximized when both healthy exercise and nutrition life-styles are adopted.

- Success in sports is primarily dependent on genetic endowment and proper training, but nutrition also can be an important contributing factor.

- Studies reveal that although athletes desire to eat a diet that may enhance sport performance, their knowledge of nutrition is inadequate. Surveys indicate athletes are consuming less than the RDA for several nutrients, particularly those attempting to lose weight for competition, and many are not meeting the recommendations of sports nutritionists.

- A dietary supplement is a food product, added to the total diet, that may contain a number of ingredients, including vitamins, minerals, herbs or botanicals, amino acids, metabolites, constituents, extracts, or any combination of the above.

KEY TERMS

A Healthy North American Diet
antipromoters
chronic-training effect
dietary supplement
doping
ergogenic aids
epidemiological research
exercise
experimental research
health-related fitness
malnutrition
meta-analysis
nutraceutical
nutrient
nutrition
physical activity
physical fitness
promoters
quackery
risk factor
sports nutrition
sports-related fitness
structured physical activity
unstructured physical activity

- Although some people may need dietary supplements for various reasons, the use of supplements should not be routine practice for most individuals. Obtain nutrients through natural foods.
- Probably the most prevalent ergogenic aids used to increase sport performance are those classified as nutritional, for theoretical nutritional aids may be found in all six classes of nutrients.
- There appears to be no sphere of nutrition in which faddism, misconceptions, ignorance, and quackery are more obvious than in athletics.
- Nutritional quackery persists in sports for a variety of reasons, including the imitation of dietary practices of star athletes, misleading articles in sports magazines, inadequate nutritional knowledge of coaches, and direct advertising.
- There are a number of guidelines to help identify false claims of dietary supplements, but one of the critical points to consider is if the claim simply appears to be too good to be true.
- The best means to counteract nutritional quackery in sports is to possess a good background in nutrition.
- Prudent nutritional recommendations for enhancement of health or athletic performance are based on reputable research.

INTRODUCTION

There are two major focal points of this book. One is the role that nutrition, complemented by physical activity and exercise, may play in determining one's health status. The other is the role that nutrition may play in the enhancement of fitness and sports performance.

Nutrition, fitness, and health. At a national level, the health care of Americans and Canadians has improved tremendously over the past century. Primarily because of the dedicated work of medical researchers, we no longer fear the scourge of acute infectious diseases such as polio, smallpox, or tuberculosis. However, we have become increasingly concerned with the treatment and prevention of chronic diseases. Six of the ten leading causes of death in the United States are chronic diseases. Given with rank in parentheses, they include: (1) diseases of the heart, (2) cancer, (3) stroke, (4) chronic lung diseases, (7) diabetes, and (10) chronic liver disease and cirrhosis. These diseases cause over 80 percent of all deaths and this figure is destined to rise as the U.S. population becomes increasingly older, particularly during the first quarter of the twenty-first century when the baby boomers of the 1940s and 1950s reach their senior years.

The two primary factors that influence one's health status are genetics and life-style. Most diseases have a genetic basis, but whether or not an individual develops a particular disease may be dependent more upon his or her life-style. For example, cancer is a disease with a strong genetic link, but bad habits and an unhealthy life-style, such as smoking, poor diet, and lack of exercise cause about two-thirds of cancer deaths.

Although the treatment of these major chronic diseases has greatly improved through techniques such as coronary artery bypass surgery, radiation treatment, and drug therapy, the healing process may be prolonged and very expensive. Foreseeing a financial health care crisis for the government in the twenty-first century, most health professionals have advocated prevention as the best approach to address this potential major health problem. In this regard, the Public Health Service of the United States Department of Health and Human Services has published a report entitled *Healthy People 2000: National Health Promotion/Disease Prevention Objectives.* One of the major sections of this report deals with health promotion, which includes a number of life-style factors that are basically under the control of the individual. C. Everett Koop, the former Surgeon General of the United States, has noted that the best way to decrease the demand for health care is for each one of us to take charge of our own health.

Over the years, scientists in the field of epidemiology have identified a number of life-style factors considered to be health risks; these life-style factors are known as risk factors. A **risk factor** is a health behavior that has been associated with a particular disease, such as cigarette smoking being linked to lung cancer. As we shall see, exercise and proper nutrition, both individually and combined, may reduce many of the risk factors associated with the development of chronic diseases. These healthful benefits will be addressed at appropriate points throughout the book.

Nutrition, fitness, and sport. Sport is now most commonly defined as a competitive athletic activity requiring skill or physical prowess, for example, baseball, basketball, soccer, football, racing, wrestling, tennis, and golf. As with health status, athletic ability and subsequent success in sport are based primarily upon two factors: natural genetic endowment and state of training. To be successful at high levels of competition, the athlete must possess the appropriate biomechanical, physiological, and psychological genetic characteristics associated with success in a given sport, and these genetic characteristics must be developed maximally through proper biomechanical, physiological, and psychological coaching and training.

Specialized exercise training is the major means to improve athletic performance. Athletes at all levels of competition, whether for an Olympic gold medal or an age-group award in a local road race, are always interested in ways to improve their performance and gain an edge on the competition. There is nothing an athlete can do to modify his or her genetic endowment, but training programs have become more intense and individualized, resulting in significant performance gains.

Proper nutrition is also an important component in the total training program of the athlete. Certain nutrient deficiencies can seriously impair performance, while supplementation of other nutrients may help delay fatigue and improve performance. Over the past three decades, research has provided us with many answers about the role of nutrition in athletic performance, but unfortunately some findings have been misinterpreted or exaggerated so that a number of misconceptions still exist.

The purpose of this chapter is to provide a broad overview of the role that nutrition may play relative to health, fitness, and sport, and how prudent recommendations may be determined. More detailed information regarding specific relationships of nutritional practices to health and sports performance is provided in the following chapters.

Nutrition, Exercise, and Health-Related Fitness

Physical fitness may be defined, in general terms, as a set of abilities individuals possess to perform specific types of physical activity. The development of physical fitness is an important concern of many professional health organizations, including the American Alliance for Health, Physical Education, Recreation, and Dance (AAHPERD), which has categorized fitness components into two different categories. In general, these two categories may be referred to as health-related fitness and sports-related fitness. Both types of fitness may be influenced by nutrition and exercise.

Exercise and Health-Related Fitness

What is health-related fitness?

As mentioned above, one's health status is influenced strongly by hereditarian predisposition and life-style behaviors, particularly appropriate physical activity and a high-quality diet. As we shall see in various sections of this book, one of the key factors in preventing the development of chronic disease is maintaining a healthful body weight.

Proper physical activity may certainly improve one's health status by helping to prevent excessive weight gain, but it may also enhance other facets of health-related fitness as well. **Health-related fitness** includes not only a healthy body weight and composition, but also cardiovascular-respiratory fitness, adequate muscular strength and endurance, and sufficient flexibility (Figure 1.1). Several health professional organizations, such as the American College of Sports Medicine (ACSM), have indicated that various forms of physical activity may be used to enhance health.

In general, **physical activity** involves any bodily movement caused by muscular contraction that results in the expenditure of energy. For purposes of studying its effects on health, epidemiologists classify physical activity as either unstructured or structured.

Unstructured physical activity includes many of the usual activities of daily life, such as walking, climbing stairs, leisurely cycling, dancing, gardening and yard work, various domestic and occupational activities, and games and other childhood pursuits.

Structured physical activity, as the name implies, is a planned program of physical activities usually designed to improve physical fitness, including health-related fitness. For the purpose of this book, we shall refer to structured physical activity as **exercise,** particularly some form of planned vigorous exercise.

What is the role of exercise in health promotion?

As is for physical activity, exercise is becoming increasingly important as a means to help prevent, and even treat, many of the chronic diseases that afflict developed societies, including coronary artery disease, stroke, hypertension, cancer, diabetes, arthritis, osteoporosis, chronic lung disease, and obesity. Indeed, some physicians indicate that exercise is the best medicine of all because it offers such an array of health benefits.

Numerous scientific reports have detailed the health benefits of regular physical activity, including *Physical Activity, Fitness and Health* by Claude Bouchard, Roy Shephard, and Thomas Stephens; the World Forum International Scientific Consensus Conference on Physical Activity, Health, and Well Being; the National Institutes of Health (NIH) Consensus Development Conference on Physical Activity and Cardiovascular Health; the ACSM and Centers for Disease Control and Prevention (CDC) report on Physical Activity and Public Health; and, most notably, the recent release of *The Surgeon General's Report on Physical Activity and Health.* Collectively, as presented in Table 1.1, these reports document the significant health benefits of habitual physical activity. These benefits may accrue to males and females of all races across all age spans. You are never too young or too old to reap the health benefits of exercise.

In essence, physically active individuals enjoy a higher quality of life, a *joie de vivre,* because they are less likely to

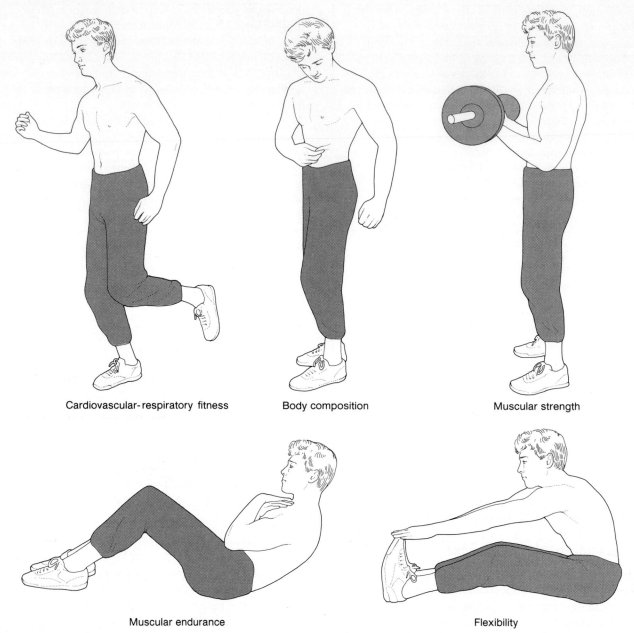

Cardiovascular-respiratory fitness

Body composition

Muscular strength

Muscular endurance

Flexibility

Figure 1.1 Health-related fitness components. The most important physical fitness components related to personal health include cardiovascular-respiratory fitness, body and composition, muscular strength, muscular endurance, and flexibility.

suffer the disabling symptoms often associated with chronic diseases, such as loss of ambulation experienced by some stroke victims. Indeed, physical activity may also increase the quantity of life. Lee and Paffenbarger estimated that a physically active life-style may add approximately two years of life by averting premature mortality.

The role that exercise may play in the prevention of some chronic diseases, such as diabetes, and other associated risk factors, such as obesity, are discussed throughout this book where relevant.

Do most of us exercise enough?

In general, no. Surveys reveal that most Americans have little or no physical activity in their daily lives. Although about 15 percent of U.S. adults engage regularly in vigorous physical activity at least three times a week during leisure time, more than 60 percent do not engage in recommended amounts of physical activity and approximately 25 percent are not active at all. Physical activity is more common among men than women, but decreases with age. Nearly half of American youths are not vigorously active on a regular basis, and participation in all types of physical activity declines strikingly as age or grade in school increases.

In *Healthy People 2000*, the Public Health Service has established various physical activity and fitness objectives to increase both unstructured and structured physical activity for children, adolescents, and adults in order to develop cardiovascular fitness, to increase muscular

Table 1.1 Possible health benefits of physical activity
Reduces the risk of dying prematurely
Reduces the risk of dying from heart disease
Reduces the risk of developing diabetes
Reduces the risk of developing high blood pressure
Helps reduce blood pressure in people who already have high blood pressure
Reduces the risk of developing colon cancer
Reduces feelings of depression and anxiety
Helps control body weight
Helps build and maintain healthy bones, muscles, and joints
Helps older adults become stronger and better able to move about without falling
Promotes psychological well-being and self-efficacy

Adapted from U.S. Department of Health and Human Services. *The Surgeon General's Report on Physical Activity and Health.*

Table 1.2 Some examples of moderate amounts of physical activity*
Washing and waxing a car for 45–60 minutes
Washing windows or floors for 45–60 minutes
Playing various team sports for 45 minutes
Gardening for 30–45 minutes
Wheeling self in wheelchair for 30–40 minutes
Walking 2 miles in 40 minutes (20 minutes/mile)
Bicycling 5 miles in 30 minutes (10 miles/hour)
Dancing (social) fast for 30 minutes
Walking 2 miles in 30 minutes (15 minutes/mile)
Water aerobics for 30 minutes
Swimming laps for 20 minutes
Bicycling 4 miles in 15 minutes (3.75 minutes/mile)
Jumping rope for 15 minutes
Running 1.5 miles in 15 minutes (10 minutes/mile)
Stairwalking for 15 minutes

*A moderate amount of physical activity is roughly equivalent to physical activity that uses 150 Calories per day, or 1,000 Calories per week. Note that exercising at lower intensity levels requires more time (walking 2 miles in 40 minutes) than exercising at higher intensity levels (running 1.5 miles in 15 minutes).

Adapted from U.S. Department of Health and Human Services. *The Surgeon General's Report on Physical Activity and Health.*

strength, muscular endurance, and flexibility, and to attain an appropriate body weight. Details of these objectives may be found in Appendix M.

What are some general guidelines for exercising properly for someone who wants to be more physically active?

One of the key points of the *Surgeon General's Report on Physical Activity and Health* is that physical activity need not be strenuous to achieve health benefits. Children, adolescents, and men and women of all ages may benefit from a moderate amount of daily physical activity. This physical activity may be unstructured, such as washing the car or raking leaves, or structured, such as brisk walking or running. The benefits of moderate activity may be obtained in longer sessions of moderately intense activities (such as 40 minutes of walking) or in shorter sessions of somewhat more strenuous activities (such as 15–20 minutes of running). You should try to average 30 minutes of moderate exercise per day most, and preferably all, days of the week. You may accumulate 30 minutes per day in several sessions, such as three 10-minute brisk walks interspersed throughout the day. Some examples of moderate amounts of physical activity are presented in Table 1.2.

The Surgeon General's report also indicates that additional health benefits can be gained through greater amounts of physical activity. Adults who maintain a regular routine of physical activity that is of longer duration or of greater intensity are likely to derive greater benefit.

Lee and Paffenbarger also note a dose-response relation of exercise to longevity, with the most active or fit individuals experiencing mortality rates that are up to one-half lower than the rates among those least active or fit. However, the Surgeon General's report indicates that care should be taken to avoid excessive amounts of high-intensity exercise because of increased risk of injury or other health problems, such as menstrual abnormalities. This is particularly true for individuals who are exercising solely for health improvement.

The American College of Sports Medicine has developed recommendations for the quantity and quality of exercise for developing and maintaining health-related fitness, including exercise programs for the development of cardiovascular fitness, muscular strength and endurance, and flexibility. These ACSM recommendations, along with some guidelines provided by the President's Council on Physical Fitness and Sports, underlie the basics of designing an aerobics program for cardiovascular-respiratory fitness and proper weight control presented in Chapter 11 and the principles of resistance training for muscular strength and endurance presented in Chapter 12.

Nutrition and Health-Related Fitness

What is nutrition?

Nutrition usually is defined as the sum total of the processes involved in the intake and utilization of food substances by living organisms, including ingestion, digestion, absorption, and metabolism of food. This definition stresses the biochemical or physiological functions of the food we eat, but the American Dietetic Association notes that nutrition may be interpreted in a broader sense and be affected by a variety of psychological, sociological, and economic factors.

Although our food selection may be influenced by these latter factors, particularly economic ones in the case of many college students, the biochemical and physiological roles of many different types of food are similar. From a standpoint of health and sport performance, it is the biochemical and physiological role or function of food that is important.

The primary purpose of the food we eat is to provide us with a variety of nutrients. A **nutrient** is a specific substance found in food that performs one or more physiological or biochemical functions in the body. There are six major classes of nutrients found in foods: carbohydrates, fats, proteins, vitamins, minerals, and water.

As illustrated in Figure 1.2, these nutrients perform three major functions. First, they provide energy for human metabolism (see Chapter 3). Carbohydrates and fats are the prime sources of energy. Protein may also provide energy, but this is not its major function. Vitamins, minerals, and water are not energy sources. Second, nutrients are used to promote growth and development by building and repairing body tissue. Protein is the major building material for muscles, other soft tissues, and enzymes, while certain minerals such as calcium and phosphorus make up the skeletal framework. Third, nutrients are used to help regulate metabolism, or body processes. Vitamins, minerals, and proteins work closely together to maintain the diverse physiological processes of human metabolism. For example, hemoglobin in the red blood cell (RBC) is essential for the transport of oxygen to muscle tissue via the blood. Hemoglobin is a complex combination of protein and iron, but other minerals and vitamins are needed for its synthesis and for full development of the RBC.

As detailed in Chapter 2, in order for our bodies to function effectively we need more than forty specific essential nutrients, and we need these nutrients in various amounts as specified by the Recommended Dietary Allowances (RDA). Nutrient deficiencies or excesses may cause various health problems, some very serious.

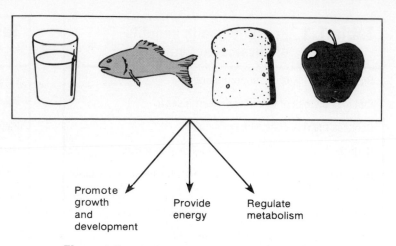

Promote growth and development

Provide energy

Regulate metabolism

Figure 1.2   Three major functions of nutrients in food. Many nutrients have only one key role (e.g., glucose provides energy), whereas others have multiple roles (e.g., protein is necessary for growth and development and regulation of metabolism, but it may also be used as a source of energy).

What is the role of nutrition in health promotion?

Let food be your medicine and medicine be your food. This statement has been attributed to Hippocrates for over two thousand years, and it is becoming increasingly meaningful as the preventative and therapeutic health values of food relative to the development of chronic diseases are being unraveled.

Most chronic diseases have a genetic basis; if one of your parents has had coronary heart disease or cancer, you have an increased probability of contracting that disease. Such diseases may go through three stages: initiation, promotion, and progression. Your genetic predisposition may lead to the initiation stage of the disease, but factors in your environment promote its development and eventual progression. In this regard, some nutrients are believed to be **promoters** that lead to the progression of the disease, while other nutrients are believed to be **antipromoters** that deter the initiation process from progressing to a serious health problem.

What you eat plays an important role in the development or progression of a variety of chronic diseases, such as coronary heart disease, diabetes, high blood pressure, osteoporosis, obesity, and a variety of different cancers (see Figure 1.3). For example, the National Cancer Institute estimates that one-third of all cancers are linked in some way to diet, ranking just behind tobacco smoking as one of the major causes of cancer.

Do we eat right?

Surveys indicate that most people are aware of the role of nutrition in health and want to eat better for healthful purposes, but they do not translate their desires into appropriate action. Although some small progress has been

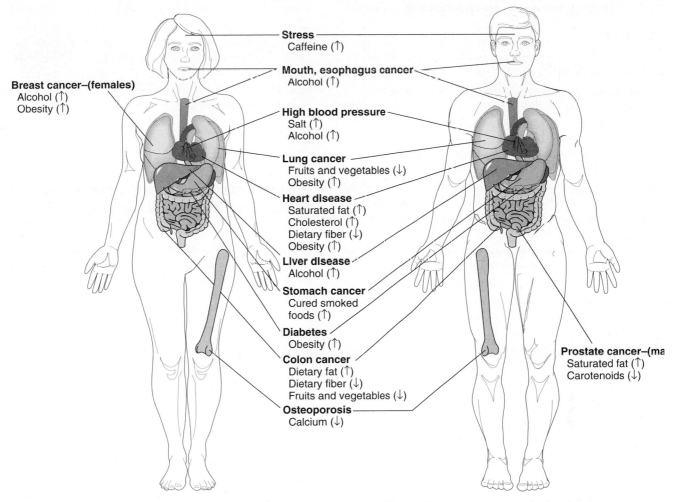

Stress
Caffeine (↑)

Mouth, esophagus cancer
Alcohol (↑)

Breast cancer–(females)
Alcohol (↑)
Obesity (↑)

High blood pressure
Salt (↑)
Alcohol (↑)

Lung cancer
Fruits and vegetables (↓)
Obesity (↑)

Heart disease
Saturated fat (↑)
Cholesterol (↑)
Dietary fiber (↓)
Obesity (↑)

Liver disease
Alcohol (↑)

Stomach cancer
Cured smoked
foods (↑)

Diabetes
Obesity (↑)

Colon cancer
Dietary fat (↑)
Dietary fiber (↓)
Fruits and vegetables (↓)

Osteoporosis
Calcium (↓)

Prostate cancer–(ma
Saturated fat (↑)
Carotenoids (↓)

Figure 1.3 Some possible health problems associated with poor dietary habits. An upward arrow (↑) indicates excessive intake while downward arrow (↓) indicates low intake or deficiency.

made in meeting the nutrition goals of *Healthy People 2000* since they were established in 1992, such as a slight decrease in total and saturated fat intake, intermediate reviews suggest that most nutrition objectives will not likely be realized. In fact, progress toward some objectives is moving in the opposite direction. For example, the prevalence of overweight people in the population is increasing, not decreasing.

Poor eating habits span all age groups. The Centers for Disease Control and Prevention and the American Dietetic Association noted that most young people do not have healthy eating habits. They eat too much total fat and saturated fat (derived mainly from fast-food diets and high-fat snacks), many are overweight, and many are chronically dieting. Other health professionals have reiterated this point for the general population. For example, the Public Health Service, in their report *Healthy People 2000*, note that poor nutrition is one of the major health problems in our country. As a nation, many Americans are overweight, eat too much fat and salt, and eat too few complex-carbohydrate and fiber-containing foods such as fruits and vegetables; many women and children do not consume enough foods rich in calcium and iron.

To relate these nutrition findings to health in simplistic terms, most Americans eat more food than they need and eat less of the food that they need more. In essence, the major nutrition goal of *Healthy People 2000* is to get more Americans to change their faulty dietary habits. The specific nutrition objectives of *Healthy People 2000* are listed in Appendix M.

What are some general guidelines for healthy eating?

Because the prevention of chronic diseases is of critical importance, thousands of studies have been and are being conducted to discover the intricacies of how various nutrients may affect our health. Particular interest is focused on nutrient function in body cells at the molecular level, the interaction effect of various nutrients, and the identification of other protective factors in certain foods. All of the answers are not in, but sufficient evidence is available to provide us with some useful, prudent guidelines for healthful eating practices.

Over the past two decades, in response to the need for healthier diets, a variety of public and private health organizations analyzed the research relating diet to health and developed some basic guidelines for the general public. The details underlying these recommendations may be found in several voluminous governmental reports, including *Diet and Health: Implications for Reducing Chronic Disease Risk* by the National Research Council, the *Surgeon General's Report on Nutrition and Health* by the Office of the Surgeon General, and the fourth edition of *Nutrition and Your Health: Dietary Guidelines for Americans* released by the U.S. Departments of Agriculture and Health and Human Services in 1996. Recommendations offered by other professional health groups, such as the American Cancer Society, the American Dietetic Association, and the American Heart Association complement these reports. Although most of the guidelines are directed to the general population, there is increasingly strong support for developing separate guidelines for children.

The following dozen guidelines represent the essence of the recommendations emanating from these reports, which collectively might be called simply **A Healthy North American Diet.**

1. Balance the food you eat with physical activity to maintain or improve your weight.

2. Eat a nutritionally adequate diet consisting of a wide variety of foods.

3. Choose a diet low in total fat, saturated fat, and cholesterol.

4. Choose a diet with plenty of whole grain products, legumes, fruits, and vegetables, which are rich in complex carbohydrates and fiber.

5. Choose a diet moderate in sugars.

6. Choose a diet moderate in salt and sodium.

7. If you drink alcoholic beverages, do so in moderation. Pregnant women should not drink any alcohol.

8. Maintain protein intake at a moderate, yet adequate level, obtaining much of your daily protein from plant sources.

9. Choose a diet adequate in calcium and iron.

10. Children and others susceptible to tooth decay should obtain adequate fluoride.

11. In general, avoid taking dietary supplements in excess of the RDA in any one day.

12. Eat fewer foods with questionable additives.

An expanded discussion of these guidelines along with practical recommendations to help you implement them is presented in Chapter 2. Additional details on how each specific recommendation may affect your health status is presented in appropriate chapters throughout this book. For example, inadequate dietary intake of calcium and iron may cause, respectively, osteoporosis and anemia. These topics are covered in Chapter 8, Minerals: The Inorganic Regulators.

You may wish to take the brief dietary inventory in Appendix I to provide you with a general analysis of your current eating habits.

Are there additional health benefits when both exercise and diet habits are improved?

Most chronic diseases are caused by the interaction of many factors, including genetic factors and multiple independent life-style behaviors. To decrease our risk of developing any given disease, we should attempt to reduce as many risk factors as possible that are associated with the development of that disease. In several recent articles, Steven Blair and his associates have noted that although numerous studies have demonstrated the beneficial effects of nutrition and physical activity separately to help reduce various risk factors associated with chronic diseases, there are fewer studies available that describe the synergistic effects of exercise and diet to promote health.

Nevertheless, although both proper exercise and sound nutrition habits may confer health benefits separately, the reduction in the sum total of risk factors would appear to be maximized when both exercise and nutrition are part of a healthy life-style. As indicated in Table 1.3, which highlights risk factors for heart disease, the key life-style behaviors that may be effective in favorably modifying heart disease risk factors are proper nutrition and exercise. Moreover, several of the risk factors for heart disease are diseases themselves, such as diabetes, obesity, and high blood pressure, all of which may benefit from the combination of proper nutrition and exercise.

As shall be noted in Chapter 11, a combination diet-exercise regimen is the favored approach for prevention and treatment of obesity, a disease unto itself and a major risk factor for other chronic diseases. The possible complementary effect of exercise and nutrition on other chronic diseases, such as osteoporosis, will be presented in later chapters as appropriate.

Nutrition, Exercise, and Sports-Related Fitness

As with health, genetic endowment plays an important underlying role in the development of success in sport, but so too do life-style behaviors, such as appropriate sports training and sports nutrition.

Table 1.3 Risk factors associated with coronary heart disease

Risk factors	Classification	Positive health life-style modification
High blood pressure	Major	Proper nutrition, aerobic exercise
High blood lipids	Major	Proper nutrition, aerobic exercise
Smoking	Major	Stop smoking
ECG abnormalities	Major	Proper nutrition, aerobic exercise
Obesity	Major	Low-Calorie diet, aerobic exercise
Diabetes	Major	Proper nutrition, weight loss, aerobic exercise
Stressful life-style	Contributory	Stress management
Dietary intake	Contributory	Proper nutrition
Sedentary life-style	Contributory	Aerobic exercise
Oral contraceptives	Contributory	Alternative methods of birth control
Family history	Major	Not modifiable
Gender	Contributory	Not modifiable
Race	Contributory	Not modifiable
Age	Contributory	Not modifiable

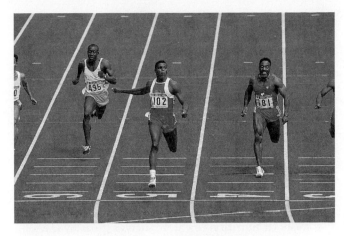

Figure 1.4 Elite athletes are exposed to state-of-the-art physiological, psychological, and biomechanical training that may mean the difference between the gold and silver medal in world-class competition.

What is sports-related fitness?

One of the key factors determining success in sport is the ability to maximize your genetic potential with appropriate physical and mental training to prepare both mind and body for intense competition. In this regard, athletes develop **sports-related fitness,** that is, fitness components such as strength, power, speed, endurance, and neuromuscular motor skills specific to their sport.

Training of elite athletes at the United States Olympic Training Center (USOTC) focuses on three attributes: physical power, mental strength, and mechanical edge. Coaches and scientists work with athletes to maximize physical power production for their specific sport, to optimize mental strength in accordance with the psychological demands of the sport, and to provide the best mechanical edge by improving specific sport skills, sportswear, and sports equipment. Jay Kearney, senior sports scientist at the USOTC, has noted that sports sci-

ence and technology are today providing elite competitors with the tiny margins needed to win in world-class competition (Figure 1.4).

Athletes at all levels of competition, whether an elite international competitor, a college wrestler, a high school baseball player, or a youth league soccer player, can best improve their performance by intense training appropriate for their age, physical and mental development, and sport. As the saying goes, "Do the best with what you got." However, as mentioned previously, sports and exercise scientists have investigated a number of means to improve athletic performance beyond that attributable to training, and one of the most extensively investigated areas has been the effect of nutrition.

What is sports nutrition?

As noted above, state-of-the-art physical and mental training is one of the most important factors underlying success in sports. At high levels of athletic competition, athletes generally receive excellent coaching to enhance their biomechanical skills, sharpen their psychological focus, and maximize physiological functions essential for optimal performance.

As we shall see, there are various dietary factors that may influence biomechanical, psychological, and physiological considerations in sport. For example, losing excess body fat will enhance biomechanical efficiency, consuming carbohydrates during exercise may maintain normal blood sugar levels and prevent psychological fatigue, and providing adequate dietary iron may ensure optimal oxygen delivery to the muscles, all sports nutrition factors that may impact favorably upon athletic performance.

Sports nutrition is a relatively new area of study involving the application of nutritional principles to enhance sports performance. Although investigators have studied the interactions between nutrition and various forms of sport or exercise for more than a hundred years, it is only within the past few decades that extensive research has been undertaken regarding specific recommendations to athletes.

Several factors suggest that sport nutrition is becoming increasingly important for optimal athletic performance, and is a viable career opportunity.

1. Probably the most important factor is the amount of research conducted over the past 30 years concerning the interactions of nutrition and physical performance. Numerous studies have been conducted world-wide in exercise science laboratories dedicated to sports nutrition research, such as those by David Costill and his associates at Ball State University and those by Wim Saris and Fred Brouns at the University of Maastrict, Netherlands.

2. Another indication is that national and international food product corporations are manufacturing sports drinks, sports bars, and other food products specifically for the athlete or physically active individual. Although smaller companies have marketed nutritional products for athletes for years, international firms such as Quaker Oats, M&M Mars, Wander Limited, Coca-Cola, and PepsiCo have become increasingly involved in marketing sports nutrition products, sponsoring sports nutrition–related research, and funding international meetings and publications that focus on the importance of sports nutrition.

3. A third factor is the formation of SCAN (Sports and Cardiovascular Nutritionists), a subsection within the American Dietetic Association concerned with the application of nutrition to sport and health. SCAN members include registered dieticians who have taken special courses and are marketing their services as sports nutritionists, some being employed by professional and university athletic teams.

4. Still another factor is the development of courses in sports nutrition at many colleges and universities throughout the world to help prepare future coaches, athletic trainers, and other sports medicine personnel to better advise athletes on sound nutritional practices. Some universities that have departments of nutrition and sports/exercise science have developed complete curricular programs of study in sports nutrition.

5. Finally, the published literature about nutrition for sport has become voluminous. The *International Journal of Sport Nutrition*, a research publication, has been initiated. Almost every scientific journal in sport/exercise science contains at least one study or review in each issue that is sport nutrition–related. Numerous magazines have been developed for specific groups of athletes pursuing almost every kind of sport, such as runners, swimmers, triathletes, bodybuilders, and weight lifters. Invariably each issue contains a nutrition-related article, and several magazines, such as *Runner's World*, employ nutrition editors with Ph.D.s in nutrition. In addition, many excellent books have recently been written on sports nutrition, several of which are mentioned later in this chapter. Because of the demand for information, the Food and Nutrition Information Center of the National Agricultural Library has developed a bibliographic resource, *Nutri-Topic*, in sports nutrition for the health professional/researcher, the educator, or the consumer.

Sports nutrition as we know it today has a relatively short history, but it appears to be an important aspect in the total preparation of the athlete, as documented by the developments cited above and the position stand entitled "Nutrition for Physical Fitness and Athletic Performance for Adults" issued jointly by the American and Canadian Dietetic Associations.

Are athletes today receiving adequate nutrition?

The dietary habits of athletes may vary tremendously, particularly when different sports are compared. Surveys conducted with several different groups of athletes reveal that some athletes may be obtaining an adequate intake of nutrients while others may not. An excellent review is presented by Sarah Short of Syracuse University who provides a critique of the validity and usefulness of various survey techniques used to assess average nutrient intake. The usual method in these studies was to obtain a three- to seven-day record of the food intake of the athletes and then use computer analyses to compare their intake with the RDA for a variety of nutrients. Although not all studies are in agreement, certain athletic groups, such as football players and strength athletes, appear to obtain adequate nutrition, while inadequate nutrient intakes have been reported in other athletic groups, including ballet dancers, basketball players, bodybuilders, gymnasts, runners, skiers, swimmers, triathletes, and wrestlers.

These nutrient deficiencies were noted in athletes of abilities ranging from the high school level to Olympic caliber. Females were much more likely than males to incur nutrient deficiencies. The most significant nutrient deficiency in most studies was iron, although zinc, calcium, protein, and several of the B vitamins also were found to be deficient by several investigators. In many of these reports, the nutrient deficiencies were due to a very low caloric intake. Several studies also noted that the percentage of Calories derived from carbohydrate was lower than that recommended for endurance athletes.

The athletic groups most susceptible to a nutrient deficiency are those attempting to lose weight for sports competition, notably dancers, gymnasts, bodybuilders, runners, and wrestlers. In one nationwide survey of the nutritional habits of elite athletes, the investigators noted that in sports in which body weight and composition are important, such as gymnastics and ballet, nutrient intake may be marginal. In addition, several studies have revealed a high incidence of eating disorders in these groups of athletes as they adopted bizarre techniques in attempts to control body weight. Although a small percentage of male athletes exhibit disordered eating behaviors, this problem is more prevalent in females. This topic is addressed in Chapter 10.

Compared with the recommendations of sports nutritionists, many endurance athletes consume a diet which may be considered deficient in carbohydrates. Although Hawley and others indicate that such diets have not been shown to impair athletic performance, they suggest that an increased carbohydrate intake would probably improve an athlete's training capacity, especially when rapid recovery between intense exercise bouts is required. Theoretically, this enhanced training would lead to improved performance in competition.

This brief review indicates that some athletic groups are not receiving the RDA for a variety of essential nutrients or may not be meeting certain recommended standards. It should be noted, however, that these surveys have only analyzed the diets of the athletes in reference to a standard, such as the RDA, and have not analyzed performance capacity or the effects that the dietary deficiency exerted on athletic performance. The RDA for vitamins and minerals incorporates a safety factor, so an individual with a dietary intake of essential nutrients below the RDA will not necessarily suffer a true nutrient deficiency. On the other hand, if the athlete does develop a nutrient deficiency, then athletic performance may deteriorate, and some deficiencies may lead to injuries.

Many athletes do not appear to be getting adequate nutrition for a number of reasons. In a recent report, several international sports nutrition experts indicated that although athletes may be making conscious efforts to eat an appropriate diet, they may be confused about the nutrient content of the foods they eat. These feelings have been reinforced by Short in her extensive review and subsequent studies that have shown that the nutritional knowledge of athletes is relatively poor; hence, the athlete may not have the basis to select and prepare nutritious meals. Other constraints, such as finances and time, may limit food selection and preparation.

Moreover, athletes may not be receiving sound nutritional information from their coaches or trainers. Several surveys cited by Short revealed that many coaches at the high school and college levels have poor backgrounds in nutrition, with approximately 60 to 80 percent of the coaches noting that they had not had a formal course in nutrition or were in need of a better background. However, this situation appears to be changing as many coaches and athletic trainers are taking college level courses in nutrition, some courses specifically in sports nutrition. The National Athletic Trainers Association requires a course in nutrition for certification.

How important is nutrition to athletic performance?

As mentioned previously, the ability to perform well in an athletic event is dependent primarily upon two factors: genetic endowment and state of training. First and foremost is genetic endowment. The individual athlete must possess the characteristics that are necessary for success in his or her chosen sport. For example, a world-class male marathoner must have a high aerobic capacity and a low body fat percentage in order to run over 26 sub-five-minute miles. However, unless he has undergone a strenuous training program and maximized his genetic potential, his performance will be suboptimal. The state of training is the most important factor differentiating athletes of comparable genetic endowment. The better-trained athlete has the advantage. No matter at what level the athlete is competing, be it a world championship or a high school swimming meet, genetic endowment and state of training are the two most critical factors determining success. Nevertheless, the nutritional status of the athlete may also exert a significant impact upon athletic performance. An internationally renowned Olympic sports medicine physician, L. Prokop, has noted that again and again he has seen a minor, seemingly negligible mistake in the diet ruin many months and years of hard training at the critical moment.

Malnutrition represents unbalanced nutrition and may exist as either undernutrition or overnutrition, that is, an individual does not receive an adequate intake (undernutrition) or consumes excessive amounts of single or multiple nutrients (overnutrition). Either condition can hamper athletic performance. As noted previously, the three major functions of foods are to supply energy, regulate metabolism, and build and repair body tissues. Thus, an inadequate intake of certain nutrients may impair athletic performance due to an insufficient energy supply, an inability to regulate exercise metabolism at an optimal level, or a decreased synthesis of key body tissues or enzymes. On the other hand, excessive intake of some nutrients may also impair athletic performance, and even the health of the athlete, by disrupting normal physiological processes or leading to undesirable changes in body composition.

Nutrition for the physically active person may be viewed from two aspects: nutrition for competition and nutrition for training. Of the three basic purposes of food—to provide energy, to regulate metabolic processes, and to support growth and development—the first two are of prime importance during athletic competition, while all three need to be considered during the training period in preparation for competition.

Nutrition for Competition In competition an athlete will utilize specific body energy sources and systems, depending upon the intensity and duration of the exercise. The three human energy systems will be discussed in detail in Chapter 3. Briefly, however, high energy compounds stored in the muscle are utilized during very short, high-intensity exercise; carbohydrate stored in the muscle as glycogen may be used without oxygen for intense exercise lasting about 1 to 3 minutes; and the oxidation of glycogen and fats becomes increasingly important in endurance activities lasting longer than 5 minutes. The release of energy in each of these three systems may require certain vitamins and minerals for optimal efficiency.

If an individual is well nourished, athletic competition will not impose any special demands for any of the six major classes of nutrients. Body energy stores of carbohydrate and fat are adequate to satisfy the energy demands of most activities lasting less than 1 hour. Protein is not generally considered a significant energy source during exercise. The vitamin and mineral content of the body will be sufficient to help regulate the increased levels of metabolic activity, and body-water supply will be adequate under normal environmental conditions.

However, certain dietary modifications may enhance performance when used prior to or during competition. For example, on the basis of the available research evidence, carbohydrate intake prior to and during exercise bouts of long duration at moderate to high intensity and adequate fluid intake prior to and during similar endurance events conducted in warm or hot environmental conditions are two dietary practices that have consistently been shown to increase performance capacity. Specific dietary recommendations will be presented in Chapters 4 and 9.

Although not all research findings are in agreement, a number of well-designed studies with several other nutrients or related compounds have documented beneficial effects upon laboratory and field exercise tasks comparable to competitive athletic events. With some of these compounds, such as sodium bicarbonate, the scientific evidence supportive of a beneficial effect is somewhat strong whereas with others, such as sodium phosphate, the data are less conclusive. The potential for all nutrients to enhance competitive performance will be discussed where relevant in the remaining chapters, as will the efficacy of various commercial nutritional supplements targeted for athletes.

Nutrition for Training Proper nutrition during training is one of the keys to success in competition. Because energy expenditure increases during a training period, the caloric intake needed to maintain body weight may increase considerably—an additional 500–1,000 Calories or more per day in certain activities. By selecting these additional Calories wisely from a wide variety of foods, you should obtain an adequate amount of all nutrients essential for the formation of new body tissues and proper functioning of the energy systems that work harder during exercise. A balanced intake of carbohydrate, fat, protein, vitamins, minerals, and water is all that is necessary. For endurance athletes, dietary carbohydrates should receive even greater emphasis.

During the early phases of training, the body will begin to make adjustments in the energy systems so that they become more efficient. This is the so-called **chronic-training effect,** and many of the body's adjustments incorporate specific nutrients. For example, one of the chronic effects of long distance running is an increased hemoglobin content in the blood and increased myoglobin and cytochromes in the muscle cells; all three compounds need iron in order to be formed. Hence, the daily diet would need to contain adequate amounts of iron to make effective body adjustments due to the chronic effects of training.

Based on the available scientific data, nutrient supplementation does not appear to be necessary for the well-nourished athlete during training. However, there are a number of viable theories suggesting certain nutrients may be helpful. For example, during strenuous training vitamin E has been theorized to help prevent tissue damage, and various amino acid supplements have been hypothesized to strengthen the immune system. Although the underlying theory may be viable with these and other nutrients, the research data are usually limited or controversial, and additional research is needed.

However, nutrient supplementation may be warranted in some cases. For example, in activities where excess body weight may serve to handicap performance, a loss of some body fat may be helpful. Recommended procedures for such weight losses will be presented in Chapter 11. Although the use of a very low-Calorie diet to achieve a desirable competitive weight is not advised, vitamin-mineral supplements may be recommended to athletes who use such a procedure.

What should I eat to help optimize my athletic performance?

The importance of nutrition to your athletic performance may depend on a variety of factors, including your gender, your age, your body weight status, your eating and life-style patterns, the environment, the type of training you do, and the type of sport or event in which you participate. As an example of the latter point, the nutrient needs of a golfer or baseball player may vary little from those of the nonathlete, whereas those of a marathon runner or ultraendurance triathlete may be altered significantly during training and competition.

The opinions offered by researchers in the area of exercise and nutrition relative to optimal nutrition for the athlete run the gamut. At one end, certain investigators note that the daily food requirement of athletes is quite similar to the nutritionally balanced diet for everyone else, and therefore no special recommendations are needed. On the other extreme, some state that it is almost impossible to obtain all the nutrients the athlete requires from the normal daily intake of food, and for that reason nutrient supplementation is absolutely necessary. Other reviewers advocate a compromise between these two extremes, recognizing the importance of a nutritionally balanced diet but also stressing the importance of increased consumption or supplementation of specific nutrients for athletes under certain situations.

The review of the scientific literature presented in this book supports the latter point of view. In general, athletes who consume enough Calories to meet their energy needs and who meet the RDA for essential nutrients should be obtaining adequate nutrition. The dietary guidelines for better health, as discussed previously and expanded upon in Chapter 2, are the same for better physical performance. The key to sound nutrition for the athletic individual is to eat a wide variety of healthful foods.

The need for sound nutrition is especially important for all females and for young males who engage in strenuous physical training. Females need to pay special attention to the iron and calcium content of their diet because of possible problems, which will be noted in Chapter 8. During the growth and development years of childhood and adolescence, the need for protein, calcium, and iron, as well as many other nutrients, is relatively high because the muscle, bone, and other body tissues are growing rapidly. Strenuous exercise may increase these needs slightly, but obtaining adequate caloric intake from healthful foods should easily provide the nutrients needed.

A nutritionally balanced diet is still the keystone of sports nutrition, but some athletes may benefit from dietary modifications. The implications of specific nutrients for optimization of physical performance will be addressed in the following chapters where applicable.

Dietary Supplements and Ergogenic Aids

Although the Healthy North American Diet is the cornerstone of nutrition to ensure optimal health and sport performance, numerous dietary supplements are marketed to the general public for improved health and to athletes for enhanced sport performance. As research in nutritional biochemistry advances, the distinction between a substance being classified as either a nutrient or a drug is becoming increasingly obscure. The term **nutraceutical** has emerged to classify those nutrients or food substances that may have pharmaceutical properties when taken in appropriate dosages. As shall be noted in later chapters, a few nutritional substances may possess qualities that may enhance health status or sport performance.

Dietary Supplements and Health

What are dietary supplements?

In the United States, the Dietary Supplement Health and Education Act (DSHEA) defines a **dietary supplement** as a food product, added to the total diet, that contains at least one of the following ingredients: a vitamin, mineral, herb or botanical, amino acid, metabolite, constituent, extract, or combination of any of these ingredients (Figure 1.5). It is important to note that the DSHEA stipulates that a dietary supplement cannot be represented as a conventional food or as the sole item of a meal or diet.

As noted by this definition, dietary supplements may contain essential nutrients such as essential vitamins, minerals, and amino acids, but also other nonessential substances such as ginseng, ginkgo, yohimbe, ma huang, and other herbal products. The definition of a supplement is something added, particularly to correct a deficiency. Theoretically then, dietary supplements should be used to correct a deficiency of a specific nutrient, such as vitamin C. Most Americans, however, do not suffer nutrient deficiencies, so excess intake of essential nutrients is generally not warranted. Moreover, we have no specific requirement for various herbal products as they are not essential for normal physiological functioning. Thus, most dietary supplements marketed in the United States are sold not to correct a deficiency, but rather to increase the total dietary intake of some food substance.

Will dietary supplements improve my health?

The dietary supplement industry is a multi-billion dollar business. Dietary supplements are usually advertised to the general public as a means to improve some facet of their health, particularly to lose weight and prevent some of the adverse effects of aging. They are often referred to

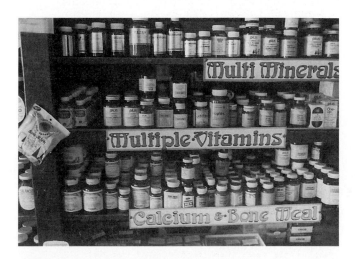

Figure 1.5 Dietary supplements are marketed as a means to enhance both health and physical performance.

as "miracle products" that can produce "magical results" in a short time, or provide insurance against a poor diet.

Unfortunately, most advertisements are based on theory alone, testimonials or anecdotal information, or on the exaggeration or misinterpretation of research findings relative to the health effects of specific nutrients or other food constituents. Moreover, although advertisers may not make unsubstantiated health claims, the 1994 DSHEA stipulates that the burden of proving the claims false rests with the government, which unfortunately may not have the resources to investigate every false claim made. Nevertheless, the government has taken action to determine if there are any health benefits associated with various dietary supplements by establishing the Office of Dietary Supplements at the National Institutes of Health, and holding a conference on how supplements might influence physically active people.

In a recent review regarding health claims for dietary supplements, Thomas indicated that although some people may need dietary supplements for specific purposes, the use of supplements should not be routine practice for most individuals. Some of his key points are:

1. No scientific body of nutrition experts recommends the routine use of dietary supplements. However, some individuals may benefit from supplements. For example, women of child-bearing age may reduce the risk of neural-tube defects in their infants by complementing their natural diet with folate supplements.

2. Nutrition is only one factor that influences health, well-being, and resistance to disease. Individuals who rely on dietary supplements to guarantee their health may disregard other very important life-style behaviors, such as appropriate exercise and a healthy diet.

3. Food is more than the sum of its nutrients. Although we may be able to identify specific constituents of food which may confer certain health benefits, consuming isolates of those substances will not provide other beneficial substances that may be present in the food.

4. Taking supplements of single nutrients in large doses may have detrimental effects on nutritional status and health. Although large doses of some vitamins may be taken to prevent some conditions, excesses may lead to other health problems.

5. Dietary supplements vary tremendously in quality. For example, chemical analysis of various commercial ginseng supplements revealed that some brands contained zero levels of the alleged active ingredient.

6. Dietary supplements may provide a false sense of security to some individuals who may use them as substitutes for a healthy diet, believing they are eating healthfully and not attempting to eat right.

Again, to reiterate the point, dietary supplements may exert some beneficial healthful effects in certain cases, but as Thomas points out, for most of us they are readily available in familiar and attractive packages called fruits, vegetables, legumes, and other healthy foods. Although the Healthy North American Diet is the optimal means to obtain the nutrients we need, dietary supplements may be recommended under certain circumstances. When deemed to be prudent behavior, such recommendations will be provided at specific points in this text.

Ergogenic Aids and Sports Performance

What is an ergogenic aid?

As mentioned previously, the two key factors important to athletic success are genetic endowment and state of training. At certain levels of competition, the contestants generally have similar genetic athletic abilities and have been exposed to similar training methods, and thus they are fairly evenly matched. Given the emphasis placed on winning, many athletes training for competition are always searching for the ultimate method or ingredient to provide that extra winning edge. Indeed, one report suggests that two of the key factors leading to better athletic records in recent years are improved diet and ergogenic aids.

The word *ergogenic* is derived from the Greek words *ergo* (meaning work) and *gen* (meaning production of), and is usually defined as *to increase potential for work output*. In sports, various **ergogenic aids,** or ergogenics, have been used for their theoretical ability to improve sports performance by enhancing physical power, mental strength, or mechanical edge. There are several different classifications of ergogenic aids, grouped according to the general nature of their application to sport. Listed below are several major categories with an example of one theoretical ergogenic aid for each.

Mechanical Aids   Mechanical, or biomechanical, aids are designed to increase energy efficiency, to provide a mechanical edge. Lightweight racing shoes may be used by a runner in place of heavier ones so that less energy is needed to move the legs and the economy of running increases.

Psychological Aids   Psychological aids are designed to enhance psychological processes during sport performance, to increase mental strength. Hypnosis, through posthypnotic suggestion, may help remove psychological barriers that may limit physiological performance capacity.

Physiological Aids   Physiological aids are designed to augment natural physiological processes to increase physical power. Blood doping, or the infusion of blood into an athlete, may increase oxygen transport capacity and thus increase aerobic endurance.

Pharmacological Aids Pharmacological aids are drugs designed to influence physiological or psychological processes to increase physical power or mental strength. Anabolic steroids, drugs that mimic the actions of the male sex hormone, testosterone, may increase muscle size and strength. The potential dangers of anabolic steroids, as well as several other drugs, are discussed in later chapters.

Nutritional Aids Nutritional aids are nutrients designed to influence physiological or psychological processes to increase physical power or mental strength. Protein supplements may be used by strength-trained athletes in attempts to increase muscle mass because protein is the major dietary constituent of muscle.

Why are nutritional ergogenics so popular?

Probably the most used ergogenic aids are those that are classified as nutritional. Because athletes may believe that certain foods possess magical qualities, it is no wonder that a wide array of nutrients or special food preparations have been used since time immemorial in attempts to run faster, jump higher, or throw farther. Additionally, as drug testing in sports becomes more sophisticated, leading to greater detection of pharmacological ergogenics, increasing numbers of athletes are relying on nutritional ergogenics in attempts to get that competitive edge.

There are a number of theoretical nutritional ergogenic aids in each of the six major classifications of nutrients, and athletes have been known to take supplements of almost every nutrient in attempts to improve performance.

Special carbohydrate compounds have been developed to facilitate absorption, storage, and utilization of carbohydrate during exercise.

Special fatty acids have been used in attempts to provide an alternative fuel to carbohydrate.

Special amino acids derived from protein have been developed and advertised to be more potent than anabolic steroids in stimulating muscle growth and strength development.

Special vitamin mixtures and even "nonvitamin vitamins," such as vitamin B_{15}, have been ascribed ergogenic qualities ranging from increases in strength to improved vision for sport.

Special mineral supplements, such as chromium, vanadium and boron, have been advertised to be anabolic in nature.

Special waters have been developed specifically for athletes.

In addition to essential nutrients derived from foods, there are literally hundreds of nonessential substances or compounds that are classified as food supplements and targeted to athletes as potent ergogenics, such as creatine, L-carnitine, coenzyme Q_{10}, inosine, octacosonal, and ginseng. Most of the popular nutritional ergogenics, including the food drugs caffeine and alcohol, will be covered in this book, but several books cited in the reference list at the end of this chapter may provide additional information.

Nutrient supplementation above and beyond the RDA is not necessary for the vast majority of athletes. In general, consumption of specific nutrients above the RDA has not been shown to exert any ergogenic effect on human physical or athletic performance. However, there are some exceptions. As noted in Chapters 4 through 10, there may be some justification for nutrient supplementation or dietary modification in certain athletes under specific conditions, particularly in cases where nutrient deficiencies may occur. Some specific dietary supplements and food drugs may also possess ergogenic potential under certain circumstances. For a broad overview, the interested reader is referred to recent reviews by Clarkson and Williams.

Are nutritional ergogenics legal?

The use of pharmaceutical agents to enhance performance in sport has been prohibited by the governing bodies of most organized sports. The use of drugs in sports is known as **doping,** and the Medical Commission of the International Olympic Committee has provided an extensive list of drugs and doping techniques that have been prohibited. In earlier pronouncements, the IOC also defined doping as follows:

> **Doping is the administration of or the use by a competing athlete of any substance foreign to the body or of any physiological substance taken in abnormal quantity . . . with the sole intention of increasing in an artificial and unfair manner his performance in competition.**

At the present time, all essential nutrients are not classified as drugs and are considered to be legal for use in conjunction with athletic competition. Most other food substances and constituents sold as dietary supplements are also legal. However, some dietary supplements are prohibited, such as DHEA (dehydroepiandrosterone), because they may exert effects similar to anabolic steroids, which are prohibited. Other dietary supplements may contain substances that are prohibited; for example, Chinese Ephedra and some forms of ginseng may contain ephedrine, a prohibited stimulant drug.

As shall be noted in later chapters, a few nutritional substances may possess ergogenic qualities when taken in dosages substantially greater than normally consumed. If the ergogenic effects of these nutritional substances are confirmed, then their use to enhance sports performance may violate one principle of the IOC doping rule, that is, taking a physiological substance in abnormal quantities with the primary intent of enhancing performance.

Nutritional Quackery in Health and Sports

Increasing numbers of dietary supplements are being marketed to the general population as health enhancers and to athletes as performance enhancers. Unfortunately many of the products that advertise extravagant claims of enhanced health or performance have no legitimate basis and may be regarded as quackery.

What is nutritional quackery?

According to the Food and Drug Administration (FDA), **quackery,** as the term is used today, refers not only to the fake practitioner but also to the worthless product and the deceitful promotion of that product. Untrue or misleading claims that are deliberately or fraudulently made for any product, including food products, constitute quackery.

Knowledge relative to all facets of life, the science of nutrition included, has increased phenomenally in recent years. Thousands of studies have been conducted, revealing facts to help unravel some of the mysteries of human nutrition. Certain individuals may capitalize on these research findings for personal financial gain. For example, isolated nutritional facts may be distorted or the results of a single study will be used to market a specific nutritional product. Health hustlers will use this information to capitalize on people's fears and hopes, be it the fear that the nutritional quality of our food is being lessened by modern processing methods or the hope of improved athletic performance capacity.

Quackery is big business. It has been estimated that over twenty-five billion dollars a year are spent on questionable health practices in the United States. A substantial percentage of this amount has been spent on unnecessary nutritional products. Authorities in this area have noted that the amount of misinformation about nutrition is overwhelming, and it is circulated widely, particularly by those who may profit from it. Although we may still think of quacks as sleazy individuals selling patent medicine from a covered wagon, the truth is quite different. Nutritional quacks today are super salespeople, using questionable scientific information to give their products a sense of authenticity and credibility and using sophisticated advertising and marketing techniques.

As noted previously, there are some bona fide health benefits associated with the foods we eat, but as shall be noted in Chapter 2, federal legislation provides strict guidelines regarding the placement of health claims on food labels for most of the packaged foods that we buy. Such may not be the case, however, with dietary supplements.

Before the passage of the 1994 Dietary Supplements Health and Education Act (DSHEA) many extravagant health claims were made by some unscrupulous companies in the food supplement industry. As an example, the label of one secret formula noted that it would help you lose excess body fat while sleeping, which is untrue. Although the DSHEA was designed to eradicate such fraudulent health claims, dietary supplements appear to have more leeway than packaged foods to infer health benefits. Technically, labels on dietary supplements are not permitted to display scientifically unsupported claims. However, because the DHSEA specifies that the responsibility of disproving advertising claims rests with the FDA, such claims are increasing. Moreover, companies are allowed to make general claims like "boosts the immune system" if, for example, the product contains a nutrient that has been deemed important in some way to immune functions in the body. Although companies may not claim that the product prevents diseases associated with impaired immune functions, such as the common cold, cancer, or AIDS, the consumer may erroneously make such an assumption.

Many companies now use a disclaimer on their labels, indicating that the effectiveness of their products has not been evaluated by the FDA. They may also provide information in the form of a reprint of an article, a brochure with highlighted research, or other printed materials that are distributed in connection with the sale of the product. Many dietary supplement companies have developed infomercials for television or home pages on the Internet to provide comparable biased advertising information to potential consumers.

Although these advertising strategies may contain fraudulent information, the federal agencies that monitor such practices are understaffed and cannot litigate every case of misleading or dishonest advertising. Thus, unsuspecting consumers may be lured into buying an expensive health-food supplement that has no scientific support of its effectiveness.

Nutritional quackery is widespread as documented in the recent position stand on food and nutrition misinformation by the American Dietetic Association. Years ago J. V. Durnin, an international authority on nutrition and exercise, stated that there is still no sphere of nutrition in which faddism, misconceptions, ignorance, and quackery are more obvious than in athletics, a situation which continues today.

Why is nutritional quackery so prevalent in athletics?

As with nutritional quackery in general, hope and fear are the motivating factors underlying the use of nutritional supplements by athletes. They hope that a special nutrient concoction will provide them with a slight competitive edge, and they fear losing if they do not do everything possible to win. In this regard, there are four factors within the athletic environment that help nurture these hopes and fears.

First, eating behavior may be patterned after some star athlete who is successful in a given sport. If an Olympic champion or professional athlete revealed that part of their success was due to a vegetarian diet, to sauerkraut juice, or to the milk of a cow in heat, you may be assured these dietary practices would be adopted by some aspiring young athletes.

Second, many coaches may suggest to their athletes that certain foods or food supplements are essential to success. Surveys reveal that many athletes still receive nutritional information from their coaches, but these surveys also reveal that many coaches have poor backgrounds in nutrition. Thus, misconceptions adopted by coaches in the past may be perpetuated in their athletes. Fortunately this situation is being rectified as more colleges and universities preparing future coaches and athletic trainers require courses in nutrition. Nevertheless, recent surveys indicate that athletes still engage in nutritional practices counter to the general recommendations of sports nutritionists and sports scientists.

Third, misinformation also may be found in leading sports magazines and books, which often present articles on nutrition for the athlete based upon very questionable research. For example, a magazine for bodybuilders published a study suggesting that amino acid supplements would help individuals lose body fat and gain muscle mass. Unfortunately, the study design contained too many flaws to allow such a conclusion. Moreover, a study by Jacobson and Gemmell reported that college athletes derive most of their nutrition information from such popular magazines. One training manual for health food products notes that books are a silent sales force. If you sell a box of bee pollen to an athlete, you have satisfied the customer's immediate need. If you sell the athlete a book, you create a whole new set of needs.

Fourth, and probably the most significant factor contributing to nutritional quackery in sports, is direct advertising of nutritional products marketed specifically for the athlete, as suggested by the fabricated example presented in Figure 1.6. Literally hundreds of nutritional supplements are advertised for athletic consumption. For example, in a recent survey of only five magazines targeted to bodybuilding athletes, Grunewald and Bailey reported that over 800 performance claims were made for 624 commercially available supplements ranging from amino acids to yohimbine. The authors noted that most claims were not supported by research.

Direct advertising is often combined with several of the methods above for perpetuating nutritional information. Often star athletes are hired to endorse a particular product. One advertisement pictured one of America's leading marathoners with the name of a nutritional supplement emblazoned across his running shirt and the statement that this product was an important part of his training program. Also, many sports magazines will run

To get an **ENERGY EDGE** on the competition
all athletes need

SUPERMIN

A balanced mixture of 20 minerals

Selenium
Uitopium
Phosphorus
Ergonium
Radium
Magnesium
Iron
Nickel
and 12 other minerals

SUPERMIN contains all the essential minerals to
help your energy systems exercise in high gear.
MORE POWER. RUN FASTER. LEAP HIGHER.
CONTAINS *NO* KRYPTONITE
HURRY! ORDER YOUR SUPPLY TODAY!
ONLY $50.00 FOR A MONTH OF SUPER ENERGY

Figure 1.6 Simulated nutritional supplement advertisement for athletes.

articles on the ergogenic benefits of a particular nutrient, and in close proximity to the article place an advertisement for a product that contains that nutrient. Freedom of speech guaranteed by the First Amendment permits the author of the article to make sensational and deceptive claims about the nutrient. However, freedom of speech does not extend to advertising, so that fraudulent or deceptive claims may be grounds for prosecution by the FDA or the Federal Trade Commission (FTC). Thus, by cleverly positioning the article and the advertisement, the promoter can make the desired claims about the value of the product and yet avoid any illegality. Classic examples of this technique may be found with protein and amino acid supplement advertising in magazines for bodybuilders. For the interested reader the reviews by Butterfield and by Lightsey and Attaway of the National Council Against Health Frauds Task Force on Ergogenic Aids provide detailed coverage of the deceptive tactics used in marketing purported ergogenic aids.

Most of these advertised products are economic frauds. The prices are exorbitant in comparison to the same amount of nutrients that may be obtained in ordinary foods. Besides being an economic fraud, these products are an intellectual fraud, for there is very little scientific evidence to support their claims. Simple basic facts about the physiological functions of the nutrients in these products are distorted, magnified, and advertised in such a way as to make one believe they will increase athletic performance. Unfortunately, in the area of nutrition and sport, it is very easy to distort the truth and appeal to the psychological emotions of the athlete. Dr. Robert Voy, former chief medical officer of the United States Olympic Training Center, has noted that we have abandoned athletes to the hucksters and charlatans. Athletes are wasting their money on worthless, and sometimes harmful, substances.

How do I recognize nutritional quackery in health and sports?

It is often difficult to differentiate between quackery and reputable nutritional information. Promoters of nutritional supplements can be rather sophisticated. They may appear to be legitimate with imposing titles and degrees listed after their names, but these usually have been obtained from a diploma mill or through their own accrediting agencies. Refer to the brief review by Kleiner and the excellent books by S. Barrett and V. Herbert for a thorough discussion of health quackery and how to recognize it. Specific questions may be addressed to the National Council against Health Fraud, whose Web site address may be found in Appendix N.

The following may be used as guidelines in evaluating the claims made for a nutritional supplement or nutritional practice advertised or recommended to athletes and others. If the answer to any of these questions is yes, then one should be skeptical of such supplements and investigate their value before investing any money.

1. Does the product promise quick improvement in health or physical performance?

2. Does it contain some secret or magical ingredient or formula?

3. Is it advertised mainly by use of anecdotes, case histories, or testimonials?

4. Are currently popular personalities or star athletes featured in its advertisements?

5. Does it take a simple truth about a nutrient and exaggerate that truth in terms of health or physical performance?

6. Does it question the integrity of the scientific or medical establishment?

7. Is it advertised in a health or sports magazine whose publishers also sell nutritional aids?

8. Does the person who recommends it also sell the product?

9. Does it use the results of a single study or dated and poorly controlled research to support its claims?

10. Is it expensive, especially when compared to the cost of equivalent nutrients that may be obtained from ordinary foods?

11. Is it a recent discovery not available from any other source?

12. Is its claim too good to be true? Does it promise the impossible?

Where can I get sound nutritional information to combat quackery in health and sports?

The best means to evaluate claims of enhanced health or sport performance made by dietary supplements or other nutritional practices is to possess a good background in nutrition and a familiarity with related high-quality research. Unfortunately, most individuals, including most athletes, coaches, athletic trainers, and physicians, have not been exposed to such an educational program, so they must either take formal course work in nutrition or sport nutrition, develop a reading program in nutrition for health and sport, or consult with an expert in the field.

This book has been designed to serve as a text for a college course in nutrition for health-related and sports-related fitness, but it may also be read independently. It is an attempt to analyze and interpret the available scientific literature as to how nutrition may impact upon health and sports performance, and to provide some simple guidelines for physically active individuals to help improve their health or athletic performance. It should provide the essential information you need to plan an effective nutritional program, either for yourself, other physically active individuals, or athletes, and to evaluate the usefulness of many nutritional supplements or practices designed to improve health or sport performance.

Numerous books that detail the relationship of nutrition to health are available, but some of the more scientific include college textbooks in nutrition, such as *Contemporary Nutrition* by Wardlaw and *Nutrition Concepts and Controversies* by Sizer and Whitney. An excellent collection of health-related nutrition articles is presented annually in *Nutrition: Annual Editions*, published by Dushkin Publishing Group/McGraw-Hill. Other accurate information relating nutrition to health is published by governmental agencies such as the Food and Drug Administration and Councils on Physical Fitness and Sports, health professional groups such as the American Dietetic Association and the American Medical Association, consumer groups such as Consumers Union and Center for Science in the Public Interest, and other groups such as the National Dairy Council. Excellent materials relative to nutrition may be obtained free or at small cost from some of these organizations; a list of Web site addresses is provided in Appendix N.

Other popular reliable sources that focus primarily upon the applications of nutrition to physical performance and health include *Sports Nutrition for the '90s: The Health Professional's Handbook* by Berning and Steen, *Ultimate Sports Nutrition Handbook* by Coleman and Steen, *Sports Nutrition Guidebook* by Clark, and *Power*

Foods by Applegate. More technical coverage is provided in *Nutrition in Exercise and Sport* edited by Wolinsky and Hickson, *Nutrients as Ergogenic Aids* by Bucci, and *Nutrition in Sport* edited by Maughan for the IOC.

Many scientific journals publish reputable findings about nutrition, exercise, and health, but unfortunately these journals may not be readily available in public libraries and may be too technical for some. Examples of such publications include: *Medicine and Science in Sports and Exercise*, *The Journal of the American Dietetic Association*, *American Journal of Clinical Nutrition*, *Sports Medicine*, and the *International Journal of Sport Nutrition*.

Articles in popular health and sports magazines may or may not be accurate. The credentials of the author, if listed, should be a good guide to an article's authenticity. A Ph.D. listed after the author's name may not guarantee accuracy of the content of the article. Be wary of publications emanating from organizations or publishers that also sell nutritional supplements.

Several manufacturers of sports drinks, such as Sandoz (Isostar) and Quaker Oats (Gatorade), as well as other food manufacturers, such as M&M Mars, publish information based on reputable research. You may obtain free or inexpensive resource materials from The Gatorade Sports Science Institute and other organizations, whose Web site addresses are listed in Appendix N.

Nutritional consultants are another source of information. Such consultants should have a solid background in nutrition, particularly sports nutrition if they are to advise athletes. The consultant should be a registered dietician (R.D.) or clinical nutritionist (C.N.). He or she should be a member of a reputable organization of nutritionists, such as the American Dietetic Association (ADA). You may contact the ADA at the Web site address provided in Appendix N and they will provide you with the name of a local dietician. Other recognized nutritional organizations include the American Society for Nutrition Sciences and the American Society for Clinical Nutrition. Qualified nutritionists are able to provide you with nutritional advice to help you meet your health goals.

As mentioned previously, the ADA has a section of dieticians specializing in sport nutrition (SCAN) and should be able to provide you with an appropriate contact. A qualified sports nutritionist will be able to assess your nutritional status, including such variables as body composition, dietary analysis, and eating and life-style patterns, and relate these nutritional factors to the physiological and related nutritional demands of your sport or exercise program, providing you with a plan to help you reach your performance goals.

Be wary of individuals who do not possess professional degrees or appropriate certification, such as "experts" in nutrition or fitness. Many states do not have regulations restricting the use of various terms, such as "nutritionist" or "fitness professional." Although these individuals may have some practical experience to help

people change their diets and initiate exercise programs, they normally do not have the depth of knowledge required in many cases. Be certain to ask for proof of education or certification by a health professional group, such as the American College of Sports Medicine (ACSM), the American Council on Exercise (ACE), or the Association of Fitness Professionals (IDEA).

Research and Prudent Recommendations

By now you should realize that nutrition and exercise may influence our health and sport performance. But how do we know what effect a nutrient, food, or dietary supplement we consume or exercise program we undertake will have on our health or performance? To find answers to specific questions we should rely on the findings derived from scientific research. As sophisticated sciences, nutrition and exercise science have a relatively short history. Not too long ago, nutrition scientists were concerned primarily with identifying the major constituents of the foods we eat and their general functions in the human body, while those investigating exercise concentrated more on its application to enhance sports performance. More recently, however, numerous scientists have turned their attention to the possible health benefits of certain foods and various forms of exercise, and, in the case of sport scientists, the possible applications to athletic performance. These scientists are not only attempting to determine the general effects of diet and exercise on health and performance, but are also investigating the effects of specific nutrients at the cellular and molecular level to determine possible mechanisms of action to improve health or performance in sport.

Because this book makes a number of nutritional (and some exercise) recommendations relative to sports and health, it is important to review briefly the nature and limitations of nutritional and exercise research with humans. For the purpose of this discussion, our emphasis will be on nutritional research, although the same research considerations apply to exercise as well.

What types of research provide valid information?

Several research techniques have been used to explore the effect of nutrition on health or athletic performance, but the two most prevalent general categories have been epidemiological research and experimental research.

Epidemiological research involves studying large populations to find relationships between two or more variables. There are various forms of epidemiological research. One general form uses retrospective techniques. In this case, individuals who have a certain disease are identified and compared with a group of their peers, called a cohort, who do not have the disease. Researchers then trace the history of both groups through interviewing techniques to identify dietary practices that may have increased the risk for developing the disease. Another general form of epidemiological research uses prospective techniques. In this case, individuals who are free of a specific disease are identified and then followed for years, during which time their diets are scrutinized. As some individuals develop the disease and others do not, the investigators then attempt to determine what dietary behaviors may increase the risk for the disease.

Epidemiological research helps scientists identify important relationships between nutritional practices and health. For example, several epidemiological studies reported that individuals who consumed a diet high in fat were more likely to develop heart disease. One should note that such research does not prove a cause and effect relationship. Although these studies did note a deleterious association between a diet high in fat and heart disease, they did not actually prove that fat consumption (possible cause) leads to heart disease (possible effect), but only that some form of relationship between the two existed. However, in some cases the relationship between a life-style behavior and a disease is so strong that causality is inferred.

Epidemiological research is useful in identifying relationships between variables, but **experimental research** is essential to establishing a cause and effect relationship (Figure 1.7). In such studies, often called intervention studies, an independent variable (cause) is manipulated so that changes in a dependent variable (effect) can be studied. If we continue with the example of fat and heart disease, a large (and expensive) clinical intervention study could be designed to see whether a low-fat diet could help prevent heart disease. Two groups of subjects would be matched on several risk factors associated with the development of heart disease, and over a certain time, say 10 years, one group would receive a low-fat diet (cause) while the other would continue to consume their normal high-fat diet. At the end of the experiment, the differences in the incidence of heart disease (effect) between the two groups would be evaluated to determine whether or not the low-fat diet was an effective preventive strategy. If the results of such a study showed that consumption of a low-fat diet had no effect upon the incidence rate of heart disease, should you continue to consume a high-fat diet? The answer to this question, as we shall see later, is "not necessarily."

Most of the research designed to explore the effect of nutrition on sport performance is experimental in nature, and of a much shorter time frame compared to those studies investigating the relationship of nutrition and health. In later chapters, as we discuss the effects of various nutritional strategies or dietary supplements on sports performance, we will often refer to studies that have problems with their experimental methodology, but we will also note studies that are well-controlled. Fol-

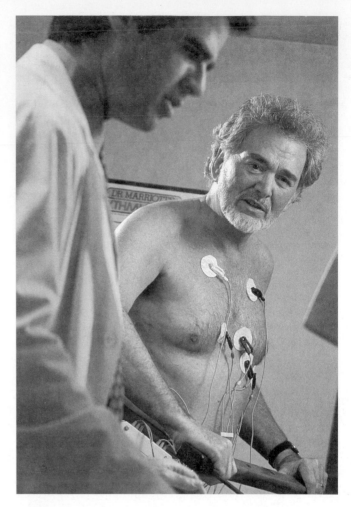

Figure 1.7 Well-controlled experimental research serves as the basis underlying recommendations for the use of nutritional strategies to enhance health status or sport performance.

lowing are some major questions you should ask when evaluating the experimental methodology of a study to see if it has been well-designed. We shall use research with creatine supplementation as an example.

1. Is there a legitimate reason for creatine supplementation? Theoretically, creatine may add to the stores of creatine phosphate in the muscle, an important energy source.

2. Were appropriate subjects used? As creatine phosphate may theoretically benefit power performance, trained strength athletes would be ideal subjects.

3. Are the performance tests valid? Validated tests should be used to collect data on the dependent variable, in this case valid power tests.

4. Was a placebo control used? A placebo similar in appearance and taste to creatine should be used in the control trial.

5. Were the subjects randomly assigned to treatments? Subjects should be randomly assigned to the treatment (creatine) or the control (placebo) group. In a repeated-measures design, in which all subjects take both the creatine and the placebo in different trials, the order of administration of the creatine and placebo are counterbalanced, which is known as a crossover design.

6. Was the study double-blind? Neither the investigators nor the subjects should know which groups received the treatment or the placebo until the conclusion of the study.

7. Were extraneous factors controlled? Investigators should try to control other factors that may influence power, such as physical training, diet, and activity prior to testing.

8. Were the data analyzed properly? Appropriate statistical techniques should be used to reduce the risk of statistical error. Using a reasonable number of subjects also helps to minimize statistical error.

Most experienced contemporary investigators generally use similar sophisticated research designs to generate meaningful data. However, some researchers do not apply such strict protocols, and thus may produce erroneous conclusions.

Why do we often hear contradictory advice about the effects of nutrition on health or physical performance?

It is very difficult to conduct nutritional research about health and athletic performance with human subjects. For example, many diseases such as cancer and heart disease are caused by the interaction of multiple risk factors and may take many years to develop. It is not an easy task to control all of these risk factors in freely-living human beings so that one independent variable, such as dietary fat, could be isolated to study its effect on the development of heart disease over 10 or 20 years. In a similar manner, numerous physiological, psychological, and biomechanical factors also influence athletic performance on any given day. Why can't athletes match their personal records day after day, such as the 19.32 second 200-meter dash performance by Michael Johnson? Because their physiology and psychology vary from day to day, and even within the day.

Although well-designed studies in peer-reviewed (reviewed by several other experts) scientific journals serve as the basis for making an informed decision as to whether or not to use a particular nutritional strategy or dietary supplement to enhance health or sport performance, it is important to realize that the results of one study with humans does not prove anything. Although most investigators attempt to control extraneous factors that may interfere with the interpretation of the results of their study, there may be some unknown factor that leads to an erroneous conclusion. For example, early epidemiological studies investigating the role of dietary fat in heart disease may not have adjusted their findings for the type of fat or intake of dietary fiber, which may help retard the development of heart disease. Thus, the results of such a study may lead to the conclusion that diets high in fat do not contribute to the development of heart disease. Consequently, for this and other reasons, the results of single studies, whether epidemiological or experimental, should be taken with a grain of salt, figuratively speaking of course.

Unfortunately, all too often the media makes bold headlines based on the findings of an individual study, and often these headlines may inadvertently exaggerate the findings of the study and their importance to health or physical performance. For example, a newspaper headline might blare that "Coffee drinking causes heart disease" after a study is published that indicated coffee drinking could increase blood cholesterol levels slightly. The study did not show coffee drinking caused heart disease, but only that it may have adversely affected one of its risk factors. A year or so later one may read headlines that report "Coffee drinking does not cause heart disease" because a more recent individual study did not find an association between coffee use and serum cholesterol levels. Is it no wonder consumers are often confused about nutrition and its effects on health or sport performance?

To evaluate the effects of nutritional strategies or dietary supplements on health or sport performance, individual studies need to be repeated by other scientists and, if possible, a consensus developed. Reviews and meta-analyses provide a stronger foundation than the results of an individual study. In reviews, an investigator analyzes most or all of the research on a particular topic, and usually offers a summarization and conclusion. However, the conclusion may be influenced by the studies reviewed or by the reviewer's orientation. There have been instances in which different reviewers evaluated the same studies and came up with diametrically opposed conclusions.

Meta-analysis, a review process that involves a statistical analysis of previously published studies, may actually provide a quantification and the strongest evidence available relative to the effect of nutritional strategies or dietary supplements on health or sport performance. However, a recent report by LeLorier and others indicates that the meta-analysis procedure, when combining many small studies into a single data base, produced conclusions at variance with subsequent single large studies. Thus, although meta-analysis is a valuable review technique, conclusions based on small studies may be inaccurate. The more studies and the larger the studies included in the meta-analytic data base, the more reliable will be the conclusion. Unfortunately, few such meta-analyses are available, although the number is increasing as the value of this literature review technique becomes more appreciated.

What is the basis for the dietary recommendations presented in this book?

Within the lifetime of many students a tremendous amount of both epidemiological and experimental research has been concerned with the effect nutrition may have upon health and athletic performance. Although in many cases we still do not have absolute proof that a particular nutritional practice will produce the desired effect, we do have sufficient information to make a recommendation that is prudent, meaning that it is likely to do some good and cause no harm. Thus, the recommendations offered in this text should be considered prudent; they are based upon a careful analysis and evaluation of the available scientific literature, primarily comprehensive reviews and meta-analyses of the pertinent research by various scientists or public and private health or sports organizations. In cases where the research data are limited, recommendations may be based on several individual studies if they have been well-designed.

Nevertheless, remember that we all possess biological individuality and thus might react differently to a particular nutritional intervention. For example, relative to health, most of us have little or no reaction to an increase in dietary salt, but some individuals are very sensitive to salt intake and will experience a significant rise in blood pressure with increased dietary salt. Relative to athletic performance, some, but not all, individuals experience gastrointestinal distress when they ingest certain forms of carbohydrate before performing. Such individual reactions have been noted in some research studies, and are discussed where relevant in the following chapters.

References

Books

Applegate, L. 1991. *Power Foods: High-Performance Nutrition for High-Performance People.* Emmaus, PA: Rodale Press.

Barrett, S., and Herbert, V. 1994. *The Vitamin Pushers: How the 'Health Food' Industry is Selling America a Bill of Goods.* Amherst, NY: Prometheus Books.

Berning, J., and Steen, S. N. 1991. *Sports Nutrition for the '90s: The Health Professional's Handbook.* Gaithersburg, MD: Aspen Publishers.

Bonner, F. (Ed.). 1995. *Nutrition and Health: Topics and Controversies.* Boca Raton, FL: CRC Press.

Bouchard, C., et al. (Eds.). 1994. *Physical Activity, Fitness, and Health.* Champaign, IL: Human Kinetics.

Bucci, L. 1993. *Nutrients as Ergogenic Aids for Sports and Exercise.* Boca Raton, FL: CRC Press.

Clark, N. 1997. *Nancy Clark's Sports Nutrition Guidebook: Eating to Fuel Your Active Lifestyle.* Champaign, IL: Human Kinetics.

Coleman, E., and Steen, S. 1996. *Ultimate Sports Nutrition Handbook.* Palo Alto, CA: Bull Publishing.

Devlin, J., and Williams, C. (Eds.). 1991. *Journal of Sport Sciences: Foods, Nutrition and Sports Performance.* London, England: E. & F. N. Spon Ltd.

Lamb, D., and Williams, M. (Eds.). 1991. *Perspectives in Exercise Science and Sports Medicine: Volume 4: Ergogenics-Enhancement of Performance in Exercise and Sport.* Dubuque, IA: Brown & Benchmark.

National Research Council. 1989. *Diet and Health: Implications for Reducing Chronic Disease Risk.* Washington, DC: National Academy Press.

National Research Council. 1989. *Recommended Dietary Allowances.* Washington, DC: National Academy Press.

Shils, M., et al. (Eds.). 1994. *Modern Nutrition in Health and Disease.* Philadelphia: Lea and Febiger.

Simopoulous, A., and Pavlou, K. (Eds.). 1993. *Nutrition and Fitness for Athletes.* Basel, Switzerland: Karger.

Sizer, F., and Whitney, E. 1997. *Nutrition: Concepts and Controversies.* Belmont, CA: West/Wadsworth.

U.S. Department of Agriculture and U.S. Department of Health and Human Services. 1990. *Nutrition and Your Health: Dietary Guidelines for Americans.* Washington, DC: U.S. Government Printing Office.

U.S. Department of Health and Human Services. Public Health Service. 1996. *The Surgeon General's Report on Physical Activity and Health.* Washington, DC: U.S. Government Printing Office.

U.S. Department of Health and Human Services. Public Health Service. 1988. *The Surgeon General's Report on Nutrition and Health.* Washington, DC: U.S. Government Printing Office.

U.S. Department of Health and Human Services Public Health Service. 1991. *Healthy People 2000: National Health Promotion and Disease Prevention Objectives.* Washington, DC: U.S. Government Printing Office.

Voy, R. 1991. *Drugs, Sports, and Politics.* Champaign, IL: Leisure Press.

Wardlaw, G. 1997. *Contemporary Nutrition: Issues and Insights.* Dubuque: Brown & Benchmark.

Watson, R., and Mufti, S. (Eds.). 1996. *Nutrition and Cancer Prevention.* Boca Raton, FL: CRC Press.

Williams, M. 1998. *The Ergogenics Edge: Pushing the Limits of Sports Performance.* Champaign, IL: Human Kinetics.

Wolinsky, I. (Ed.). 1998. *Nutrition in Exercise and Sport.* Boca Raton, FL: CRC Press.

Wolinsky, I., and Hickson, J. 1994. *Nutrition in Exercise and Sport.* Boca Raton, FL: CRC Press.

Reviews

American Dietetic Association. 1996. Position of the American Dietetic Association: Child and adolescent food and nutrition programs. *Journal of the American Dietetic Association* 96:913–916.

American Dietetic Association. 1995. Position of the American Dietetic Association: Food and nutrition misinformation. *Journal of the American Dietetic Association* 95:705–707.

American Dietetic Association and Canadian Dietetic Association. 1993. Position of the American Dietetic Association and the Canadian Dietetic Association. Nutrition for physical fitness and athletic performance in for adults. *Journal of the American Dietetic Association* 93:691–696.

American College of Sports Medicine. 1990. The recommended quantity and quality of exercise for developing and maintaining cardiorespiratory and muscular fitness in healthy adults. *Medicine and Science in Sports and Exercise* 22:265–274.

Barrett, S., and Herbert, V. 1994. Fads, fraud, and quackery. In *Modern Nutrition in Health and Disease,* eds. M. Shils, et al. Philadelphia: Lea and Febiger.

Blair, S. 1995. Diet and activity: The synergistic merger. *Nutrition Today* 30 (May/June):108–112.

Blair, S., and Connelly, J. 1996. How much physical activity should we do? The case for moderate amounts and intensities of physical activity. *Research Quarterly for Exercise and Sport* 67:193–205.

Blair, S., and Morrow, M. 1997. Surgeon General's Report on Physical Fitness: The inside story. *ACSM's Health & Fitness Journal* 1 (January/February):14–18.

Blair, S., et al. 1996. Physical activity, nutrition, and chronic disease. *Medicine and Science in Sports and Exercise* 28:335–349.

Blumberg, J. 1993. Nutraceuticals: A taste of the future. *Nestle Worldview* 5:(1), 8.

Brown, J., and Pollitt, E. 1996. Malnutrition, poverty and intellectual development. *Scientific American* 274 (February):38–43.

Burke, L., and Read, R. 1993. Dietary supplements in sport. *Sports Medicine* 15: 43–65.

Butterfield, G. 1996. Ergogenic aids: Evaluating sport nutrition products. *International Journal of Sport Nutrition* 6:191–197.

Clarkson, P. 1996. Nutrition for improved sports performance. *Sports Medicine* 21:393–401.

Cowart, V. 1992. Dietary supplements: Alternatives to anabolic steroids? *The Physician and Sportsmedicine* 20 (March): 189–198.

Durnin, J. V. 1967. The influence of nutrition. *Canadian Medical Association Journal* 96:715–20.

Economos, C., et al. 1993. Nutritional practices of elite athletes. *Sports Medicine* 16:381–399.

Elrick, H. 1996. Exercise is medicine. *The Physician and Sportsmedicine* 24 (February):72–76.

Fentem, P. 1992. Exercise in prevention of disease. *British Medical Bulletin* 48:638–50.

Gabel, L., et al. 1992. Dietary prevention and treatment of disease. *American Family Physician* 46(5 Suppl):41S–48S.

Gatorade Sports Science Institute. 1995. Nutrition and health of physically active people: An international perspective. *Sports Science Exchange* 6 (4):1–4.

Gisis, F. 1992. Nutrition in women across the life span. *Nursing Clinics in North America* 27:971–82.

Grandjean, A. 1989. Macronutrient intake of US athletes compared with the general population and recommendations made for athletes. *American Journal of Clinical Nutrition* 49:1070–76.

Grunewald, K., and Bailey, R. 1993. Commercially marketed supplements for bodybuilding athletes. *Sports Medicine* 15:90–103.

Hawley, J., et al. 1995. Nutritional practices of athletes: Are they sub-optimal? *Journal of Sports Sciences* 13:S75–S87.

Hoffman, C., and Coleman, E. 1991. An eating plan and update on recommended dietary practices for the endurance athlete. *Journal of the American Dietetic Association* 91:325–330.

International Society of Sport Psychology Position Statement. 1992. Physical activity and psychological benefits. *The Physician and Sportsmedicine* 20 (October):179–83.

Kearney, J. 1996. Training the Olympic athlete. *Scientific American* 274 (June):52–63.

Kleiner, S. 1991. Performance-enhancing aids in sport: Health consequences and nutritional alternatives. *Journal of the American College of Nutrition* 10:163–76.

Kriska, A. 1997. Physical activity and the prevention of type II (non-insulin dependent) diabetes. *President's Council on Physical Fitness and Sports Research Digest* 2 (10):1–8.

Lakin, J., et al. 1990. Eating behaviors, weight loss methods and nutrition practices among high school wrestlers. *Journal of Community Health Nursing* 7:223–34.

LeLorier, J., et al. 1997. Discrepancies between meta-analyses and subsequent large, randomized, controlled trials. *New England Journal of Medicine* 337:559–61.

Lee, I-Min., and Paffenbarger, R. 1996. Do physical activity and physical fitness avert premature mortality? *Exercise and Sport Sciences Reviews* 24:135–172.

Levine, G. 1993. The benefits and risks of exercise training: the exercise prescription. *Advances in Internal Medicine* 38:57–79.

Lewis, C., et al. 1994. Healthy People 2000: Report on the 1994 Nutrition Progress Review. *Nutrition Today* 29 (November/December):6–13.

Lightsey, D., and Attaway, J. 1992. Deceptive tactics used in marketing purported ergogenic aids. *National Strength and Conditioning Association Journal* 14(2):26–31.

Lindeman, A. 1992. Eating for endurance or ultraendurance. *The Physician and Sportsmedicine* 20 (March):87–104.

Macdonald, I. 1992. Food and drink in sport. *British Medical Bulletin* 48:605–14.

National Dairy Council. 1996. Teens at risk: Nutrition issues for the '90s. *Dairy Council Digest* 67:13–18.

National Institutes of Health. 1996. Physical activity and cardiovascular health. *Journal of the American Medical Association* 276:241–246.

Pate, R., et al. 1995. Physical activity and public health: A recommendation from the Centers for Disease Control and Prevention and American College of Sports Medicine. *Journal of the American Medical Association* 273:402–406.

Prokop, L. 1989. International Olympic Committee Medical Commission's policies and programs in nutrition and physical fitness. *American Journal of Clinical Nutrition* 49:1065.

Rejeski, W. J., et al. 1996. Physical activity and health-related quality of life. *Exercise and Sport Sciences Reviews* 24:71–108.

Sharp, N. 1992. Sport and the overtraining syndrome: immunological aspects. *British Medical Bulletin* 48:518–33.

Sherman, W. M., and Lamb, D. 1995. Proceedings of the Gatorade Sports Science Institute Conference on Nutritional Ergogenic Aids. *International Journal of Sport Nutrition* 5:Sii–S131.

Short, S. 1994. Surveys of dietary intake and nutrition knowledge of athletes and their coaches. In *Nutrition in Exercise and Sport,* eds. I. Wolinsky and J. Hickson. Boca Raton, FL: CRC Press.

Singh, V. 1992. A current perspective on nutrition and exercise. *Journal of Nutrition* 122:760–65.

Sternfeld, B. 1992. Cancer and the protective effect of physical activity: the epidemiological evidence. *Medicine and Science in Sports and Exercise* 24:1195–209.

Storlie, J. 1991. Nutrition assessment of athletes: A model for integrating nutrition and physical performance indicators. *International Journal of Sport Nutrition* 1:205–207.

Thomas, P. 1996. Food for thought about dietary supplements. *Nutrition Today* 31 (March/April):46–54.

Trichopoulos, D., et al. 1996. What causes cancer? *Scientific American* 275 (September):80–87.

Williams, M. 1997. The gospel truth about dietary supplements. *ACSM's Health & Fitness Journal* 1 (January/February):24–29.

Williams, M. 1996. Ergogenic aids: A means to citius, altius, fortius, and Olympic gold? *Research Quarterly for Exercise and Sport* 67.S58–S64.

Williams, M. 1995. Nutritional ergogenics in athletics. *Journal of Sports Sciences* 13:S63–S74.

Williams, M. 1994. The use of nutritional ergogenic aids in sports: Is it an ethical issue? *International Journal of Sport Nutrition* 4:120–131.

Williams, M. 1993. Nutritional supplements for strength trained athletes. *Sports Science Exchange* 6 (6): 1–6.

Willett, W., et al. 1996. Strategies for minimizing cancer risk. *Scientific American* 275 (September):88–95.

Specific Studies

Barr, S., and Costill, D. 1992. Effect of increased training volume on nutrient intake of male collegiate swimmers. *International Journal of Sports Medicine* 13:47–51.

Blair, S., et al. 1996. Influences of cardiorespiratory fitness and other precursors on cardiovascular disease and all-cause mortality in men and women. *Journal of the American Medical Association* 276:205–10.

Corley, G., et al. 1990. Nutrition knowledge and dietary practices of college coaches. *Journal of the American Dietetic Association* 90:705–709.

Frusztajer, N., et al. 1990. Nutrition and the incidence of stress fractures in ballet dancers. *American Journal of Clinical Nutrition* 51:779–83.

Graves, K., et al. 1991. Nutrition training, attitudes, knowledge, recommendations, responsibility, and resource utilization of high school coaches and trainers. *Journal of the American Dietetic Association* 91:321–24.

Hawley, J., and Williams, M. 1991. Dietary intakes of age-group swimmers. *British Journal of Sports Medicine* 25:154–58.

Jacobson, B., and Gemmell, H. 1991. Nutrition information sources of college varsity athletes. *Journal of Applied Sport Science Research* 5:204–207.

Katzel, L., et al. 1995. Effects of weight loss vs aerobic exercise training on risk factors for coronary disease in healthy, obese, middle-aged and older men. *Journal of the American Medical Association* 274:1915–1921.

Kleiner, S., et al. 1990. Metabolic profiles, diet, and health practices of championship male and female bodybuilders. *Journal of the American Dietetic Association* 90:962–67.

Kushi, L., et al. 1997. Physical activity and mortality in postmenopausal women. *Journal of the American Medical Association* 277:1287–92.

Manson, J. et al. 1992. A prospective study on exercise and incidence of diabetes among US male physicians. *Journal of the American Medical Association* 268:63–67.

Massad, S., et al. 1995. High school athletes and nutritional supplements: A study of knowledge and use. *International Journal of Sport Nutrition* 5:232–45.

Niekamp, R., and Baer, J. 1995. In-season dietary adequacy of trained male cross-country runners. *International Journal of Sport Nutrition* 5:56–61.

Paffenbarger, R. Jr. 1993. The association of changes in physical activity level and other lifestyle characteristics with mortality among men. *New England Journal of Medicine* 328:538–45.

Philen, R., et al. 1992. Survey of advertising for nutritional supplements in health and bodybuilding magazines. *Journal of the American Medical Association* 268:1008–1011.

Popkin, B., et al. 1996. A comparison of dietary trends among racial and socioeconomic groups in the United States. *New England Journal of Medicine* 335:716–20.

Posner, B., et al. 1995. Secular trends in diet and risk factors for cardiovascular disease: The Framingham study. *Journal of the American Dietetic Association* 95:171–79.

Pratt, C., and Walberg, J. 1988. Nutrition knowledge and concerns of health and physical education teachers. *Journal of the American Dietetic Association* 88:840–41.

van Erp-Baart, A., et al. 1989. Nationwide survey on nutritional habits in elite athletes. *International Journal of Sports Medicine* 10:S11–S16.

Webster, B., and Barr, S. 1995. Calcium intake of adolescent female gymnasts and speed skaters: Lack of association with dieting behavior. *International Journal of Sport Nutrition* 5:2–11.

Wiita, B., and Stombaugh, I. 1996. Nutrition knowledge, eating practices, and health of adolescent female runners: A 3-year longitudinal study. *International Journal of Sport Nutrition* 6:414–425.

CHAPTER 2

Healthful Nutrition for Fitness and Sport

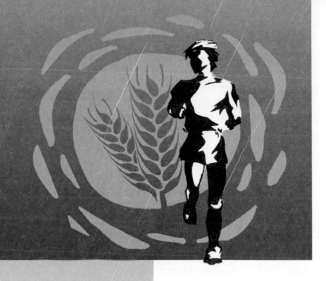

KEY CONCEPTS

- The principal purposes of the nutrients in the food we eat are to provide energy, build and repair body tissues, and regulate metabolic processes in the body.

- More than forty specific nutrients are essential to life processes. They may be obtained in the diet through consumption of the six major nutrient classes: carbohydrates, fats, proteins, vitamins, minerals, and water.

- The Recommended Dietary Allowances (RDA) should not be construed to be an ideal diet plan, but they can provide us with a set of standards for our nutritional needs. New RDA are being developed with the goal of promoting optimal health.

- If most healthy individuals in a given population consume wholesome, natural foods in amounts adequate to meet their RDA, there will be very little likelihood of nutritional inadequacy or impairment of health.

- The Food Guide Pyramid and the related Food Exchange System—meat, milk, starch, fruit, vegetable, and fat—should be viewed as an educational approach to help individuals obtain proper nutrition. Foods of similar nutrient value are found in each of the six exchanges.

- There are eight key nutrients (protein, vitamin A, thiamin, riboflavin, niacin, vitamin C, calcium, and iron) that, if adequate in the diet and obtained from wholesome foods, should provide an ample supply of all nutrients essential to human nutrition.

- Some foods contain a greater proportion of these key essential nutrients than other foods and thus have a greater nutrient density or nutritional value.

- Twelve general recommendations for healthier nutrition include: (1) maintain or improve your weight, (2) consume a wide variety of foods, (3) choose a diet low in total fat, saturated fats, and cholesterol, (4) choose a diet with plenty of whole-grain products, legumes, fruits, and vegetables, (5) choose a diet moderate in sugars, (6) choose a diet moderate in salt and sodium, (7) drink alcoholic beverages in moderation, if at all, (8) eat protein at a moderate, yet adequate level, (9) choose a diet adequate in calcium and iron, (10) obtain enough fluoride, (11) avoid excess dietary supplements, and (12) eat fewer foods containing questionable additives.

- Vegetarians must be careful in selecting foods in order to obtain a balanced mixture of amino acids and adequate amounts of B_{12}, calcium, iron, and zinc.

- Vegetarian diets are based on healthful nutritional concepts, but nonvegetarian diets may confer the same health and performance benefits if animal foods are carefully chosen.

- Those interested in becoming vegetarians may do so on a gradual basis, but conversion to a total vegetarian diet will require some extensive reading.

- Information provided through nutritional labeling on most food products may serve as a useful guide in finding foods that have a high nutrient density and are healthful choices.

KEY TERMS

complementary proteins
Daily Reference Values (DRVs)
Daily Value (DV)
essential nutrients
Estimated Safe and Adequate Daily Dietary Intakes (ESADDI)
food additives
food allergy
Food Exchange System
Food Guide Pyramid
food intolerance
food poisoning
generally recognized as safe (GRAS)
key-nutrient concept
lactovegetarians
liquid meals
macronutrient
micronutrient
nonessential nutrient
nutrient density
nutritional labeling
organic foods
ovolactovegetarians
ovovegetarians
pescovegetarians
phytochemicals
Recommended Dietary Allowances (RDA)
Reference Daily Intakes (RDIs)
semivegetarians
sports bars
standards of identity
vegan

INTRODUCTION

What you eat can have a significant effect on your health. Hippocrates, the Greek physician known as the father of medicine, recognized the value of nutrition and the power of food to enhance health when he declared that you should let food be your medicine and medicine be your food. As noted in Chapter 1, the foods we eat contain various nutrients to sustain life by providing energy, promoting growth and development, and regulating metabolic processes. Basically, healthful nutrition is designed to optimize these life-sustaining properties of nutrients and other substances found in food.

As the human race evolved over the aeons a natural diet of plant and animal foods provided the nutrients necessary to sustain the lives of our hunter/gatherer ancestors. As human civilization developed, however, human food consumption patterns gradually changed as the emerging food industry developed newer and increasingly more technological methods to plant, grow, process, and prepare foods. Overall, modern developments in the food industry have improved food quality and safety, but there are still some practices that are cause for consumer concern. For example, provision of a wide variety of foods has helped to eradicate most nutrient-deficiency diseases in industrialized nations, but provision of many high-fat, low-fiber foods appears to have increased the possibility of the development of various chronic diseases.

The three keys to a healthful diet are balance, variety, and moderation. In general, a healthful diet is simply one that provides a balanced proportion of foods from different food groups, a variety of foods from within the different food groups, and moderation in the consumption of any food. Such a diet should provide us with the nutrients we need to sustain life. In this regard, several governmental and professional health organizations have developed guidelines to help us obtain the nutrients we need.

Additionally, the current major focus of nutrition research, both epidemiological and experimental, is how our diets—and even specific foods or nutrients in our diets—affect our health, primarily as related to the development of chronic diseases. Again, specific dietary guidelines have been recommended as a means to enhance one's health status, and these recommendations underlie the Healthy North American Diet. In essence, the basic premise of the Healthy North American Diet is to consume foods in as natural a state as possible, primarily relying on plant foods and a movement toward a vegetarian diet.

Although the basic guidelines underlying the Healthy North American Diet are rather simple, selecting the appropriate foods in modern society may be somewhat confusing. Fortunately, nutrition labels should provide the knowledgeable consumer with sufficient information to make intelligent choices and select high-quality foods. Food safety is also another consumer concern, and appropriate food selection and preparation practices may help minimize most of the health risks associated with certain foods.

The Healthy North American Diet also serves as the basic diet for those interested in optimal physical performance, although it may be modified somewhat for specific types of athletic endeavors as shall be noted as appropriate throughout the book.

Essential Nutrients and the RDA

"You are what you eat" is a popular phrase, and we are becoming increasingly aware of its implications for both health and athletic performance. Careful selection of wholesome, natural foods will provide you with the proper amount of nutrients to optimize energy sources, to build and repair tissues, and to regulate body processes. However, as we shall see in later chapters, poor food selection with an unbalanced intake of some nutrients may contribute to the development of significant health problems.

What are essential nutrients?

As noted in Chapter 1, six classes of nutrients are considered necessary in human nutrition: carbohydrates, fats, proteins, vitamins, minerals, and water. Within several of these general classes (notably protein, vitamins, and minerals) are a number of specific nutrients necessary for life. For example, more than a dozen vitamins are needed for optimal physiological functioning.

In relation to nutrition, the term **essential nutrients** describes nutrients that the body needs but cannot produce at all or cannot produce in adequate quantities. Thus, in general, essential nutrients must be obtained from the food we eat. Essential nutrients also are known as indispensable nutrients.

Table 2.1 lists the specific nutrients currently known to be essential or probably essential to humans. Some of the nutrients listed have been shown to be essential for various animals and are theorized to be essential for humans. It is possible that this list may be expanded in the future as more accurate analytical methods are developed to study the effects of certain nutrients in human nutrition. Although carbohydrate is not an essential nutrient in the strictest sense, many nutritionists consider dietary fiber, which is primarily carbohydrate, a specific necessity in the diet for prevention of certain health problems.

Some foods, such as whole wheat bread, may contain all six general classes of nutrients, whereas others, such as table sugar, contain only one nutrient class. However, whole wheat bread cannot be considered a complete food because it does not contain a proper balance of all essential nutrients.

The human body requires substantial amounts of some nutrients, particularly those that may provide energy and support growth and development of the body tissues, namely carbohydrate, fat, and protein, as well as water. These nutrients are referred to as **macronutrients** because the daily requirement is greater than a few grams. Most nutrients that help to regulate metabolic processes, particularly vitamins and minerals, are needed in much smaller amounts (usually measured in milligrams or micrograms) and are referred to as **micronutrients,** although as noted in Chapter 8, minerals may be classified by other terminology according to the daily requirement.

Essential nutrients are necessary for human life. An inadequate intake may lead to disturbed body metabolism, certain disease states, or death. Conversely, an excess of certain nutrients may also disrupt normal metabolism and may even be lethal (see Figure 2.1).

What are nonessential nutrients?

Those nutrients that may be formed in the body are known as **nonessential nutrients,** or dispensable nutrients. A good example of a nonessential nutrient is glucose, a simple carbohydrate. Although we may obtain glucose from food, the body can also manufacture glucose from protein and parts of fats when necessary. As we shall see later, glucose is a very important nutrient for energy production during exercise, and although the body may produce some glucose during exercise, the rate of production is not adequate to meet the energy demands during moderate to heavy exertion. Thus, glucose may be a vital nutrient for certain types of physical activity, but dietary glucose is not essential for life.

Other than essential and nonessential nutrients, a wide variety of non-nutrients may be involved in various

Table 2.1	Nutrients essential or probably essential to humans

Carbohydrates
Fiber*

Fats (essential fatty acids)
Linoleic fatty acid

Alpha linolenic fatty acid

Protein (essential amino acids)

Histidine	Phenylalanine
Isoleucine	Threonine
Leucine	Tryptophan
Lysine	Valine
Methionine	

Vitamins

Water soluble	*Fat soluble*
B_1 (thiamin)	A (retinol)
B_2 (riboflavin)	D (calciferol)
Niacin	E (tocopherol)
B_6 (pyridoxine)	K
Pantothenic acid	
Folacin	
B_{12} (cyanocobalamin)	
Biotin	
C (ascorbic acid)	

Minerals

Major	*Trace*	
Calcium	Chromium	Molybdenum
Chloride	Cobalt	Nickel
Magnesium	Copper	Selenium
Phosphorus	Fluorine	Silicon
Potassium	Iodine	Tin
Sodium	Iron	Vanadium
Sulfur	Manganese	Zinc

Water

*See text for qualification.

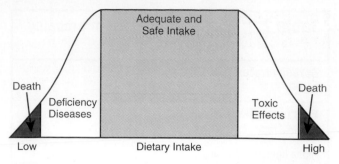

Figure 2.1 One model of the possible relationship between nutrient intake and health status. An inadequate intake may lead to nutrient-deficiency diseases, while excessive amounts may cause various toxic reactions. Both deficiencies and excesses may be fatal if carried to extremes.

metabolic processes in the body. These non-nutrients include those found naturally in foods and those added either intentionally or inadvertently during the various phases of food preparation. Some non-nutrients, such as carnitine, may be marketed as dietary supplements for health or sport performance enhancement. Table 2.2 provides some examples of nonessential nutrients and other substances that will be covered in various sections of this text.

What are the RDA?

As noted in Table 2.1, humans have an essential requirement for more than forty specific nutrients. A number of countries, as well as the Food and Agriculture and World Health Organizations (FAO/WHO), have calculated the amount of each nutrient that individuals should consume in their diets. In the United States, the amounts of certain of these nutrients have been established by the Food and Nutrition Board, National Academy of Sciences–National Research Council. The **Recommended Dietary Allowances (RDA)** represent the levels of intake of essential nutrients considered in the judgment of the Food and Nutrition Board on the basis of available scientific knowledge to be adequate to meet the known nutritional needs of practically all healthy persons in the United States. However, the RDA are not appropriate for individuals with special nutrient needs. RDA have been established for energy intake (Calories), protein, eleven vitamins, and seven minerals. Although technically not an RDA, **Estimated Safe and Adequate Daily Dietary Intakes (ESADDI)** have been developed for two additional vitamins and five minerals. The current RDA and ESADDI are found in Appendix A-1, the tenth revision issued in 1989; the first edition appeared in 1943. In the United States, the RDA are revised periodically.

The National Academy of Sciences is currently working on the eleventh edition of the RDA that will be

Table 2.2 Nonessential nutrients and other substances found in foods
Nonessential nutrients
Carnitine
Creatine
Glycerol
Drugs
Caffeine
Ephedrine
Phytochemicals
Indoles
Isoflavones
Polyphenols
Extracts
Bee pollen
Ginseng
Yohimbe
Antinutrients
Oxalates
Phytates

released to help guide nutrition practices into the twenty-first century. In the past, the RDA have been developed to help prevent nutrient-deficiency diseases, but the current revision establishes the RDA with the intent of optimizing health by reducing the risk of chronic diseases. The new RDA are being introduced in stages, and the first step involves those nutrients important to bone metabolism, especially calcium. For example, the calcium RDA has been increased from 800 mg to 1,000 mg for adults aged 19–50 and 1,200 to adults 51 and over. For the first time, the new RDA also makes recommendations for individuals over age 70. The new RDA will be incorporated in appropriate chapters as they become available.

In a recent review, Hudnall indicated that the new RDA are designed to provide the amount of a nutrient that should decrease the risk of chronic disease for almost all healthy individuals of a specific age and gender. Also, some new terms have been introduced. Adequate intake (AI), is similar to ESADDI, being similar to the RDA but without enough scientific evidence to set an RDA. The Tolerable Upper Intake Level (UL) represents an upper safety limit, which if exceeded could produce adverse health effects. The Dietary Reference Intake (DRI) is an umbrella term incorporating the RDAs, SIs, and ULs. These new terms will become increasingly familiar as the current RDA are updated.

It should be noted that the RDA are based on the median heights and weights for specific age groups. The average male aged 25–50 weighs 174 pounds, or in metric terms, 79 kilograms (kg). One kg equals 2.2 pounds. The average female aged 25–50 weighs 138 pounds, or 63 kg. Hence, in general, adults who weigh more than these average weights will require a slightly higher RDA, while those who weigh less will require a slightly lower amount. RDA established for children of various ages would also have to be adjusted accordingly.

An individual does not necessarily have a deficient diet if the full RDA for a given nutrient is not received daily. The daily RDA should average over a five- to eight-day period, so that one may be deficient in iron consumption one day but compensate for this one-day deficiency during the remainder of the week. Nutritionists generally become concerned when the dietary intake of a specific nutrient is consistently below 67 percent, or about two-thirds, of the RDA.

The RDA are a set of standards designed to ensure adequate nutrition. If individuals in a population consume foods in amounts adequate to meet their RDA, there will be very little likelihood of nutritional inadequacy or impairment of health. In fact, the RDA are not minimum recommendations, but actually exceed the requirements of most individuals because a safety factor is incorporated in the RDA for protein, vitamins, and minerals in order to provide the known benefits of such nutrients to most healthy people in the United States.

The RDA are not designed to be used for the requirements of specific individuals. Only a clinical and biochemical evaluation can reveal an individual's nutritional status in regard to any specific nutrient. Nevertheless, comparison of an individual's nutrient intake to the RDA over a sufficient period may be useful in estimating that individual's risk for deficiency.

Similar philosophies underlie the development and application of specific nutrient recommendations in other countries, but the use and interpretation of the available scientific data may vary, and in some cases the RDA may be established rather arbitrarily. For example, in Canada the term used is *Nutrient Recommendations*, and the recommended amounts are somewhat different compared to those in the United States. The Nutrient Recommendations for Canadians are presented in Appendix A-2.

Although the RDA are useful because they state approximately how much of all the essential nutrients we need, they are not designed to inform us as to which specific foods we may need to consume to obtain these nutrients. Other dietary guidelines have been developed to help us select foods that will provide us with the RDA for all essential nutrients.

The Balanced Diet and Nutrient Density

One of the major concepts advanced by nutritionists over the years to teach proper nutrition is that of the balanced diet, stressing variety and moderation. In order to obtain the nutrients that we need, guides to food selection have been developed, establishing various food groups with key nutrients, and in more recent years focusing on the concept of nutrient density.

What is a balanced diet?

As noted in Chapter 1, the human body needs more than forty different nutrients to function properly. The concept of the balanced diet is that by eating a wide variety of foods in moderation you will obtain all the nutrients you need to support growth and development of all tissues, regulate metabolic processes, and provide adequate energy for proper weight control. (See Figure 2.2.) You should obtain the RDA for all essential nutrients and adequate food energy to achieve a healthy body weight.

Although everyone's diet requires the essential nutrients and adequate energy, the proportions differ at different stages of the life cycle. The infant has needs differing from his grandfather, and the pregnant or lactating woman has needs differing from her adolescent daughter. There also are differences between the needs of the sexes, particularly in regard to the iron content of the diet. Moreover, individual variations in life-style may impose different nutrient requirements. A long-distance runner in training for a marathon has some distinct nutritional needs compared to a sedentary colleague. The individual trying to lose weight needs to balance Calorie losses with nutrient adequacy. The diabetic individual needs strict nutritional counseling for a balanced diet. Thus, there are a number of different conditions that may influence nutrient needs and the concept of a balanced diet.

The food supply in the United States is extremely varied, and most individuals who consume a wide variety of foods do receive an adequate supply of nutrients. However, there appears to be some concern that many Americans are not receiving optimal nutrition because they consume excessive amounts of highly processed foods. This may be true, as improper food processing may lead to depletion of key nutrients and the addition of high-Calorie and low-nutrient ingredients, such as fat and sugar. Three out of every five Calories that the average American eats are derived from fat and sugar.

An unbalanced diet is due not to the unavailability of proper foods but rather to our choice of foods. To improve our nutritional habits we need to learn to select our foods more wisely.

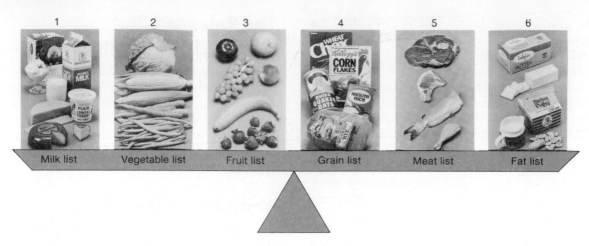

Figure 2.2 The key to sound nutrition is a balanced diet that is high in nutrients and low in Calories. For balance, select a wide variety of foods from among and within the Exchange Lists (Appendix F) or food groups in the Food Guide Pyramid.

Table 2.3 Major nutrients found in the six food categories of the Food Guide Pyramid

Milk, Yogurt, Cheese	Meat, Poultry, Fish, Dry beans, Eggs, Nuts	Bread, Cereal, Rice, Pasta	Vegetables	Fruits	Fats, Oils, Sweets*
Calcium	Protein	Thiamin	Vitamin A (carotene)	Vitamin A (carotene)	Vitamin A
Protein	Thiamin	Niacin	Vitamin C	Vitamin C	Vitamin D
Riboflavin	Niacin	Riboflavin			Vitamin E
Vitamin A	Iron	Iron			

*Mainly contains Calories. Fat-soluble vitamins found in some foods.

What foods should I eat to obtain the nutrients I need?

Although the Recommended Dietary Allowances (RDA) provide us with information relative to the nutrients we need, it is not an effective mechanism to guide us in appropriate food selection. Thus, over the years a number of different educational approaches have been used to convey the concept of a balanced diet to help individuals select foods that will provide sufficient amounts of all essential nutrients. In essence, foods with similar nutrient content were grouped into categories. For the interested reader, Welsh and others provide an excellent historical perspective on the evolution of food guides in the United States from 1916 through the present day development of the Food Guide Pyramid.

In the past, foods were grouped into the Basic Seven or the Basic Four Food Groups, but today there is some consensus that six general categories of foods may be used to represent the grouping of various nutri-

ents. Although different terminology may be used with various food guides, the six categories are: (1) milk, yogurt, and cheese; (2) meat, poultry, fish, eggs, dry beans, and nuts; (3) bread, cereal, rice, and pasta; (4) vegetables; (5) fruits; and (6) fats, oils, and sweets. Table 2.3 lists some of the major nutrients found in each of these six food categories.

Two contemporary food guides using a six-food classification system are the Food Guide Pyramid and the Food Exchange System.

What is the Food Guide Pyramid?

The most recent food guide designed to provide sound nutritional advice for daily food selection is the **Food Guide Pyramid,** developed by the United States Department of Agriculture (USDA). The Food Guide Pyramid is designed to provide a visual image of the variety of foods that Americans should eat, the proportion of Calories that should come from each of the food groups, and the use of

Food Guide Pyramid
A Guide to Daily Food Choices

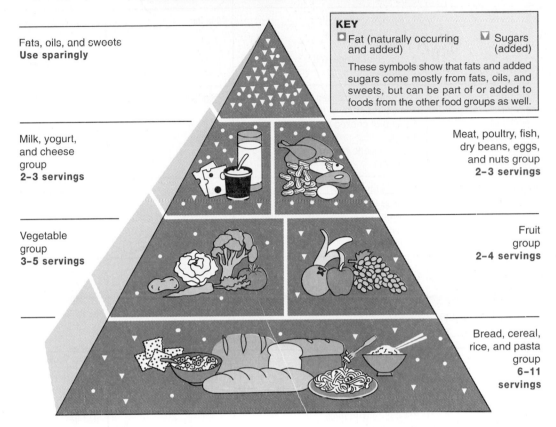

KEY
- ◻ Fat (naturally occurring and added)
- ▽ Sugars (added)

These symbols show that fats and added sugars come mostly from fats, oils, and sweets, but can be part of or added to foods from the other food groups as well.

Fats, oils, and sweets
Use sparingly

Milk, yogurt, and cheese group
2–3 servings

Meat, poultry, fish, dry beans, eggs, and nuts group
2–3 servings

Vegetable group
3–5 servings

Fruit group
2–4 servings

Bread, cereal, rice, and pasta group
6–11 servings

Figure 2.3   Use the Food Guide Pyramid to help you eat better every day . . . the Dietary Guidelines way. Start with plenty of breads, cereals, rice, pasta, and vegetables and fruits. Add two to three servings from the milk group and two to three servings from the meat group. Each of these food groups provides some, but not all, of the nutrients you need. No one food group is more important than another—for good health you need them all. Go easy on fats, oils, and sweets, the foods in the small tip of the pyramid.

Source: U.S. Department of Agriculture/U.S. Department of Health and Human Services.

moderation in consumption of fats, oils, and sweets. The Food Guide Pyramid is the result of years of deliberation by renowned scientists.

Although there are six categories of foods in the Food Guide Pyramid, the USDA does not regard the fats, oils, and sweets group as an actual food group; thus, officially there are only five food groups in the Food Guide Pyramid.

The base of the pyramid, which should constitute the majority of daily Calories, is represented by the bread, cereal, rice, and pasta group (6–11 servings), as well as the vegetable group (3–5 servings) and the fruit group (2–4 servings). These three food groups are derived from grains and plants. Fewer servings are recommended from the milk, yogurt, and cheese group (2–3 servings) and the meat, poultry, fish, dry beans, eggs, and nuts group derived primarily from animals. Fats, oils, and sweets (not classi-

fied as a group) should be used sparingly. Figure 2.3 depicts the food pyramid graphic.

Typical serving sizes are presented in Table 2.4, and Table 2.5 provides general recommendations for various segments of the population. The daily number of servings are based on caloric needs of different individuals.

What is the Food Exchange System?

A food guide similar to the Food Guide Pyramid is the **Food Exchange System,** a grouping of foods developed by the American Dietetic Association, American Diabetes Association, and other professional and governmental health organizations. Foods in each of the six exchanges contain approximately the same amount of Calories, carbohydrate, fat, and protein. As with the Food Guide Pyramid, eating a wide variety of foods from the

Table 2.4 Serving sizes for the Food Guide Pyramid and the Food Exchange System

Pyramid food group	Serving size	Food exchange	Serving size*
Milk, yogurt, and cheese	1 cup of milk or yogurt 1 1/2 ounces natural cheese 2 ounces of processed cheese	Milk list	1 cup milk or yogurt
Meat, poultry, fish, dry beans, eggs, and nuts	2–3 ounces of cooked lean meat, poultry, or fish 1/2 cup of cooked dry beans 1 egg 2 tablespoons peanut butter	Meat list	1 ounce meat, poultry, or fish 2 ounces crab, shrimp, scallops, or lobster 1 ounce cheese 1 egg
Bread, cereal, rice, and pasta	1 slice of bread 1 ounce of ready-to-eat cereal 1/2 cup of cooked cereal, rice, or pasta	Starch list	1 ounce of bread 1/2 cup of cereal, grain, or pasta
Vegetable	1 cup of raw, leafy vegetables 1/2 cup of other vegetables, cooked or chopped raw 3/4 cup vegetable juice	Vegetable list	1 cup of raw vegetables 1/2 cup of cooked vegetables or vegetable juice
Fruit	1 medium apple, banana, or orange 1/2 cup of chopped, cooked, or canned fruit 3/4 cup of fruit juice	Fruit list	1/2 cup of fresh fruit or fruit juice 1/4 cup of dried fruit 1 apple, orange, or peach 1/2 banana
Fats, oils, and sweets (Not an official food group)	No serving size	Fat list	1 teaspoon butter, margarine, or oil 1 teaspoon mayonnaise 1 tablespoon nuts 1 tablespoon salad dressing

*Serving sizes vary; see Appendix F for more specific serving sizes.

Table 2.5 Daily number of servings with the Food Guide Pyramid

	Many women, older adults	Children, teenage girls, active women, most men	Teenage boys, active men
Calorie level*	About 1,600	About 2,200	About 2,800
Bread group servings	6	9	11
Vegetable group servings	3	4	5
Fruit group servings	2	3	4
Milk group servings	2–3+	2–3+	2–3+
Meat group servings	2, for a total of 5 ounces	2, for a total of 6 ounces	3, for a total of 7 ounces
Total fat (grams)	53	73	93

*These are the Calorie levels if you choose low-fat, lean foods from the five major food groups and use foods from the fats, oils, and sweets group sparingly.
+Women who are pregnant or breastfeeding, teenagers, and young adults to age 24 need 3 servings.
Source: U.S. Department of Agriculture.

Table 2.6 Carbohydrate, fat, protein, and Calories in the six food exchanges

Food exchange	Carbohydrate	Fat	Protein	Calories
Milk				
Skim/very low fat	12	0–3	8	90
Low fat	12	5	8	120
Whole	12	8	8	150
Meat and meat substitutes				
Very lean	0	0–1	7	35
Lean	0	3	7	55
Medium fat	0	5	7	75
High fat	0	8	7	100
Starch	15	0–1	3	80
Fruit	15	0	0	60
Vegetable	5	0	2	25
Fat	0	5	0	45

Carbohydrate, fat, and protein in grams (g).
1 g carbohydrate = 4 Calories
1 g fat = 9 Calories
1 g protein = 4 Calories

six food exchanges will help guarantee that you receive the RDA for essential nutrients. The basic content of each food exchange is presented in Table 2.6, and serving sizes are presented in Table 2.4. A detailed list of common foods in the various exchanges may be found in Appendix F. The Food Exchange System was developed for diabetics and for weight control, and it will be covered in greater detail in Chapter 11.

What is the key-nutrient concept for obtaining a balanced diet?

As already noted, humans require many diverse nutrients, including twenty amino acids, thirteen vitamins, and more than fifteen minerals. To plan our daily diet to include all of these nutrients would be mind-boggling, so simplified approaches to diet planning have been developed.

The nutritional composition of foods varies tremendously. If you examine a food-composition table, you will quickly see that no two foods are exactly alike in nutrient composition. However, certain foods are similar enough in nutrient content to be grouped accordingly. This fact is the basis for approaching nutrition education by way of the Food Guide Pyramid and the Food Exchange Lists. In essence, foods are grouped or listed according to approximate caloric content and nutrients in which they are rich.

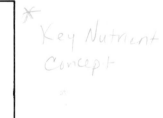

Protein
Vitamin A
Thiamin
Riboflavin
Niacin
Vitamin C
Iron
Calcium

Figure 2.4 The key-nutrient concept. Obtaining the RDA for these eight key nutrients from a balanced diet of wholesome, natural foods among the six food exchanges will most likely support your daily needs for all other essential nutrients.

Eight nutrients are central to human nutrition: protein, thiamin, riboflavin, niacin, vitamins A and C, iron, and calcium (Figure 2.4). When found naturally in plant and animal sources, these nutrients are usually accompanied by other essential nutrients. The central theme of the **key-nutrient concept** is simply that if these eight key nutrients are adequate in your diet, you will probably receive an ample supply of *all* nutrients essential to humans. It is important to note that in order for the key-nutrient concept to work, you must obtain the nutrients from a wide variety of wholesome, natural

Table 2.7 Eight key nutrients and significant food sources from plants and animals

Nutrient	RDI*	Plant source	Animal source	Food exchange
Protein	56 g	Dried beans and peas, nuts	Meat, poultry, fish, cheese, milk	Meat, milk
Vitamin A	5000 IU	Dark-green leafy vegetables, orange-yellow vegetables, margarine	Butter, fortified milk, liver	Fruit, vegetable, fat
Vitamin C	60 mg	Citrus fruits, broccoli, potatoes, strawberries, tomatoes, cabbage, dark-green leafy vegetables	Liver	Fruit, vegetable
Thiamin (vitamin B_1)	1.5 mg	Breads, cereals, pasta, nuts	Pork, ham	Starch, meat
Riboflavin (vitamin B_2)	1.7 mg	Breads, cereals, pasta	Milk, cheese, liver	Starch, milk
Niacin	20 mg	Breads, cereals, pasta, nuts	Meat, fish, poultry	Starch, meat
Iron	18 mg	Dried peas and beans, spinach, asparagus, dried fruits	Meat, liver	Meat, starch
Calcium	1000 mg	Turnip greens, okra, broccoli, spinach, kale	Milk, cheese, sardines, salmon	Milk, vegetable

*Recommended Daily Intake

foods. For example, highly processed foods to which some vitamins have been added will not contain all of the trace elements, such as chromium, that were removed during processing.

Table 2.7 presents the eight key nutrients and some significant plant and animal sources. You can see that the Food Exchange Lists can be a useful guide to securing these eight key nutrients. Keep in mind, however, that there is some variation in the proportion of the nutrients, not only between the food exchanges but also within each food exchange. For example, the starch exchange does contain some protein, but it is not as good a source as the meat or milk exchange. Within the fruit exchange, oranges are an excellent source of vitamin C, but peaches are not, although peaches are high in vitamin A. If you select a wide range of foods within each group, the nutrient intake should be balanced over time. Table 2.8 presents a daily diet based upon the exchange lists. An example of a low-Calorie diet plan based upon the Food Exchange Lists is presented in Chapter 11, together with methods for planning a diet based upon a specific number of Calories.

What is the concept of nutrient density?

As mentioned before, the nutrient content of foods varies considerably, and the differences between food groups are more distinct than the differences between foods in the same group. **Nutrient density** is an important concept relative to the proportions of essential nutrients such as protein, vitamins, and minerals that are found in specific foods. In essence, a food with high nutrient density possesses a significant amount of a specific nutrient or nutrients per serving compared to its caloric content. We refer to these as quality Calories.

Let's look at an extreme example between two different food groups. Consider the nutrient differences between a 6-ounce can of tuna fish packed in water and a piece of Boston cream pie. The tuna fish would provide you with over 100 percent of your RDA for two key nutrients (protein and niacin) along with substantial amounts of several other vitamins and minerals, but very little fat. The caloric content would be only 220. For 220 Calories of Boston cream pie, you would receive little protein, few vitamins, and few minerals, with greater amounts of fat and refined carbohydrates. Hence, the tuna fish has greater

Table 2.8 Example of a daily menu based on the food exchanges

Exchange	Food selections	Exchange	Food selections
Breakfast		**Dinner**	
Meat	Canadian bacon	Meat	Baked beans
Starch	English muffin	Starch	Rice or pasta
Milk	Skim milk		Bagel
Fruit	Orange juice	Milk	Yogurt
Fat	Low-fat margarine	Fruit	Sliced peaches (in yogurt)
Lunch		Vegetable	Mixed salad
Meat	Tuna fish (water pack)	Fat	Low-fat salad dressing
Starch	Whole wheat bread	**Snacks**	
Milk	Skim milk	Fruit	Banana
Fruit	Apple		
Vegetable	Lettuce and tomato		
Fat	Low-fat mayonnaise		

Note: This table presents some common examples of foods within each of the six food exchanges. As discussed in the text, however, you should select food wisely among exchanges and within each exchange. For example, to avoid excessive amounts of Calories, cholesterol, and saturated fats, you should select skim milk, lean meats such as skinless turkey and chicken, water-packed tuna fish, low-fat yogurt, and corn-oil margarine.

nutrient density and considerably greater nutritional value. Another example is presented in Figure 2.5, which compares the nutrient density of several fluids.

Let's also look at a comparison of two foods within the same group, the meat group. Consider the following nutritional data for three ounces of tuna fish and three ounces of clams:

	Calories	Protein	Iron
3 oz. tuna:	110	24 g	1.6 mg
3 oz. clams:	65	11 g	5.2 mg

The protein density is similar in the two foods, as you get approximately 1 gram of protein for 5 Calories of tuna fish (110/24) and 1 gram of protein for 6 Calories of clams (65/11). However, clams contain more than three times the amount of iron per serving, and if you consider the fact that the caloric content of the clams is less than that of the tuna fish, the nutrient density of iron is over five times greater in the clams than in the tuna fish. Both foods are excellent sources of protein for the amount of Calories consumed, and although tuna fish is also a good source of iron, clams are a much superior source. This illustrates the need to consume a wide variety of foods within each food group to satisfy your nutrient needs.

Will use of the Food Guide Pyramid or the Food Exchange System guarantee me optimal nutrition?

If you use the key-nutrient and nutrient density concepts, the Food Guide Pyramid or the Food Exchange System may be an effective means to obtain optimal nutrition and help sustain a healthful body weight. However, although the Food Guide Pyramid and the Food Exchange System represent a significant improvement over previous food guides to help ensure proper nutrition, both have some flaws if foods are not selected carefully. For example, the Center for Science in the Public Interest, a public interest organization concerned primarily with nutrition issues, has criticized the Food Guide Pyramid, noting that there is only a hint that meat and dairy products are the largest sources of fat and saturated fat in the average American diet. In addition, the pyramid lacks appropriate information on dietary fiber, because it fails to distinguish between refined-grain products with little fiber, such as white bread, and whole wheat products with high fiber content, such as whole wheat bread. The pyramid also places dry beans and meat in the same category, which may be interpreted as a recommendation to eat less beans. As shall be noted later in the text, beans are one of the healthiest food choices. Although the Food Exchange System does provide some classification for high-fat and

Amount	8 ounces	8 ounces	8 ounces	8 ounces
Calories	120	150	90	100
Protein (grams)	0	8*	8*	0
Fat (grams)	0	8	Trace	0
Carbohydrates (grams)	30	12	12	25
Calcium (milligrams)	27	352*	352*	0
Iron (milligrams)	0.5	0.1	0.1	0
Vitamin A (IU)	500*	500*	500*	0
Thiamin (milligrams)	0.2*	0.1	0.1	0
Riboflavin (milligrams)	0.07	0.5*	0.5*	0
Niacin (milligrams)	1.0	0.2	0.2	0
Vitamin C (milligrams)	152*	2	2	0
	Orange juice	Milk, whole	Milk, skim	Cola

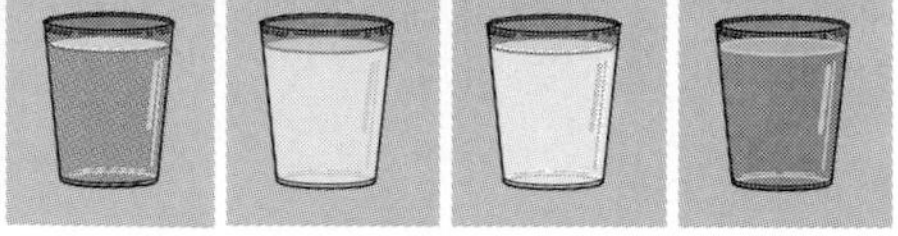

*Significant source of this key nutrient, over 10% of the RDA.

Figure 2.5 The concept of nutrient density. The key principle is to select foods that are high in nutrients and low in Calories. Compare the nutrient value of the four beverages in this figure. As you can see, orange juice and milk are significant sources of several key nutrients, whereas cola contains only Calories in the form of simple carbohydrates. Compared to whole milk, skim milk contains similar nutrient value but 60 fewer Calories due to lower fat content.

$$Ca^{2+}$$
$$OJ = \frac{150\ cal}{27\ mg} = 5.6\ cal/mg\ Ca^{2+}$$

$$Milk = \frac{90\ cal}{352\ mg} = 0.25\ cal/mg\ Ca^{2+}$$

$$\frac{\#\ Cal}{g\ or\ mg\ of\ nutrient} = \frac{Kcal}{g\ or\ mg\ nutrient}$$

low-fat foods in the milk and meat exchanges, and does indicate good sources of dietary fiber in its food lists, individuals who predominantly choose the high-fat, low-fiber foods from among the food lists may be more susceptible to the development of chronic health problems.

Other food pyramids have been developed in attempts to improve on the Food Guide Pyramid. For example, one version of the Mediterranean Food Guide Pyramid, primarily a Greek or Southern Italian diet, puts beans and nuts on the same level as fruits and vegetables, separates fish, poultry, and red meat into their own levels, and specifies olive oil as the major source of dietary fat on its own level. Although these changes may be favorable because they may change the type of fat we eat, again improper selection of specific foods could lead to a diet conducive to the development of chronic diseases. Simopoulos notes that the Mediterranean diet may be healthful, but she indicates that each society should develop its own pyramid guide based on its diverse genetic patterns and culture.

The Food Guide Pyramid and the Food Exchange System have been developed for the United States, but we are a land of multiple cultures and different dietary patterns and, in general, these guides do not specifically address ethnic diets. As a result, several ethnic versions stressing more healthful food choices have already appeared, including the Mexican Pyramid for our Hispanic constituency and the Soul Food Pyramid for the African American population.

Basically, all modifications to the Food Guide Pyramid attempt to reduce the consumption of or modify the type of fat, to increase the consumption of whole-grain products, and to increase the consumption of plant products, particularly beans and other legumes, fruits, and vegetables. A modification of the food choices in the Food Guide Pyramid designed by the Center for Science in the Public Interest is presented in Table 2.9. It lists examples of foods that should be eaten anytime (these foods should be the backbone of the diet), sometimes (these foods should be limited to two or three a day or used in small portions), and seldom (these foods, if eaten, should be in small portions and limited to two or three times per week).

Although these guides may help us select healthful foods, education in proper food selection is essential. The major guidelines for healthier food choices within these systems are presented in the following section.

Healthful Dietary Guidelines

In the past most morbidity and mortality in industrialized nations were caused by nutrient-deficiency diseases and infectious diseases, but advances in nutritional and medical science have almost eliminated most of the adverse health consequences associated with these diseases. Today, most morbidity and mortality are associated with various chronic diseases (e.g., coronary heart disease, stroke, cancer, diabetes, osteoporosis, obesity), and most dietary guidelines for healthful nutrition are targeted to prevent these chronic diseases.

Nutrition scientists are using both epidemiological and experimental research in attempts to determine what types of diet, specific foods, and specific nutrients or food

Table 2.9 Modifications to the Food Guide Pyramid by the Center for Science in the Public Interest

Food group	Anytime*	Sometimes**	Seldom***
Bread, cereal, rice, pasta, and baked goods	Bread, English muffins, bagels (whole wheat or whole-grain); breakfast cereals, whole-grain, cold, low-sugar, such as Cheerios, Grape-Nuts; breakfast cereals, whole-grain, hot, such as oatmeal; bulgur; corn tortillas; low-fat, whole-grain crackers; pasta; whole-grain pretzels; rice; no-oil tortilla chips	Angelfood cake; biscuits; bread, bagels, English muffins, not whole grain; heavily sweetened breakfast cereals, such as Honey Nut Cheerios; cakes; cookies; crackers, not low-fat or whole-grain; croissants; tortilla chips; white rice; pretzels	Apple pie, fried; bread stuffing, from mix; cake with frosting; chocolate chip cookies; cream pie; Danish; doughnuts; granola bars; shortbread cookies; lemon meringue pie; peanut butter cookies; pecan pie
Vegetables and beans	Vegetables, fresh, frozen, or canned; vegetable juice, no-salt or light; beans, e.g., black, garbanzo, pinto, great northern, kidney, and other beans; split peas, lentils, black-eyed peas	Avocado; coleslaw; corn chips; french fries; guacamole; hash browns; potato chips; potato salad; canned tomato juice; tofu	Onion rings; potatoes au gratin; vegetables with hollandaise sauce
Fruits	Fruit, fresh, frozen, dried, or canned with juice; fruit juice	Cranberry sauce, canned; fruit canned in syrup; fruit drinks and blends	Coconut
Dairy foods	Milk, skim and 1% fat; fat-free cheese; cottage cheese, fat-free or low-fat; nonfat plain yogurt; buttermilk	Milk, 2% fat; frozen yogurt, nonfat or regular; fruit yogurt, nonfat or low-fat; cheese, light; ice cream, nonfat; ice milk; sherbet	Milk, whole; yogurt, whole milk; cheese; cream cheese; ice cream, regular or gourmet; cheesecake
Fish, poultry, meat, nuts, and eggs	All fish; clams; low-fat fishsticks; lobster; shrimp cocktail; tuna canned in water; chicken breast; turkey; beef, top or eye of round (select); ground beef (96% fat-free); hot dogs (97% fat-free); egg white; egg substitutes	Fish sticks; tuna canned in oil; chicken or turkey with skin; chicken nuggets; beef, tenderloin or top loin; nuts; peanut butter	Chicken thigh or wing, with skin; turkey hot dog; beef steaks and roasts, most types; beef ribs; ground beef, regular or lean; ham; hot dog; bologna; salami; liver; eggs
Fats, sweets, and condiments	Catsup; mustard; fat-free mayonnaise; fat-free salad dressing; olives	Fruit snack candies; hard candies; jelly; syrup; mayonnaise; margarine, diet, tub; vegetable oils; pickles; salad dressing; soy sauce	Butter; candy bars; chocolate; lard; margarine, stick
Mixed foods	Bean burrito; cheeseless pizza; grilled chicken sandwich; spaghetti with tomato sauce; low-sodium canned soups; turkey sandwich; vegetable pita sandwich	Baked potato with cheese; beef or chicken burrito; cheese pizza; chicken taco; lasagna with meat; McLean Deluxe; macaroni and cheese; peanut butter and jelly sandwich; spaghetti with meatballs; tuna or chicken salad sandwich	Beef taco; chef salad with regular dressing; double hamburger or cheeseburger; grilled cheese sandwich; bologna sandwich; hot dog on bun; nachos with cheese; pepperoni or sausage pizza; quarter-pound hamburger or cheeseburger

*Make anytime foods the backbone of your diet.
**Limit sometimes to two or three a day or use small portions.
***If you eat any seldom foods, keep the portions small and/or limit them to two or three times a week.

Source: Copyright 1993, CSPI. Adapted from *Healthy Eating Pyramid* which is available from CSPI, 1875 Conn. Ave., N. W. #300, Washington, DC 20009–5728, for $5.00.

constituents may either cause or prevent the development of chronic diseases. Such research may provide simple dietary guidelines to help us select the most healthful diet and foods to eat.

What is the basis underlying the development of healthful dietary guidelines?

In general, healthful dietary guidelines are based on appropriate research. Over the years, epidemiologists have attempted to determine the relationship between diet and the development of chronic diseases. In early research, the focus was simply on the overall diet and its relationship to disease, such as comparing the typical American diet to the Mediterranean (Greece, Italy, Spain) or Japanese diet. If a significant relationship was found between the diets of two nations, say more heart disease among Americans compared to those consuming the Mediterranean diet, scientists then attempted to determine what specific foods, particularly which macronutrients (carbohydrate, fat, and protein) in those foods, may have been related to either an increased or decreased risk for heart disease. In more recent years, scientists have been investigating the roles of specific nutrients or food constituents, especially certain vitamins and nutraceuticals, and their potential to prevent or deter chronic diseases. Although most of the research relating diet to disease is epidemiological in nature, a number of experimental studies have been conducted and are underway to evaluate the effect of specific nutrient interventions, particularly studies involving the use of various vitamins and nutraceuticals.

Based on the evaluation of current research findings, nutritional scientists believe that the development of most chronic diseases may be associated with either deficiencies or excesses of various nutrients or food constituents in the diet. As mentioned previously, most Americans eat more food than they need and eat less of the food they need more.

In general, many Americans eat too many Calories, consume too much fat, saturated fat, cholesterol, refined sugars, and salt and sodium, and drink too much alcohol. Such dietary practices may predispose one to several chronic diseases, including obesity, heart disease, hypertension, and cancer.

Conversely, possibly because they rely more on highly processed foods, many Americans do not consume a diet rich in whole grain products, legumes, fruits, and vegetables, foods that are rich in dietary fiber and nutraceuticals known as phytochemicals. Some may not obtain adequate amounts of calcium and iron. These dietary practices may lead to such chronic diseases as cancer, osteoporosis, and anemia.

To help prevent chronic diseases, numerous governmental and professional health organizations have developed general dietary guidelines for good health. Some specific guidelines have been criticized, possibly because they may not be based on the best science or they may not apply to everyone in the population. The interested reader is referred to the articles by Harper and Callaway for more information. Nevertheless, the scientists involved in the development of healthful dietary guidelines believe that they are prudent recommendations. The guidelines are not considered to be static, and may be modified somewhat as we gain more knowledge through research.

What are the recommended dietary guidelines for reducing the risk of chronic disease?

Although there is no absolute proof that dietary changes will enhance the health status of every member of the population, the guidelines presented below appear to be prudent recommendations for most individuals and are based upon the available scientific evidence. These recommendations represent a synthesis of various recent reports from both professional health and governmental organizations such as the American Heart Association, the American Cancer Society, the National Cancer Institute, the U.S. Department of Agriculture, and the U.S. Department of Health and Human Services, including the comprehensive sources *Diet and Health: Implications for Reducing Chronic Disease Risk* and the *Surgeon General's Report on Nutrition and Health.*

Taken together, these recommendations may be helpful in preventing most chronic diseases, including cardiovascular diseases and cancer. The rationale as to how these dozen healthful dietary recommendations may promote good health is presented in later chapters where appropriate. These guidelines do, however, come with several caveats.

Remember, diet is only one factor that may influence the development of chronic diseases. Exercise, as discussed in Chapter 1 is also important, as are other positive life-style behaviors, such as avoiding tobacco use.

Most dietary guidelines have been developed for Americans over age 2, but many health professionals are advocating the development of separate dietary guidelines for children. Children and adolescents need energy to support growth and development, so it is important that adequate Calories be provided if dietary fat is restricted. Several of the guidelines presented below have special implications for children.

Although research may show that some foods, such as fruits and vegetables, may be protective against the development of chronic diseases, it is the total diet that is important. The benefits that may accrue from adhering to a few healthful eating recommendations may be negated if most dietary guidelines are ignored. You can maximize your health benefits by adopting as many of the healthful dietary guidelines as possible.

1. *Balance the food you eat with physical activity to maintain or improve your weight.* Preventing obesity helps to reduce the risk of numerous chronic diseases,

such as heart disease and cancer. To avoid becoming overweight, you should consume only as many Calories as you expend daily. Methods of regulating your body weight are presented in detail in Chapter 11. An aerobic exercise program and adherence to the concept of nutrient density, which includes a number of the following recommendations, could serve as the basis for a sound weight-control program.

2. *Eat a nutritionally* _adequate diet_ *consisting of a wide variety of foods*. Eating a wide variety of natural foods from within and among the Food Guide Pyramid or the Food Exchange Lists will assure you of obtaining a balanced and adequate intake of all essential nutrients. Stress foods that are high in the key nutrients.

3. *Choose a diet low in total fat, saturated fats, and cholesterol.* There is no specific requirement for fat in the diet. However, a need exists for essential fatty acids (linoleic and alpha-linolenic fatty acids) and vitamins that are components of fat. Since almost all foods contain some fat, sufficient amounts of the essential fatty acids and related vitamins are found in the average diet. Even on a vegetarian diet of fruits, vegetables, and grain products, about 5 to 10 percent of the Calories are derived from fat, thus supplying enough of these essential nutrients. Fat, however, currently comprises almost 35 percent of our Calories; the recommended dietary goal is to obtain less than 30 percent of Calories from fat. In addition, the amount of saturated fat in the diet should be 10 percent or less, and cholesterol intake should be limited to 300 milligrams or less per day. However, it should be noted that some healthful diet plans recommend lower values, such as 10–20 percent total fat, less than 7 percent saturated fat, and less than 200 milligrams of cholesterol.

The following practical suggestions will help you meet the recommended dietary goal.

a. Eat less meat with a high-fat content. Avoid hot dogs, luncheon meats, sausage, and bacon. Trim off excess fat before cooking. Eat only lean red meat and more white meat, such as turkey and chicken, which have less fat. Remove the skin from poultry. Eat more fish. Many fish, such as sardines, salmon, tuna, and mackerel, are rich in omega-3 fatty acids. White fish, such as flounder, is very low in fat Calories. Eat no more than 6 ounces of animal meat per day.

b. Eat only two to three eggs per week. One egg yolk contains about 220–250 milligrams of cholesterol, close to the limit of 300 milligrams per day. Egg whites have no cholesterol and are an excellent source of high-quality protein. You may use commercially prepared egg substitutes, particularly those that are low in fat.

c. Eat fewer dairy products that are high in fat. Switch from whole milk to skim milk. Eat other dairy products made from skim or nonfat milk, such as yogurt and cottage cheese. If you like cheese, switch from hard cheeses to soft cheeses, although most cheeses, except low-fat cottage cheese, are still high in fat and Calories. Some fat-free cheeses are now available.

d. Eat less butter, which is high in saturated fats, by substituting soft margarine made from liquid oils that are monounsaturated or polyunsaturated, such as corn oil. Avoid margarine made from hydrogenated or partially hydrogenated oils, which basically are metabolized like saturated fats. Eat butter and margarine sparingly. Some fat-free margarines are also available.

e. Eat fewer commercially prepared baked goods made with eggs and saturated or hydrogenated fats.

f. Limit your consumption of fast foods. Although fast-food chains generally serve grade A foods, many of their products are high in fat. The average fast-food sandwich contains approximately 50 percent of its Calories in fat. Appendix G provides a breakdown of the fat Calories and milligrams of cholesterol in products served by popular fast-food restaurants. Some fast-food restaurants do serve nutrient-dense foods. Wise choices, such as baked fish, grilled skinless chicken, lean meat, baked potatoes, and salads can provide healthy nutrition.

g. Use food labels to help you select foods low in total fat, saturated fat, and fat Calories, all of which are listed on the food label for most products. In the ingredients list, look for the terms presented in Figure 2.6, all of which are other names for fat.

h. Broil, bake, or microwave your foods. Limit frying. If you must use oil in your cooking, try to use monounsaturated oils such as olive or peanut oil.

In general, decrease your intake of cholesterol, total fat, and saturated fat by substituting monounsaturated, polyunsaturated, and omega-3 fatty acids for saturated or hydrogenated fats.

4. *Choose a diet with plenty of whole-grain products, legumes, fruits, and vegetables, foods which are rich in complex carbohydrates and fiber.* (See Figure 2.7.) In general, about 60 percent or more of your daily Calories should come from carbohydrates, about 50 percent from complex carbohydrates, and the other 10 percent from simple, naturally occurring carbohydrates. To accomplish this, you need to eat more whole-grain products (breads and cereals), legumes (beans and peas), and vegetables and fruits.

Sugars	Fats
Sucrose	Oil
Glucose	Lard
Fructose	Palm oil
Corn syrup	Coconut oil
Honey	Monoglycerides
Molasses	Diglycerides
Sorbitol	Triglycerides
Mannitol	Stearate
Brown sugar	Palmitate
Dextrose	Vegetable shortening
Levulose	Hydrogenated oils
Invert sugar	
Malt Sugar	

Figure 2.6 Nutritional labeling as a guide to sugar and fat in processed foods. Refined sugar and fats may appear in processed foods in a variety of forms. Check for these terms on nutrition labels.

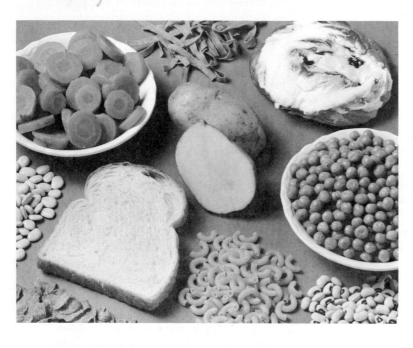

Figure 2.7 Include in your diet foods high in plant starch and fiber. Eat more fruits, vegetables, and whole-grain products.

In particular, eat vegetables. Stress vegetables and fruits high in beta-carotene and vitamin C (the antioxidant vitamins), such as carrots, peaches, squash, and sweet potatoes. Deep yellow and orange fruits and vegetables, as well as dark-green leafy vegetables are usually good sources of these vitamins. Also increase your intake of cruciferous vegetables, those from the cabbage family, such as broccoli, cauliflower, brussels sprouts, and all cabbages. These fruits and vegetables contain various phytochemicals that appear to protect you against several forms of cancer, as discussed in the next section on vegetarianism.

Another benefit of complex carbohydrates is their high fiber content. Whole-grain products and numerous vegetables are excellent sources of water-insoluble fiber. Fruits, beans, and products derived from oats, such as oatmeal and oat bran, are rich in the water-soluble type of fiber. The high fiber content of these foods is believed to be important in the prevention of diseases such as cancer of the colon and coronary heart disease. Food labels list the total carbohydrate and the amount of dietary fiber per serving.

5. *Choose a diet moderate in sugars.* The recommended dietary goal is to reduce consumption of refined sugar from the current level of 24 percent of daily Calories to 10 percent or less. Excessive consumption of refined sugar has been associated with high blood triglyceride levels. Sticky sugars are a major contributing factor to dental cavities. Sugars also significantly increase the caloric content of foods without an increase in nutritional value, so they may contribute to body weight problems.

To meet this goal you should reduce your intake of common table sugar and products high in refined sugar. Sugar is one of the major additives to processed foods, so check the labels. If sugar is listed first, it is the main ingredient. Also look for terms such as corn syrup, dextrose, fructose, and malt sugar, which are also primarily refined sugars (Figure 2.6). Food labels list the total amount of sugar per serving.

Use naturally occurring sugars to satisfy your sweet tooth. Most fruits have a high sugar content, but also contain vitamins, minerals, and fiber as well.

6. *Choose a diet moderate in salt and sodium.* Restrict sodium intake to less than 2,400 mg daily, which is the equivalent of 6,000 milligrams, or 6 grams, of table salt. This lower amount will provide sufficient sodium for normal physiological functioning.

Sodium is found naturally in a wide variety of foods, so it is not difficult to get an adequate supply. Several key suggestions may help you reduce the sodium content in your diet.

a. Get rid of your salt shaker. One teaspoon of salt is 2,000 mg of sodium; the average well-salted meal contains about 3,000 to 4,000 mg. Put less salt on your food both in your cooking pot and on your table.

b. Reduce the consumption of obviously high-salt foods such as most pretzels and potato chips, pickles, and other such snacks.

c. Check food labels for sodium content. If salt or sodium is one of the ingredients listed, you have a high-sodium food. Salt is a major additive in many processed foods, often disguised by terms such as monosodium glutamate and others. Food labels list the sodium content per serving.

d. Eat more fresh fruits and vegetables, which are very low in sodium. Fruits, both fresh and canned, have less than 8 mg of sodium per serving. Fresh and frozen vegetables may have 35 mg or less, but if canned may contain up to 460 mg.

e. Use fresh herbs, spices that do not contain sodium, or lite salt as seasoning alternatives.

7. *If you drink alcoholic beverages, do so in moderation.* The current available scientific evidence does not suggest that light to moderate daily alcohol consumption will cause any health problems to the healthy, nonpregnant adult. Light to moderate drinking is based upon a limit of one drink for every 50 pounds of body weight. A drink is defined as one 12-ounce bottle of beer, one 4-ounce glass of wine, or 1.5 ounces of 80-proof distilled spirits. Thus, for an average-size male of 150 pounds, light to moderate drinking would be three drinks daily. However, excessive alcohol consumption is one of the most serious health problems in our society today, and even small amounts may pose health problems to some individuals. An expanded discussion is presented in Chapter 4.

8. *Maintain protein intake at a moderate, yet adequate level, obtaining much of your daily protein from plant*

sources. The recommended dietary intake is 0.8 grams of protein per kilogram body weight, which averages out to about 50 to 60 grams per day, or 10–12 percent of daily Calories. The National Research Council recommends an upper limit of 1.6 grams per kilogram body weight. Since the average daily American intake of protein is about 100 grams, we appear to be staying within the guidelines. However, most of the protein Americans eat is of animal origin. Although animal products are an excellent source of complete protein, they tend to be higher in saturated fats and cholesterol compared with foods high in plant protein. On the other hand, animal protein is usually a better source of dietary iron and other minerals like zinc and copper than plant protein is.

Four ounces of meat, fish, or poultry, together with two glasses of skim milk, will provide the average individual with the daily RDA for protein, totaling about 45 grams of high-quality protein. Combining this animal protein intake with plant foods high in protein, such as whole-grain products, beans and peas, and vegetables, will substantially increase your protein intake and more than meet your needs.

9. *Choose a diet adequate in calcium and iron.* This is particularly important for women and children. Skim or low-fat milk and other low-fat dairy products are excellent sources of calcium. For example, one glass of skim milk provides nearly one-third the RDA for calcium. Certain vegetables, such as broccoli, are also good sources of calcium. Iron is found in good supply in the meat and starch exchanges. Lean or very-lean meats should be selected so as to limit fat intake, and whole-grain or enriched products should be chosen over those made with bleached, unenriched white flour. Some foods rich in calcium and iron are listed in Table 2.10.

10. *Children and others susceptible to tooth decay should obtain adequate fluoride.* This is particularly important during childhood when the primary and secondary teeth are developing, for fluoride helps prevent tooth decay by strengthening the tooth enamel. Your water supply may contain sufficient fluoride—naturally or artificially—to provide an adequate amount, but if not, fluoride supplements or use of fluoride toothpaste is recommended.

11. *In general, avoid taking dietary supplements in excess of the RDA in any one day.* As noted in Chapters 7 through 9, dietary supplements of most vitamins and minerals are not necessary for individuals consuming a balanced diet. If you adhere to the recommendations listed here, you are not likely to need any supplementation at all, for the consumption

Table 2.10	Foods rich in calcium and iron
Mineral	**Food source**
Calcium	All dairy products: milk, cheese, ice milk, yogurt; egg yolk; dried peas and beans; dark-green leafy vegetables such as beet greens, spinach, and broccoli; cauliflower
Iron	Organ meats such as liver; meat, fish, and poultry; shellfish, especially oysters; dried beans and peas; whole-grain products such as breads and cereals; dark-green leafy vegetables such as spinach and broccoli; dried fruits such as figs, raisins, apricots, and dates

of nutrient-dense foods should guarantee adequate vitamin and mineral nutrition. If you feel a supplement is needed, the ingredients should not exceed 100 percent of the daily RDA for any vitamin or mineral. Many one-a-day vitamin-mineral supplements do adhere to this standard. Excess supplementation with some vitamins and minerals may elicit some serious adverse health effects. However, as noted in Chapter 7, some data suggest that supplementation with the antioxidant vitamins may confer some health benefits, and some health professionals suggest there is now sufficient evidence to warrant people taking supplements on top of an excellent diet. However, additional research is necessary to strengthen the scientific base underlying this recommendation as noted in later chapters.

12. *Eat fewer foods with questionable additives.* The general consensus is that most additives used in processed foods are safe, but several health agencies, such as the Center for Science in the Public Interest, recommend caution with additives such as saccharin and nitrates, which have been linked to the development of cancer in laboratory animals, and other substances such as sulfites and certain food colors, which may cause allergic reactions in some individuals. Eating fresh, natural foods is one of the best approaches to avoiding additives.

It is important to note that you can eat whatever you want with the Healthy North American Diet. There are no unhealthy foods, only unhealthy diets. The dietary advice to moderate intake of certain foods, such as high-fat meats and ice cream, does not mean that they have to be eliminated from the diet, but that their intake be limited and balanced with other nutrient-dense foods in the total diet. It is balance, variety, and moderation in the overall diet that is important, not any single food.

Your health depends on a variety of factors such as heredity and certain aspects of your environment. Adher-

ence to these twelve simple guidelines will not guarantee you good health; however, the available data indicate that these dietary changes have the potential to keep you healthy or even to improve upon your current health status.

A Dietary Guidelines Alliance, with representatives from several leading health, government, and food industry organizations has proposed five simple messages to motivate you into positively changing your eating and physical activity routines. They are:

- Be realistic. Make small changes over time in what you eat and the level of activity you do. Small steps work better than giant leaps.

- Be adventurous. Expand your tastes to enjoy a variety of foods.

- Be flexible. Balance what you eat and the physical activity you do over several days. No need to worry about just one meal or one day.

- Be sensible. Enjoy all foods, just don't overdo it.

- Be active. Start moving, even in small steps. Walk the dog, don't just watch the dog walk.

Although it may not appear obvious, the general nature of the Healthy North American Diet is a shift toward vegetarianism, so it may be important to address the nature of this dietary regimen.

Vegetarianism

Many individuals have been changing their diets to improve their health. One of the major changes has been a shift toward a vegetarian-type diet.

What types of foods does a vegetarian eat?

There are a variety of ways to be a vegetarian. A strict vegetarian, known also as a **vegan,** eats no animal products at all. Most nutrients are obtained from fruits, vegetables, breads, cereals, legumes, nuts, and seeds. **Ovovegetarians** include eggs in their diet, while **lactovegetarians** include foods in the milk group such as cheese and other dairy products. An **ovolactovegetarian** eats both eggs and milk products. These latter classifications are not strict vegetarians, because eggs and milk products are derived from animals.

Others may call themselves **semivegetarians** because they do not eat red meat such as beef and pork products, although they may eat fish and poultry. Those who eat fish, but not poultry, are known as **pescovegetarians.** In practice, then, vegetarians range on a continuum from those who eat nothing but plant foods to those who eat a typical American diet with the exception of red meat. The concern over obtaining a balanced intake of nutrients depends upon where the vegetarian is on that continuum. The more you restrict your food groups, the more difficult it is to get the nutrients you need.

Table 2.11 Daily food guidelines for a vegetarian diet

Starch exchange
Servings: 4 or more daily

Note: Use whole wheat or other whole grains.
Products made of oats, rice, rye, corn, and whole wheat are good sources of protein, vitamin B, and iron, more so if they are enriched products.

Food examples:

Barley	Oatmeal
Bran flakes	Potatoes
Bread, whole wheat	Rice, brown
Buckwheat pancakes	Rye wafers
Corn	Spaghetti, enriched
Corn muffins	Sweet potatoes
Farina, cooked	Wheat, shredded
Macaroni, enriched	

Legumes (meat exchange substitute)
Servings: 2 or more daily

Note: Good sources of protein, niacin, iron, and Calories.

Food examples:

Great northern beans	Soybeans
Navy beans	Black-eyed peas
Red kidney beans	Split peas
Pinto beans	Chickpeas
Lima beans	Lentils

Nuts and seeds (fat exchange)
Servings: 2 or more daily

Note: Good sources of Calories, protein, niacin, and iron. May be excellent snack foods.

Food examples:

Almonds	Pecans
Brazil nuts	Walnuts
Cashew nuts	Sesame seeds
Peanuts	Sunflower seeds
Peanut butter	Pumpkin seeds

Fruit exchange
Servings: 3 or more daily

Note: Fruits are generally good sources of vitamins and minerals. At least one fruit should come from the citrus group and one from the high-iron group.

Food examples:

Regular	Citrus	High iron
Apples	Oranges	Dried apricots
Bananas	Orange juice	Dried prunes
Grapes	Grapefruit	Dried dates
Peaches	Grapefruit juice	Dried figs
Pears	Lemon juice	Dried peaches
Pineapple		Raisins
		Prune juice

Vegetable exchange or free foods
Servings: 2 or more daily

Note: Vegetables are good sources of vitamins and minerals. At least one serving should come from the dark-green or deep-yellow vegetables.

Food examples:

Regular	Dark-green or deep-yellow
Artichokes	Beet greens
Asparagus	Broccoli
Beans, green	Carrots
Cabbage	Collard greens
Cauliflower	Lettuce
Cucumbers	Spinach
Eggplant	Squash
Radishes	
Tomatoes	

Vegans consume most of their food from the lower levels of the Food Guide Pyramid—the pasta, rice, bread, and cereal group, and the fruit and vegetable groups—but do obtain some plant foods from the meat, fish, poultry, dry beans, nuts, and egg group, as well as the fats and sweets group. Other classes of vegetarians, particularly semivegetarians, may obtain foods from all food groups.

As a general guide to vegetarians, Table 2.11 presents the amounts of food that should help meet daily nutrient requirements for the vegan. The amounts may be increased to provide additional Calories. Foods rich in iron, calcium, zinc, and riboflavin should be included daily.

What are some of the nutritional concerns with a vegetarian diet?

The American Dietetic Association, in a position paper devoted to vegetarian diets, noted that such diets are healthful and nutritionally adequate, but deficiencies may occur if the diet is not planned appropriately. If foods are not selected carefully, the vegetarian may suffer nutritional deficiencies involving Calories, vitamins, minerals, and protein. Vegetarian diets, particularly vegan diets, should be well-planned for children.

Calories   Caloric deficiency is one of the lesser concerns of a vegetarian diet. However, because plant products are generally low in caloric content, a vegetarian may be on a diet with insufficient Calories for proper body weight maintenance. This may be particularly true for the active individual who may be expending over 1,000 Calories per day through exercise. The solution is to eat greater quantities of the foods that constitute the diet, and to include some of the higher-Calorie foods like nuts, beans, corn, green peas, potatoes, sweet potatoes, avocados, orange juice, raisins, dates, figs, whole wheat bread, and pasta products. These foods may be used in main meals and as snacks. On the other hand, the low caloric content of vegetarian diets may be a desirable attribute, as it may be useful in weight-reduction programs or helpful in maintenance of proper body weight.

Vitamins   Strict vegetarians may incur a vitamin B_{12} deficiency because this vitamin is not found in plant foods. Vitamin B_{12} is found in many animal products such as meat, eggs, fish, and dairy products, so the addition of these foods to the diet will help prevent a deficiency state. An ovolactovegetarian should have no problem getting the required amounts. A vegan will need a source of B_{12}, such as fortified soy milk, fortified breakfast cereal, or a B_{12} supplement. If not exposed to sunlight, vegans will also need dietary supplements of vitamin D, which is not found in plant foods.

Minerals   Mineral deficiencies of iron, calcium, and zinc may occur. During the digestion process, some plant foods form compounds known as phytates and oxalates that can bind these minerals so that they cannot be absorbed into the body. Avoidance of unleavened bread helps reduce this effect, as does thorough cooking of legumes such as beans. However, research has revealed that a balanced intake of grains, legumes, and vegetables will not significantly impair mineral absorption. Foods rich in iron, calcium, and zinc should also be included in the vegetarian diet. Iron-rich plant foods include nuts, beans, split peas, dates, prune juice, raisins, green leafy vegetables, and many iron-enriched grain products. Semivegetarians may obtain high-quality iron in fish and poultry. Calcium-rich plant foods include many green vegetables like broccoli, cabbage, mustard greens, and spinach. Dairy products added to the diet supply very significant amounts of calcium. Zinc-rich plant foods include whole wheat bread, peas, corn, and carrots. Egg yolk and seafood also add substantial zinc to the diet.

Protein   The major concern of the vegetarian is to obtain adequate amounts of the right type of protein, particularly in the case of young children. Generally speaking, consuming enough Calories to maintain an optimal body weight will provide adequate amounts of protein.

As will be noted in Chapter 6, proteins are classified as either complete or incomplete. A protein is complete if it contains all of the essential amino acids that the human body cannot manufacture. Animal products generally contain complete proteins, whereas plant proteins are incomplete. However, certain vegetable products may also provide good sources of protein. Grain products such as wheat, rice, and corn, as well as beans (particularly soybeans), peas, and nuts, have a substantial protein content. However, most vegetable products lack one or more essential amino acids in sufficient quantity. They are incomplete proteins and, eaten individually, are not generally adequate for maintaining proper human nutrition. But, if certain plant foods are eaten together, they may supply all the essential amino acids necessary for human nutrition and may be as good as animal protein. (See Figure 2.8.)

The strict vegetarian must receive nutrients from breads and cereals, nuts and seeds, legumes, fruits, and vegetables. To receive a balanced distribution of the essential amino acids, the vegan must eat plant foods that possess **complementary proteins.** In essence, a vegetable product that is low in a particular amino acid is eaten with a food that is high in that same amino acid. For example, grains and cereals, which are low in lysine, are complemented by legumes, which have adequate amounts of lysine. The low level of methionine in the legumes is offset by its high concentration in the grain products. These types of food combinations are practiced throughout the world. Mexicans eat beans and corn while the Chinese eat soybeans and rice. Through the proper selection of foods that contain complementary proteins, the vegan can get an adequate intake of the essential amino acids. Because all amino acids need to be present for tissue formation, a deficiency of one or two essential amino acids will limit the proper development of protein structures in the body.

In their position statement regarding vegetarian diets, the American Dietetic Association stated that complementary proteins should be consumed over the course of the day. The ADA noted that since endogenous sources of amino acids are available, it is not necessary that com-

Figure 2.8 It is important for the vegetarian to eat protein foods that complement each other (e.g., nuts and bread, rice and beans) so that all the essential amino acids are obtained in the diet.

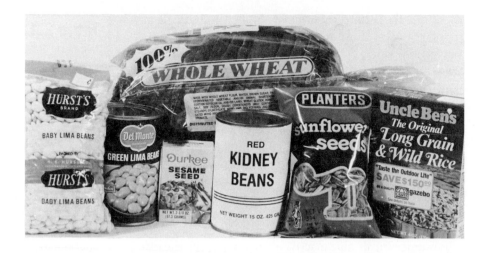

[handwritten annotations: lysine, methionine, grain(cereal) (legumes), cereal grains + legumes seeds]

plementation of amino acids occur at the same meal. Nevertheless, eating them at one meal will help guarantee that they are utilized by the body.

Table 2.12 provides some examples of food combinations that achieve protein complementarity. Milk is included because it is a common means to enhance the quality of plant protein, but eggs could also be substituted where appropriate. The two most common plant foods that are combined to achieve protein complementarity are grains and legumes. Grains such as wheat, corn, rice, and oats are combined with legumes such as soybeans, peanuts, navy beans, kidney beans, lima beans, black-eyed peas, and chickpeas.

Is a vegetarian diet more healthful than a nonvegetarian diet?

To help in the prevention of some degenerative diseases common to industrialized society, the vegetarian diet is based on certain nutritional concepts, including the following.

Low Fat and Cholesterol   The total fat and saturated fat content in a vegetarian diet is usually low because the small amounts of fats found in plant foods are generally polyunsaturated. Plants also do not contain cholesterol; this compound is found only in animal products. These two factors account for the finding that vegetarians generally have lower blood triglycerides and cholesterol than meat eaters, and these lower levels may be important to the prevention of coronary heart disease.

High Dietary Fiber   Plant foods possess a high content of fiber, which may help reduce levels of serum cholesterol and prevent certain disorders in the intestinal tract. More details on the health benefits of dietary fiber are presented in Chapter 4.

Low Calorie   If the proper foods are selected, the vegetarian diet supplies more than an adequate amount of nutrients and is rather low in caloric content. Plant foods can be high in nutrient density, providing bulk in the diet without the added Calories of fat. Hence, the vegetarian

Table 2.12	**Combining foods for protein complementarity**
Milk and grains	
Pasta with milk or cheese	
Rice and milk pudding	
Cereal with milk	
Macaroni and cheese	
Cheese sandwich	
Cheese on nachos*	
Milk and legumes	
Creamed bean soups*	
Cheese on refried beans*	
Grains and legumes	
Rice and bean casserole	
Wheat bread and baked beans	
Corn tortillas and refried beans*	
Pea soup and toast	
Peanut-butter sandwich	

[handwritten annotations: Dairy - a complete protein; grains: wheat, corn, rice, oats; legumes: soybeans, peanuts, navy beans, kidney beans, lima beans, black-eye pea, chickpea]

*Low-fat, low-sodium versions should be selected to minimize excessive saturated fat and sodium intake.

diet can be an effective dietary regimen for losing excess body weight. However, vegetarians who consume dairy products need to select low-fat versions instead of high-fat cheeses and whole milk.

Antioxidants and Phytochemicals   Plant foods are rich in antioxidant vitamins, particularly vitamin C and beta-carotene, a precursor to vitamin A. Polyunsaturated plant oils provide substantial amounts of vitamin E. Selenium, an antioxidant mineral, is found in other plant foods. Other than nutrients, plants also contain numerous **phy-**

tochemicals (plant chemicals), compounds, such as indoles, isoflavones, and polyphenols, which have no nutritional value but may still influence various metabolic processes in the body. Collectively, these antioxidant nutrients and phytochemicals are referred to as nutraceuticals, parts of food that may provide a medical or health benefit, as suggested in a recent position stand of the American Dietetic Association on phytochemicals. Table 2.13 provides a list of some antioxidant nutrients and phytochemicals and their common plant sources.

Although the exact mechanisms whereby antioxidant nutrients and phytochemicals may help prevent chronic diseases such as cancer or heart disease have not been identified, several hypotheses are being studied. Various nutraceuticals may inactivate enzymes, block the formation of carcinogenic compounds, prevent the formation of oxygen-free radicals, alter cell membrane structure and integrity, compete with natural hormones for cell receptors, or suppress DNA and protein synthesis. Some of these actions may favorably affect health, as in the following two examples. Antioxidants, such as vitamin E, may block the oxidation of certain forms of serum cholesterol, reducing their potential to cause atherosclerosis and possible heart disease. Also, phytochemicals known as phytoestrogens may compete with natural forms of estrogen in the body for estrogen receptors in various tissues, blocking estrogen's natural proliferative activity and possibly suppressing cancer development.

Some research has suggested that certain nutrients or phytochemicals may possess therapeutic value. However, experimental research in this area is still in its infancy, although increasing rapidly as indicated by the initiation of *The Journal of Nutraceuticals, Functional and Medical Foods*. Most nutrition scientists indicate that many of these nutrients and phytochemicals share the same food sources, so the protective health effect associated with a plant-rich diet may not be attributed to a single food constituent, but may be due to the collective effect of multiple nutraceuticals. Thus, consuming natural plant foods, rather than supplements, is the best way to obtain these purported nutraceuticals.

Although a vegetarian diet is more healthful than a typical high-fat diet, it should be emphasized that the nonvegegtarian who carefully selects foods from the meat and milk group, including lean red meat, may attain the same health benefits as the vegetarian. The major nutritional difference between a vegetarian and a nonvegetarian diet appears to be the higher content of saturated fats and cholesterol in the latter. Selection of animal products with a low-fat and low-cholesterol content helps avoid this problem and also assures consumption of very high-quality proteins. The National Research Council, in *Diet and Health: Implications for Reducing Chronic Disease Risk*, did not recommend against eating meat, but advised eating leaner meat in smaller and fewer portions than is customary in the United States.

Table 2.13 Some antioxidant nutrients and phytochemicals with common food sources

Antioxidant nutrients	Common plant sources
Vitamin C	Citrus fruits
	Potatoes
	Strawberries
Vitamin E	Dark-green leafy vegetables
	Margarine
	Vegetable oils
	Wheat germ
	Whole grains

Phytochemicals	Common plant sources
Allium sulfides	Garlic
Organosulfides	Onions
	Scallions
Capsaicin	Hot peppers
Carotenoids	Carrots
Beta-carotene	Dark-green leafy vegetables
Lycopene	Sweet potatoes
Lutein	Tomatoes
Glycyrrhiza	Licorice root
Indoles	Cruciferous vegetables
	Broccoli
	Brussels sprouts
	Cabbage
	Cauliflower
	Kale
Isoflavones	Soybeans
Phytoestrogens	Peanuts
Genistein	Soy milk
Isothiocyanates	Cruciferous vegetables
	Broccoli
	Brussels sprouts
	Cabbage
	Cauliflower
	Kale
Phenolic acids	Carrots
	Citrus fruits
	Tomatoes
	Whole grains
Polyphenols	Grapes
Rutin	Green tea
Quercitin	Wine
Saponins	Beans
	Legumes
Terpenes	Cherries
	Citrus fruits

How can I become a vegetarian?

People become vegetarians for a number of reasons, including religion, love for all animals, and taste preferences. Choosing to adopt a vegetarian diet is up to the individual and represents a significant change in dietary habits. Anyone desiring to make an abrupt change to a vegetarian diet should do some serious reading on the matter beforehand. Once you have done some reading on vegetarianism, there may be several ways to gradually phase yourself into a vegetarian diet.

- You may become a partial vegetarian simply by eating less red meat. For example, you may have several meatless meals each day by skipping the ham or sausage at breakfast and having a big salad for lunch. Eventually, you may move toward having several meatless days per week, possibly incorporating vegetarian "meats" such as meatless chicken or meatless smoked turkey in your meals.

- You may become a semivegetarian, substituting white meat such as chicken and turkey breast, with its generally lower fat content, for red meat. You may become a pescovegetarian, eating fish as your main animal food.

- You may wish to become an ovolactovegetarian, eating eggs and dairy products. These excellent sources of complete protein can be blended with many vegetable products or eaten separately.

- You may use the above methods as forerunners to a strict vegan diet, gradually phasing out animal products altogether as you learn to select and prepare vegetable foods to obtain protein complementarity and adequate intake of essential nutrients.

The following simple suggestions may help you incorporate more fruits, vegetables, and whole grains in your diet.

- Buy only bread products that list whole wheat as the first ingredient on the food label.

- Keep a variety of fruit handy for snacks, such as bananas, grapes, apples, and oranges. *Kiwi*

- Keep a bowl of vegetables in the refrigerator, such as small carrots, cut-up celery, and radishes for handy snacks.

- Use frozen vegetables for quick stir-fry meals.

- Add vegetables, such as onions, tomatoes, lettuce, spinach, and peppers to your sandwiches.

- Load up on fresh vegetables at the supermarket salad bar, putting meal-sized portions in small containers to take for lunch during the week.

- Add cut-up vegetables to canned beans and soups to increase their nutrient value.

- Use your microwave to cook sweet potatoes and baked potatoes, and to steam vegetables with a little water.

The scope of this book does not permit a discussion of food preparation. A number of excellent cookbooks for vegetarian meals are available at local bookstores, the titles of which may be obtained from a local dietician or local branch of the American Heart Association. These cookbooks provide the vegetarian with a variety of appetizing recipes that not only incorporate complementary proteins with a balance of vitamins and minerals but also make vegetarianism a gastronomical delight. An excellent example is the *Vegetarian Times Complete Cookbook*.

Ref

Will a vegetarian diet affect physical performance potential? *Can be*

As noted previously, a diet that follows vegetarian principles is considered to be more healthful than the typical American diet today. But will such a diet have any significant impact upon physical performance? Very little experimental research has investigated the value of a vegetarian diet as a means of increasing performance capacity. Moreover, most of the research that has been done was conducted nearly 80 years ago, and the research methods employed do not meet today's standards for reliability. In one rather well-designed study by Hanne and others, no differences were found in the aerobic or anaerobic capacities of vegetarian men or women compared with nonvegetarians. Other research has noted that performance in a distance run was neither improved nor impaired significantly after a 14-day diet consisting primarily of fruits, nor was endurance performance adversely affected in eight endurance athletes who consumed an ovolactovegetarian diet for 6 weeks. Although the available evidence does not support either a beneficial or a detrimental effect of a vegetarian diet upon physical performance capacity, active individuals should have a good understanding of vegetarian dietary principles before attempting an extreme diet such as the fruitarian plan, which relies primarily upon fruits and nuts to supply nutrient needs.

Some world-class athletes have been vegetarians, and on occasion their diets have been cited as a reason for their success. On the other hand, there are a far greater number of world-class athletes who eat a balanced diet including animal products. Both types of diet may supply the nutrients necessary for the physically active individual if foods are selected properly. It is especially important for female endurance athletes who are vegetarians to obtain adequate amounts of iron and calcium. Moreover, vegetarian diets have been associated with athletic amenorrhea in nonathletes and female endurance athletes and decreased testosterone levels in male endurance athletes. Additionally, vegetarian diets may be low in creatine, a compound whose role as a potential ergogenic aid is discussed in Chapter 6. However, if adequate amounts of nutrients are in the diet, the performance of either the world-class athlete or the weekend racer will not be affected one way or the other.

David Nieman notes that the vegetarian diet is usually high in carbohydrate content, which may be of importance to the individual who trains at a high level about an hour or so per day. Long-distance swimmers, runners, and bicyclists fall into this category. The carbohydrate content will help ensure replacement of body glycogen stores. However, meat eaters can also include substantial amounts of high-carbohydrate foods in their daily diets and achieve the same effect.

We noted above that if you wanted to shift toward a vegetarian diet, you would need to do some careful reading beforehand and then could initiate the process gradually. During the process, you should listen to your body—a common phrase among many athletes today. If you are active, how do you feel during your workouts? Do you have more or less stamina? Are you gaining or losing weight? Is your physical performance getting better or worse? The answers to these questions, together with other body reactions, may offer you some feedback as to whether the dietary change is beneficial.

Remember, there is nothing magical about a vegetarian diet that will increase your physical performance capacity. It can be a healthful way to obtain the nutrients your physically active body needs, but so too is a well-balanced diet containing animal products.

Consumer Nutrition

Guidelines for a healthful diet will not be effective unless people change their behavior to buy and eat healthier foods. A model often used to explain the development of a set of behaviors involves a sequence of (1) acquisition of knowledge, (2) formation of an attitude or set of values, and (3) development of a particular behavior. In this sequence, knowledge is the first step that may enhance the development of proper health behaviors. Knowing how to interpret food labels, to prepare foods, and to avoid dietary contaminants may guide you in developing a nutritious, safe, and healthful diet.

What nutrition information do food labels provide?

Food manufacturers view labels as a device for persuading you to buy their product instead of a competitor's product. Just walk down the cereal aisle next time you visit the supermarket and notice the bewildering number of choices. As manufactured food products multiplied over the years, and as competition for your food dollar intensified, food companies began to manipulate their labels to enhance sales. Unfortunately many of these practices were deceptive, and the consumer had a difficult time determining the nutritional quality of many processed foods. Thus, Congress passed a law designed to establish a set of standards to help Americans base their food choices on sound nutritional information.

This set of standards resulted in **nutritional labeling,** whereby major nutrients found in a food product must be listed on the label. It is not the total solution to the problem of poor food selection existing among many Americans, but combined with an educational program to increase nutritional awareness, it may effectively improve the nutritional health of our nation.

Initial food labeling legislation was passed in 1973, but it contained numerous flaws. Because of pressure from a variety of consumer interest groups, a major overhaul of the nutritional labeling program was signed into law as the Nutrition Labeling and Education Act in 1990, and it was in full effect in 1994. Under this law, nutrition labeling is mandatory for almost all foods regulated by the Food and Drug Administration (FDA). However, there are some exceptions. Some foods, such as milk, are exempt from the law if they meet certain **standards of identity,** that is, the ingredients are established by law. Food produced by very small businesses; food served in restaurants, hospital cafeterias, and airplanes; ready-to-eat food prepared primarily on site; and several other categories are also exempt from these regulations. Other modifications may be used for children under the age of 2, and others for children under the age of 4. Additionally, providing nutrition information is currently voluntary for many raw foods such as fresh fruits, vegetables, and fish.

The new label illustrated in Figure 2.9 is called *Nutrition Facts*, and it is designed to provide information on the nutrients that are of major concern for consumers. Food labels must contain the following information:

List of ingredients
   Ingredients will be listed in descending order by weight, even on standardized foods such as mayonnaise and bread.
Serving size
   Serving size has been standardized.
Servings per container
Amount per serving of the following:
   Total Calories
      Calories from fat
   Total fat
      Saturated fat
   Cholesterol
   Sodium
   Total carbohydrate
      Dietary fiber
      Sugars
   Protein
   Vitamin A

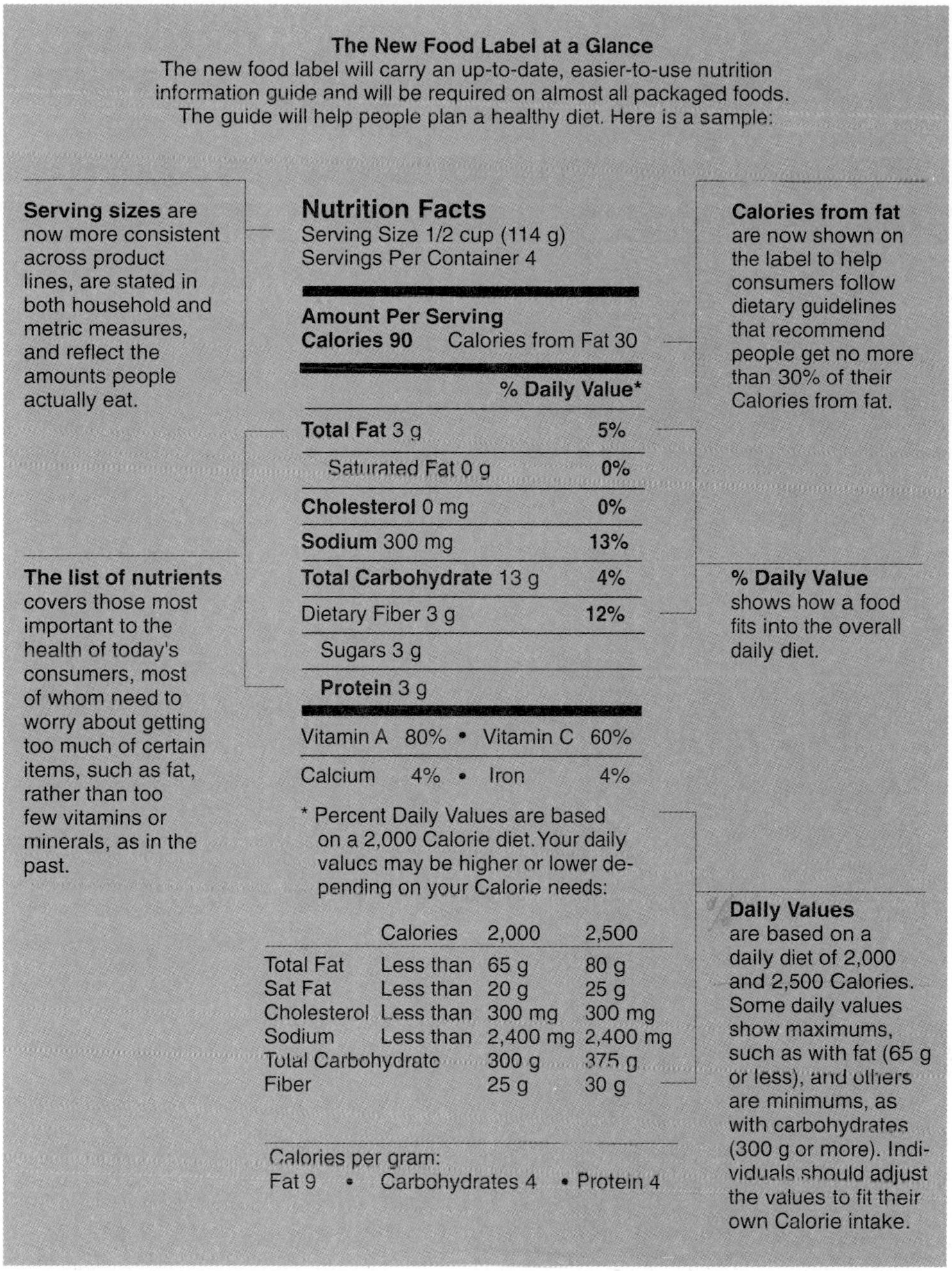

The New Food Label at a Glance

The new food label will carry an up-to-date, easier-to-use nutrition information guide and will be required on almost all packaged foods. The guide will help people plan a healthy diet. Here is a sample:

Serving sizes are now more consistent across product lines, are stated in both household and metric measures, and reflect the amounts people actually eat.

The list of nutrients covers those most important to the health of today's consumers, most of whom need to worry about getting too much of certain items, such as fat, rather than too few vitamins or minerals, as in the past.

Nutrition Facts
Serving Size 1/2 cup (114 g)
Servings Per Container 4

Amount Per Serving
Calories 90   Calories from Fat 30

	% Daily Value*
Total Fat 3 g	5%
Saturated Fat 0 g	0%
Cholesterol 0 mg	0%
Sodium 300 mg	13%
Total Carbohydrate 13 g	4%
Dietary Fiber 3 g	12%
Sugars 3 g	
Protein 3 g	

Vitamin A   80%   •   Vitamin C   60%

Calcium   4%   •   Iron   4%

* Percent Daily Values are based on a 2,000 Calorie diet. Your daily values may be higher or lower depending on your Calorie needs:

	Calories	2,000	2,500
Total Fat	Less than	65 g	80 g
Sat Fat	Less than	20 g	25 g
Cholesterol	Less than	300 mg	300 mg
Sodium	Less than	2,400 mg	2,400 mg
Total Carbohydrate		300 g	375 g
Fiber		25 g	30 g

Calories per gram:
Fat 9   •   Carbohydrates 4   •   Protein 4

Calories from fat are now shown on the label to help consumers follow dietary guidelines that recommend people get no more than 30% of their Calories from fat.

% Daily Value shows how a food fits into the overall daily diet.

Daily Values are based on a daily diet of 2,000 and 2,500 Calories. Some daily values show maximums, such as with fat (65 g or less), and others are minimums, as with carbohydrates (300 g or more). Individuals should adjust the values to fit their own Calorie intake.

Figure 2.9   An example of a Nutrition Fact food label with some explanatory material.

Source: Food and Drug Administration, 1992.

Vitamin C
Calcium
Iron
The following may be listed voluntarily:
    Calories from saturated fat
    Polyunsaturated fat
    Monounsaturated fat
    Potassium
    Soluble fiber
    Insoluble fiber
    Sugar alcohols
    Other carbohydrates

How can I use this information to select a healthier diet?

To provide information to help consumers see how foods may be part of a daily diet plan, a new label reference value, the **Daily Value (DV)** has been created. Actually, the DV is based on two other new sets of dietary standards, the **Daily Reference Values (DRVs)** and the **Reference Daily Intakes (RDIs).**

    The DRVs cover the macronutrients that are sources of energy, consisting of carbohydrate (including fiber), fat, and protein, as well as cholesterol, sodium, and potassium, which contain no Calories. The DRVs for the energy-producing nutrients are based on the number of Calories consumed daily. On the food label, the percent of the DV that a single serving of a food contains is based on a 2,000 Calorie diet, which has been selected because it is believed to have the greatest public health benefit for the nation. However, the DV may be higher or lower depending on your Calorie needs. Values for some of the macronutrients are also provided for a 2,500 Calorie diet on the food label.

The DRVs are based on certain minimum and maximum allowances, including the following for a 2,000 Calorie diet:

Total fat: Maximum of 30 percent of Calories, or less than 65 grams.

Saturated fat: Maximum of 10 percent of Calories, or less than 20 grams.

Carbohydrate: Minimum of 60 percent of Calories, or more than 300 grams.

Protein: Based on 10 percent of Calories. Applicable only to adults and children over age 4.

Fiber: Based on 12.5 grams of fiber per 1,000 Calories.

Cholesterol: Less than 300 milligrams.

Sodium: Less than 2,400 milligrams.

The Reference Daily Intakes (RDIs) replace the old United States Recommended Daily Allowances (U.S. RDAs), which were used prior to 1994 as the label reference value for vitamins, minerals, and protein. Although the name has been changed, the values for the RDIs are the same as the old U.S. RDAs but may be modified in the near future. The DVs on the food label for vitamins A and C, calcium, and iron are based on the RDIs. Table 2.14 presents the current RDIs for various nutrients.

Some important points to consider in reading the new food labels are as follows:

1. The DV for a nutrient represents the percentage contribution one serving of the food makes to the daily diet for that nutrient based on current recommendations for healthful diets. A lower DV is desirable for total fat, saturated fat, cholesterol, and sodium, while a higher DV is desirable for total carbohydrates, dietary fiber, iron, calcium, vitamins A and C, and other vitamins and minerals that may be listed.

2. To calculate the percentage of fat Calories in one serving, divide the value for Calories from fat by the total Calories and multiply by 100. For example, if one serving contains 70 Calories from fat and the total number of Calories is 120, the food consists of 58 percent fat Calories ($70/120 \times 100$).

3. Related to carbohydrates, sugars include both natural and added sugars. Dietary fiber is total

Table 2.14 RDIs for various nutrients

Key nutrients	
Protein	56 grams
Vitamin A	5,000 IU; 1 milligram
Vitamin C	60 milligrams
Thiamin	1.5 milligrams
Riboflavin	1.7 milligrams
Niacin	20 milligrams
Calcium	1,000 milligrams
Iron	18 milligrams
Other nutrients	
Vitamin D	400 IU
Vitamin E	30 IU
Vitamin B_6	2 milligrams
Folic acid	400 micrograms
Vitamin B_{12}	6 micrograms
Zinc	15 milligrams
Copper	2 milligrams
Magnesium	400 milligrams

dietary fiber, but may be listed as soluble and insoluble. Other carbohydrates represent total carbohydrates minus sugars and dietary fiber.

Labels also must disclose certain ingredients, such as sulfites, certain food dyes, and milk proteins, so food-sensitive consumers may avoid foods that may cause allergic responses.

In the past, many terms used on food labels, such as "lean" and "light," had no definite meaning. However, under the new regulations, most terms used have specific definitions, and a summary of these terms is presented in Table 2.15. Additionally, new milk labels may be based on fat content, expressed as percent or grams of fat, as follows: fat-free, skim, or nonfat milk (0 grams); lowfat or light milk (1% or 2.5 grams); reduced fat milk (2% or 5 grams); and whole milk (8 grams).

What health claims are allowed on food products?

The FDA permits food manufacturers to make health claims on food labels if the food meets certain minimum standards. These health claims are permitted because the FDA believes there may be sufficient scientific data supporting a relationship between consumption of a specific

Table 2.15 Definitions of terms for food labels

The following terms refer to one serving. A reference food is a standard food containing set proportions of nutrients.

Free (None or trivial amount; if the product is inherently free of the ingredient, it must be noted so on the label.)

Fat free: Less than 0.5 gram per serving

Saturated fat free: Less than 0.5 gram per serving

Cholesterol free: Less than 2 milligrams per serving

Sugar free: Less than 0.5 gram per serving

Sodium free: Less than 5 milligrams per serving

Calorie free: Less than 5 Calories per serving

Low (very little, or low source of)

Fat: No more than 3 grams

Sodium: Fewer than 40 milligrams

Calories: Fewer than 40

Saturated fat: No more than 1 gram

Cholesterol: Less than 20 milligrams

High or Good Source

Based on daily reference value (DRV), high is 20% or more of the DRV; good source is 10–19%. For example, to be high in fiber, a cereal must have 5 grams because the DRV is 25 grams

Reduced, Less, or Fewer

At least 25% less of a nutrient per serving compared to the particular nutrient in the reference food

More or Added

Must be 10% or more of the daily value for the particular nutrient in the reference food

Light or Lite

If a food normally derives 50% or more of its Calories from fat, it can be labeled light or lite if it is reduced in fat by 50%. If it derives less than 50% of its Calories from fat, the food must be reduced in fat by at least 50% or reduced in Calories by at least one-third.

Light foods must carry the percentage reduction. Light in sodium may be used if the sodium content is reduced by 50%

Lean (meat, fish, and game)

Contains fewer than 10 grams of fat, 4 grams of saturated fat, and 95 milligrams of cholesterol per 100 grams

Extra lean

Contains fewer than 5 grams of fat, 2 grams of saturated fat, and 95 milligrams of cholesterol per 100 grams

Fresh

If the food is unprocessed, it must be in its raw state, having not been frozen or subjected to other forms of processing. Fresh does not apply to processed foods such as fresh milk or fresh bread

Meals and Main Dishes (per 100 grams)

Low Calorie is defined as fewer than 120 Calories. To be called light, the meal must meet the definition for a low-Calorie or a low-fat meal, and it must signify which, e.g., a low-Calorie meal. A low-cholesterol meal must contain less than 20 milligrams of cholesterol and no more than 2 grams of saturated fat

Source: Data from The Food and Drug Administration, United States Department of Agriculture.

nutrient and possible prevention of a certain chronic disease. However, there are several requirements, such as not stating the degree of risk reduction, using only terms such as "may" or "might" in reference to reducing health risks, and indicating that other foods may provide similar benefits. Currently, nine health claims are allowed on food labels. Although additional constraints may be required before a food can carry a health claim, the following are the conditions that must be met:

1. Calcium and osteoporosis: A food must contain 20 percent or more of the DV for calcium.

2. Fat and cancer: A food must meet the definition for low fat. *(no more than 3gm fat per svg)*

3. Saturated fat and cholesterol and coronary heart disease: A food must meet the definition for low saturated fat, low cholesterol, and low fat.

4. Fiber containing grain products, fruits and vegetables and cancer: A food must meet the definition for low fat and be, without fortification, a good source of fiber.

5. Fruits, vegetables, and grain products that contain fiber and risk of coronary heart disease: Fruits and vegetables must meet the definition for low saturated fat, low cholesterol, low fat, and contain, without fortification, at least 0.6 grams of soluble fiber.

6. Sodium and hypertension: A food must meet the description for low sodium.

7. Fruits and vegetables and cancer: Fruits and vegetables must meet the definition for low fat and, without fortification, be a good source of at least one of the following: dietary fiber, vitamin A, or vitamin C.

8. Oats and heart disease: A food must be low fat and contain at least 0.75 gram of soluble fiber.

9. Folic acid, or folate, and neural tube defects: A food, including fortified foods, must be a good or rich source of folic acid.

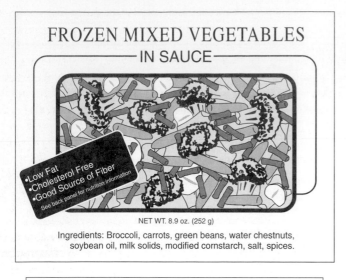

"While many factors affect heart disease, diets low in saturated fat and cholesterol may reduce the risk of this disease."

Figure 2.10   An example of a Nutrition Fact food label with an approved health claim.

Source: Food and Drug Administration, 1992.

An example of a food label containing a health claim is illustrated in Figure 2.10.

Does food processing impair food quality?

One of the major features of the Healthy North American Diet is the consumption of wholesome, natural, low-fat foods. But most of us do consume a wide variety of packaged foods, some of which may be highly processed and may be of questionable nutritional value. There has been increasing concern over the years that the nutritional quality of our food has been declining because many of our foods are overprocessed. They contain too much refined sugar, extracted oils, or white flour, all products of a refinement process. Refined sugar is pure carbohydrate with no nutritional value except Calories. The same can be said for extracted oils, which are pure fat. In the bleaching and processing of wheat to white flour, at least twenty-two known essential nutrients are removed, including the B vitamins, vitamin E, calcium, phosphorus, potassium, and magnesium. In addition, many fruits and vegetables are artificially ripened before they have reached maturity and contain smaller quantities of vitamins and minerals than naturally ripened ones do. We also consume many totally synthetic products such as artificial orange juice, nondairy creamers, and imitation ice cream, which do not possess the same nutrient value as their natural counterparts. Concern about the declining nutritional value of our food supply appears to be legitimate. Much of the blame is assigned to the processing of food, but this is not necessarily so.

In the mind of the public, processed foods more and more are thought to be inferior foods as compared with natural sources—for example, frozen peas versus fresh peas. The major purpose of food processing is to prevent waste through deterioration or spoilage. There are a variety of ways to do this, including heat, irradiation, dehydration, refrigeration, freezing, and the use of chemicals. Food is processed by companies preparing their products for sale, but food processing also occurs at home in the preparation of a meal. You may wash, cut, cook, and freeze a variety of foods at home. Food processing, both at home and by commercial organizations, results in the loss of some nutrients. However, Erdman and Poneros-Schneier note that commercial preservation techniques in common use today do not cause major nutrient losses in the foods we eat. Commercial food processing may actually cause less nutrient loss than home processing. In addition, food companies may enrich or fortify certain products before marketing. Examples include the addition of some B vitamins and iron to grain products, vitamins A and D to milk, vitamin A to margarine, and iodine to table salt. In some cases not all of the nutrients that were removed in processing are returned, but in some products a greater amount is returned or added.

A few nutrients may be susceptible to loss through processing. Borenstein and Lachance have noted with some reservations that carbohydrates, lipids, protein, niacin, vitamin K, and minerals are relatively stable during food processing and storage. Vitamins A, D, E, B_2, B_6, B_{12}, pantothenic acid, and folacin are a little less stable, while B_1 and vitamin C may be seriously depleted by commercial and home food processing.

You can minimize nutrient losses and preserve the healthful quality of foods by following these procedures in the preparation of food at home.

- Keep most fruits and vegetables chilled in the refrigerator to prevent enzymic destruction of nutrients. For similar reasons, keep frozen foods in the freezer until ready for preparation to eat.

- After cutting, wrap most fruits and vegetables tightly to prevent exposure to air, which may accelerate oxidation and spoiling, and store them in the refrigerator.

- Buy milk in cardboard or opaque plastic containers to prevent light from destroying riboflavin, a B vitamin. For similar reasons, keep most grain products stored in opaque containers or dark cupboards.

- Steam or microwave vegetables in very little water to prevent the loss of water-soluble vitamins and some minerals. Microwaving is very effective in preserving the nutrient value of food.

- Avoid cooking with high temperatures and prolonged cooking of foods, particularly in water, which may increase nutrient losses.

- Avoid grilling or broiling foods, especially meats, over open flames on a daily basis. In particular, avoid charring meats, which may lead to the formation of various carcinogens known as heterocyclic amines (HCA). Frying foods may also produce HCA, but steaming, boiling and microwaving meat is much safer because these techniques produce fewer HCA that may cause cancer.

The key point is that both commercial and home processing of food will not necessarily lead to a nutritionally inferior product. Even if commercial food processing does cause a slight decrease in nutritional quality, it helps provide a greater and more varied food supply with adequate amounts of dietary nutrients. Nutrient losses incurred with home food processing are also minimal, and an adequate nutrient intake will be obtained if you consume a wide variety of foods.

The major problem with food processing is the excessive use of highly refined products like sugar, oils, fats, unenriched white flour, and salt. Wise food selection can help avoid these problems, though this may be somewhat tricky in today's food marketplace. It requires careful reading of food labels.

Are food additives safe?

Do you ever read the list of ingredients on the labels of highly processed food products? If not, check one out soon. My guess is you will not know what half the ingredients are or why they are there (unless the reason is listed). A recently purchased box of Long Grain & Wild Rice with Herb Seasoning, thought to be totally natural, had the main ingredients of enriched parboiled long grain rice, wild rice, and dehydrated vegetables (onion, parsley, spinach, garlic, celery) as the herb seasoning—along with hydrolyzed vegetable protein, salt, sugar, monosodium glutamate, autolyzed yeast, sodium silicoaluminate, disodium inosinate, disodium guanylate, and sodium sulfite. The rice was delicious, but were all the additives necessary?

The Food and Drug Administration (FDA) classifies a **food additive** as any substance added directly to food. There are more than forty different purposes for the additives in the foods we eat, but the four most common are to add flavor, to enhance color, to improve texture, and to preserve the food. For example, vanilla extract may be added to ice cream to impart a vanilla flavor, vitamin C (ascorbic acid) may be added to fruits and vegetables to prevent discoloration, emulsifiers may be added to help blend oil evenly throughout a product, and sodium propionate may be used to prolong shelf life.

To earn FDA approval, additives must be **generally recognized as safe (GRAS).** They may be added only to specific foods for specific purposes, and in general must improve the quality of the food without posing any hazards to humans. Only the minimum amount necessary to achieve the desired purpose may be added.

Although we realize that absolute safety does not exist in anything we do, including eating, we do have a right to expect that the food we purchase is generally safe for consumption. The government and food manufacturers must take utmost care to ensure that food additives do not create any appreciable health risks. On the other hand, we as consumers also have a responsibility to select foods necessary for good nutrition. Food product labeling has helped us in this regard, for we now can tell what ingredients we are eating, although we may not always know why they are there.

In the past, the major concern with most additives was the possibility that they could cause cancer. The Delaney Clause to the Food, Drug, and Cosmetic Act prohibits the addition of any additive to foods if it has been shown to cause cancer in animals or humans at any dose. Saccharin, which has been shown to cause cancer in laboratory animals when given in high doses, was exempted from the Delaney Clause by an act of Congress. More recently, in its position statement on food and water safety, the American Dietetic Association cited a National Research Council report indicating that people should worry less about the risk of cancer from food additives and be more concerned about the carcinogenic effects of excess macronutrients, evidenced by the linkage of obesity to various cancers.

In general, the additives in today's food are regarded safe. Nevertheless, there is concern that some additives may increase health risks for certain individuals. For example, some individuals are allergic to sulfites, a preservative used in a variety of foods. Dietary supplements also may contain substances that increase health risks.

Are dietary supplements safe?

Literally thousands of different dietary supplements are available in the marketplace, including vitamin and mineral supplements, various herbal extracts, and synthetic compounds. Some dietary supplements consist of a single substance, while others may contain a dozen or more so-called ingredients. Buzz words such as "antioxidants," "phytochemicals," and "active enzymes" are used to promote health benefits, along with marketing ploys using names such as "UpTime Food Supplement" and "SuperPep" to suggest enhanced sport performance. Where appropriate, the effectiveness and safety of various dietary supplements will be discussed in later sections of this book, but a general discussion of safety will be presented at this point.

Although dietary supplements are not classified as drugs, many of them, particularly herbal preparations, may be regarded as drugs in disguise. Some potent medicinal drugs, such as the heart medication digitalis, are extracted from plants. Other plant extracts also may elicit pharmacological effects in the body, possibly conferring some therapeutic benefits. Unfortunately, for several reasons, there is little well-controlled research documenting the

Delaney Clause

effectiveness of most plant products or other dietary supplements intended to improve health or sport performance. First, major pharmaceutical companies do not fund research with herbal products, primarily because herbal products cannot be patented to ensure profits to the company. Second, for synthetic products that are patented, companies may not sponsor well-controlled research because of the possibility of negative results—that is, their product was found to be ineffective in producing the desired results. Concomitantly, there are few data relative to the safety of most dietary supplements.

Nonetheless, some research suggests that use of several herbal products may have some healthful effects. In some countries, such as Germany, herbs are approved for medical use by agencies comparable to the U.S. FDA. For example, tea made from the herb chamomile may be used to suppress muscle spasms, such as menstrual cramps, and use of the herb echinacea may relieve symptoms of upper respiratory tract infections. However, use of either herb may elicit reactions in individuals allergic to the daisy family, to which both herbs belong.

As mentioned in Chapter 1, the burden of proof of safety rests with the FDA, although manufacturers must provide reasonable assurance that no ingredient presents a significant or unreasonable risk of illness or injury. One would like to believe that most dietary supplements are safe, and that may be the case for most vitamins, minerals, and other nutrient-related dietary supplements when consumed in reasonable doses. However, although the adverse effects of nutrient megadoses will be discussed in later chapters as appropriate, there are very few data regarding health risks associated with the chronic intake of most dietary supplements. The President's Commission on Dietary Supplement Labels recently recommended swift enforcement action by the FDA to ensure the safety of dietary supplements, including herbal preparations, but safety regulations may take several years to be implemented.

Most data regarding adverse health effects of dietary supplements are usually case reports released by public health agencies, often documenting serious health problems. For example, in a recent Consumers Union report various herbal preparations, including chaparral, comfrey, and yohimbe, were associated with stomach disorders, nonviral hepatitis (rapid liver damage), obstructed blood flow to the liver and possible cirrhosis, and even death. Many dietary supplements promoted for weight control or energy production contain potent stimulants, such as caffeine (guarana) and ephedrine (ma huang); excess consumption may increase blood pressure, cause heart palpitations, or be fatal.

Use of some dietary supplements may increase health risks. The Consumers Union recommends these safeguards to protect your health:

- Before trying a dietary supplement to treat a health problem, try changing your diet or life-style first.

- Check with your doctor before taking any dietary supplement, particularly herbal preparations. This is especially important for pregnant and nursing women.

- Buy standardized products. Most dietary supplements in the United States should be standardized according to federal regulations. Dietary supplement manufacturers have until March, 1999 to provide "Supplement Facts" labels on their products that will provide information comparable to the "Nutrition Facts" food label.

- Use only single-ingredient dietary supplements. Use of combination supplements may make it difficult to determine the cause of any side effects.

- Be alert to both the positive and negative effects of the supplement. Try to keep an objective record of the effects.

- Stop taking the supplement immediately if you experience any health-related problems. Contact your physician and local health authorities to report the problem. This may help establish a data base for the safety of dietary supplements.

Do foods contain enough pesticides to cause health concerns?

As noted previously, plants contain substances called phytochemicals, which may contribute to various health benefits associated with a diet high in fruits, vegetables, and other wholesome plant foods. Many of these phytochemicals also help the plant survive, primarily by acting as herbicides or pesticides to prevent damage from naturally occurring weeds and insects. Nevertheless, over two thousand insects, weeds, or plant diseases damage nearly one-third of our nation's farm crop each year. To help minimize crop damage from these pests, agriculturalists have developed synthetic herbicides and pesticides to augment plants' natural defenses.

Although synthetic herbicides and pesticides may effectively control weeds and pests harmful to plants, they appear to function differently in the human body than do natural plant phytochemicals. Synthetic chemicals may cause health problems. A number of illnesses including cancer and nervous system disorders, along with genetic mutations, birth defects, miscarriages, and deaths, have been attributed to prolonged exposure to these chemicals. On the one hand, we need to control those pests destructive to our food supply, but on the other hand, the health of the public should not be harmed by the chemicals being used. This is the dilemma concerning the use of pesticides and similar chemicals.

Most of the serious diseases from pesticide use have been among farm workers who may be exposed to high concentrations on a daily basis or in people who live near sprayed areas. However, direct exposure to even small amounts of household insect spray has been known to alter brain function, causing irritability, insomnia, and reduced concentration. The prudent individual should avoid direct contact with these substances as much as possible, for even thorough washing with soap and water has little effect upon the absorption through the skin of some insect sprays.

Pesticides may also be on the food we eat and in the water we drink. The FDA and state government agencies conduct spot surveys to analyze the pesticide content of produce for sale. The Delaney Clause applied to pesticides, but Congress recently passed the Food Quality Protection Act replacing the Delaney Clause with a reasonable certainty of no harm standard. In a recent report that analyzed data on more than 200 known carcinogens in foods, the National Research Council of the National Academy of Sciences concluded that both synthetic and naturally-occurring pesticides are consumed at such low levels that they pose little threat to human health. However, meat products may contain higher amounts of pesticides, as pesticides become more concentrated in animals that consume large quantities of plants containing pesticide residue. Fish from contaminated waters may also contain high levels of pesticides. There is increasing concern that children may be exposed to higher levels of pesticides because the current acceptable standards for pesticide residuals are based on adult body size and food intake; children are smaller and normally consume greater amounts of fruits and vegetables per unit of body weight. Under the 1996 Food Quality Protection Act, revised lower limits for pesticides in foods are due to be completed in 1999.

Government agencies are attempting to reduce pesticide residues in the food we eat, and more farmers are turning to pesticide-free farming, producing more organic foods certified to be free of any pesticide residue. Unfortunately, at the present time there is little understanding of how varying levels of pesticide exposure will affect human health. Based on current knowledge, the following points appear to be sound advice to help reduce, but may not completely eliminate, the pesticide content in the foods we eat.

1. Avoid direct skin contact or breathing exposure to pesticides.

2. Food preparation may reduce pesticide residues. Wash produce thoroughly; some, but not all, pesticides on fruits and vegetables are water soluble. Washing may be particularly helpful to remove pesticide residues from apples, bananas, corn, grapes, lettuce, peaches, and tomatoes. Peeling some fruits and vegetables also helps. Peeling is effective for apples, carrots, cucumbers, grapes, oranges, peaches, and potatoes. Cooking may also help, particularly with broccoli, green beans, potatoes, and tomatoes.

3. Eat less animal fat and seafood from contaminated waters. Pesticides may concentrate in animal fat.

4. Buy fruits and vegetables locally and in season. Farmers are less likely to use pesticides if the food is to be sold locally.

5. Eat a wide variety of foods. If a food contains pesticides, it will only contribute a small amount as part of your overall diet.

6. Buy certified **organic foods.** Although there is currently no national definition of organic foods, certain states and independent groups have certification programs. The United States Department of Agriculture is considering a set of national standards for organic foods to help the consumer make informed choices. In general, certified organic foods are not anymore nutritious than nonorganic foods, but they are grown in soil without artificial fertilizers, and no pesticides are used in the growing process.

Why do some people experience adverse reactions to some foods?

Although most food we eat is safe and causes no acute health problems, some individuals may experience mild to severe reactions, or possibly death, from eating certain foods. These reactions may be attributed to food intolerance, food allergy, or food poisoning.

Food intolerance, the most common problem, is a general term for any adverse reaction to a food or food component that does not involve the immune system. The body cannot properly digest a portion of the food because it lacks the appropriate enzyme, resulting in gastrointestinal distress such as nausea and diarrhea. For example, many African Americans lack lactase, the enzyme needed to digest lactose (milk sugar), and thus suffer from lactose intolerance, a topic that is covered in Chapter 4.

Food allergy, also known as food hypersensitivity, involves an adverse immune response to an otherwise harmless food substance. Many foods contain allergens, usually proteins, that may stimulate the immune system to manufacture antibodies (immunoglobulin E, or IgE) specific to that food. When individuals who have inherited a food allergy are first exposed to that food, their immune system produces millions of IgE antibodies. These antibodies reside in some white blood cells and mast cells in the body, particularly in the skin, respiratory tract, and gastrointestinal tract, the parts of the body that come into contact with air and the food we eat. These cells also contain substances, such as histamine, that are released when the antibodies are exposed again to the offending food allergen. Histamine and other chemicals cause the allergic reaction, which may involve the skin (swelling, hives, itchy skin and eyes), gastrointestinal tract (nausea, vomiting, abdominal cramps, diarrhea), or respiratory tract (runny nose, sneezing, coughing). In severe cases, an allergic response may involve anaphylactic shock and death. Although allergens may be found in many foods, 90 percent of the offenders are proteins found in milk, eggs, fish and seafood, nuts, peanuts, soy protein, and wheat. Some additives also may cause allergic responses, particularly sulfites used as preservatives.

If you experience problems when you consume certain foods, you may be able to make a self-diagnosis by simply avoiding that food and noting whether or not you experience a recurrence. But, because there may be many causes of food-related illness, you should consult an allergist or other appropriate physician to determine whether you have either food intolerance or food allergy. Once the offending food is determined, you may need to eliminate that food from your diet or reduce the amount you consume. In some cases this is relatively simple. For example, if you develop a reaction to clams, a common problem, you should have no difficulty finding other sources of high-quality protein. However, if you react to milk, it may be more difficult to obtain an adequate dietary intake of calcium. A dietician will be able to assist you in planning a diet that compensates for the reduced intake of calcium. Some suggestions are presented in Chapter 8.

Food poisoning is caused primarily by consuming foods contaminated with bacteria. Historically, bacteria such as Salmonella, Escherichia, Staphylococcus, and Clostridium accounted for most foodborne illness, but more recent strains include Campylobacter and Listeria. The most common symptoms of food poisoning include nausea, vomiting, or diarrhea, which normally clear up in a day or two. However, the Center for Science in the Public Interest indicates that individuals should seek medical help in cases involving headache, stiff neck, and fever occurring together; bloody diarrhea; diarrhea lasting longer than three days; fever that lasts more than 24 hours; or sensations of weakness, numbness and tingling in the arms and legs. Some cases of food poisoning may be fatal if not treated properly.

Waites and Arbuthnott indicate that individuals living in developed countries may be at greater risk for foodborne illness because of changing dietary habits, such as consuming foods with fewer preservatives and eating more meals outside the home. Although governmental health agencies attempt to control the spread of bacteria to food through appropriate regulations governing the food industry, occasional outbreaks do occur because of food contamination during industrial processing. For example, 25 million pounds of ground meat was recently recalled because of possible contamination with the bacteria Escherichia coli (E. coli). Many cases also occur because of improper food handling in the home. Indeed, the USDA estimates that up to 2.5 million Americans may become ill every year after eating poultry or meat contaminated with Salmonella bacteria, while the Centers for Disease Control and Prevention estimate that about 9,000 Americans die each year from contaminated food.

At the minimum, the following guidelines should be helpful in preventing the spread of bacteria in food prepared at home.

1. Treat all raw meat, poultry, fish, seafood, and eggs as if they were contaminated. Prevent juices from getting on other foods.

2. Wash hands thoroughly before preparing any food.

3. Thoroughly clean all utensils used in food preparation with hot soapy water. Microwaving your sponges for about 30 to 60 seconds may help kill bacteria.

4. Use a clean preparation surface. After preparing poultry or other animal foods, clean the preparation surface thoroughly before using it to prepare other foods. When using the same surface, prepare animal foods last.

5. Do not use canned foods that are extensively dented or bulging.

6. Cook all meat, poultry, seafood, and eggs thoroughly according to directions. However, do not overcook or char meats, as this process may produce carcinogens.

7. Store heated foods promptly in the refrigerator or freezer.

8. Reheat foods thoroughly.

9. Use leftovers within a few days. When in doubt, throw it out.

Healthful Nutrition Recommendations for Better Physical Performance

Articles about nutrition for athletes in popular sports magazines, and food supplements advertised therein, give the impression that athletes have special nutritional requirements above those of nonathletes. Special vitamin and mineral supplements, protein and amino acid mixtures, fat mobilizing substances, and specific "sport nutritional compounds" often are highly recommended as means to improve athletic performance, but these products are not needed by the vast majority of athletes. In general, the diet that is optimal for health is also optimal for physical or sport performance. The Healthy North American Diet will provide adequate Calories and nutrients to meet the needs of almost all athletes in training.

Nevertheless, modifications to the Healthy North American Diet may help enhance performance for certain athletic endeavors, and subsequent chapters will focus on specific recommendations relative to the use of various nutrients and dietary supplements to enhance physical performance. The purpose of this section is to provide some general recommendations regarding the use of the Healthy North American Diet by the athlete before, during, and after competition or a hard training session.

When and what should I eat prior to competition?

In Chapter 4 we cover the special pre-event nutrition needs of athletes involved in prolonged exercise tasks, such as the marathon. Dietary practices such as carbohydrate loading and substantial intake of carbohydrates in the pre-event meal are designed to maximize body stores of muscle and liver glycogen. Although most athletic events are not prolonged endurance events, there may be some important points to consider regarding the timing and composition of the meal eaten prior to competition.

It is a well-established fact that the ingestion of food just prior to competition will not benefit physical performance in most athletic events, yet the pregame meal, so to speak, is one of the major topics of discussion among athletes. A number of special meals have been utilized throughout the years because of their alleged benefits to physical performance, and special products have been marketed as pre-event nutritional supplements. Although research has not substantiated the value of any one particular precompetition meal, some general guidelines have been developed from practical experience over the years.

There are several major goals of the precompetition meal that may be achieved through proper timing and composition. In general, the precompetition meal should do the following:

1. Allow for the stomach to be relatively empty at the start of competition.

2. Help to prevent or minimize gastrointestinal distress.

3. Help avoid sensations of hunger, lightheadedness, or fatigue.

4. Provide adequate fuel supplies, primarily carbohydrate, in the blood and muscles.

5. Provide an adequate amount of body water.

In general, a solid meal should be eaten about 3 to 4 hours prior to competition. This should allow ample time for digestion to occur so that the stomach is relatively empty, and yet hunger sensations are minimized. However, pre-event emotional tension or anxiety may delay digestive time, as will a meal with a high-fat or high-protein content. Hence, the composition of the meal is critical. It should be high in carbohydrate and low in fat and protein, providing for easy digestibility.

The composition of the precompetition meal should not contribute to any gastrointestinal distress, such as flatulence, increased acidity in the stomach, heartburn, or increased bulk that may stimulate the need for a bowel movement during competition. In general, foods to be avoided include gas formers like beans, spicy foods that may elicit heartburn, and bulk foods like bran products. High-sugar compounds may delay gastric emptying or create a reverse osmotic effect, possibly increasing the fluid content of the stomach, which may lead to a feeling of distress, cramps, or nausea. High-sugar loads, particularly fructose, may also lead to other forms of gastrointestinal distress, such as diarrhea. Large amounts of concentrated sugar can cause a reactive drop in blood sugar in susceptible individuals. Through experience, you should learn what foods disagree with you during performance, and of course, you should avoid these prior to competition.

Adequate fluid intake should be assured prior to an event, particularly if the event will be of long duration or conducted under hot environmental conditions. Diuretics such as alcohol, which increase the excretion of body water, should be avoided. Large amounts of protein increase the water output of the kidneys and thus should be avoided. Fluids may be taken up to 15 to 30 minutes prior to competition to help ensure adequate hydration. Details are provided in Chapter 9.

A wide variety of foods may be selected for the precompetition meal. The meal should consist of foods that are high in complex carbohydrates with moderate to low amounts of protein. Examples of such foods are presented in later chapters and also may be found in Appendix F, particularly those in the starch list. The foods should be agreeable to you. You should eat what you like within the guidelines presented above.

Two examples of precompetition meals, each containing about 500–600 Calories with substantial amounts of carbohydrate, are presented in Table 2.16.

One important last point. Meals other than the precompetition meal eaten on the same day should not be skipped. They should adhere to the basic principles set forth earlier in this chapter. Follow these general recommendations.

1. For events in the morning, eat a precompetition meal similar to breakfast; for example, meal A in Table 2.16.

Table 2.16 Two examples of precompetition meals containing 500–600 Calories	
Meal A	**Meal B**
Glass of orange juice	One cup low-fat yogurt
One bowl of oatmeal	One banana
Two pieces of toast with jelly	One toasted bagel
Sliced peaches with skim milk	One ounce of turkey breast
	One-half cup of raisins

2. For events in early to mid-afternoon, eat breakfast and lunch. You might consume a more substantial breakfast, along with meal B in Table 2.16 as a precompetition meal for lunch.

3. For events in the late afternoon, eat breakfast, lunch, and a snack. Again, eat a substantial breakfast and lunch and consume snacks that appeal to you, such as fruit, bagels with jelly, or other easily digestible foods.

4. For events in the evening, eat breakfast, lunch, and a precompetition meal for dinner.

How about the use of liquid meals, sports bars, and dietary supplements?

Liquid meals have some advantages over solid meals for precompetition nutrition. The available **liquid meals** are well balanced in nutrition value, have a high-carbohydrate content, have no bulk, are easily digested and assimilated, and may be more practical and economical than a solid meal.

A number of different liquid meal products are available commercially, including Nutrament, GatorPro, Ensure, Ensure-Plus, and others associated with weight loss programs, such as Slim-Fast. The composition of each may vary somewhat, but checking the label will reveal the exact nutrient content. The energy content is usually about 250–400 Calories. Most liquid meals are high in carbohydrates, moderate in protein, and low in fat. Vitamins and minerals may be added in varying amounts.

Because a liquid meal may be assimilated more readily than a solid meal, it may be taken closer to competition, say 2 to 3 hours before. Research has shown that there is no difference between a liquid meal and a solid meal relative to subsequent hunger, nausea, diarrhea, or weight changes prior to competition. In addition, liquid meals will not affect physical performance any differently than a well-planned solid precompetition meal.

From a practical standpoint, liquid meals may save time and money. The time and expense of stopping for a solid meal prior to an event may be avoided by the proper use of liquid meals. Although they are rather economically priced in comparison to a solid meal, liquid meals may be prepared even more economically at home. Nonfat dry milk powder can be purchased in any supermarket, while various glucose polymer powders can be obtained at stores specializing in sports merchandise, particularly running and cycling shops. The following formula will provide one quart of a tasty liquid meal:

1/2 cup water

1/2 cup of nonfat dry milk powder

1/4 cup of a glucose polymer

3 cups of skim milk

1 teaspoon of flavoring for palatability (cherry, vanilla, or chocolate extract)

Sports bars have become increasingly popular in recent years, and over a dozen products are targeted to physically active individuals. Most **sports bars** are good sources of carbohydrate, and most contain some protein and fat, but the actual content will vary. As with liquid meals, the food label on the sports bar will describe its contents. When compared to comparable energy sources from ordinary food, sports bars do not possess any magical qualities to enhance physical performance, but they possess some advantages similar to liquid meals, such as convenience. Because the major ingredient in sports bars is carbohydrate, an expanded discussion is presented in Chapter 4.

It is important to note that liquid meals and sports bars should be used primarily as a substitute for precompetition nutrition and should not be used on a long-term basis to replace the Healthy North American Diet concept.

Numerous dietary supplements are marketed to athletes as a means to enhance sport performance, but, with few exceptions, have not been shown to exert any potent ergogenic effects. Research evaluating the effectiveness of purported sport ergogenics is presented throughout the book. Pertinent discussion topics include the following:

Chapter 4: Alcohol and carbohydrate ergogenics

Chapter 5: Caffeine and ergogenics that affect fat metabolism

Chapter 6: Amino acids, creatine, and other protein-related ergogenics

Chapter 7: Vitamins and other vitamin-related ergogenics, such as ginseng

Chapter 8: Mineral ergogenics

Chapter 9: Sodium bicarbonate, glycerol

Chapter 12: Anabolic ergogenics for strength-trained athletes

How important is breakfast for the physically active individual?

Breakfast may be especially important. A balanced breakfast provides a significant amount of Calories and other nutrients in the daily diet of the physically active person. A breakfast of skim milk, a poached egg, whole-grain toast, fortified high-fiber cereal, and orange juice will help provide a substantial part of the RDA for protein, calcium, iron, fiber, vitamin C, and other nutrients and is also relatively high in complex carbohydrates. A balanced breakfast high in fiber with an average amount of protein also will help prevent the onset of mid-morning hunger. The fiber and protein may help maintain a feeling of satiety throughout the morning, whereas a breakfast of refined carbohydrates, like doughnuts, may trigger an insulin response and produce hypoglycemia (low blood sugar) in the middle of the morning. The resultant hunger is typically satisfied by eating other refined carbohydrates, which will satisfy the hunger urge only until about lunch time. A balanced breakfast having a high nutrient density is therefore preferable to a breakfast based on refined carbohydrate products. Nontraditional breakfast foods, such as pizza, may also provide a balanced meal for breakfast.

Skipping breakfast would be comparable to a small fast, as the individual might not eat for 12 to 14 hours. This could conceivably produce hypoglycemia with resultant symptoms of weakness and possible impairment of training. Although individual preferences should be taken into account, a balanced breakfast could provide a good source of some major nutrients to the individual who is involved in a physical conditioning program. For those on a tight time schedule, a bowl of ready-to-eat, fortified high-fiber cereal with skim milk and fruit may be an ideal choice. Nancy Clark notes that this breakfast is not only quick, easy, and convenient but also rich in carbohydrate, fiber, iron, calcium, and vitamins, and low in fat, cholesterol, and Calories.

What should I eat during competition?

There is no need to consume anything during most types of athletic competition with the possible exception of carbohydrate and water. Carbohydrate may provide additional supplies of the preferred energy source during prolonged exercise, while water intake may be critical for regulation of body temperature when exercising in warm environments. In very rare cases, such as ultradistance competition, a hypotonic salt solution may be recommended. Appropriate details are presented in Chapters 4 and 9.

What should I eat after competition or a hard training session?

In general, a balanced diet is all that is necessary to meet your nutrient needs and restore your nutritional status to normal following competition or daily, hard physical training. Carbohydrate and fat are the main nutrients used during exercise and can be replaced easily from foods among the food exchange lists. The increased caloric intake that is needed to replace your energy expenditure also will help provide you with the additional small amounts of protein, vitamins, minerals, and electrolytes that may be necessary for effective recovery. Thirst will normally help replace water losses on a day-to-day basis; you can check this by recording your body weight each morning to see if it is back to normal.

Those individuals involved in daily physical activity of a prolonged nature, such as long-distance running and swimming or prolonged tennis bouts, should stress complex carbohydrate foods in their daily diet. This will help

replenish muscle glycogen, which is necessary for continued daily workouts at high intensity. Complex carbohydrates are also rich in the vitamins and minerals necessary for their metabolism in the body. Simple sugars eaten immediately after a hard workout may help restore muscle glycogen fairly rapidly, but the addition of protein to the carbohydrate source may be even more effective. Specific guidelines are presented in Chapter 4.

For those who must compete several times daily and eat between competitions, such as in tennis tournaments or swim meets, the principles relative to pregame meals may be relevant.

How can I eat more nutritiously while traveling for competition?

Athletes who must travel to compete are often faced with the problem of obtaining proper pre-event and postevent nutrition. After reading this chapter, you should be aware of how to select foods that are high in carbohydrate, low in fat, and moderate in protein. More guidelines are presented in Chapters 4 through 6. One possible solution is to pack your own food and fluids in a traveling bag or cooler. Foods from each of the Food Exchange Lists can be easily packed or kept on ice, such as skim milk; precooked low-fat meats; bagels and cereal; fruits, juices, and vegetables; sports drinks; and high-carbohydrate snacks including whole wheat crackers and pretzels, and low-fat cookies such as Fig Newtons and vanilla wafers. Small containers of condiments can also be easily transported in the cooler, along with proper eating utensils. Taking your own food means you can eat your pre-event or postevent meal as planned, and you may save money as well. Such an approach may be very effective for short, one-day trips and may also be used to complement other meals on longer journeys. Some easily packed snack foods are presented in Table 2.17.

While traveling, you have a variety of eating places from which to select your food, including full-service restaurants, restaurants with all-you-can-eat buffets, steakhouses and fishhouses, fast-food restaurants, pizza parlors, sub shops, supermarkets, convenience stores, and even vending machines. With a solid background on the nutritional principles presented in this chapter, you should be able to select healthful, high-carbohydrate and low-fat foods at any of these establishments, but of course the variety of food choices will vary depending on the place you choose.

Although all fast foods can be part of a healthy diet when consumed in moderation, many are relatively high in fat content, and their intake should be restricted. Some fast-food restaurants attempted to provide foods with less fat, such as McDonald's McLean Deluxe hamburger, which has been removed from the menu because of poor sales. Nevertheless, many restaurants do provide a few healthier choices with individual sandwiches containing less than

Table 2.17 Easily packed snacks for traveling or brown bag lunches

Starch exchange	Meat exchange	Vegetable exchange
Bagels	Small can of baked beans	Sliced carrots
Pita bread	Cooked chicken or turkey, small 2-ounce commercial packages, packed in airtight plastic bags	Broccoli stalks
Muffins		Cauliflower pieces
Fig Newtons		Tomatoes
Vanilla wafers		Canned vegetable juices
Whole wheat crackers	Small can of sardines	
Graham crackers	Peanut butter	
Dry cereals	Reduced-fat cheese slices	
Wheat Chex	String cheese	
Grapenuts		
Plain popcorn		
Fruit exchange	**Milk exchange**	**Fat exchange**
Small cans of fruit in own juice	Small containers of skim or low-fat milk, aseptic packaging if available	Nuts
Small containers of fruit juice, aseptic packages		Peanuts
Oranges	Dried skim milk powder, to be reconstituted	
Apples	Packaged yogurt	
Other raw fruits		
Dried fruits		

30 percent of their Calories from fat, including McDonald's McGrilled Chicken Classic and Arby's Roast Beef Deluxe. In some cases, particularly with grilled, skinless chicken sandwiches, much of the fat content is in the sauce added to the sandwich, so ordering the sauce on the side allows you to control the amount added. Other sandwich shops, such as Au Bon Pain and Subway may serve healthful sandwiches, but unwise selections in these stores may also contain substantial amounts of fat.

In a recent review article, Marion Franz noted that you can eat fast food and stay within the recommended nutrition guidelines for a healthy diet, but obtaining a healthful diet requires careful selection of foods. Almost all fast-food restaurants provide materials detailing the nutrient content of each of their products. In some cases the materials may be obtained in the restaurant, while in other cases you must contact regional or national headquarters. McDonald's has even developed a nutrition facts menu for athletes, with meals containing 60–70 percent of Calories from carbohydrates. See Appendix G for the fat percentages of specific fast-food products.

The following suggestions may be helpful if you are dining in a fast-food or budget-type restaurant, such as McDonald's, Wendy's, Arby's, Pizza Hut, Denny's, Chi-Chi's, Bamboo Hut, or the Olive Garden. Many supermarkets also have takeout departments or salad bars from which to select lunch or dinner.

Breakfast selections
    English muffins, unbuttered, with jelly
    English muffins with Canadian bacon
    Whole wheat pancakes with syrup
    French toast
    Bran muffins, fat-free or low-fat
    Hot whole-grain cereal, oatmeal
    Ready-to-eat fortified, high-fiber cereal
    Skim or low-fat milk
    Orange juice
    Hot cocoa
Lunch or dinner selections
    Any low-fat sandwiches, no mayonnaise or high-fat sauces
    Grilled chicken breast sandwich, on whole-grain bun

Baked or broiled fish sandwich

Lean roast beef sandwich, on whole-grain bun

Single, plain hamburger, on whole-grain bun

Baked potato, with toppings on the side (add sparingly)

Pasta dishes, spaghetti, and macaroni, with low-fat sauces

Rice dishes

Lo mein noodles, not chow mein (fried noodles)

Soups, rice and noodle

Salsas, made with tomatoes

Chicken or seafood tostadas, made with cornmeal tortillas

Bean and rice dishes

All whole-grain and other breads

Salads, low-fat dressing

Salad bar, focus on vegetables and high-carbohydrate foods; avoid high-fat items

Pizza, thick crust, vegetable type with minimum cheese topping

Skim or low-fat milk

Orange juice

Frozen yogurt, fat-free or low-fat

Sherbet

With any of these selections, it is always a good idea to order toppings, for example, mayonnaise, salad dressing, etc., on the side so that you can control portions. When selecting sandwiches, ask for those that are either baked, broiled, or grilled.

For the most part, research supports the general finding that the diet that is optimal for your health is also the optimal diet for your performance. Eating right, both for health and performance, does not mean you need to eat bland foods because all foods, some in moderation, can be tastefully prepared and blended into The Healthy North American Diet.

How does gender and age influence nutritional recommendations for enhanced physical performance?

The diet that is optimal for health is the optimal diet for physical performance. This is the key principle of sports nutrition and it applies to physically active males and females of all ages. However, as shall be noted at certain points in this text, specific nutrient needs may vary by gender and age, and various forms of exercise training may influence nutrient requirements as well.

For example, adolescent and adult premenopausal females need more dietary iron than males. Female athletes, especially those participating in aerobic endurance sports such as distance running, must include iron-rich foods in their diet or risk incurring iron-deficiency anemia and impaired running ability. Also, disordered eating in female athletes may contribute to the development of premature osteoporosis, prompting the American College of Sports Medicine to develop a position stand on the Female Athlete Triad, an important issue discussed in Chapter 8.

Relative to sports participation, the American Dietetic Association recognizes that children are not little adults. For example, compared to adults children experience different responses to exercise under hot environmental conditions. The ADA has published two timely statements, written by Suzanne Steen, providing nutrition guidance for child and adolescent athletes involved in organized sports. On the other end of the age spectrum, older athletes may experience decreases in their resting metabolic rate. In order to obtain an adequate dietary supply of nutrients, they must focus more on nutrient density.

The special nutrient requirements of females, the young, and the elderly, as they relate to physical activity, will be incorporated in the text where relevant. However, most of the nutritional principles underlying exercise and sport performance that are presented in this text apply to most physically active individuals.

References

Books

American Academy of Allergy and Immunology. 1993. *Understanding Food Allergy.* Milwaukee: American Academy of Allergy and Immunology.

American Dietetic Association and American Diabetes Association. 1995. *Exchange Lists for Meal Planning.* Chicago: American Dietetic Association.

Editors of Vegetarian Times. 1995. *Vegetarian Times Complete Cookbook.* New York: Macmillan.

International Center for Sports Nutrition and the United States Olympic Committee. 1990. *Vegetarianism—Implications for Athletes.* Omaha: International Center for Sports Nutrition.

Jaret, P. 1997. *30 Foods that Fight Disease.* San Francisco: Time Publishing Ventures.

National Dairy Council. 1992. *Guide to Good Eating.* 6th ed. Rosemont, IL: National Dairy Council.

National Research Council. 1989. *Diet and Health: Implications for Reducing Chronic Disease Risk.* Washington, DC: National Academy Press.

Shils, M., et al. (Ed.) 1994. *Modern Nutrition in Health and Disease.* Philadelphia: Lea and Febiger.

Simopoulos, A., and Pavlou, K. (Eds.) 1993. *Nutrition and Fitness for Athletes.* Basel, Switzerland: Karger.

Tyler, V. 1993. *The Honest Herbal.* New York: Haworth Press.

U.S. Department of Agriculture and U.S. Department of Health and Human Services. 1995. *Nutrition and Your Health: Dietary Guidelines for Americans.* Washington, DC: U.S. Government Printing Office.

U.S. Department of Agriculture, Human Nutrition Information Service. 1992. *The Food Guide Pyramid.* Home and Garden Bulletin Number 252. Washington, DC: U.S. Government Printing Office.

U.S. Department of Health and Human Services. 1988. *The Surgeon General's Report on Nutrition and Health.* Washington, DC: U.S. Government Printing Office.

U.S. Department of Health and Human Services Public Health Service. 1991. *Healthy People 2000: National Health Promotion and Disease Prevention Objectives.* Washington, DC: U.S. Government Printing Office.

Review Articles

American Dietetic Association. 1997. Position of the American Dietetic Association: Food and water safety. *Journal of the American Dietetic Association* 97:184–89.

American Dietetic Association. 1995. Position of the American Dietetic Association: Phytochemicals and functional foods. *Journal of the American Dietetic Association* 95:493–95.

American Dietetic Association. 1993. Final food labeling regulations. *Journal of the American Dietetic Association* 93:146–48.

American Dietetic Association. 1988. Position of the American Dietetic Association: Vegetarian diets. *Journal of the American Dietetic Association* 88:351–55.

American Institute for Cancer Research. 1997. Pesticides and cancer risk. *American Institute for Cancer Research Newsletter* 55: 5.

Anderson, J., and Geil, P. 1994. Nutrition management of diabetes mellitus. In *Modern Nutrition in Health and Disease,* eds. M. Shils, et al. Philadelphia: Lea and Febiger.

Applegate, L. 1996. Going organic. *Runner's World* 31 (August): 30–31.

Beaton, G. 1988. Criteria of an adequate diet. In *Modern Nutrition in Health and Disease,* eds. M. Shils and V. Young. Philadelphia: Lea and Febiger.

Berning, J. 1993. Food on the fly. *Running Times* 199 (August):38–41.

Bialostosky, K., and St. Jeor, S. 1996. The 1995 dietary guidelines for Americans. *Nutrition Today* 31 (1):6–12.

Bland, J. 1996. Phytonutrition, phytotherapy, and phytopharmacology. *Alternative Therapy in Health and Medicine* 2:73–76.

Borenstein, B., and Lachance, P. 1988. Effects of processing and preparation on the nutritional value of foods. In *Modern Nutrition in Health and Disease,* eds. M. Shils and V. Young. Philadelphia: Lea and Febiger.

Burke, L. 1995. Practical issues in nutrition for athletes. *Journal of Sports Sciences* 13:S83–S90.

Callaway, W. 1994. Reexamining cholesterol and sodium recommendations. *Nutrition Today* 29 (5):32–36.

Center for Science in the Public Interest. 1992. Pyramid scheme foiled. *Nutrition Action Health Letter* 19 (July/August):3.

Clark, N. 1987. Breakfast of champions. *Physician and Sportsmedicine* 15(January):209–12.

Consumers Union. 1995. Herbal roulette. *Consumer Reports* 60:698–705.

Consumers Union. 1996. Looking for a good meal? *Consumer Reports* 61:10–17.

Consumers Union. 1996. The food pyramid: How to make it work for you. *Consumer Reports on Health* 8:102–104.

Consumers Union. 1996. Fast food: Fatter than ever. *Consumer Reports on Health* 8:85–88.

Consumers Union. 1997. Food poisoning: How to protect yourself from pathogens. *Consumer Reports* 62:64–65.

Consumers Union. 1998. Greener greens: The truth about organic food. Consumer Reports 63:12–18.

Davis, D., and Bradlow, H. 1995. Can environmental estrogens cause breast cancer? *Scientific American* 273 (October):165–72.

Doyle, M. 1991. A new generation of foodborne pathogens. *Contemporary Nutrition* 16 (6):1–2.

Editor, Nutrition Reviews. 1993. The FDA's final regulations on health claims for foods. *Nutrition Reviews* 51:90–93.

Erdman, J., and Poneros-Schneier, A. 1994. Factors affecting nutritive values of food. In *Modern Nutrition in Health and Disease,* eds. M. Shils, et al. Philadelphia: Lea and Febiger.

Finn, R. 1992. Food allergy—fact or fiction: A review. *Journal of the Royal Society of Medicine* 85(9):560–64.

Food and Drug Administration. 1992. The new food label. *FDA Backgrounder* December 4, 1–8.

Franz, M. 1991. A new look for fast food. *Diabetes Forecast* 44(4):32–38.

Gershoff, S. 1992. Fifty ways to improve your diet. *Tufts University Diet and Nutrition Newsletter* 10 (June):3–6.

Harper, A. 1996. Dietary guidelines in perspective. *Journal of Nutrition* 126:1042S–48S.

Hathcock, J., and Rader, J. 1994. Food additives, contaminants, and natural toxins. In *Modern Nutrition in Health and Disease,* eds. M. Shils, et al. Philadelphia: Lea and Febiger.

Hotchkiss, J. 1989. Assessment and management of food safety risks. *Contemporary Nutrition* 14:1–2.

Houtkooper, L. 1992. Food selection for endurance sports. *Medicine and Science in Sports and Exercise* 24(9; Supplement): S349–S359.

Hudnall, M. 1997. Optimal health becomes goal of revolutionary new RDA's. *Environmental Nutrition* 20:1, 4.

Johnson, K., and Klingman, E. 1992. Preventive nutrition: An 'optimal' diet for older adults. *Geriatrics* 47 (October):56–60.

Kleiner, S. 1993. Sidestepping food sensitivities. *The Physician and Sportsmedicine* 21(March):59–60.

Kleiner, S. 1996. Fruits and veggies: Are you getting enough of a good thing? *Physician and Sportsmedicine* 24(11):97–98.

Krauss, R. et al. 1996. Dietary guidelines for healthy American adults. *Circulation* 94:1795–1800.

Lachance, P., and Langseth, L. 1994. The RDA concept: Time for a change? *Nutrition Reviews* 52:266–70.

Lefferts, L. 1993. A commonsense approach to pesticides. *Nutrition Action Health Letter* 20 (September):5–7.

Liebman, B. 1995. Dodging cancer with diet. *Nutrition Action Health Letter* 22 (1):4–7.

Liebman, B. 1996. Plants for supper? 10 reasons to eat more like a vegetarian. *Nutrition Action Health Letter* 23 (8):10–12.

Liu, J., and Guthrie, H. 1992. Nutrient labeling—A tool for nutrition education. *Nutrition Today* 27 (March/April):16–21.

Marston, W. 1997. What's best for breakfast? *Health* 11:34–38.

McMahon, K. 1996. Consumer nutrition and food safety trends. 1996. *Nutrition Today* 31 (1):19–23.

McMann, M. 1997. Unfriendly foods: How great is the threat of food allergy? *Environmental Nutrition* 20 (3):1, 6.

McNutt, K. 1995. Medicinals in food. *Nutrition Today* 30 (6): 261–63.

Mertz, W. 1995. Risk assessment of essential trace elements: New approaches to setting recommended dietary allowances and safety limits. *Nutrition Reviews* 53:179–85.

Messina, M., and Messina, V. 1996. Nutritional implications of dietary phytochemicals. *Advances in Experimental Medicine and Biology* 401:207–12.

National Dairy Council. 1997. Interpreting the dietary guidelines: It's all about you. *Dairy Council Digest* 68 (1):1–6.

Nestle, M. 1996. Fruits and vegetables: Protective or just fellow travelers? *Nutrition Reviews* 54:255–57.

Nieman, D. 1988. Vegetarian dietary practices and endurance performance. *American Journal of Clinical Nutrition* 48:754–61.

Porter, D. 1996. Health claims on food products: NLEA. *Nutrition Today* 31 (1):35–38.

Shardt, D., and Schmidt, S. 1996. How to avoid food poisoning. *Nutrition Action Health Letter* 23 (6):6–9.

Sherman, W. M. 1989. Pre-event nutrition. *Sports Science Exchange* 1 (February):1–4.

Simopoulos, A. 1995. The Mediterranean food guide. *Nutrition Today* 30 (2):54–61.

Steen, S. 1996. Timely statement of the American Dietetic Association: Nutrition guidance for child athletes in organized sports. *Journal of the American Dietetic Association* 96:610–11.

Steen, S. 1996. Timely statement of the American Dietetic Association: Nutrition guidance for adolescent athletes in organized sports. *Journal of the American Dietetic Association* 96:611–12.

Waites, W., and Arbuthnott, J. 1990. Foodborne illnesses. *The Lancet* 336 (September):722–25.

Weinhouse, S., et al. 1991. American Cancer Society guidelines on diet, nutrition, and cancer. *Ca-A Cancer Journal for Clinicians* 41 (November/December):334.

Welsh, S., et al. 1992. Development of the food guide pyramid. *Nutrition Today* 27 (November/December):12–23.

Welsh, S., et al. 1992. A brief history of food guides in the United States. *Nutrition Today* 27 (November/December):6–11.

Specific Studies

Deleeuw, E., et al. 1992. Developing menus to meet current dietary recommendations: Implications and applications. *Journal of Nutrition Education* 24:136–44.

Dorant, E., et al. 1996. Consumption of onions and reduced risk of stomach carcinoma. *Gastroenterology* 110:12–20.

Gillman, M., et al. 1995. Protective effect of fruits and vegetables on development of stroke in men. *Journal of the American Medical Association* 273:1113–17.

Hanne, N., et al. 1986. Physical fitness, anthropometric, and metabolic parameters in vegetarian athletes. *Journal of Sports Medicine* 26:180–85.

Key, T., et al. 1996. Dietary habits and mortality in 11,000 vegetarians and health conscious people: Results of a 17-year follow up. *British Medical Journal* 313:775–79.

Levine, A., et al. 1989. Effect of breakfast cereals on short-term food intake. *American Journal of Clinical Nutrition* 50:1303–7.

Nathan, I., et al. 1996. The dietary intake of a group of vegetarian children aged 7–11 years compared with matched omnivores. *British Journal of Nutrition* 75:533–44.

Pederson, A., et al. 1991. Menstrual differences due to vegetarian and nonvegetarian diets. *American Journal of Clinical Nutrition* 53:879–85.

Raben, A., et al. 1992. Serum sex hormones and endurance performance after a lacto-ovovegetarian and a mixed diet. *Medicine and Science in Sports and Exercise* 24:1290–97.

Resnicow, K., et al. 1991. Diet and serum lipids in vegan vegetarians: a model for risk reduction. *Journal of the American Dietetic Association* 91:447–53.

Sabate, J., et al. 1992. Lower height of lacto-ovovegetarian girls at preadolescence: An indicator of physical maturation delay? *Journal of the American Dietetic Association* 92:1263–65.

Willit, W., et al. 1987. Dietary fats and the risk of breast cancer. *New England Journal of Medicine* 316:22–28.

CHAPTER 3

Human Energy

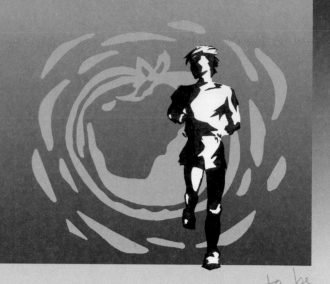

KEY TERMS

adenosine triphosphate (ATP)
aerobic glycolysis
anaerobic glycolysis
aerobic lipolysis
ATP-PC system
basal metabolic rate (BMR)
Calorie (kilocalorie)
calorimeter
dietary-induced thermogenesis (DIT)
electron transfer system
energy
exercise metabolic rate (EMR)
fatigue
glycolysis
joule
kilojoule
Krebs cycle
lactic acid system
maximal oxygen uptake
metabolic aftereffects of exercise
metabolism
METS
mitochondrion
onset of blood lactic acid (OBLA)
oxygen system
phosphocreatine (PC)
power
resting energy expenditure (REE)

KEY CONCEPTS

• Energy represents the capacity to do work, and food is the source of energy for humans.

• The Calorie, or kilocalorie, is a measure of chemical energy stored in foods; this chemical energy can be transformed into heat and mechanical work energy in the body. A related measure is the kilojoule. One Calorie is equal to 4.2 kilojoules.

• Carbohydrates and fats are the primary energy nutrients, but protein may also be an energy source. In the human body one gram of carbohydrate = 4 Calories, one gram of fat = 9 Calories, and one gram of protein = 4 Calories. Alcohol is also a source of Calories; one gram = 7 Calories.

• The potential energy sources in the body include ATP and PC; serum glucose; glycogen in the liver and muscle; serum free fatty acids (FFA); triglycerides in the muscle and in adipose tissue; and muscle protein.

• Three human energy systems have been classified on the basis of their ability to release energy at different rates of speed; they are the ATP-PC, lactic acid, and oxygen systems.

• Human metabolism represents the sum total of all physiological processes in the body, and the metabolic rate reflects the speed at which the body utilizes energy.

• The basal metabolic rate (BMR) represents the energy requirements necessary to

BMR — suppose to be measured fasting no exercise

maintain physiological processes in a resting, postabsorptive state, while the resting energy expenditure (REE) is a little higher due to prior muscular activity. The terms BMR and REE are often used interchangeably because of small differences between them.

• A number of different factors may affect the REE, including body composition, drugs, climatic conditions, and prior exercise.

• Eating a meal increases the metabolic rate as the digestive system absorbs, metabolizes, and stores the energy nutrients, a process termed the thermic effect of food (TEF).

• The thermic effect of exercise (TEE), or exercise metabolic rate (EMR), provides us with the most practical means to increase energy expenditure.

• The metabolic rate during exercise is directly proportional to the intensity of the exercise, and the exercise heart rate may serve as a general indicator of the metabolic rate.

• Activities that use the large muscle groups of the body, such as running, swimming, bicycling, and aerobic dance, facilitate energy expenditure.

• The total daily energy expenditure (TDEE) is accounted for by REE (60–75%), TEF (5–10%), and TEE (15–30%), although these percentages may vary.

- The ATP-PC and lactic acid energy systems are used primarily during fast, anaerobic, power-type events, while the oxygen system is used primarily during aerobic, endurance-type events.
- Fats serve as the primary source of fuel during mild levels of exercise intensity, but

Untrained persons

- carbohydrates begin to be the preferential fuel as the exercise intensity increases.
- A sound training program and proper nutrition are important factors in the prevention of fatigue during exercise.

2° anaerobic

resting metabolic rate (RMR)
steady-state threshold
thermic effect of exercise (TEE)
thermic effect of food (TEF)
total daily energy expenditure (TDEE)
VO_2 max
work

INTRODUCTION

As noted in Chapter 1, the body uses the food we eat to provide energy, to build and repair tissues, and to regulate metabolism. Of these three functions, the human body ranks energy production first and will use food for this purpose at the expense of the other two functions in time of need. Energy is the essence of life.

Through technological processes, humans have harnessed a variety of energy sources such as wind, waterfalls, the sun, wood, and oil to operate the machines invented to make life easier. However, humans cannot use any of these energy sources for their own metabolism but must rely on food sources found in nature. The food we eat must be converted into energy forms that the body can use. Thus, the human body is equipped with a number of metabolic systems to produce and regulate energy for its diverse needs, such as synthesis of tissues, movement of substances between tissues, and muscular contraction.

Sport energy! The underlying basis for the control of movement in all sports is human energy, and successful performance depends upon the ability of the athlete to produce the right amount of energy and to control its application to the specific demands of the sport. Sports differ in their energy demands. In some events, such as the 100-meter dash, success is dependent primarily upon the ability to produce energy very rapidly. In others, such as the 26.2-mile marathon, energy need not be produced so rapidly but must be sustained for a much longer period. In still other sports, such as golf, the athlete need not only

produce energy at varying rates (compare the drive with the putt) but must carefully control the application of that energy. Thus each sport imposes specific energy demands upon the athlete.

A discussion of the role of nutrition as a means to help provide and control human energy is important from several standpoints. First, inadequate supplies of necessary energy nutrients, such as muscle glycogen or blood glucose, may cause fatigue. Fatigue also may be caused by the inability of the energy systems to function optimally because of a deficiency of other nutrients, such as selected vitamins and minerals. In addition, the human body is capable of storing energy reserves in a variety of body forms, including body fat and muscle tissue. Excess body weight in the form of fat or decreased body weight due to losses of muscle tissue may adversely affect some types of athletic performance.

One purpose of this chapter is to review briefly the major human energy systems and how they are used in the body under conditions of exercise and rest. The following six chapters discuss the role of each of the major classes of nutrients as they relate to energy production in the human body, with the primary focus on prevention of fatigue caused by impaired energy production. Another purpose of this chapter is to discuss the means by which humans store and expend energy. Chapters 10 through 12 focus on weight control methods and expand on some of the concepts presented in this chapter.

Measures of Energy

What is energy?

For our purposes, **energy** represents the capacity to do work. **Work** is one form of energy, often called mechanical energy. When we throw a ball or run a mile, we have done work; we have produced mechanical energy.

Energy exists in a variety of other forms in nature, such as the light energy of the sun, nuclear energy in uranium, electrical energy in lightning storms, heat energy in fires, and chemical energy in oil. The six forms of

energy—mechanical, chemical, heat, electrical, light, and nuclear—are all interchangeable according to various laws of thermodynamics. We take advantage of these laws every day. One such example is the use of the chemical energy in gasoline to produce mechanical energy, or the movement of our cars.

In the human body, four of these types of energy are important. Our bodies possess stores of chemical energy that can be used to produce electrical energy for creation of electrical nerve impulses, to produce heat to help keep our body temperature at 37° C (98.6° F) even on cold

• Mechanical
• Chemical
• heat
• electrical
• light
• nuclear

Humans – • chemical
• mechanical
• heat
• electrical

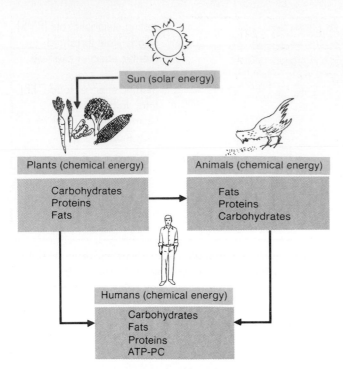

Figure 3.1 Through photosynthesis, plants utilize solar energy and convert it to chemical energy in the form of carbohydrates, fats, or proteins. Animals eat plants and convert the chemical energy into their own stores of chemical energy—primarily fat and protein. Humans ingest food from both plant and animal sources and convert the chemical energy for their own stores and use.

days, and to produce mechanical work through muscle shortening so that we may move about.

The sun is the ultimate source of energy. Solar energy is harnessed by plants, through photosynthesis, to produce either plant carbohydrates, fats, or proteins, all forms of stored chemical energy. When humans consume plant and animal products, the carbohydrates, fats, and proteins undergo a series of metabolic changes and are utilized to develop body structure, to regulate body processes, or to provide a storage form of chemical energy (Figure 3.1).

The optimal intake and output of energy is important to all individuals, but especially for the active person. To perform to capacity, body energy stores must be used in the most efficient manner possible.

How do we measure work and energy?

Energy has been defined as the ability to do work. According to the physicist's definition, work is simply the product of force times vertical distance, or in formula format, Work = Force × Distance. When we speak of how fast work is done, the term **power** is used. Power is simply work divided by time, or Power = Work/Time.

Two major measurement systems have been used in the past to express energy in terms of either work or power.

The metric system has been in use by most of the world, while England, its colonies, and the United States have used the English system. In an attempt to provide some uniformity in measurement systems around the world, the International Unit System (*Systeme International d'Unites*, or SI) has been developed. Most of the world has adopted the SI. Although legislation has been passed by Congress to convert the United States to the SI, and terms such as gram, kilogram, milliliter, liter, and kilometer are becoming more prevalent, it appears that it will take some time before this system becomes part of our everyday language.

The SI is used in most scientific journals today, but the other two systems appear in older journals. Terms that are used in each system are presented in Table 3.1. For our purposes in this text, we shall use several English terms that are still in common usage in the United States, but if you read scientific literature, you should be able to convert values among the various systems if necessary. For example, work may be expressed as either foot-pounds, kilogram-meters (KGM), joules, or watts. If you weigh 150 pounds and climb a 20-foot flight of stairs in one minute, you have done 3,000 foot-pounds of work. One KGM is equal to 7.23 foot-pounds, so you would do about 415 KGM. One **joule** is equal to about 0.102 KGM, so you have done about 4,062 joules of work. One watt is equal to one joule per second, so you have generated about 68 watts of power. Some basic interrelationships among the measurement systems are noted in Table 3.2. Other equivalents may be found in Appendix B.

In general, exercise scientists and nutritionists are interested in measuring work output under two conditions. One condition involves specific exercise tasks. Various laboratory techniques have been developed to accurately record work output during exercise, such as measurement of KGM or watts on a cycle ergometer. The other condition involves measurement of work output during normal daily activities over prolonged periods of time, such as a 24-hour period. Various devices, such as small accelerometers attached to the body, detect motion throughout the day and provide an approximation of daily work output.

To measure work we need to know the weight of an object and the vertical distance through which it is moved. This is fine according to the formal definition of work, but are you doing work while holding a stationary weight out in front of your body? According to the formal definition, the answer is no, because the distance the weight moved is zero. How about when you come down stairs as compared to going up? It is much easier to descend the stairs, and yet according to the formula you have done the same amount of work. Also, how about when you run a mile? You know you have worked, but most of the distance you covered was horizontal, not vertical. Therefore, we need to have means to express the energy expenditure of the human body other than simply the amount of work done.

Table 3.1   Terms in the English, metric, and international systems

Unit	English system	Metric system	International system
Mass	slug	kilogram (kg)	kilogram (kg)
Distance	foot (ft)	meter (m)	meter (m)
Time	second (s)	second (s)	second (s)
Force	pound (lb)	newton (N)	newton (N)
Work	foot-pound (ft-lb)	kilogram-meter (kgm)	joule (J)
Power	horsepower (hp)	watt (W)	watt (W)

Table 3.2   Some interrelationships between work measurement systems

Weight	Distance	Work	Power
1 kilogram = 2.2 pounds	1 meter = 3.28 feet	1 KGM = 7.23 foot-pounds	1 watt = 1 joule per second
1 kilogram = 1,000 grams	1 meter = 1.09 yards	1 KGM = 9.8 joules	1 watt = 6.12 KGM per minute
454 grams = 1 pound	1 foot = 0.30 meter	1 foot-pound = 0.138 KGM	1 horsepower = 550 foot-pounds per second
1 pound = 16 ounces	1,000 meters = 1 kilometer	1 foot-pound = 1.35 joules	1 horsepower = 33,000 foot-pounds per minute
1 ounce = 28.4 grams	1 kilometer = 0.6215 mile	1 newton = 0.102 KG	
3.5 ounces = 100 grams	1 mile = 1.61 kilometers	1 joule = 1 newton meter	
	1 inch = 2.54 centimeters	1 kilojoule = 1,000 joules	
	1 centimeter = 0.39 inch	1 megajoule = 1,000,000 joules	
		1 joule = 0.102 KGM	
		1 joule = 0.736 foot-pound	
		1 kilojoule = 102 KGM	

The other means of measuring energy in the body deal with chemical and heat energy. Without going into much detail, look briefly at two different methods for measuring energy production in humans. First, a device known as a **calorimeter** may be used to measure the energy content of a given substance. Figure 3.2 shows how a bomb calorimeter works. For example, a gram of fat contains a certain amount of chemical energy. When placed in the calorimeter and oxidized completely, the heat it gives off can be recorded. We then know the heat energy of one gram of fat and can equate it to chemical or work units of energy if needed. Large, expensive whole-room calorimeters are available that can accommodate human beings and measure their heat production under normal home activities and some conditions of exercise. This technique is known as direct calorimetry.

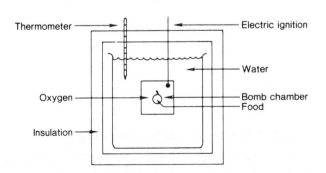

Figure 3.2   A bomb calorimeter. The food in the calorimeter is combusted via electrical ignition. The heat (Calories) given off by the food raises the temperature of the water, thereby providing data about the caloric content of specific foodstuffs.

measurement of human body under some physical activities

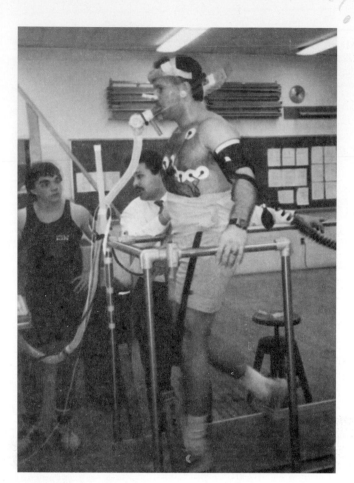

Figure 3.3 Indirect calorimetry may be used to measure metabolism by determining the amount of oxygen consumed and the carbon dioxide produced. The test may also be used to measure VO₂ max and other measures of cardiovascular and respiratory function.

A second, more commonly used method of measuring energy is to determine the amount of oxygen an individual consumes, an indirect calorimetric technique. This procedure is normally done under laboratory conditions (see Figure 3.3), but lightweight portable oxygen analyzers are also available. The volume of oxygen one uses is usually expressed in liters (L) or milliliters (ml); one L is equal to 1,000 ml. One liter is slightly larger than a quart. In general, humans need oxygen, which helps metabolize the various nutrients in the body to produce energy. It is known that when oxygen combines with a gram of carbohydrate, fat, or protein, a certain amount of energy is released. If we can accurately measure the oxygen consumption (and carbon dioxide production) of an individual, we can get a pretty good measure of energy expenditure. The amount of oxygen used can be equated to other forms of energy, such as work done in foot-pounds or heat produced in Calories.

Another method is the doubly labeled water technique in which stable isotopes of hydrogen and oxygen in water ($^2H_2{}^{18}O$) are ingested. This is a safe procedure as the isotopes are stable and emit no radiation. Analysis of urine and blood samples provide data on ^2H and ^{18}O excretion. The labeled oxygen is eliminated from the body as water and carbon dioxide, whereas the hydrogen is eliminated only as water. Subtracting the hydrogen losses from the oxygen losses provides a measure of carbon dioxide fluctuation, which may be converted to energy expenditure. Although expensive, the advantage of this technique is that it may be used with individuals while they perform their normal daily activities, and they need not be confined to a metabolic chamber or be attached to equipment to measure oxygen consumption.

Although all of these techniques to measure energy expenditure have limitations, they do provide useful data relative to the energy cost of exercise and normal diary activities.

What is the most commonly used measure of energy?

Although there are a number of different ways to express energy, the most common term used in the past and still most prevalent and understood in the United States by most people is **Calorie.** This term is used as the energy requirement in the 1989 RDA.

A calorie is a measure of heat. One small calorie represents the amount of heat needed to raise the temperature of one gram of water one degree Celsius; it is sometimes called the gram calorie. A large Calorie, or kilocalorie, is equal to 1,000 small calories. It is the amount of heat needed to raise 1 kg of water (1 L) one degree Celsius. In human nutrition, because the gram calorie is so small, the kilocalorie is the main expression of energy. It is usually abbreviated as kcal, kc, or C, or capitalized as Calorie. Throughout this book, *Calorie* or C will refer to the kilocalorie.

According to the principles underlying the first law of thermodynamics, energy may be equated from one form to another. Thus, the Calorie, which represents thermal or heat energy, may be equated to other forms of energy. Relative to our discussion concerning physical work such as exercise and its interrelationships with nutrition, it is important to equate the Calorie with mechanical work and the chemical energy stored in the body. As will be explained later, most stored chemical energy must undergo some form of oxidation in order to release its energy content as work.

The following represents some equivalent energy values for the Calorie in terms of mechanical work and oxygen utilization. Some examples illustrating several of the interrelationships will be used in later chapters.

1 C = 3,086 foot-pounds
1 C = 427 KGM
1 C = 4.2 kilojoules (kJ) or 4,200 joules
1 C = 200 ml oxygen (approximately)

Although the Calorie is the most commonly used expression for energy, work, and heat in the United States, **kilojoule** is the proper term in the SI. It is important for you to be able to convert from Calories to kilojoules, and vice versa. To convert Calories to kilojoules, multiply the number of Calories by 4.2 (4.186 to be exact); to convert kilojoules to Calories, divide the number of kilojoules by 4.2. Simply multiplying or dividing by 4 for each respective conversion will provide a ballpark estimate. In some cases megajoules (MJ), a million joules, are used to express energy. One MJ equals about 240 Calories, or 4.2 MJ is the equivalent of about 1,000 Calories.

Through the use of a calorimeter, the energy contents of the basic nutrients have been determined. Energy may be derived from the three major foodstuffs—carbohydrate, fat, and protein—plus alcohol. The caloric value of each of these three nutrients may vary somewhat, depending on the particular structure of the different forms. For example, carbohydrate may exist in several forms—as glucose, sucrose, or starch—and the caloric value of each will differ slightly. In general, one gram of each of the three nutrients, measured in a calorimeter, yields the following Calories:

from calorimeter

1 gram carbohydrate = 4.30 C
1 gram fat = 9.45 C
1 gram protein = 5.65 C
1 gram alcohol = 7.00 C

Unfortunately, or fortunately if one is trying to lose weight, humans do not extract all of this energy from the food they eat. The human body is not as efficient as the calorimeter. For one, the body cannot completely absorb all the food eaten. Only about 97 percent of ingested carbohydrate, 95 percent of fat, and 92 percent of protein are absorbed. In addition, a good percentage of the protein is not completely oxidized in the body, with some of the nitrogen waste products being excreted in the urine. In summary, then, the caloric value of food is reduced somewhat in relation to the values given above. Although the following values are not exactly precise, they are approximate enough to be used effectively in determining the caloric values of the foods we eat. Thus, the following caloric values are used throughout this text as a practical guide:

1 gram carbohydrate = 4 C
1 gram fat = 9 C
1 gram protein = 4 C
1 gram alcohol = 7 C

For our purposes, the Calories in food represent a form of potential energy to be used by our bodies to produce heat and work (Figure 3.4). However, the fact that alcohol and fat have about twice the amount of energy per gram as either carbohydrate or protein does not mean they are

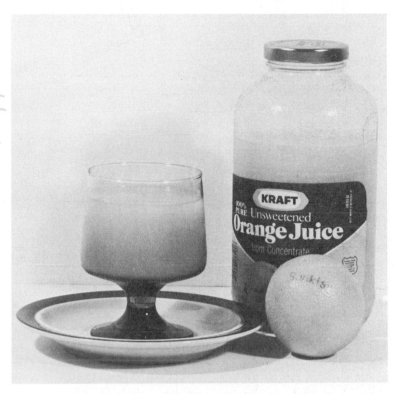

Figure 3.4   Eight ounces of orange juice will provide enough chemical energy to enable an average man to produce enough mechanical energy to run about one mile.

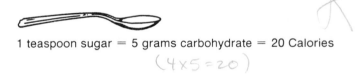

1 teaspoon sugar = 5 grams carbohydrate = 20 Calories
(4 × 5 = 20)

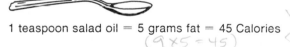

1 teaspoon salad oil = 5 grams fat = 45 Calories
(9 × 5 = 45)

Figure 3.5   The Calorie as a measure of energy.

better energy sources for the active individual (Figure 3.5). These important issues are discussed in later chapters when we talk of the efficient utilization of body fuels.

Human Energy Systems

How is energy stored in the body?

The ultimate source of all energy on earth is the sun. Solar energy is harnessed by plants, which take carbon, hydrogen, oxygen, and nitrogen from their environment and manufacture either carbohydrate, fat, or protein. These foods possess stored energy. When we consume these foods, our digestive processes break them down into

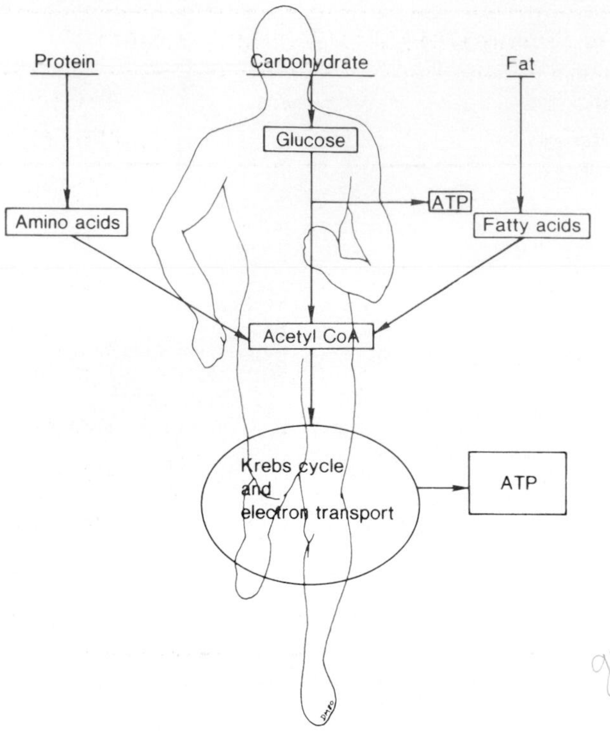

Figure 3.6 Simplified schematic of ATP formation from carbohydrate, fat, and protein. All three nutrients may be used to form ATP, but carbohydrate and fat are the major sources via the aerobic metabolism of the Krebs cycle. Carbohydrate may be used to produce small amounts of ATP under anaerobic conditions, thus providing humans with the ability to produce energy rapidly without oxygen for relatively short periods. For more details, see Appendix K.

simple compounds that are absorbed into the body and transported to various cells. One of the basic purposes of body cells is to transform the chemical energy of these simple compounds into forms that may be available for immediate use or other forms that may be available for future use.

Energy in the body is available for immediate use in the form of **adenosine triphosphate (ATP).** It is a complex molecule constructed with high-energy bonds, which, when split by enzyme action, can release energy rapidly for a number of body processes, including muscle contraction. ATP is classified as a high-energy compound and is stored in the tissues in small amounts. It is important to note that ATP is the immediate source of energy for all body functions, and the other energy stores are used to replenish ATP at varying rates.

Another related high-energy phosphate compound, **phosphocreatine (PC),** is also found in the tissues in small amounts. Although it cannot be used as an immediate source of energy, it can rapidly replenish ATP.

ATP may be formed from either carbohydrate, fat, or protein after those nutrients have undergone some complex biochemical changes in the body. Figure 3.6 represents

a basic schematic of how ATP is formed from each of these three nutrients. PC is actually derived from excess ATP.

Because ATP and PC are found in very small amounts in the body and can be used up in a matter of seconds, it is important to have adequate energy stores as a backup system. Your body stores of carbohydrate, fat, and protein can provide you with ample amounts of ATP, enough to last for many weeks even on a starvation diet. The digestion and metabolism of carbohydrate, fat, and protein are discussed in their respective chapters, so it is unnecessary to present that full discussion here. However, you may wish to preview Figure 3.12 in order to visualize the metabolic interrelationships between the three nutrients in the body. For those who desire more detailed schematics of energy pathways, Appendix K provides some of the major metabolic pathways for carbohydrate, fat, and protein.

It is important to note that parts of each energy nutrient may be converted to the other two nutrients in the body under certain circumstances. For example, protein may be converted into carbohydrate during prolonged exercise, whereas excess dietary carbohydrate may be converted to fat in the body during rest.

Table 3.3 summarizes how much energy is stored in the human body as ATP, PC, and various forms of carbohydrate, fat, and protein. The total amount of energy, represented by Calories, is approximate and may vary considerably between individuals. Carbohydrate is stored in limited amounts as blood glucose, liver glycogen, and muscle glycogen. The largest amount of energy is stored in the body as fats. Fats are stored as triglycerides in both muscle tissue and adipose (fat) tissue; triglycerides and free fatty acids (FFA) in the blood are a limited supply. The protein of the body tissues, particularly muscle tissue, is a large reservoir of energy but is not used under normal circumstances. Table 3.3 also depicts how far an individual could run using each of these energy sources as the sole supply. The role of each of these energy stores during exercise is an important consideration that is discussed briefly in this chapter and more extensively in their respective chapters.

What are the human energy systems?

Why does the human body store chemical energy in a variety of different forms? If we look at human energy needs from an historical perspective, the answer becomes obvious. Sometimes humans needed to produce energy at a rapid rate, such as when sprinting to safety to avoid dangerous animals. Thus, a fast rate of energy production was an important human energy feature that helped ensure survival. At other times, our ancient ancestors may have been deprived of adequate food for long periods, and thus needed a storage capacity for chemical energy that would sustain life throughout these times of deprivation. Hence, the ability to store large amounts of energy

Table 3.3 Major energy stores in the human body with approximate total caloric value*

Energy source	Major storage form	Total body Calories	Total body kilojoules	Distance covered**
ATP	Tissues	1	4.2	17.5 yards
PC	Tissues	4	16.8	70 yards
Carbohydrate	Serum glucose	20	88	350 yards
	Liver glycogen	400	1,680	4 miles
	Muscle glycogen	1,500	6,300	15 miles
Fat	Serum free fatty acids	7	29.2	123 yards
	Serum triglycerides	75	315	0.75 mile
	Muscle triglycerides	2,500	10,500	25 miles
	Adipose tissue triglycerides	80,000	336,000	800 miles
Protein	Muscle protein	30,000	126,000	300 miles

*These values may have extreme variations depending on the size of the individual, amount of body fat, physical fitness level, and diet.
**Running at an energy cost of 100 Calories per mile (1.6 kilometers).

was also important for survival. These two factors—rate of energy production and energy capacity—appear to be determining factors in the development of human energy systems.

One need only watch weekend television programming for several weeks to realize that a diversity of sports are popular throughout the world. Each of these sports imposes certain requirements on humans who want to be successful competitors. For some sports, such as weight lifting, the main requirement is brute strength, while for others such as tennis, quick reactions and hand/eye coordination are important. A major consideration in most sports is the rate of energy production, which can range from the explosive power needed by a shot-putter to the tremendous endurance capacity of an ultramarathoner. The physical performance demands of different sports require specific sources of energy.

As noted above, the body stores energy in a variety of ways—in ATP, PC, muscle glycogen, and so on. In order for this energy to be used to produce muscular contractions and movement, it must undergo certain biochemical reactions in the muscle. These biochemical reactions serve as a basis for classifying human energy expenditure by three energy, or power, systems: the ATP-PC system, the lactic acid system, and the oxygen system.

The **ATP-PC system** is also known as the phosphagen system because both adenosine triphosphate (ATP) and phosphocreatine (PC) contain phosphates. ATP is the immediate source of energy for almost all body processes, including muscle contraction. This high-energy compound, stored in the muscles, rapidly releases energy when an electrical impulse arrives in the muscle. No matter what you do, scratch your nose or lift 100 pounds, ATP breakdown makes the movement possible. ATP must be present for the muscles to contract. The body has a limited supply of ATP and must replace it rapidly if muscular work is to continue. See Figure 3.7 for a graphical representation of ATP breakdown.

PC, which is also a high-energy compound found in the muscle, can help form ATP rapidly as ATP is used. Energy released when PC splits is used to form ATP from ADP and P. PC is also in short supply and needs to be replenished if used. PC breakdown to help resynthesize ATP is illustrated in Figure 3.8.

The ATP-PC system is critical to energy production. Because these phosphagens are in short supply, any all-out exercise for 5 to 10 seconds could deplete the supply in a given muscle. Hence, the phosphagens must be replaced, and this is the function of the other energy sources. Although some supplements, such as creatine, discussed in later chapters are theorized to facilitate ATP or PC replenishment, we cannot eat ATP-PC per se, but we can produce it from the other nutrients stored in our body. PC replenishment will not be discussed, but keep in mind that when ATP is being regenerated, so is some PC. In summary, the value of the ATP-PC system is its ability to provide energy rapidly, for example, in sport events such as competitive weight lifting or sprinting 100 meters. Anaerobic power is a term often associated with the ATP-PC energy system.

The **lactic acid system** cannot be used directly as a source of energy for muscular contraction, but it can help

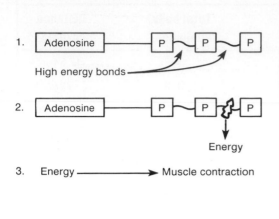

1. Adenosine ——[P]~[P]~[P]

High energy bonds

2. Adenosine ——[P]~[P]~⟨ P]

↓

Energy

3. Energy ——————→ Muscle contraction

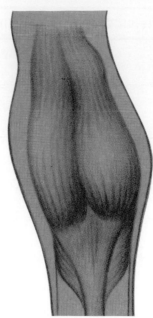

Figure 3.7 ATP, adenosine triphosphate. (1) ATP is stored in the muscle in limited amounts. (2) Splitting of a high-energy bond releases adenosine diphosphate (ADP), inorganic phosphate (P), and energy, which (3) can be used for many body processes including muscular contraction. The ATP stores are used for fast, all-out bursts of power that last about one second. ATP must be replenished from other sources for muscle contraction to continue.

(Phosphate)

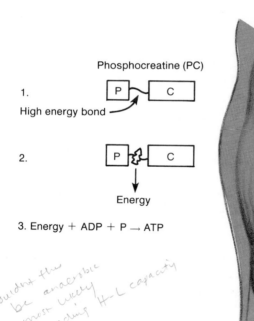

Phosphocreatine (PC)

1. [P]~[C]

High energy bond

2. [P]⟨ C]

↓

Energy

3. Energy + ADP + P → ATP

Figure 3.8 Phosphocreatine (PC). (1) PC is stored in the muscle in limited amounts. (2) Splitting of the high-energy bond releases energy, which (3) can be used to rapidly synthesize ATP from ADP and P. ATP and PC are called phosphagens and together represent the ATP-PC energy system. This system is utilized primarily for quick, maximal exercises lasting about 1 to 6 seconds, such as sprinting.

? hum - wouldn't this be anaerobic - most likely exceeding H-L capacity

replace ATP rapidly when necessary. If you are exercising at a high intensity level, the next best source of energy besides ATP-PC is muscle glycogen. To be used for energy, muscle glycogen must be broken down to glucose, which undergoes a series of reactions to eventually form ATP, a process called **glycolysis.** One of the major factors controlling the metabolic fate of muscle glycogen is the availability of oxygen in the muscle cell. In simple terms, if oxygen is available, a large amount of ATP is formed. This is known as **aerobic glycolysis.** If inadequate oxygen is available, then little ATP is formed and lactic acid is a by-product. This is known as anaerobic, or without oxygen, glycolysis; **anaerobic glycolysis** is the scientific term for

Glycogen

the lactic acid energy system. The lactic acid system is diagrammed in Figure 3.9. It is used in sport events in which energy production is near maximal for 1 to 2 minutes, such as a 400- or 800-meter run. Anaerobic capacity is a term often associated with the lactic acid energy system.

The lactic acid system has the advantage of producing ATP rapidly. Its capacity is limited in comparison to aerobic glycolysis, for only about 5 percent of the total ATP production from muscle glycogen can be released. Moreover, the lactic acid produced as a by-product may be involved in the onset of fatigue. Lactic acid releases a hydrogen ion that increases the acidity within the muscle cell and disturbs the normal cell environment. The

ATP : aerobic = 38 anaerobic = 2

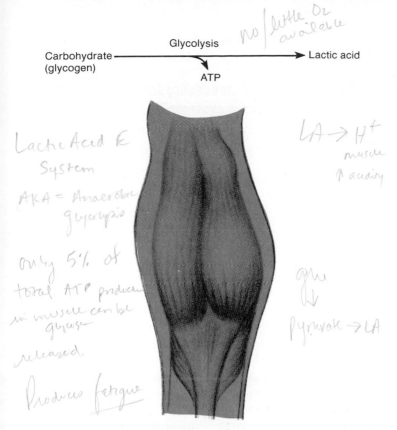

Glycolysis

Carbohydrate
(glycogen) ———————————→ Lactic acid

ATP

Handwritten annotations:
- no/little O₂ available
- Lactic Acid E System
- AKA = Anaerobic glycolysis
- only 5% of total ATP produced in muscle can be glucose released.
- Produces fatigue
- LA → H⁺ muscle ↑ acidity
- glu ⇓⇓ Pyruvate → LA

Figure 3.9 The lactic acid energy system. Muscle glycogen can break down without the utilization of oxygen. This process is called anaerobic glycolysis. (See Appendix K, Figure K.1, for more details.) ATP is produced rapidly, but lactic acid is the end product. Lactic acid may be a major cause of fatigue in the muscle. The lactic acid energy system is utilized primarily during exercise bouts of very high intensity, those conducted at maximal rates for about 1 to 3 minutes.

processes of energy release and muscle contraction in the muscle cell are controlled by enzymes whose functions may be impaired by the increased acidity in the cell. The lactate present after loss of the hydrogen ion still has considerable energy content, which may be used by other tissues for energy or converted back into glucose in the liver.

The third system is the **oxygen system.** It is also known as the aerobic system. Aerobics is a term used by Dr. Kenneth Cooper in 1968 to describe a system of exercising that created an exercise revolution in this country. In essence, aerobic exercises are designed to stress the oxygen system and provide benefits for the heart and lungs. Figure 3.10 represents the major physiological processes involved in the oxygen system. The oxygen system, like the lactic acid system, cannot be used directly as a source of energy for muscle contraction, but it does produce ATP in rather large quantities from other energy sources in the body. Muscle glycogen, liver glycogen, blood glucose, muscle triglycerides, blood FFA and triglycerides, adipose cell triglycerides, and body protein all may be ultimate sources of energy for ATP production and subsequent muscle contraction. To do this, glycogen and fats

Handwritten margin notes:
- #3
- oxygen system
- AA = aerobic system

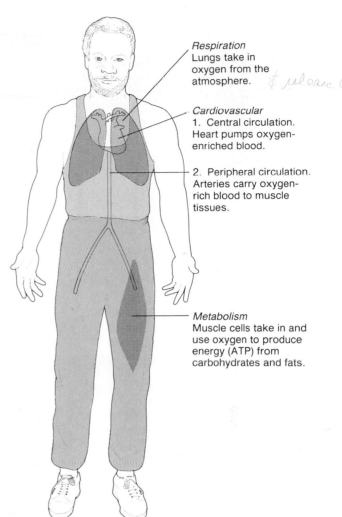

Labels:
Respiration
Lungs take in oxygen from the atmosphere. *(handwritten: & release CO₂)*

Cardiovascular
1. Central circulation. Heart pumps oxygen-enriched blood.

2. Peripheral circulation. Arteries carry oxygen-rich blood to muscle tissues.

Metabolism
Muscle cells take in and use oxygen to produce energy (ATP) from carbohydrates and fats.

Figure 3.10 Physiological processes involved in oxygen uptake.

must be present within the muscle cell or must enter the muscle cell as glucose, FFA, or amino acids. Through a complex series of reactions metabolic by-products of carbohydrate, fat, or protein combine with oxygen to produce energy, carbon dioxide, and water. These reactions occur in the energy powerhouse of the cell, the **mitochondrion.** The whole series of events of oxidative energy production primarily involves aerobic processing of carbohydrates and fats (and small amounts of protein) through the **Krebs cycle** and the **electron transfer system.** The oxygen system is depicted in Figure 3.11. The Krebs cycle and the electron transfer system represent a highly structured array of enzymes designed to remove hydrogen, carbon dioxide, and electrons from substrates such as glucose. At different steps in this process energy is released and ATP is formed. The hydrogen and electrons eventually combine with oxygen to form water.

The major advantage of the oxygen system is the production of large amounts of energy in the form of ATP. However, oxygen from the air we breathe must be delivered

Handwritten margin notes:
- Mito
- Krebs ETS
- ↑ ATP

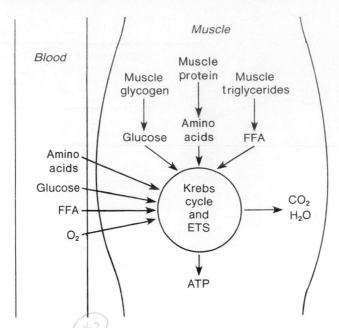

Figure 3.11 *#3* The oxygen energy system. The muscle stores of glycogen and triglycerides, along with blood supplies of glucose and free fatty acids (FFA), as well as small amounts of muscle protein and amino acids, undergo complex biochemical changes for entrance into the Krebs cycle and the associated electron transfer system (ETS). In this process in which oxygen is the final acceptor to the electron, large amounts of ATP may be produced. The oxygen energy system is utilized primarily during endurance-type exercises, those lasting longer than 4 or 5 minutes. (See Appendix K for more details.)

to the muscle cells deep in the body and enter the mitochondria to be used. This process may be adequate to handle mild and moderate levels of exercise but may not be able to meet the demand of very strenuous exercise. The oxygen system is used primarily in sports emphasizing endurance, such as distance runs ranging from 5 kilometers (3.1 miles) to the 26.2-mile marathon and beyond.

Hawley and Hopkins recently proposed that the oxygen energy system be subdivided into two systems. The scientific terms for these two subdivisions are aerobic glycolysis, which uses carbohydrates (muscle glycogen and blood glucose) for energy production, and **aerobic lipolysis,** which uses fats (muscle triglycerides, blood FFA). As discussed in the next two chapters, carbohydrate is the more efficient fuel during high-intensity exercise, whereas fat becomes the predominant fuel used at lower levels of exercise intensity. Thus, aerobic glycolysis provides most of the energy in high-intensity aerobic running events such as 5 kilometers (3.1 miles) and 10 kilometers (6.2 miles), while aerobic lipolysis may contribute significant amounts of energy in more prolonged aerobic events, such as ultramarathons of 50 to 100 kilometers (31 to 62 miles). Aerobic glycolysis and aerobic lipolysis may respectively be referred to as aerobic power and aerobic capacity.

Figure 3.12 presents a simplified schematic reviewing the three human energy systems.

What nutrients are necessary for the operation of the human energy systems?

Although the energy for the formation of ATP is derived from the energy stores in carbohydrate, fat, and sometimes protein, this energy transformation and utilization would not occur without the participation of the other major nutrients—water, vitamins, and minerals. These three classes of nutrients function very closely with protein in the structure and function of numerous enzymes, many of which are active in the muscle-cell energy processes.

Water is used to help break up and transform some energy compounds by a process known as hydrolysis.

Several vitamins are needed for energy to be released from the cell sources. For example, niacin serves an important function in glycolysis, thiamin is needed to convert glycolytic end products to acetyl CoA for entrance into the Krebs cycle, and riboflavin is essential to forming ATP through the Krebs cycle and electron transfer system. A number of other B vitamins are also involved in facets of energy transformation within the cell.

Minerals, too, are essential for cellular energy processes. Iron is one of the more critical compounds. Aside from helping hemoglobin deliver oxygen to the muscle cell, it is also a component of myoglobin and the cytochrome part of the electron transfer system. It is needed for proper utilization of oxygen within the cell itself. Other minerals such as zinc, magnesium, potassium, sodium, and calcium are involved in a variety of ways, either as parts of active enzymes, in energy storage, or in the muscle-contraction process.

Proper utilization of body energy sources requires attention not only to the major energy nutrients but also to the regulatory nutrients—water, vitamins, and minerals.

Human Energy Metabolism during Rest

What is metabolism?

Human **metabolism** represents the sum total of all physical and chemical changes that take place within the body. The transformation of food to energy, the formation of new compounds such as hormones and enzymes, the growth of bone and muscle tissue, the destruction of body tissues, and a host of other physiological processes are parts of the metabolic process.

Metabolism involves two fundamental processes, anabolism and catabolism. Anabolism is a building-up process, or constructive metabolism. Complex body components are synthesized from the basic nutrients. For the active individual, this may mean an increased muscle

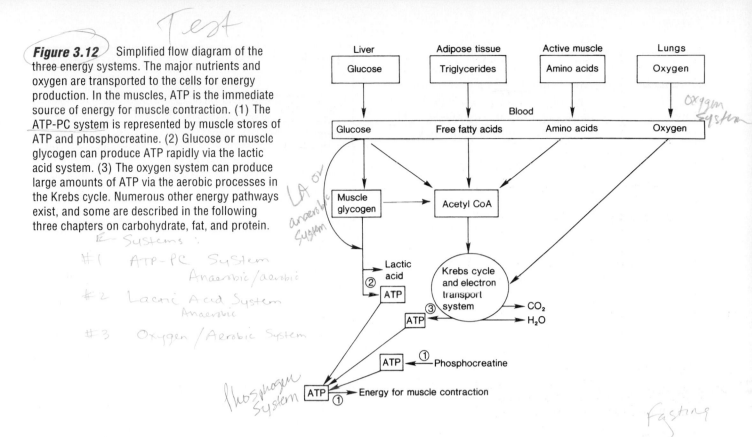

Figure 3.12 Simplified flow diagram of the three energy systems. The major nutrients and oxygen are transported to the cells for energy production. In the muscles, ATP is the immediate source of energy for muscle contraction. (1) The ATP-PC system is represented by muscle stores of ATP and phosphocreatine. (2) Glucose or muscle glycogen can produce ATP rapidly via the lactic acid system. (3) The oxygen system can produce large amounts of ATP via the aerobic processes in the Krebs cycle. Numerous other energy pathways exist, and some are described in the following three chapters on carbohydrate, fat, and protein.

[Handwritten annotations: "Test" at top; labels "Oxygen System", "LA or Anaerobic System", "Phosphagen System"; "3 Systems:", "#1 ATP-PC System Anaerobic/aerobic", "#2 Lactic Acid System Anaerobic", "#3 Oxygen/Aerobic System"]

mass through weight training or an increased amount of cellular enzymes to better use oxygen following endurance-type training. Energy is needed for anabolism to occur. Catabolism is the tearing-down process. This involves the disintegration of body compounds into their simpler components. The breakdown of muscle glycogen to glucose and eventually CO_2, H_2O, and energy is an example of a catabolic process. The energy released from some catabolic processes is used to support the energy needs of anabolism.

Metabolism is life. It represents human energy. The metabolic rate reflects how rapidly the body is using its energy stores, and this rate can vary tremendously depending upon a number of factors. For all practical purposes, the **total daily energy expenditure (TDEE)** may be accounted for by three factors: resting energy expenditure, increases due to eating a meal, and physical activity. We shall examine resting energy expenditure and the effect of eating in this section, while the role of physical activity, or exercise, will be covered in the following section.

What factors account for the amount of energy expended during rest?

The body is constantly using energy to build up and tear down substances within the cells. Certain automatic body functions such as contraction of the heart, breathing, secretion of hormones, and the constant activity of the nervous system also are consuming energy.

Basal metabolism, or the **basal metabolic rate (BMR),** represents the energy requirements of the many different cellular and tissue processes that are necessary to continuing physiological activities in a resting, postabsorptive state throughout most of the day. Other than sleeping, it is the lowest rate of energy expenditure. The determination of the BMR is a clinical procedure conducted in a laboratory or hospital setting. The individual fasts for 12 hours. Then, with the subject in a reclining position, the individual's oxygen consumption and carbon dioxide production are measured. Through proper calculations, the BMR is determined.

The **resting metabolic rate (RMR)** is slightly higher than the BMR. It represents the BMR plus small amounts of additional energy expenditure associated with previous muscular activity. According to the National Research Council, the BMR and RMR differ by less than 10 percent. Consequently, although there are some fine differences in the two terms, they are often used interchangeably. Additionally, the National Research Council uses the term **resting energy expenditure (REE)** to account for the energy processes at rest; REE and RMR are also considered to be equivalent terms.

What effect does eating a meal have on the metabolic rate?

The significant elevation of the REE that occurs after ingestion of a meal was previously known as the specific dynamic action of food but is now often referred to as **dietary-induced thermogenesis (DIT)** or **thermic effect of food (TEF).** This elevation is usually highest about 1 hour after a meal and lasts for about 4 hours, and it is due to the energy necessary to absorb, transport, store, and metabolize the food consumed. The greater the caloric content of the meal, the greater this TEF effect. Also, the type of food ingested may affect the magnitude of the TEF. Protein and carbohydrates significantly increase the TEF, whereas the effect of fat is minimal. Alcohol intake also causes a modest rise in the REE.

The normal increase in the REE due to TEF from a mixed meal of carbohydrate, fat, and protein is about 8–10 percent, although some studies have reported increases ranging from 6–16 percent. The TEF effect accounts for approximately 5–10 percent of the total daily energy expenditure.

A number of studies have reported that the TEF is significantly higher in lean subjects compared to obese ones, suggesting that the obese are more efficient in storing fat. The composition of some diets for weight-loss purposes has been based upon this TEF effect; this topic is discussed in Chapters 10 and 11 concerning diets for weight control.

How can I estimate my daily resting energy expenditure (REE)?

There are several ways to estimate your REE, but whichever method is used, the value obtained is an estimate and will have some error associated with it. To get a truly accurate value you would need a clinical evaluation, such as a standard BMR test. However, a number of formula estimates may give you an approximation of your daily REE.

Table 3.4 provides a simple method for calculating the REE of males and females of varying ages. Examples are provided in the table along with calculation of a 10 percent variability. Keep in mind that this is only an estimate of the daily REE, and additional energy would be expended during the day through the TEF effect and the effect of physical activity.

A very simple, rough estimate of your REE is one Calorie per kilogram body weight per hour. Using this procedure, the estimated value for the male in Table 3.4 is 1,680 Calories per day (1 × 70 kg × 24 hours) and for the female is 1,320 Calories (1 × 55 kg × 24 hours), values which are not substantially different than those calculated by the table procedure.

What genetic factors affect my REE?

Your REE is directly related to the amount of metabolically active tissue that you possess. At rest, tissues such as the heart, liver, kidneys, and other internal organs are more metabolically active than muscle tissue, but muscle tissue is more metabolically active than fat. Changes in the proportion of these tissues in your body will therefore cause changes in your REE.

Table 3.4 Estimation of the daily resting energy expenditure (REE)

Age (years)	Equation
Males	
3–9	(22.7 × body weight*) + 495
10–17	(17.5 × body weight) + 651
18–29	(15.3 × body weight) + 679
30–60	(11.6 × body weight) + 879
> 60	(13.5 × body weight) + 487

Example
154-lb male, age 20
154 lbs/2.2 = 70 kg
(15.3 × 70) + 679 = 1,750

Age (years)	Equation
Females	
3–9	(22.5 × body weight*) + 499
10–17	(12.2 × body weight) + 746
18–29	(14.7 × body weight) + 496
30–60	(8.7 × body weight) + 829
> 60	(10.5 × body weight) + 596

Example
121-lb female, age 20
121 lbs/2.2 = 55 kg
(14.7 × 55) + 496 = 1,304

To get a range of values, simply add or subtract a normal 10-percent variation to the RMR estimate.

Male example: 10 percent of 1,750 = 175 Calories
Normal range = 1,575–1,925 Calories/day
Female example: 10 percent of 1,304 = 130 Calories
Normal range = 1,174–1,434 Calories/day

*Body weight is expressed in kilograms (kg).

Many factors influencing the REE, such as age, sex, natural hormonal activity, body size and surface area, and to a degree, body composition, are genetically determined. The effect of some of these factors on the REE is generally well known. Because infants have a large proportion of metabolically active tissue and are growing rapidly, their REE is extremely high. The REE declines through childhood, adolescence, and adulthood as full growth and maturation are achieved. Individuals with naturally greater muscle mass in comparison to body fat have a higher REE; the REE of women is about 10–15 percent lower than that of men, mainly because women have a higher proportion of fat to muscle tissue. Genetically lean individuals have a higher REE than do stocky individuals because their body surface area ratio is larger in proportion to their weight and they lose more body heat through radiation.

How does body composition affect my REE?

Body composition may be changed so as to alter REE. Losing body weight, including both body fat and muscle tissue, generally lowers the total daily REE. The REE may be decreased significantly in obese individuals who go on a very low-Calorie diet of less than 800 Calories per day. The decrease in the REE, which is greater than would be due to weight loss alone, may be caused by lowered levels of thyroid hormones. In one study, the REE of obese subjects dropped 9.4 percent on a diet containing only 472 Calories per day. This topic is covered in more detail in Chapters 10 and 11. The possibility of decreased REE in some athletes who maintain low body weight through exercise, such as female distance runners and male wrestlers, has been the subject of recent debate and will be covered in Chapter 10 when we discuss body composition.

On the other hand, maintaining normal body weight while reducing body fat and increasing muscle mass may raise the REE because muscle tissue has a higher metabolic level than fat tissue or because the ratio of body surface area to body weight is increased. The decline in the REE that occurs with aging may be attributed partially to physical inactivity with a consequent loss of the more metabolically active muscle tissue and an accumulation of body fat. Methods to lose body fat and increase muscle mass are covered in Chapters 11 and 12.

What environmental factors may also influence the REE?

Although caffeine is not a food, it is a common ingredient in some of the foods we may eat or drink. Caffeine is a stimulant and may elicit a significant rise in the REE. One study reported that the caffeine in 2–3 cups of regular coffee increased the REE 10–12 percent.

Smoking cigarettes also raises the REE. Apparently the nicotine in tobacco stimulates the metabolism similarly to caffeine. This may be one of the reasons why some individuals gain weight when they stop smoking.

Climatic conditions, especially temperature changes, may also raise the REE. Exposure to the cold may stimulate the secretion of several hormones and muscular shivering, which may stimulate heat production up to 400 percent. Exposure to warm or hot environments will increase energy expenditure through greater cardiovascular demands and the sweating response. Altitude exposure will also increase REE due to increased ventilation.

Many of these factors influencing the REE are important in themselves but may also be important considerations relative to weight control programs and body temperature regulation. Thus, they are discussed further in later chapters.

The most important factor that can increase the metabolic rate in general is exercise. As we shall see in a later section, exercise also may exert some effects upon the REE.

What energy sources are used during rest?

The vast majority of the energy consumed during a resting situation is used to drive the automatic physiological processes in the body. Because the muscles expend little energy during rest, there is no need to produce ATP rapidly. Hence, the oxygen system is able to provide the necessary ATP for resting physiological processes.

The oxygen system can use carbohydrates, fats, and protein as energy sources. However, as noted in Chapter 6, protein is not used as a major energy source under normal dietary conditions. Carbohydrates and fats, when combined with oxygen in the cells, are the major energy substrates during rest. Several factors may influence which of the two nutrients is predominantly used. In general, though, on a mixed diet of carbohydrate, protein, and fat, about 40 percent of the energy expenditure at rest is derived from carbohydrate and about 60 percent comes from fat.

Human Energy Metabolism during Exercise

What effect does muscular exercise have on the metabolic rate?

As noted above, the REE is measured with the subject at rest in a reclining position. Any physical activity will raise metabolic activity above the REE and thus increase energy expenditure. Accounting for changes in physical activity over the day may provide a reasonable, although imprecise, estimate of the total daily energy expenditure. Very light activities such as sitting, standing, playing cards, cooking, and typing all increase energy output above the REE, but we normally do not think of them as exercise. For purposes of this discussion, the **exercise metabolic rate (EMR),** represents the increase in metabolism brought about by moderate or strenuous physical activity such as brisk walking, climbing stairs, cycling, dancing, running, and other such activities. The EMR is known more appropriately as the **thermic effect of exercise (TEE).**

Exercise is a stressor to the body, and almost all body systems respond. If the exercise is continued daily, the body systems begin to adapt to the stress of exercise. As we shall see in later chapters, these adaptations may have significant health benefits. The two body systems most involved in exercise are the nervous system and the muscular system. The nervous system is needed to activate muscle contraction, but it is in the muscle cell itself that the energetics of exercise occur. Most other body systems are simply designed to serve the needs of the muscle cell during exercise.

The muscle cell, or muscle fiber, is a rather simple machine in design but extremely complex in function. It is a tube-like structure containing filaments that can slide by one another to shorten the total muscle. The shortening of the muscle moves bones, and hence work is accomplished, be it simply the raising of a barbell as in weight training or moving the whole body as in running. Like most other machines, the muscle cell has the capability of producing work at different rates, ranging from very low levels of energy expenditure during sleep to nearly a ninety-fold increase during maximal, short-term anaerobic exercise.

The human body possesses several different types of muscle fibers, and their primary differences are in the ability to produce energy. Type I is called a slow-twitch red fiber, and it can produce energy primarily by aerobic processes, the oxygen system. It is also referred to as the slow-oxidative fiber (SO). Type IIa is known as a fast-twitch red fiber; it also can produce energy by aerobic processes but in addition can produce energy anaerobically via the lactic acid system. It is also known as the fast-oxidative glycolytic fiber (FOG). The third fiber type, IIb, is a fast-twitch white fiber that produces energy primarily by anaerobic processes and is also known as the fast glycolytic fiber (FG). Type II fibers may use the ATP-PC system at a faster rate than Type I fibers.

The most important factor affecting the metabolic rate is the intensity or speed of the exercise. To move faster, your muscles must contract more rapidly, consuming proportionately more energy. Use of type I muscle fibers predominates during low-intensity exercise, and type II fibers are increasingly recruited with more intense exercise. The following represents approximate energy expenditure in Calories per minute for increasing levels of exercise intensity for an average-sized adult male. However, for most of us it would be impossible to sustain the higher levels of energy expenditure for a minute, and the highest level could be sustained for only a second or so.

Level of intensity	Caloric expenditure per minute
Resting metabolic rate	1.0
Sitting and writing	2.0
Walking at 2 mph	3.3
Walking at 3 mph	4.2
Running at 5 mph	9.4
Running at 10 mph	18.8
Running at 15 mph	29.3
Running at 20 mph	38.7
Maximal power weightlift	>90.0

Although the intensity of the exercise is the most important factor affecting the magnitude of the metabolic rate, there are some other important considerations. In some activities the increase in energy expenditure is not directly proportional to speed, for the efficiency of movement will affect caloric expenditure. Very fast walking becomes more inefficient, so the individual burns more Calories per mile compared to more leisurely walking. A beginning swimmer wastes a lot of energy, whereas one who is more accomplished may swim with less effort, saving Calories when swimming a given distance. Swimming and cycling at very high speeds exponentially increase water or air resistance, so caloric expenditure also increases exponentially. Moreover, the individual with a greater body weight will burn more Calories for any given amount of work in which the body has to be moved, as in walking, jogging, or running. It simply costs more total energy to move a heavier load.

How is exercise intensity measured?

The intensity of a given exercise may be measured in two general ways. One way is to measure the actual work output or power of the activity, such as foot-pounds per second, kilojoules per second, or watts. In some cases this is rather easy to do because some machines, such as bicycle ergometers, are designed to provide an accurate measure of work output. However, the actual work output of a basketball player during a game is more difficult to measure, although use of accelerometers and other motion-detection devices help.

A second way is to measure the physiological cost of the activity by monitoring the activity of the three human energy systems. There are highly sophisticated laboratory techniques to measure the activity of the ATP-PC system, but they are not commonly used.

Laboratory techniques are also available to measure the role of the lactic acid system in exercise, primarily by measuring the concentration of lactic acid in the blood or in muscle tissues. One measure of exercise intensity is the so-called anaerobic threshold, or that point where the metabolism is believed to shift to a greater use of the lactic acid system. This point is often termed the **onset of blood lactic acid (OBLA),** or lactate threshold. The anaerobic threshold may also be referred to as the **steady-state threshold,** indicating that endurance exercise may continue for prolonged periods if you exercise below this threshold value. Exercise physiologists disagree about which is the better term, but all terms may be found in scientific literature.

Laboratory tests also are necessary to measure the contribution of the oxygen system during exercise, and this is the most commonly used technique for measuring exercise intensity (see Figure 3.3). The most commonly used measurement is the **maximal oxygen uptake,**

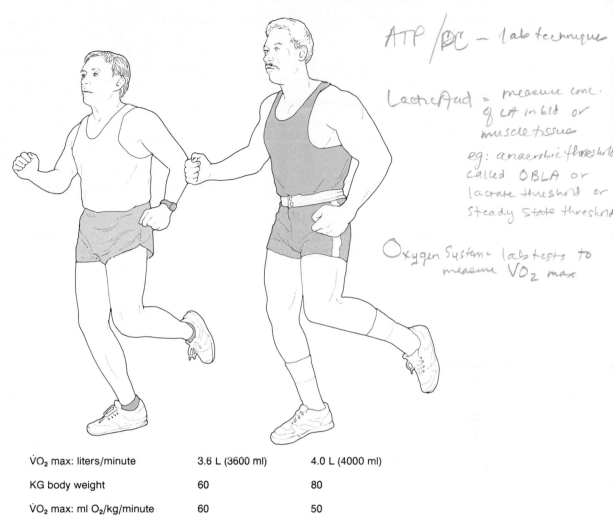

V̇O₂ max: liters/minute	3.6 L (3600 ml)	4.0 L (4000 ml)
KG body weight	60	80
V̇O₂ max: ml O₂/kg/minute	60	50

Figure 3.13 Maximal oxygen uptake (VO₂ max). The best way to express VO₂ max is in milliliters of oxygen per kilogram (kg) of body weight per minute (ml O₂/kg/min). As noted in the figure, the smaller individual has a lower VO₂ max in liters but a higher VO₂ max when expressed relative to weight. In this case, the smaller individual has a higher degree of aerobic fitness, at least as measured by VO₂ max.

which represents the highest amount of oxygen that an individual may consume under exercise situations. In essence, the technique consists of monitoring the oxygen uptake of the individual while the exercise intensity is increased in stages. When oxygen uptake does not increase with an increase in workload, the maximal oxygen uptake has been reached. Maximal oxygen uptake is usually expressed as **VO₂ max,** which may be stated as liters per minute or milliliters per kilogram body weight per minute. An example is provided in Figure 3.13. A commonly used technique to indicate exercise intensity is to report it as a certain percentage of an individual's VO₂ max, such as 50 or 75 percent. In summary, measurement of the three energy systems during exercise provides us with a measure of the energy cost of the physical activity.

Figure 3.14 illustrates the effects of training on VO₂ max and the steady-state threshold.

How is the energy expenditure of exercise metabolism expressed?

A number of research studies have been conducted to determine the energy expenditure of a wide variety of sports and other physical activities.

The energy costs have been reported in a variety of ways, including Calories per minute based upon body weight, kilojoules (kJ), oxygen uptake, and **METS.** The MET is a unit that represents multiples of the resting metabolic rate (see Figure 3.15). These concepts are, of course, all interrelated, so an exercise can be expressed in any one of the four terms and converted into the others.

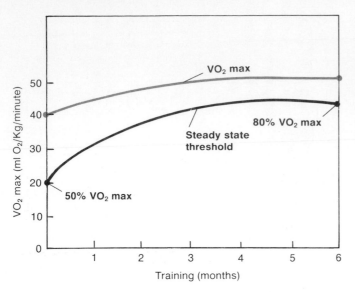

Figure 3.14 The effect of training upon VO$_2$ max and the steady-state threshold. Training increases both your VO$_2$ max and your steady-state threshold, which is the ability to work at a greater percentage of your VO$_2$ max without producing excessive lactic acid—a causative factor in fatigue. For example, before training the VO$_2$ max may be 40 ml while the steady-state threshold is only 20 ml (50% of VO$_2$ max). After training, VO$_2$ max may rise to 50 ml, but the steady-state threshold may rise to 40 ml (80% of the VO$_2$ max).

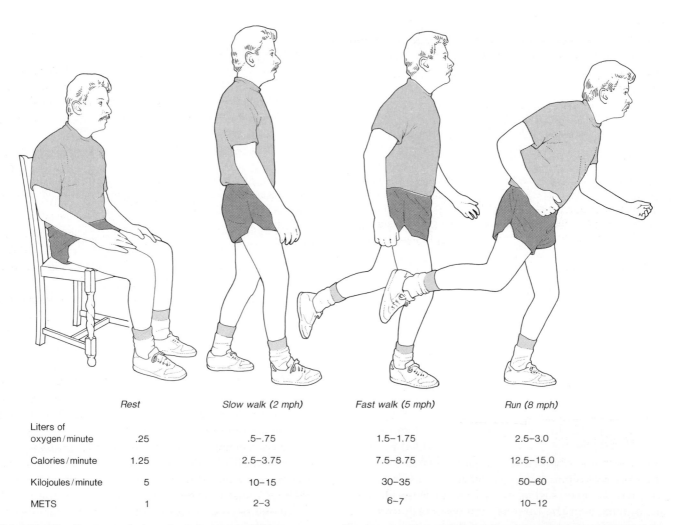

	Rest	Slow walk (2 mph)	Fast walk (5 mph)	Run (8 mph)
Liters of oxygen / minute	.25	.5–.75	1.5–1.75	2.5–3.0
Calories / minute	1.25	2.5–3.75	7.5–8.75	12.5–15.0
Kilojoules / minute	5	10–15	30–35	50–60
METS	1	2–3	6–7	10–12

Figure 3.15 Energy equivalents in oxygen consumption, Calories, Kilojoules, and METS. This figure depicts four means of expressing energy expenditure during four levels of activity.

These approximate values are for an average male of 154 pounds (70 kg). If you weigh more or less, the values will increase or decrease accordingly.

For our purposes, we will express energy cost in Calories per minute based upon body weight, as that appears to be the most practical method for this book. However, just in case you see the other values in another book or magazine, here is how you may simplify the conversion. We know the following approximate values:

1 C = 4 kJ
1 L O_2 = 5 C
1 MET = 3.5 ml O_2/kg body weight/min
(amount of oxygen consumed during rest)

These values are needed for the following calculations:
Example: Exercise cost = 20 kJ/minute
To get Calorie cost, divide kJ by the equivalent value for Calories.

$$20 \text{ kJ/min}/4 = 5 \text{ C/min}$$

Example: Exercise cost = 3 L of O_2/min
To get Calorie cost, multiply liters of O_2 × Calories per liter.

$$\text{Caloric cost} = 3 \times 5 = 15 \text{ C/min}$$

Example: Exercise cost = 25 ml O_2/kg body weight/min
You need body weight in kg, which is weight in pounds divided by 2.2. For this example 154 lbs=70 kg. Determine total O_2 cost/min by multiplying body weight times O_2 cost/kg/min.

$$70 \times 25 = 1,750 \text{ ml } O_2$$

Convert ml to L: 1,750 ml = 1.75 L

Multiply liters O_2 × Calories per liter

$$\text{Caloric cost} = 1.75 \times 5 = 8.75 \text{ C/min}$$

Example: Exercise cost = 12 METS
You need body weight in kg—for this example, 70 kg. Multiply total METS times O_2 equivalent of 1 MET.

$$12 \times 3.5 \text{ ml } O_2/\text{kg/min} = 42.0 \text{ ml } O_2/\text{kg/min}$$

Multiply body weight times this result.

$$70 \times 42 \text{ ml } O_2/\text{kg/min} = 2,940 \text{ ml } O_2/\text{min}$$

Convert ml to L: 2,940 ml O_2/min = 2.94 L O_2/min

Multiply liters O_2 × Calories per liter

$$\text{Caloric cost} = 2.94 \times 5 = 14.70 \text{ C/min}$$

How can I tell what my metabolic rate is during exercise?

The human body is basically a muscle machine designed for movement. Almost all of the other body systems serve the muscular system. The nervous system causes the muscles to contract. The digestive system supplies nutrients. The cardiovascular system delivers these nutrients along with oxygen in cooperation with the respiratory system. The endocrine system secretes hormones that affect mus-

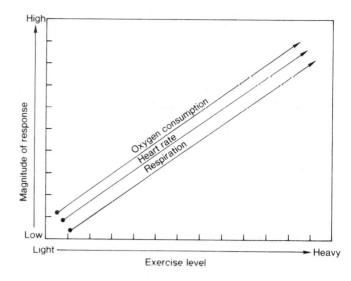

Figure 3.16   Relationships between oxygen consumption, heart rate, and respiration responses to increasing exercise rates. In general, as the intensity of exercise continues, there is a rise in oxygen consumption, which is accompanied by proportional increases in heart rate and respiration.

cle nutrition. The excretory system removes waste products. When humans exercise, almost all body systems increase their activity to accommodate the increased energy demands of the muscle cell. In most types of sustained exercises, however, the major demand of the muscle cells is for oxygen.

As noted previously, the major technique for evaluating metabolic rate is to measure the oxygen consumption of an individual during exercise. Athletes may benefit from such physiological testing. Measurements of VO_2 max, maximal heart rate, and the anaerobic threshold may help in planning an optimal training program, and subsequent testing may illustrate training effects. Such testing is becoming increasingly available at various universities and comprehensive fitness/wellness centers.

Unfortunately, this may not be practical for most of us. However, because of some interesting relationships among exercise intensity, oxygen consumption, and heart rate, the average individual may be able to get a relative approximation of the metabolic rate during exercise. A more or less linear relationship exists between exercise intensity and oxygen uptake. As the intensity level of work increases, so does the amount of oxygen consumed. The two systems primarily responsible for delivering the oxygen to the muscles are the cardiovascular and respiratory systems. There is also a fairly linear relationship between their responses and oxygen consumption. A simplified schematic is presented in Figure 3.16.

Because the heart rate (HR) generally is linearly related to oxygen consumption (the main expression of metabolic rate), and because it is easy to measure this physiological response during exercise either at the wrist or neck pulse, it may prove to be a practical guide to your metabolic rate. However, a number of factors may influence your specific heart rate response to exercise, such as the type of exercise (running vs. swimming), your level of physical fitness, sex, age, skill efficiency, percentage of body fat, and a number of environmental conditions. Thus, it is difficult to predict your exact metabolic rate from your exercise HR. As we shall see in Chapter 11, however, the HR data during exercise may be used as a basis for establishing a personal fitness program for health and weight control.

How can I determine the energy cost of exercise?

To facilitate the determination of the energy cost of a wide variety of physical activities, Appendix C has been developed. This is a composite table of a wide variety of individual reports in the literature. When using this appendix, keep the following points in mind.

1. The figures include the REE. Thus, the total cost of the exercise includes not only the energy expended by the exercise itself, but also the amount you would have used anyway during that same period. Suppose you ran for 1 hour and the calculated energy cost was 800 Calories. During that same time at rest you may have expended 75 Calories as your REE. The net cost of the exercise is only 725 Calories.

2. The figures in the table are only for the time you are doing the activity. For example, in an hour of basketball you may exercise strenuously for only 35–40 minutes, as you may take timeouts and rest during foul shots. In general, record only the amount of time that you are actually moving during the activity.

3. The figures may give you some guidelines to total energy expenditure, but actual caloric cost might vary somewhat because of such factors as your skill level, running against the wind or uphill, and so forth.

4. Not all body weights could be listed, but you may approximate by going to the closest weight listed.

5. There may be small differences between men and women, but not enough to make a marked difference in the total caloric value for most exercises.

As one example, suppose we calculate the energy expenditure of a 154-pound individual who ran 5 miles in 30 minutes. You must calculate either the minutes per mile or miles per hour (mph).

1. 30 minutes / 5 miles = 6 min/mile
2. 60 minutes / 6 minutes/mile = 10 mph

Consult Appendix C and find the caloric value per minute for a body weight of 155 lbs and a running speed of 10 mph, a value of 18.8 Calories/minute. Multiply this value times the number of minutes of running, and you get the total caloric cost of that exercise. In this example, $30 \times 18.8 = 564$ total C expended.

If the activity you do does not appear in Appendix C, try to find one you think closely matches the movements found in your activity. Then check the caloric expenditure for the related activity.

What are the best types of activities to increase energy expenditure?

Activities that use the large muscle groups of the body and are performed continuously usually will expend the greatest amount of Calories. Intensity and duration are the two key determinants of total energy expenditure. Activities in which you may be able to exercise continuously at a fairly high intensity for a prolonged period will maximize your total caloric loss. Although this may encompass a wide variety of different physical activities, those that have become increasingly popular include walking, running, swimming, bicycling, and aerobic dance. A few general comments about these common modes of exercising would appear to be in order.

Walking and running are popular exercises because they are so practical to do. All you need is a good pair of shoes. As a general rule, the caloric cost of running a given distance does not depend on the speed. It will take you a longer time to cover the distance at a slower speed, but the total caloric cost will be similar to that expended at a faster speed. However, walking is more economical than running, and hence you generally expend fewer Calories for a given distance walking than you do running. Slow, leisurely walking uses about half the number of Calories per mile as compared to running. This does not hold true, however, if you walk vigorously at a high speed. A study by Thomas and Londeree has shown that the caloric cost of jogging at 4.7 mph is only about 5 percent higher than walking at the same speed. At high walking speeds (above 5 mph), you may possibly expend more energy than if you jogged at the same speed. Fast, vigorous walking, known as aerobic walking, can be an effective means to expend Calories. However, as with other exercise activities, it takes practice to become a fast walker.

Climbing stairs, at home, at work, in an athletic stadium, or on step machines, is one means to make walking more vigorous. Skipping is also more vigorous but may lead to injuries.

Many individuals use small weights in conjunction with their walking or running programs either by carrying them or strapping them to the ankles or waist. The most popular technique is to carry small weights of 1–3 pounds. A number of research studies have reported that this technique, particularly if the arms are swung vigorously through a wide range of motion during walking, may increase the energy expenditure about 5–10 percent or higher above unweighted walking at the same speed. Use of walking poles, similar to ski poles, may increase caloric expenditure by 15 percent. Increases in energy expenditure greater than 30 percent have been reported with vigorous pumping of 1-pound hand weights as compared with just running at the same speed. The heart rate response also increases, and using hand weights with fast walking is an adequate stimulus to promote a training effect on the cardiovascular system. However, use of hand weights exaggerates the blood pressure response, and thus should be used with caution by individuals with blood pressure problems. Since some researchers have noted that simply walking a little faster without weights will have the same effect on energy cost and heart rate response, this may be a good alternative. Nevertheless, at any given walking speed, hand weights will increase energy expenditure. Addition of weights to the ankle also will increase energy expenditure, but it may also change the normal running style and may predispose one to injury.

Because of water resistance, swimming takes more energy to cover a given distance than does either walking or running. Although the amount of energy expended depends somewhat on the type of swimming stroke used and the ability of the swimmer, swimming a given distance takes about four times as much energy as running. For example, swimming a quarter-mile is the energy equivalent of running a mile. Water aerobics and water running (doing aerobics or running in waist-deep, chest-deep, or deep water) may be effective exercise regimens that help prevent injuries due to impact.

Bicycling takes less energy, about one-third the cost, to cover a given distance in comparison to running on a level surface. The energy cost of bicycling depends on a number of factors such as body weight, the type of bicycle, hills, and body position on the bike (assuming a streamlined position to reduce air resistance). Owing to rapidly increasing air resistance at higher speeds such as 20 mph, the energy cost of bicycling increases at a much faster rate at such speeds. A detailed method for calculating energy expenditure during bicycling is presented in the article by Hagberg and Pena.

For a simplified procedure, you may calculate the approximate caloric expenditure for running a given distance by either one of the following formulas:

Caloric cost = 1 C/kg body weight/kilometer

Caloric cost = 0.73 C/pound body weight/mile

If you are an average-sized male of about 154 lbs (70 kg), or an average-sized female of about 121 lbs (55 kg), you would burn approximately the following amounts of Calories for a kilometer or a mile.

	Male (154 lbs, 70 kg)	Female (121 lbs, 55 kg)
Kilometer	70	55
Mile	112	88

Slow, leisurely walking would burn a little more than half this amount of Calories per mile. Swimming a mile would use approximately four times this amount, whereas bicycling a mile would burn about one-third. In-line skating at about twice the speed of running would use about the same number of Calories per mile.

Aerobic dance, as now known, has been a popular form of exercise for over 20 years. There is a variety of styles of aerobic dance varying in intensity and the degree of impact with the floor. Several studies have shown that high-intensity, high-impact aerobic dancing approximates 10 Calories per minute in women, which is indicative of strenuous exercise. Unfortunately, other research has shown that high-impact dancing is more traumatic and may lead to a higher incidence of leg injuries. Thus, the low-impact, or soft-impact, technique in which one foot usually remains in contact with the floor was introduced. Several studies have also shown that if done at a high intensity, low-impact aerobic dance may also use approximately 9–10 Calories per minute and be less likely to induce injuries to the legs. The use of step benches may also increase exercise intensity.

Home exercise equipment may also provide a strenuous aerobic workout. Recent research suggests that for any given level of perceived effort, treadmill running burned the most Calories. Exercising on cross-country ski machines, rowing ergometers, and stair-climbing apparatus also expended significant amounts of Calories, more so than bicycling apparatus.

Table 3.5 provides a classification of some common physical activities based upon rate of energy expenditure. The implications of these types of exercises in weight control programs are discussed later.

Does exercise affect my resting energy expenditure (REE)?

Exercise not only raises the metabolic rate during exercise but, depending upon the intensity and duration of the activity, will also keep the REE elevated during the recovery period. The increase in body temperature and in the amounts of circulating hormones such as adrenaline (epinephrine) will continue to influence some cellular activity, and some other metabolic processes, such as circulation and respiration, will remain elevated for a limited time. This effect, which has been labeled the **metabolic aftereffects of exercise,** is calculated by monitoring the oxygen consumption for several hours during the recovery period after the exercise task. The amount of oxygen in excess of the preexercise REE, often called excess postexercise

Table 3.5   Classification of physical activities based upon rate of energy expenditure*

Light, mild aerobic exercise (< 7 Calories/min)

Archery	Billiards	Horseback riding
Badminton, social	Bowling	Nautilus weight training
Baseball	Dancing, mild square	Swimming (20–25 yards/min)
Bicycling (5–10 mph)	Golf	Walking (2–4 mph)

Moderate to heavy aerobic exercise (8–12 Calories/min)

Badminton, competitive	Handball, moderate	Soccer
Basketball	In-line skating (9–12 mph)	Squash
Bicycling (11–14 mph)	Racquetball	Swimming (30–50 yards/min)
Circuit weight training, vigorous	Rope skipping (60–80 rpm)	Tennis, competitive
Dancing, aerobic	Running (5–6 mph)	Volleyball, competitive
Field hockey	Skiing, cross-country (4–6 mph)	Walking (4.5–5.5 mph)

Maximal aerobic exercise (> 13 Calories/min)

Bicycling (15–20 mph)	Running (7–9 mph)
Calisthenics, vigorous	Skiing, cross-country (7–9 mph)
Handball, competitive	Swimming (55–70 yards/min)
In-line skating (14–18 mph)	Walking (5.8–6.0 mph)
Rope skipping (120–140 rpm)	

*Calories per minute based upon a body weight of 70 kg, or 154 pounds. Those weighing more or less will expend more or fewer Calories, respectively, but the intensity level of the exercise will be the same. The actual amount of Calories expended may also depend on a number of other factors, depending on the activity. For example, bicycling into or with the wind will increase or decrease, respectively, the energy cost.

Source: Modified from M. H. Williams, *Nutritional Aspects of Human Physical and Athletic Performance*, 1985, Charles C Thomas Publishers, Springfield, IL.

oxygen consumption (EPOC), reflects the additional caloric cost of the exercise above and beyond that expended during the exercise task itself.

Some older research noted that the average number of additional Calories expended after each exercise session would be about 45–50. However, in a series of more recent studies with more appropriate controls, although most investigators did report an increased REE following exercise of varying durations and intensities, the magnitude of the response was generally lower. Depending on the intensity and duration of the exercise bout in these studies, the REE during the recovery period ranged from 4–16 percent higher than the preexercise REE, and it remained elevated for only 15–20 minutes in some studies but up to 4–5 hours in others. Both aerobic and resistance-type exercises increase EPOC, with greater increases associated with high-intensity, long duration exercise. Using the oxygen consumption values presented in these studies, the additional energy expenditure ranged from 3–30 Calories.

Although the metabolic aftereffects of exercise would not appear to make a significant contribution to weight loss, exercise may help mitigate the decrease in the REE often seen in individuals on very low-Calorie diets. This point is explored further in Chapter 11.

Does exercise affect the thermic effect of food (TEF)?

Many studies have been conducted to investigate the effect of exercise on the thermic effect of food (TEF). Unfortunately, no clear answer has been found. Some studies have reported an increase in TEF when subjects exercise either before or after the meal, while others revealed little or no effects. Some research even suggests that exercise training decreases the TEF. Other studies have investigated differences between exercise-trained and untrained individuals relative to TEF, and although some preliminary research noted a decreased TEF in endurance-trained athletes, Tremblay and others also

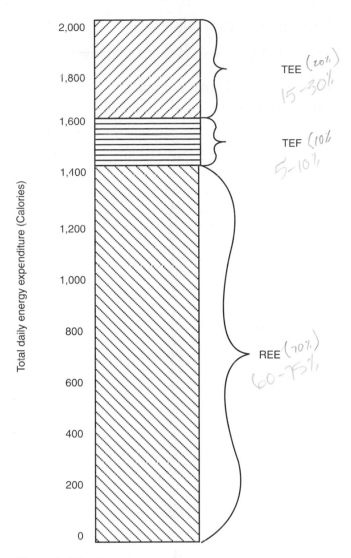

Handwritten annotations on figure: TEE (20%) 15-30%; TEF (10% 5-10%); REE (70%) 60-75%

Figure 3.17 Total daily energy expenditure. Three major factors account for the total daily energy expenditure. Resting energy expenditure (REE) accounts for 60–75 percent, the thermic effect of food (TFF) accounts for 5–10 percent, and 15–30 percent is accounted for by the thermic effect of exercise (TEE). However, all of these percentages are variable in different individuals, with exercise being the most modifiable component. In the figure, the REE is 70 percent, the TEF is 10 percent, and the TEE is 20 percent.

noted that it is still unclear if training causes any significant alterations in TEF. In any case, the increases or decreases noted in the TEF due to either exercise or exercise training were minor, averaging about 5–9 Calories for several hours.

What role does the thermic effect of exercise (TEE) play in my total daily energy expenditure?

Your total daily energy expenditure is the sum of your REE, your TEF, and your TEE. Figure 3.17 provides some approximate values for the typical individual, indicating that REE accounts for 60–75 percent of the total daily energy expen-

(handwritten) TDEE = REE + TEF + TEE

Table 3.6	Physical activity factor classification system	
Activity		**Multiple of REE**
1. **Resting:** Sleeping, reclining while watching TV		1.0
2. **Very light:** Sitting and standing activities, such as driving, playing cards, typing		1.5
3. **Light:** Activities comparable to walking at a leisurely pace, light housework, sports such as golf, bowling, archery		2.5
4. **Moderate:** Walking at a pace of 3.5–4.0 mph, active gardening, sports such as cycling, tennis, dancing		5.0
5. **Heavy:** Faster walking, stair and hill climbing, more active sports such as basketball, soccer		7.0

Source: Adapted with permission from *Recommended Dietary Allowances: 10th Edition.* Copyright 1989 by the National Academy of Sciences. Courtesy of the National Academy Press, Washington, D. C.

diture, TEF represents 5–10 percent, and TEE explains 15–30 percent. These values are approximate and may vary tremendously, particularly TEE, which may range from near 0 percent in the totally sedentary individual to 50 percent or more in ultraendurance athletes.

In order to illustrate the effect that TEE may have on total daily energy expenditure, the National Research Council has developed a five-category physical activity factor as a means to determine an individual's daily caloric needs. The scale used is based upon an REE value of 1.0, and increasing levels of physical activity are multiples of the REE, somewhat comparable to the MET system discussed earlier. For example, an individual doing light activity, such as walking at 2.5 mph, would be expending Calories at approximately 2.5 times the REE. Table 3.6 briefly summarizes this classification system, although it should be mentioned that this is an arbitrary system and could be affected greatly by factors previously discussed in this chapter. Nevertheless, it is a useful tool to illustrate an answer to the question posed above.

Let us take an example of the 24-hour energy expenditure of two 20-year-old women who have the same body weight, 132 pounds or 60 kg. However, one of the women is a typical sedentary sofa spud, while the other is physically active on her job and as a competitive triathlete. Let us assume that the REE is the same for both, 1,378 Calories per day as calculated from the equation in Table 3.4. Let us further assume that, on average, the sedentary woman sleeps and rests for 12 hours, performs very light activity for 10 hours, and does light activity 2 hours per day. To calculate her total daily energy expenditure (TDEE), we need to calculate her average daily physical activity quotient. The following example should provide you with the technique:

Resting	12 hours × 1.00 = 12.00
Very light activity	10 hours × 1.5 = 15.00
Light activity	2 hours × 2.5 = 5.00
Totals	24 hours 32.00

Average physical activity quotient = 32/24 = 1.33

TDEE = 1.33 × 1,378 = 1,832 Calories

A related calculation procedure is presented in Figure 3.18.

For our physically active female, let us assume that she rests 8 hours, does very light activity for 8 hours, does light activity for 4 hours, and performs both moderate and heavy exercise for 2 hours each. Following the same procedure, we obtain a TDEE of 3,100 Calories.

Resting	8 hours × 1.0 = 8.00
Very light activity	8 hours × 1.5 = 12.00
Light activity	4 hours × 2.5 = 10.00
Moderate activity	2 hours × 5.0 = 10.00
Heavy activity	2 hours × 7.0 = 14.00
Totals	24 hours 54.00

Average physical activity quotient = 54/24 = 2.25

TDEE = 2.25 × 1,378 = 3,100 Calories

The total caloric difference between the two women is approximately 1,270 per day. It is interesting to note that over 75 percent (1,378/1,832) of the daily caloric intake of the sedentary woman is accounted for by the REE, as compared with only about 44 percent in the physically active woman.

As noted above, you may be able to modify your REE slightly by certain techniques. However, if you are interested in increasing your TDEE, for all practical purposes your best bet is to incorporate more light, moderate, and heavy physical activities into your life-style.

The importance of such physical activities, particularly exercise, in the design of a proper weight control program is explored in Chapter 11.

Human Energy Systems and Fatigue during Exercise

What energy systems are used during exercise?

The most important factor determining which energy system will be used is the intensity of the exercise, which is the rate, speed, or tempo at which you pursue a given activity. In general, the faster you do something, the higher your rate of energy expenditure and the more rapidly you must produce ATP for muscular contraction. Very rapid muscular movements are characterized by high rates of power production. If you were asked to run 100 meters as fast as you could, you would exert maximal speed for a short time. On the other hand, if you were asked to run 5 miles, you certainly would not run at the same speed as you would for the 100 meters. In the 100-meter run your energy expenditure would be very rapid, characterized by a high-power production. The 5-mile run would be characterized by low-power production, or endurance.

The requirement of energy for exercise is related to a power-endurance continuum. On the power end, we have extremely high rates of energy expenditure that a sprinter might use; on the endurance end, we see lower rates that might be characteristic of a marathon runner. The closer we are to the power end of the continuum, the more rapidly we must produce ATP. As we move toward the endurance end, our rate of ATP production does not need to be as great, but we need the capacity to produce ATP for a longer time.

It should be noted from the outset that all three energy systems—ATP-PC, lactic acid, and oxygen—are used in one way or another during most athletic activities. However, one system may predominate, depending primarily upon the intensity level of the activity. In this regard, the three human energy systems may be ranked according to several characteristics, which are displayed in Table 3.7.

Both the ATP-PC and the lactic acid systems are able to produce ATP rapidly and are used in events characterized by high intensity levels that occur for short periods, because their capacity for total ATP production is limited. Because both of these systems may function without oxygen, they are called anaerobic. Relative to physical performance, the ATP-PC system predominates in short, powerful bursts of muscular activity such as the short dashes like 100 meters, whereas the lactic acid system begins to predominate during the longer sprints and middle distances such as 400 and 800 meters. In any athletic event where maximal power production lasts about 1–10 seconds, the ATP-PC system is the major energy source. The lactic acid system begins to predominate in events lasting 30–120 seconds, but studies have noted significant

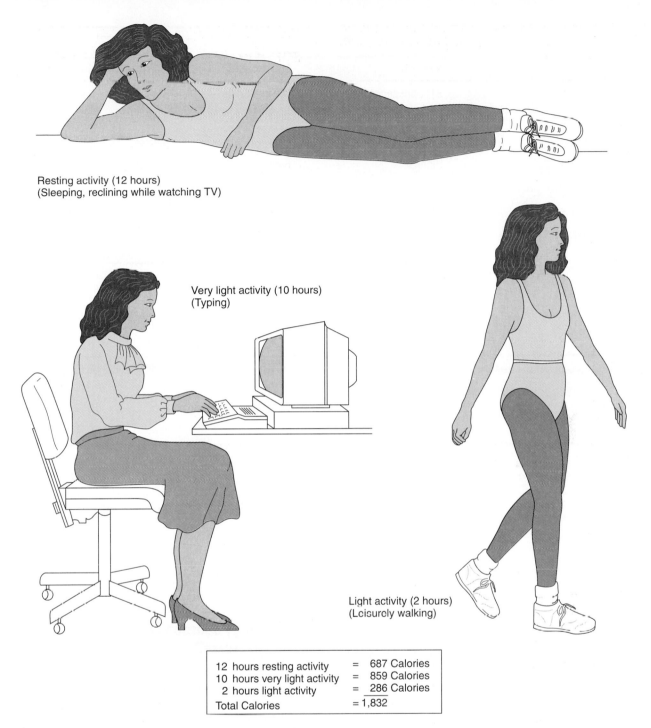

Resting activity (12 hours)
(Sleeping, reclining while watching TV)

Very light activity (10 hours)
(Typing)

Light activity (2 hours)
(Leisurely walking)

12 hours resting activity	=	687 Calories
10 hours very light activity	=	859 Calories
2 hours light activity	=	286 Calories
Total Calories	=	1,832

Figure 3.18 Total daily caloric expenditure for a sedentary, 20-year-old female who weighs 132 pounds (60 kg). Based upon calculations from the data presented in the text, she expends approximately 57 Calories per hour during resting activity (1,378/24), 86 Calories per hour during very light activity (57 × 1.5), and 143 Calories per hour during light activity (57 × 2.5).

elevations in muscle lactic acid in maximal exercise even as brief as 10 seconds.

The oxygen system possesses a lower rate of ATP production than the other two systems, but its capacity for total ATP production is much greater. Although the intensity level of exercise while using the oxygen system is by necessity lower, this does not necessarily mean that an individual cannot perform at a relatively high speed for a long time. The oxygen system can be improved through a physical conditioning program so that ATP production may be able to meet the demands of relatively high-intensity exercise, as discussed previously and highlighted in Figure 3.14. Endurance-type activities, such as those that last 5 minutes or more, are dependent primarily upon

Table 3.7 Major characteristics of the human energy systems*

	ATP-PC	Lactic acid	Oxygen	Oxygen
Main energy source	ATP; phosphocreatine	Carbohydrate	Carbohydrate	Fat
Intensity level	Highest	High	Lower	Lowest
Rate of ATP production	Highest	High	Lower	Lowest
Power production	Highest	High	Lower	Lowest
Capacity for total ATP production	Lowest	Low	High	Highest
Endurance capacity	Lowest	Low	High	Highest
Oxygen needed	No	No	Yes	Yes
Anaerobic/aerobic	Anaerobic	Anaerobic	Aerobic	Aerobic
Characteristic track event	100-meter dash	400–800 meters	5,000-meter (5 km) run	Ultradistance
Time factor	1–10 seconds	10–120 seconds	5 minutes or more	Hours

*Keep in mind that during most exercises, all three energy systems will be operating to one degree or another. However, one system may predominate, depending primarily on the intensity of the activity. See text for further explanation.

Table 3.8 Percentage contribution of anaerobic and aerobic energy sources during different time periods of maximal work

Time	10 sec	1 min	2 min	4 min	10 min	30 min	60 min	130 min
Anaerobic	85	70	50	30	15	5	2	1
Aerobic	15	30	50	70	85	95	98	99

the oxygen system, but the oxygen system makes a very significant contribution even in events as short as 30–90 seconds.

In summary, we may simplify this discussion by categorizing the energy sources as either aerobic or anaerobic. Anaerobic sources include both the ATP-PC and lactic acid systems while the oxygen system is aerobic. Table 3.8 illustrates the percentage contribution of anaerobic and aerobic energy sources, dependent upon the level of maximal intensity that can be sustained for a given time period. Thus, for a 100-meter dash covered in 10 seconds, 85 percent of the energy is derived from anaerobic sources. For a marathoner (26.2 miles) with times of approximately 130 minutes in international-level competition, the aerobic energy processes contribute 99 percent. The key point is that the longer you exercise, the less your intensity has to be, and the more you rely on your oxygen system for energy production.

What energy sources are used during exercise?

The ATP-PC system can use only adenosine triphosphate and phosphocreatine, but as noted previously, these energy sources are in short supply and need to be replaced by the other two energy systems.

The lactic acid system uses only carbohydrate, primarily the muscle glycogen stores. At high-intensity exercise levels that may be sustained for 4–6 minutes or less, such as exercising above your VO_2 max, carbohydrate will supply over 95 percent of the energy. However, the accumulation of lactic acid may cause the early onset of fatigue.

On the other hand, the oxygen system can use a variety of different energy sources, including protein, although carbohydrate and fat are the primary ones. The carbohydrate is found as muscle glycogen, liver glycogen, and blood glucose. The fats are stored primarily as triglycerides in the muscle and adipose cells. As we shall see below and in the next three chapters, a number of different factors can influence which energy source is used by the oxygen system during exercise, but exercise intensity and duration are the two most important factors.

Under normal conditions, exercise intensity is the key factor determining whether carbohydrate or fat is used. As you do mild to moderate exercise, say up to 50 percent of your VO_2 max, you will use less carbohydrate and more fat. The muscle glycogen and triglycerides in the muscle, as well as glucose delivered from the liver and free fatty acids from the adipose tissues, are your main sources. As you start to exceed 50 percent of your VO_2 max—that is, as you increase your speed or intensity—you begin to rely more and more on carbohydrate as an energy source. Apparently the biochemical processes for fat metabolism are too slow to meet the increased need for faster production of ATP, and carbohydrate utilization increases. The major source of this carbohydrate is muscle glycogen. At high levels of energy expenditure, 70–80 percent of VO_2 max, carbohydrates may contribute more than 80 percent of the energy sources. This speaks for the need of adequate muscle glycogen stores when this level of exercise is to be sustained for long periods, say in events lasting over an hour.

In events of long duration, when body stores of carbohydrate are nearly depleted, the primary energy source is fat. In the later stages of ultramarathoning events, fat may become the only fuel available. However, protein may become an important energy source in these circumstances; its role is detailed in Chapter 6.

Other than exercise intensity and duration, a number of different factors are known to influence the availability and use of human energy sources during exercise. Hormones, state of training, composition of the diet, time of eating prior to competition, nutritional status, nutrient intake during exercise, environmental temperature, and drugs are some of the more important considerations. For example, warm environmental temperatures may increase the use of carbohydrates, whereas caffeine may facilitate the use of fats. These considerations will be incorporated in the following chapters where appropriate.

What is fatigue?

Fatigue is a very complex phenomenon. It may be deemed to be psychological in nature as often noted in cases of mental depression, or it may be physiological in nature as seen in the untrained runner during the latter stages of an all-out 400-meter, or quarter-mile, dash. The site of fatigue in the human body may be classified as central, that is, in the brain or spinal cord of the central nervous system (CNS). The theory of CNS fatigue will be discussed in both Chapters 4 and 6 in relation to the effects of dietary carbohydrates and amino acids on brain neurotransmitters. Fatigue may also be peripheral, located in the muscle tissue itself or at the junction of the muscle

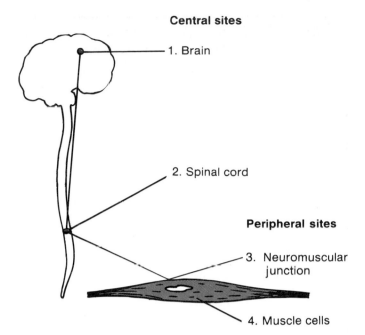

Central sites

1. Brain
2. Spinal cord

Peripheral sites

3. Neuromuscular junction
4. Muscle cells

Figure 3.19 Fatigue sites. The causes of fatigue are complex and may involve central sites such as the brain and spinal cord or peripheral sites in the muscles. Hypoglycemia, or low blood sugar, could adversely affect the functioning of the brain, while the acidity associated with the production of lactic acid could possibly interfere with optimal energy production in the muscle cells.

and nerve fibers (see Figure 3.19). The actual psychological or physiological causes of fatigue are also very complex, but they appear to be related closely to the intensity and duration of the mental or physical tasks to be accomplished. However, most instances of fatigue during exercise are believed to be related to adverse changes in the muscle itself.

For purposes of the present discussion, **fatigue** will be defined as the inability to continue exercising at a desired level of intensity. Relative to this definition, fatigue may be due to a failure of the rate of energy production in the human body to meet the demands of the exercise task. This failure may be due to an inability of the central nervous system to fully stimulate the appropriate muscles, an insufficient supply of the optimal energy source, a reduced ability to metabolize the energy source in the muscle, or inadequate support from body systems, such as blood flow, serving the muscle. In essence, for one or more of these reasons the muscle cannot produce or use ATP rapidly enough to sustain the desired level of exercise intensity. Some possible causes of fatigue during exercise are listed in Table 3.9.

How can I delay the onset of fatigue?

The most important factor in the prevention of premature fatigue is proper training, including physiological, psychological, and biomechanical training.

Table 3.9	**Some possible causes of fatigue during exercise**

Increased formation of depressant neurotransmitters
Increased serotonin levels

Decreased levels of metabolic substrates
Decrease in phosphocreatine levels

Depletion of muscle glycogen

Decrease in blood-sugar levels

Decrease in plasma branched-chain amino acids

Disturbed acid-base balance
Increase in hydrogen ions due to excess lactic acid production

Decreased oxygen transport
Decreased blood volume due to dehydration

Increased core body temperature resulting in hyperthermia
Decreased cooling effect due to dehydration

Disturbed electrolyte balance
Increased or decreased concentration due to sweat losses and water replacement

Physiologically, athletes must train specifically the energy system or systems that are inherent to their event. Under the guidance of sport physiologists and coaches, appropriate physiological training for each specific energy system may increase its energy stores, enzymic activity, and metabolic efficiency, thus enhancing energy production. Physiological training enhances physical power.

Psychologically, athletes must train the mind to tolerate the stresses associated with their specific event. Sport psychologists may help provide the athlete with various mental strategies, such as inducing either a state of relaxation or arousal, whichever may be appropriate for their sport. Physiological training may also confer some psychological advantages, such as tolerating higher levels of pain associated with intense exercise. Psychological training enhances mental strength.

Biomechanically, athletes must maximize the mechanical skills associated with their sport. For any sport, sport biomechanists can analyze the athlete's skill level and recommend modifications in movement patterns or equipment to improve energy production or efficiency. In many cases, modification of the amount of body fat and muscle mass may provide the athlete with a biomechanical advantage. Biomechanical training helps provide a mechanical edge.

Proper physiological, psychological, and biomechanical training represents the best means to help deter premature fatigue. However, what you eat may affect phys-iological, psychological, and biomechanical aspects of sport performance. Thus, nutrition is an important consideration in delaying the onset of fatigue during sport training and competition.

How is nutrition related to fatigue processes?

As noted above in our discussion of the power-endurance continuum, we can exercise at different intensities, but the duration of our exercise is inversely related to the intensity. We can exercise at a high intensity for a short time or at a low intensity for a long time. The importance of nutrition to fatigue is determined by this intensity-duration interrelationship.

In very mild aerobic activities, such as distance walking or low-speed running in a trained ultramarathoner, the body can sustain energy production by using fat as the primary fuel when carbohydrate levels diminish. Because the body has large stores of fat, energy supply is not a problem. However, low blood-sugar levels, dehydration, and excessive loss of minerals may lead to the development of both mental and physical fatigue in very prolonged activities.

In moderate to heavy aerobic exercise, the body needs to use more carbohydrate as an energy source and thus will run out of muscle glycogen faster. As we shall see later, carbohydrate is a more efficient fuel than fat, so the athlete will have to reduce the pace of the activity when liver and muscle carbohydrate stores are depleted, such as during endurance-type activities lasting over 90 minutes. Thus, energy supply may be critical. Low blood sugar, changes in blood constituents such as certain amino acids, and dehydration also may be important factors contributing to the development of mental or physical fatigue in this type of endeavor.

In very high-intensity exercise lasting only 1 or 2 minutes, the probable cause of fatigue is the disruption of cellular metabolism caused by the accumulation of hydrogen ions resulting from excess lactic acid production. There is some evidence to suggest that sodium bicarbonate (discussed in Chapter 9) may help reduce this disruptive effect of lactic acid to some extent. Furthermore, a very low supply of muscle glycogen in fast-twitch muscle fibers may impair this type of performance.

In extremely intense exercise lasting only 5–10 seconds, a depletion of phosphocreatine (PC) may be related to the inability to maintain a high force production. Although some nutritional practices, such as phosphate loading or gelatin supplements, have been used in attempts to increase PC, they have not been regarded to be effective. However, recent research involving creatine supplements has shown some promising effects, which are discussed in Chapter 6.

In summary, a deficiency of almost every nutrient may be a causative factor in the development of fatigue. A poor diet can hasten the onset of fatigue. Proper nutrition is

Table 3.10 Examples of some nutritional ergogenic aids and, theoretically, how they may influence physiological, psychological, or biomechanical processes to delay fatigue

Provide energy substrate
Carbohydrate: Energy substrate for aerobic glycolysis

Creatine: Substrate for formation of phosphocreatine (PC)

Enhance energy-generating metabolic pathways
B vitamins: Coenzymes in aerobic and anaerobic glycolysis

Carnitine: Enzyme substrate to facilitate fat metabolism

Increase cardiovascular-respiratory function
Iron: Substrate for hemoglobin formation and oxygen transport   *Blood doping*

Glycerol: Substance to increase blood volume

Increase size or number of energy-generating cells
Arginine and ornithine: Amino acids that stimulate production of human growth hormone, an anabolic hormone

Chromium: Mineral to potentiate activity of insulin, an anabolic hormone

Attenuate fatigue-related metabolic by-products
Aspartate salts: Amino acids that mitigate ammonia production   *↑ H+   ↑ fatigue*

Sodium bicarbonate: Buffer to reduce effects of lactic acid

Prevent catabolism of energy-generating cells
Antioxidants: Vitamins to prevent unwanted oxidation of cell membranes

HMB: By-product of amino acid metabolism to prevent protein degradation

Ameliorate psychological function
BCAA: Amino acids that favorably modify neurotransmitter production

Choline: Substrate for formation of acetylcholine, a neurotransmitter

essential to assure the athlete that an adequate supply of nutrients is available in the diet not only to provide the necessary energy, such as through carbohydrate and fat, but also to ensure optimal metabolism of the energy substrate via protein, vitamins, minerals, and water. The role of specific nutrients relative to fatigue processes will be discussed in later sections of the book where appropriate. Table 3.10 provides some examples of how some nutrients or dietary supplements are theorized to delay fatigue.

References

Books

Hunt, S., and Groff, J. 1990. *Advanced Nutrition and Human Metabolism.* St Paul, MN: West Publishing Company.

Lee, R., and Nieman, D. 1996. *Nutritional Assessment.* St. Louis: Mosby.

Maud, P., and Foster, C. 1995. *Physiological Assessment of Human Fitness.* Champaign, IL: Human Kinetics.

McArdle, W., Katch, F., and Katch, V. 1996. *Exercise Physiology.* Philadelphia: Lea and Febiger.

National Research Council. 1989. *Recommended Dietary Allowances.* Washington, DC: National Academy of Sciences.

Poortmans, J. 1993. *Principles of Exercise Biochemistry.* Basel, Switzerland: Karger.

Simopoulos, A., ed. 1992. *Metabolic Control of Eating, Energy Expenditure and the Bioenergetics of Obesity.* Basel, Switzerland: Karger.

Review Articles

Ainsworth, B., et al. 1993. Compendium of physical activities: Classification of energy costs of human physical activities. *Medicine and Science in Sports and Exercise* 25:71–80.

Ainsworth, B., et al. 1993. Validity and reliability of self-reported physical activity status. *Medicine and Science in Sports and Exercise* 25:92–98.

Calles-Escandon, J., and Horton, E. 1992. The thermogenic role of exercise in the treatment of obesity: A critical evaluation. *American Journal of Clinical Nutrition* 55:533S–537S.

Carpenter, W., et al. 1995. Influence of body composition and resting metabolic rate on variation in total energy expenditure: A meta-analysis. *American Journal of Clinical Nutrition* 61: 4–10.

Cerretelli, P. 1992. Energy sources for muscular exercise. *International Journal of Sports Medicine* 13:S106–S110.

Coggan, A. 1997. Symposium: Metabolic adaptations to endurance training: Recent advances. *Medicine and Science in Sports and Exercise* 29:620–76.

Dahlstrom, M., et al. 1995. Do highly physically active females have a lowered basal metabolic rate? *Scandinavian Journal of Medicine & Science in Sports* 5:81–87.

Fitts, R., and Metzger, J. 1993. Mechanisms of muscular fatigue. In *Principles of Exercise Biochemistry,* ed. J. Poortmans. Basel, Switzerland: Karger.

Hagberg, J., and Pena, N. 1989. Bicycling's exclusive calorie counter. *Bicycling* 30:100–103.

Hagerman, F. 1992. Energy, metabolism, and fuel utilization. *Medicine and Science in Sports and Exercise* 24:S309–S314.

Hawley, J., and Hopkins, W. 1995. Aerobic glycolytic and aerobic lipolytic power systems. *Sports Medicine* 19:240–50.

Hill, J., and Commerford, R. 1996. Physical activity, fat balance, and energy balance. *International Journal of Sport Nutrition* 6:80–92.

Honig, C., et al. 1992. O_2 transport and its interaction with metabolism: A systems view of aerobic capacity. *Medicine and Science in Sports and Exercise* 24:47–53.

Hultman, E., and Greenhaff, P. 1991. Skeletal muscle energy metabolism and fatigue during intense exercise in man. *Science and Progress* 75:361–70.

Katz, A., and Sahlin, K. 1990. Role of oxygen in regulation of glycolysis and lactate production in humans. *Exercise and Sport Science Reviews* 18:1–28.

Knuttgen, H. 1995. Force, work, and power in athletic training. *Sports Science Exchange* 8(4):1–6.

Korge, P., and Campbell, K. 1995. The importance of ATPase microenvironment in muscle fatigue: A hypothesis. *International Journal of Sports Medicine* 16:172–79.

Lamb, D. 1995. Basic principles for improving sport performance. *Sports Science Exchange* 8(2):1–6.

Newsholme, E. 1993. Application of knowledge of metabolic integration to the problem of metabolic limitations in sprints, middle distance and marathon running. In *Principles of Exercise Biochemistry,* ed. J. Poortmans. Basel, Switzerland: Karger.

Newsholme, E., et al. 1992. Physical and mental fatigue: Metabolic mechanisms and importance of plasma amino acids. *British Medical Bulletin* 48:477–95.

Pavlou, K. 1993. Energy needs of the elite athlete. *World Review of Nutrition and Dietetics* 71:9–20.

Poehlman, E. 1992. Energy expenditure and requirements in aging humans. *Journal of Nutrition* 122:2057–65.

Rall, J., and Wahr, P. 1993. Molecular aspects of muscular contraction. In *Principles of Exercise Biochemistry,* ed. J. Poortmans. Basel, Switzerland: Karger.

Sleivert, G., and Rowlands, D. 1996. Physical and physiological factors associated with success in the triathlon. *Sports Medicine* 22:8–18.

Spurway, N. 1992. Aerobic exercise, anaerobic exercise, and the lactate threshold. *British Medical Bulletin* 48:569–91.

Stager, J., et al. 1995. The use of doubly labelled water in quantifying energy expenditure during prolonged activity. *Sports Medicine* 19:166–72.

Thayer, R., et al. 1993. The fibre composition of skeletal muscle. In *Principles of Exercise Biochemistry,* ed. J. Poortmans. Basel, Switzerland: Karger.

Thompson, J., et al. 1996. Effects of diet and diet-plus-exercise programs on resting metabolic rate: A meta-analysis. *International Journal of Sport Nutrition* 6:41–61.

Toth, M., and Poehlman, E. 1996. Effects of exercise on daily energy expenditure. *Nutrition Reviews* 54:S140–S148.

Tremblay, A., et al. 1985. The effects of exercise-training on energy balance and adipose tissue morphology and metabolism. *Sports Medicine* 2:223–33.

Werner, J. 1993. Temperature regulation during exercise: An overview. In *Exercise, Heat, and Thermoregulation,* eds. C. Gisolfi, D. Lamb, and E. Nadel. Dubuque, IA: Brown and Benchmark.

Wolfe, R., and George, S. 1993. Stable isotopic tracers as metabolic probes in exercise. *Exercise and Sport Sciences Reviews* 21:1–31.

Young, V. 1992. Energy requirements in the elderly. *Nutrition Reviews* 50 (April):95–101.

Specific Studies

Ballor, D. 1992. Resting metabolic rate and coronary-heart-disease risk factors in aerobically and resistance-trained women. *American Journal of Clinical Nutrition* 56:968–74.

Bullough, R., et al. 1995. Interaction of acute changes in exercise energy expenditure and energy intake on resting metabolic rate. *American Journal of Clinical Nutrition* 61:473–81.

Cade, R., et al. 1992. Marathon running: Physiological and chemical changes accompanying late race functional deterioration. *European Journal of Applied Physiology* 65:485–91.

Calles-Escandon, J., et al. 1996. Exercise increases fat oxidation at rest unrelated to changes in energy balance or lipolysis. *American Journal of Physiology* 270:E1009–E1014.

Eckerson, J., and Anderson, T. 1992. Physiological response to water aerobics. *Journal of Sports Medicine and Physical Fitness* 32:255–61.

Eyestone, E., et al. 1993. Effect of water running and cycling on maximum oxygen consumption and 2-mile run performance. *American Journal of Sports Medicine* 21:41–44.

Gillette, C., et al. 1994. Postexercise energy expenditure in response to acute aerobic or resistive exercise. *International Journal of Sport Nutrition* 4:347–60.

Goss, F., et al. Energy cost of bench stepping and pumping light handweights in trained subjects. *Research Quarterly for Exercise and Sport* 60:369–72.

Graves, J., et al. 1987. The effect of hand-held weights on the physiological responses to walking exercise. *Medicine and Science in Sports and Exercise* 19:260–65.

Green, H., et al. 1991. Early muscular and metabolic adaptations to prolonged exercise training in humans. *Journal of Applied Physiology* 70:2032–38.

Horton, T., et al. 1994. Energy balance in endurance-trained female cyclists and untrained controls. *Journal of Applied Physiology* 76:1937–45.

Katzmarzyk, P., et al. 1996. Differences between observed and predicted energy costs at rest and during exercise in three subsistence-level populations. *American Journal of Physical Anthropology* 99:537–45.

Klesges, R., et al. 1994. Effects of alcohol intake on resting energy expenditure in young women social drinkers. *American Journal of Clinical Nutrition* 59:805–9.

Leblanc, J. 1992. Mechanisms of adaptation to cold. *International Journal of Sports Medicine* 13 (Supplement 1): S169–S178.

McCully, K., et al. 1992. Muscle metabolism in track athletes: Using magnetic resonance spectroscopy. *Canadian Journal of Physiology and Pharmacology* 70:1353–59.

Meijer, G. 1992. Physical activity and energy expenditure in lean and obese adult human subjects. *European Journal of Applied Physiology* 65 (6): S25–S28.

Melanson, E., et al. 1996. Exercise responses to running and in-line skating at self-selected paces. *Medicine and Science in Sports and Exercise* 28:247–50.

Melby, C. 1992. Energy expenditure following a bout of non-steady state resistance exercise. *The Journal of Sports Medicine and Physical Fitness* 32:128–35.

Melby, C., et al. 1990. Resting metabolic rate in weight-cycling collegiate wrestlers compared with physically active, noncycling control subjects. *American Journal of Clinical Nutrition* 52:409–14.

Morgan, D., et al. 1995. Variation in the aerobic demand of running among trained and untrained subjects. *Medicine and Science in Sports and Exercise* 27:404–9.

Parker, S., et al. 1989. Failure of target heart rate to accurately monitor intensity during aerobic dance. *Medicine and Science in Sports and Exercise* 21:230–34.

Poehlman, E., et al. 1992. Resting energy metabolism and cardiovascular disease risk in resistance-trained and aerobically trained males. *Metabolism* 41:1351–68.

Reed, G., and Hill, J. 1996. Measuring the thermic effect of food. *American Journal of Clinical Nutrition* 63:164–69.

Roberts, S., et al. 1993. Energy expenditure, aging, and body composition. *Journal of Nutrition* 123:474–80.

Rodgers, C., et al. 1995. Energy expenditure during submaximal walking with Exerstriders. *Medicine and Science in Sports and Exercise* 27:607–11.

Schoeller, D., and Hnilicka, J. 1996. Reliability of the doubly labeled water method for the measurement of total daily energy expenditure in free-living subjects. *Journal of Nutrition* 126:348S–354S.

Segal, K., et al. 1990. Thermic effect of a meal over 3 and 6 hours in lean and obese men. *Metabolism* 39:985–92.

Sjodin, A., et al. 1996. The influence of physical activity on BMR. *Medicine and Science in Sports and Exercise* 28:85–91.

Suter, E., et al. 1993. Muscle fiber type distribution as estimated by Cybex testing and by muscle biopsy. *Medicine and Science in Sports and Exercise* 25:363–70.

Thomas, T., and Londeree, B. 1989. Energy cost during prolonged walking vs jogging exercise. *Physician and Sportsmedicine* 17 (5):93–102.

Thompson, J., et al. 1995. Daily energy expenditure in male endurance athletes with differing energy intakes. *Medicine and Science in Sports and Exercise* 27:347–54.

Thompson, J., and Manore, M. 1996. Predicted and measured resting metabolic rate of male and female endurance athletes. *Journal of the American Dietetic Association* 96:30–34.

Tremblay, A., et al. 1990. Long-term exercise training with constant energy intake. 2: effect of glucose metabolism and resting energy expenditure. *International Journal of Obesity* 14:75–81.

Westerterp, K., et al. 1991. Physical activity and sleeping metabolic rate. *Medicine and Science in Sports and Exercise* 23:166–70.

Wibom, R., et al. 1992. Adaptation of mitochondrial ATP production in human skeletal muscle to endurance training and detraining. *Journal of Applied Physiology* 73:2004–10.

Wilmore, J., et al. 1992. Is there energy conservation in amenorrheic compared with eumenorrheic distance runners? *Journal of Applied Physiology* 72: 15–22.

Zeni, A., et al. 1996. Energy expenditure with indoor exercise machines. *Journal of the American Medical Association* 275:1424–27.

CHAPTER 4

Carbohydrates: The Main Energy Food

KEY TERMS

alcoholism
blood alcohol content (BAC)
carbohydrate loading
carbohydrates
cirrhosis
complex carbohydrates
cortisol
dietary fiber
disaccharide
epinephrine
ergolytic
ethanol
fetal alcohol effects (FAE)
fetal alcohol syndrome (FAS)
fructose
galactose
glucagon
gluconeogenesis
glucose
glucose-alanine cycle
glucose polymer
glycemic index
hyperglycemia
hypoglycemia
insoluble dietary fibers
insulin
lactose intolerance
millimole
monosaccharides
polysaccharide
proof
reactive hypoglycemia
simple carbohydrates
soluble dietary fibers

KEY CONCEPTS

• Most foods in the starch, fruit, and vegetable exchanges contain a high percentage of carbohydrates, primarily complex carbohydrates, which should constitute at least 55–60 percent, or preferably more, of the daily caloric intake of most individuals and athletes.

• The Daily Reference Value (DRV) for carbohydrate is 300 grams and for dietary fiber is 25 grams, based on a 2,000 Calorie diet.

• Most ingested carbohydrates are initially converted into blood glucose and used for energy or stored as liver and muscle glycogen, but excess carbohydrates may be converted into fat.

• The major function of carbohydrates in human metabolism is to supply energy; blood glucose is essential for optimal functioning of the nervous system, whereas muscle glycogen is essential for endurance exercise.

• The three sources of carbohydrate in the body of an average adult male are blood glucose (5 grams; 20 Calories), liver glycogen (75–100 grams; 300–400 Calories), and muscle glycogen (350–400 grams; 1,400–1,600 Calories).

• The body can make glucose from certain by-products of protein and fat.

• Carbohydrate is the most important energy source for high-intensity exercise, and the only one that can participate significantly in aerobic and anaerobic energy pathways.

• Regular training increases the ability of the muscles to store and use carbohydrate for energy production.

• Low levels of blood glucose or muscle glycogen may be contributing factors in the early onset of fatigue in prolonged exercise.

• Carbohydrate intake before and during prolonged intermittent high-intensity or continuous exercise may help delay the onset of fatigue, but such practices will not improve performance in most athletic events of shorter duration unless they correct a muscle glycogen deficiency.

• Glucose, sucrose, glucose polymers, and solid carbohydrates appear to be equally effective as a means to enhance performance, but fructose may be more likely to cause gastrointestinal distress if used alone.

• Athletes who train intensely on a daily basis should eat a diet high in complex carbohydrates to replenish muscle glycogen in order to maintain the quality of training. Carbohydrates with a high glycemic index may facilitate muscle glycogen replenishment when consumed immediately after exercise and every 2 hours thereafter. Adding protein to the carbohydrate may also help.

• Carbohydrate loading is not a technique for all types of athletes, but it appears to benefit athletes involved in long-distance competition such as marathoning.

• Various carbohydrate-loading techniques may effectively increase muscle glycogen stores, but rest and a high-carbohydrate diet are the essential points.

INTRODUCTION

One of the most important nutrients in your diet, from the standpoint of both health and athletic performance, is dietary carbohydrate.

In the past, dietary carbohydrate suffered a poor reputation in the mind of the general public, particularly in those attempting to lose body weight, and a recent popular book touting a low-carbohydrate diet to lose body fat has perpetuated this feeling. However, most dietitians and nutrition scientists consider consumption of carbohydrate-rich foods to be one of the most important components of a healthful diet, not only for its potential in preventing certain chronic diseases but also as an integral part of a proper diet to lose excess body fat. The possible health benefits of a diet high in complex carbohydrates and fiber and low in simple refined sugars were introduced in Chapter 2 and are explained further in this chapter, whereas the role of carbohydrate foods in a weight-control plan will be addressed in Chapter 11.

As noted in Chapter 3, the major role of carbohydrate in human nutrition is to provide energy, and scientists have long known that carbohydrate is one of the prime sources of energy during exercise. Of all the nutrients we consume, carbohydrate has received the most research attention in regard to a potential influence upon athletic performance, particularly in exercise tasks characterized by endurance such as long-distance running, cycling, and triathloning.

Such research is important to athletes who are concerned about optimal carbohydrate nutrition during training and competition. Indeed, continued research over the past quarter century, both in the United States and abroad, has enabled sports nutritionists to provide more specific and useful responses to athletes' questions. For example, compared to the first edition of this book published in 1983, readers of this fifth edition will note several significant differences concerning dietary carbohydrate recommendations to athletes.

In this chapter, we explore the nature of dietary carbohydrates, their metabolic fates and interactions in the human body, their possible influence upon health status, and their potential application to physical performance, including the following: the adverse effects of low-carbohydrate diets; the value of carbohydrate intake before, during, and after exercise; the efficacy of different types of carbohydrates; the role of carbohydrate loading; and carbohydrate foods or compounds, including alcohol, with alleged ergogenic properties. Although the role of sports drinks containing carbohydrate, such as Gatorade and PowerAde, is introduced in this chapter, additional detailed coverage of these fluids and their effect upon performance is presented in Chapter 9: Water, Electrolytes, and Temperature Regulation.

Dietary Carbohydrates

What are the different types of dietary carbohydrates?

Carbohydrates represent one of the least expensive forms of Calories and hence are one of the major food supplies for the vast majority of the world's peoples. They are one of the three basic energy nutrients formed when the energy from the sun is harnessed in plants through the process of photosynthesis. Although the energy content of the various forms of carbohydrate varies slightly, each gram of carbohydrate contains approximately 4 Calories.

Carbohydrates are organic compounds that contain carbon, hydrogen, and oxygen in various combinations. A wide variety of different forms exist in nature and in the human body. In general terms, the ones of importance to our discussion may be categorized as simple carbohydrates, complex carbohydrates, and dietary fiber.

Simple carbohydrates, which are usually known as sugars, can be subdivided into two categories: disaccharides and monosaccharides. Saccharide means "sugar" or "sweet." Think of saccharin, a noncaloric sweetener. The three major monosaccharides (single sugars) are glucose, fructose, and galactose. Glucose and fructose occur widely in nature, primarily in fruits, as free monosaccharides.

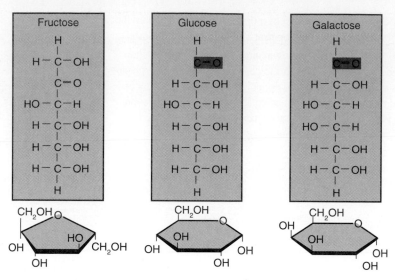

Figure 4.1 Chemical structure of the three monosaccharides is depicted in both the linear and ring configurations.

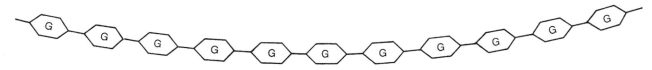

Figure 4.2 Glucose polymer. A glucose polymer is a string of glucose molecules. Muscle glycogen is a glucose polymer.

Glucose is often called dextrose or grape sugar, while fructose is known as levulose or fruit sugar. Galactose is found in milk as part of lactose. Figure 4.1 presents two methods illustrating the structure of monosaccharides.

The combination of two monosaccharides yields a **disaccharide.** The disaccharides (double sugars) include maltose (malt sugar), lactose (milk sugar), and sucrose (cane sugar or table sugar). Upon digestion these disaccharides yield the monosaccharides as follows:

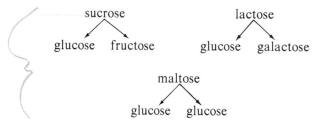

Monosaccharides and disaccharides, such as glucose and sucrose, may be isolated from foods in purified forms known as refined sugars. For example, high-fructose corn syrup, a common food additive, is derived from the conversion of glucose in corn starch to fructose. Other food additives that are primarily sugar include honey, brown sugar, corn syrup, maple syrup, molasses, and fruit juice concentrate.

Complex carbohydrates, commonly known as starches, are generally formed when three or more glucose molecules combine. This combination is known as a **polysaccharide,** or a **glucose polymer** when more than ten glucose molecules are combined (Figure 4.2). Starches,

Commercial glucose polymers also have been developed for consumption by endurance athletes.

which exist in a variety of forms such as amylose, amylopectin, and resistant starch, are the storage form of carbohydrates. The vast majority of carbohydrates that exist in the plant world are in polysaccharide form. Maltodextrin and polycose are common glucose polymers used in sports drinks. Glucose polymers are prepared commercially by controlled hydrolysis of starch. Of prime interest to us are the plant starches, through which we obtain a good proportion of our daily Calories along with a wide variety of nutrients, and the animal starch, glycogen, about which we shall hear more later in relation to energy for exercise.

Unfortunately, because of disagreements over the classification of various forms of carbohydrate, the term "complex carbohydrate" does not appear on the Nutrition Facts food label. You may obtain a rough estimate of the complex carbohydrate content by subtracting the grams of sugar from the grams of total carbohydrate. In some cases, the term "other carbohydrates" is used, which could include complex carbohydrates and other forms of carbohydrate as well.

Dietary fiber is the general term for the diverse carbohydrate polysaccharides in plant cell walls that are resistant to digestive enzymes and hence leave some residue in the digestive tract. Dietary fiber exists in two basic forms: water soluble and water insoluble. **Soluble dietary fibers** include gums and pectins, whereas the **insoluble dietary fibers** are cellulose, hemicellulose, and lignin. Although classified as fiber, technically, lignin is not a carbohydrate. Some plant fibers are both water soluble

Table 4.1   Types of dietary carbohydrates

Monosaccharides	Disaccharides	Polysaccharides
Glucose	Sucrose	Plant starch
		Amylose
Fructose	Maltose	Amylopectin
		Resistant starch
Galactose	Lactose	
		Glycogen
Insoluble fibers	**Soluble fibers**	**Other carbohydrates****
Cellulose	Gums	Sorbitol (sugar alcohol)
Hemicellulose	Pectins	Ribose (a five-carbon sugar)
Lignin*	Mucilages	

* Not technically a carbohydrate.

**Not discussed in the text.

and water insoluble, such as psyllium. Insoluble fibers pass through the entire gastrointestinal tract (mouth, esophagus, stomach, small intestine, large intestine, and rectum) unmetabolized, but soluble fibers may be metabolized in the large intestine.

Sugar substitutes are designed to provide the sweetness of sugars, but with no or fewer Calories. Two of the most commonly used sugar substitutes include saccharin, a coal tar derivative, and aspartame, a derivative of two amino acids.

A summary of the different types of carbohydrates is presented in Table 4.1, and the health effects of different forms of carbohydrate are presented later in this chapter.

What are some common foods high in carbohydrate content?

Of the six Food Exchanges, the starch, fruit, and vegetable exchanges are the three primary contributors of carbohydrate to the diet. You may recall that these three food groups represented the broad base of the Food Guide Pyramid. Some foods in the meat and milk groups contain moderate to high amounts of carbohydrate. Dried beans and peas, because their protein content is comparable to meat, may be listed in the meat group. One-half cup of navy beans contains 20 grams of carbohydrate, which is nearly 70 percent of the energy content. A glass of skim milk contains 12 grams of carbohydrate, over 50 percent of the energy content. Table 4.2 shows some foods in the different food exchanges that have high carbohydrate content. A more extensive listing is provided in Appendix F. Complex-carbohydrate foods are accentuated, as they are highly recommended in the Healthy North American Diet.

Miscellaneous foods such as pies, puddings, candy, cookies, and cake with icing are high in carbohydrates, but primarily the refined type. Reading food labels will provide you with the total amount of carbohydrate in grams, grams of sugar, and grams of dietary fiber. The label will also provide you with the percentage of your recommended Daily Value for total carbohydrate and fiber, as explained on pages 48–50.

As carbohydrates are the major fuel for most exercise tasks, several products have been marketed to athletes, particularly sports drinks, sport gels, and sports bars. Sports drinks, like Gatorade and PowerAde, usually contain about 6–8 percent carbohydrates, or about 14–18 grams of carbohydrate per 8 fluid ounces. The carbohydrate source in each varies, but usually contains a mixture of one of the following: glucose, fructose, sucrose, and glucose polymers. More details on sports drinks are presented in Chapter 9. Sports gels, such as ReLode, GU, PowerGel, and Clif-Shot, contain forms of carbohydrates similar to those used in sports drinks, but in a more solid gel form. They come in small squeeze containers (usually about 1 ounce) and contain roughly 20–30 grams of carbohydrate. Sports bars are also high in carbohydrate, usually with small amounts of protein and fats. The amount and type of carbohydrate per bar varies, ranging from 19 grams in the PR Bar, which is higher in protein and fat content, to about 50 grams in the Clif Bar. Again, Nutrition Facts food labels on sports drinks, sports gels, and sports bars provide information on the nutrient content, including amount of total carbohydrate, sugar, and fiber. By careful label reading and price comparisons, you may be able to get a better buy on some products. For example, sports bars are rather expensive, so purchasing lower-cost granola bars that contain similar nutrient value may provide some financial savings.

Foods high in dietary fiber include most vegetables and fruits, foods in the starch exchange made from whole grains, and dried beans and peas in the meat exchange. Wheat products are good sources of insoluble fiber, while

Table 4.2 Foods high in carbohydrate content

Starch exchange	Fruit exchange	Vegetable exchange	Milk exchange	Meat exchange	Sports drinks/ sports gels/ sports bars

Whole grain
  Brown rice
  Buckwheat groats
  Bulgur
  Corn tortillas
  Granola
  Oatmeal
  Ready-to-eat cereal*
  Rye crackers
  Whole wheat bread
  Whole wheat crackers
  Whole wheat pasta
 	
Enriched
  Bagels
  English muffins
  Grits
  Macaroni
  Pasta
  Ready-to-eat cereal*
  White bread
  White rice
 	
Starchy vegetables
  Baked beans
  Corn
  Green peas
  Potatoes
  Squash, winter
  Sweet potatoes
	Apples
	Applesauce
	Apricots
	Bananas
	Blackberries
	Blueberries
	Cantaloupe
	Cherries
	Dried fruits
	Figs
	Fruit juices
	Oranges
	Peaches
	Pears
	Pineapple
	Plums
	Raspberries
	Tangerines
		Asparagus
		Broccoli
		Carrots
		Mushrooms
		Radishes
		Rutabaga
		Squash, summer
		Tomatoes
		Zucchini
			Ice milk
			Skim milk
			Yogurt, fruit
				Kidney beans
				Navy beans
				Split peas
				Lentils
				Chestnuts
					Gatorade
					GatorLode
					Power Ade
					Sport Ade
					ReLode
					GU
					Power Gel
					Power Bar
					Clif Bar
					PR Bar

*May be whole wheat or enriched depending on the brand.

oats, beans, dried peas, and fruits are excellent sources of soluble fiber. Because of the purported health benefits of fiber, cereal manufacturers have released new products containing 13–14 grams of fiber per serving. Psyllium, once used primarily as a laxative, is now added to several breakfast cereals. Table 4.3 presents the average fiber content in some common foods. High-fiber foods in the six food exchanges are also highlighted in Appendix F and Figure 4.3. Food labels also document fiber content per serving.

How much carbohydrate do we need in the diet?

As we shall see below, carbohydrate serves several important functions in human metabolism. However, the National Research Council has not established an RDA for carbohydrate, probably because the body can adapt to a carbohydrate-free diet and manufacture the glucose it needs from parts of protein and fat. Nevertheless, some

Table 4.3 Fiber content in some common foods†

Beans	7–9 grams per 1/2 cup, cooked
Vegetables	3–5 grams per 1/2 cup, cooked
Fruits	1–3 grams per piece
Breads and cereals*	1–3 grams per serving
Nuts and seeds	2–5 grams per ounce

*Fiber content may vary considerably in bran-type cereals, ranging up to 13–14 grams per serving. Select whole-grain products for higher fiber content.

†Check food labels for grams of fiber per serving.

dietitians contend that carbohydrate is an essential nutrient, and the daily diet should include at least 50–100 grams to spare the catabolism of protein. Nutritionists also suggest that fiber is an essential nutrient.

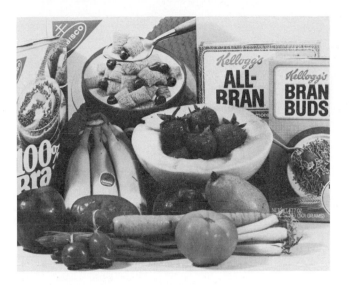

Figure 4.3 Foods high in dietary fiber.

Recent recommendations for increased consumption of carbohydrate have suggested that such a dietary change would have important health benefits. As mentioned in previous chapters, the Healthy North American Diet represents an attempt to change the nutritional habits of most individuals toward a more healthful diet. One of the recommended goals is to raise the carbohydrate content of the diet to 55–60 percent of the total caloric intake. Simple refined sugars should be limited to 10 percent, while the complex carbohydrates should comprise about 45–50 percent. The Daily Reference Value (DRV) for a 2,000 Calorie diet is 300 grams of carbohydrate, which represents 60 percent of the daily caloric intake ($4 \times 300 = 1,200$ carbohydrate Calories; $1,200/2,000 = 60$ percent). Other diet plans developed for optimal health, such as the Pritikin program, recommend that 80 percent of the dietary Calories be supplied by carbohydrates, mostly complex and unrefined.

The current average amount of fiber intake is approximately 12–14 grams per day, and the National Cancer Institute recommends that this amount be doubled, or in the range of 20–35 grams per day. The DRV for a 2,000 Calorie diet is 25 grams of fiber, or 12.5 grams per 1,000 Calories. An increased intake of complex carbohydrates would facilitate this goal.

A large percentage of the world's population subsists on this type of a high-carbohydrate diet. The health implications of a high-carbohydrate diet are discussed later in this chapter.

Sports nutritionists also recommend a high-carbohydrate diet for individuals engaged in athletic training programs. The general recommendation for most athletes parallels the recommended dietary goals noted above. For an athlete consuming 3,000 Calories per day, 55–60 percent from carbohydrate would be 1,650–1,800 Calories, or about 400–450 grams. However, even higher amounts, 70 percent or more of the dietary Calories from carbohydrate, have been recommended for those athletes involved in heavy endurance-type training programs. For an endurance athlete who consumes about 3,500 Calories per day, this would amount to about 2,450 Calories from carbohydrate (70 percent of 3,500), or about 600 grams per day. However, many recent dietary surveys conducted with athletes, including endurance athletes, often reveal a carbohydrate intake significantly lower than these recommendations.

Metabolism and Function

How do dietary carbohydrates get into the body?

Carbohydrates usually are ingested in the forms of polysaccharides (starches), disaccharides (sucrose and lactose), and monosaccharides (glucose and fructose). In addition, special carbohydrate compounds, such as glucose polymers, have been developed for athletes. In order to be useful in the body, these carbohydrates must be digested, absorbed, and transported to appropriate cells for metabolism.

Figure 4.4 represents the digestive system and some of the major associated organs that we will discuss in the following chapters. The digestive tract from the mouth to the anus is also known as the alimentary canal, which includes the mouth, pharynx, esophagus, stomach, small and large intestines, rectum, and anal canal. The most important segment for digestion and absorption includes the stomach and the intestines, known as the gastrointestinal tract (GI tract). The major area of the GI tract where the major nutrients are absorbed is also highlighted in Figure 4.4.

Digestion is the process by which food is broken down both mechanically and chemically in the digestive tract and converted into absorbable forms. It is not necessary to detail all the intricate steps of the digestive process here, but essentially, specific enzymes break down the polysaccharides and disaccharides to the monosaccharides. The key enzymes and their end products are presented in Table 4.4. The primary site of digestion is the small intestine, and the monosaccharides are then absorbed into the blood.

Some substances are absorbed in the stomach and large intestine as noted in Figure 4.4, but most absorption of nutrients occurs through the millions of villi lining the small intestine. Some substances are absorbed by passive diffusion, such as water, but others need energy supplied by the villi cells in order to be absorbed, a process known as active transport. Figure 4.5 presents a cross section of a villus and highlights some of the key nutrients and the associated process of absorption.

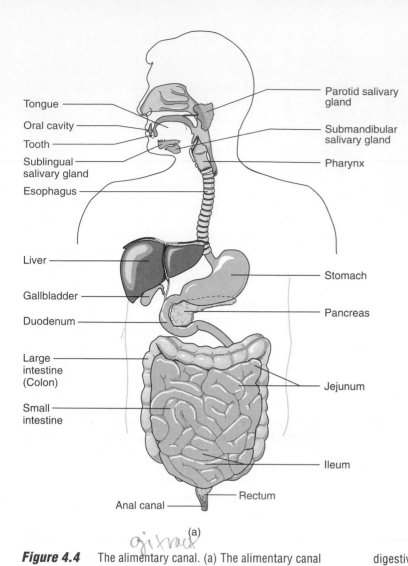

	Site of Absorption	Substance Absorbed
	Esophagus	
	Stomach	Water Alcohol
Small intestine	Duodenum	Monosaccharides Calcium Magnesium Iron Water
	Jejunum	Monosaccharides Fatty acids Peptides Amino acids Water-soluble vitamins Water
	Ileum	Peptides Amino acids Vitamin B$_{12}$ Bile salts Water
Large intestine	Colon	Sodium chloride Water Short-chain fatty acids

Tongue
Oral cavity
Tooth
Sublingual salivary gland
Esophagus
Liver
Gallbladder
Duodenum
Large intestine (Colon)
Small intestine

Parotid salivary gland
Submandibular salivary gland
Pharynx
Stomach
Pancreas
Jejunum
Ileum
Rectum
Anal canal

(a)

(b)

Figure 4.4   The alimentary canal. (a) The alimentary canal includes the mouth, the pharynx, the esophagus, the stomach, the small intestine (duodenum, jejunum, ileum), the large intestine (colon), the rectum, and the anal canal. Various glands and organs including the salivary glands, the gallbladder, and the pancreas secrete enzymes and other constituents into the digestive tract. Most blood draining from the intestines goes to the liver for processing. (b) The general sites in the digestive tract where some key nutrients and other substances are absorbed is shown, although there is some overlap in the exact site of absorption. Most absorption of nutrients occurs throughout the small intestine.

Table 4.4   Major digestive enzymes involved in carbohydrate digestion

Enzyme	Source	Effects
Salivary amylase	Salivary glands	Starts conversion of starch to disaccharides in the mouth
Pancreatic amylase	Pancreas	Converts starch to disaccharides in the small intestine
Sucrase	Intestinal cells	Converts sucrose to glucose and fructose in the small intestine
Maltase	Intestinal cells	Converts maltose to two molecules of glucose in the small intestine
Lactase	Intestinal cells	Converts lactose to glucose and galactose in the small intestine

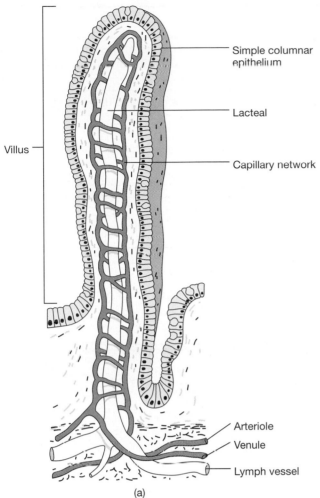

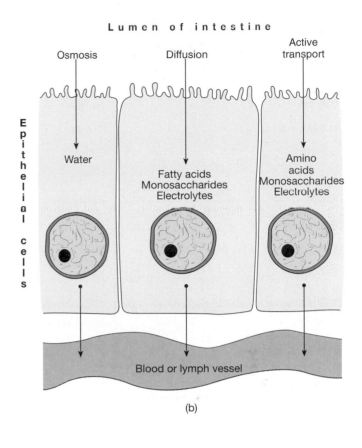

Figure 4.5 (a) Basic structure of the villus. Millions of villi in the small intestine absorb the digested nutrients. Most nutrients are absorbed into the capillaries and are transported in the blood. Fats are absorbed primarily in the lacteal, being transported to the lymph vessels and eventually into the blood. (b) Nutrients are absorbed into the body in various ways. Water enters the cell by osmosis, most fatty acids by diffusion, and amino acids enter via active transport, a process that requires energy. Monosaccharides and electrolytes may use two pathways, i.e., diffusion and active transport.

Optimal functioning of the GI tract following carbohydrate intake has been studied extensively because improper functioning may impair athletic performance. For example, although there is very little digestion of carbohydrate in the stomach, the rapidity with which carbohydrate leaves the stomach, and its impact upon the absorption of water, may be important considerations for athletes involved in prolonged exercise under warm environmental conditions. Foods containing carbohydrate and sodium may enhance water absorption via a co-transport mechanism, a topic that is discussed in Chapter 9.

Certain dietary practices may predispose individuals to gastrointestinal distress, which will compromise exercise performance. High concentrations of simple sugars, particularly fructose, may exert a reverse osmotic effect in the intestines, drawing water from the circulatory system into the intestinal lumen. The resulting symptoms are referred to as the dumping syndrome and include weakness, sweating, and diarrhea. Lactose may present a problem to some athletes, and its possible effects are discussed later in the chapter.

What happens to the carbohydrate after it is absorbed into the body?

Of the three monosaccharides, glucose is of most importance to human physiology. Most dietary carbohydrates are broken down to glucose for absorption into the blood, while the majority of the absorbed fructose and galactose are converted to glucose by the liver. Glucose is the blood sugar.

A high-carbohydrate meal will lead to a rather rapid increase in the blood sugar level, usually within an hour. Although its use is controversial, the **glycemic index** represents the effect a particular food has upon the rate and amount of increase in the blood glucose level. The glycemic index for any given food may vary considerably between

Table 4.5 Glycemic index of some common foods

The glycemic index is a measure of the rate of digestion and absorption of carbohydrate foods and the resultant effect on the blood sugar level. The baseline is 100, which is based on the response to the oral ingestion of glucose. However, the glycemic index of any food may vary among different individuals.

High glycemic index (> 85)	Medium glycemic index (60–85)	Low glycemic index (< 60)
Glucose	All-Bran cereal	Fructose
Sucrose	Banana	Apple
Maple syrup	Grapes	Applesauce
Corn syrup	Oatmeal	Cherries
Honey	Orange juice	Kidney beans
Bagel	Pasta	Navy beans
Candy	Rice	Chick-peas
Corn flakes	Whole-grain rye bread	Lentils
Carrots	Yams	Dates
Crackers	Corn	Figs
Molasses	Baked beans	Peaches
Potatoes	Potato chips	Plums
Raisins		Ice cream
Bread, white and whole wheat		Milk
Soda, with sugar		Yogurt

Sports drinks with sugar
    Power Ade
    Gatorade
		Tomato soup

Sports drinks with polymers Gatorlode		

individuals, so although some general values of the glycemic index may be given, the effects of different foods should be tested individually in those who are concerned about their blood sugar levels. In general, foods containing high amounts of refined sugars have a high glycemic index because they lead to a rapid rise in the blood sugar, but some starchy foods also have a high glycemic index. On the other hand, foods high in fiber, such as beans, generally have a low glycemic index. Interestingly, fructose has a low glycemic index, which is one of the reasons its use as the primary carbohydrate source in sports drinks had been advocated for endurance athletes. We discuss the role of fructose later in this chapter. Based on various sources in the scientific literature, Table 4.5 classifies some common foods according to their glycemic index.

Normal blood glucose levels (normoglycemia) range between 80–100 milligrams per deciliter of blood (80–100 mg/ml, or 80–100 milligram percent). The maintenance of a normal blood glucose level is very important for proper metabolism. Thus, the human body possesses a variety of mechanisms, primarily hormones, to help keep blood glucose levels under precise control. The rise in blood glucose, also known as serum glucose, stimulates the pancreas to secrete insulin into the blood. **Insulin** is a hormone that facilitates the uptake and utilization of glucose by various tissues in the body, most notably the muscles and adipose tissue. Other hormones, discussed later in this chapter, are also involved in regulating blood glucose. With normal levels of carbohydrate intake in a mixed meal, blood glucose levels remain normal.

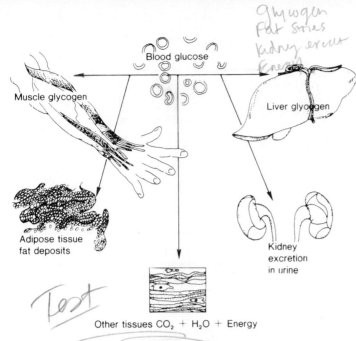

Handwritten annotations near top of figure: "Glycogen / Fat stores / kidney excret / Energy"

Blood glucose

Muscle glycogen

Liver glycogen

Adipose tissue
fat deposits

Kidney
excretion
in urine

Other tissues CO_2 + H_2O + Energy

Handwritten: "Test"

Figure 4.6 Fates of blood glucose. After assimilation into the blood, glucose may be stored in the liver or muscles as glycogen or be utilized as a source of energy by these and other tissues, particularly the nervous system. Excess glucose may be partially excreted by the kidneys, but major excesses are converted to fat and stored in the adipose tissues.

However, foods with a high glycemic index may lead rapidly to high blood glucose levels, possibly **hyperglycemia** (> 140 mg %), which will cause an enhanced secretion of insulin from the pancreas. High serum levels of insulin will then lead to a rapid, and possibly excessive, transport of blood glucose into the tissues. This may lead in turn to **hypoglycemia** (< 40–50 mg %), or low blood glucose level. This insulin response and **reactive hypoglycemia** following carbohydrate intake may be an important consideration for some athletes and is discussed later.

The fate of blood glucose is dependent upon a multitude of factors, and exercise is one of the most important. The following points represent the major fates of blood glucose. Figure 4.6 schematically represents these fates.

1. Blood glucose may be used for energy, particularly by the brain and other parts of the nervous system that rely primarily on glucose for their metabolism. Hypoglycemia can impair the normal function of the brain. Although hypoglycemia as a clinical condition is quite rare in the general population, transitory hypoglycemia may occur in very prolonged endurance exercise.

2. Blood glucose may be converted to either liver or muscle glycogen. It is important to note that liver glycogen may later be reconverted to blood glucose. However, this does not occur to any appreciable extent with muscle glycogen. In essence, glucose is

locked in the muscle once it enters, owing to the lack of a specific enzyme needed to change its form so it can cross the cell membrane. Most of the muscle glycogen is converted to this locked form of glucose during the production of energy.

3. Blood glucose may be converted to and stored as fat in the adipose tissue. This situation occurs when the dietary carbohydrate, in combination with caloric intake of other nutrients, exceeds the energy demands of the body and the storage capacity of the liver and muscles for glycogen.

4. Some blood glucose also may be excreted in the urine if an excessive amount occurs in the blood because of rapid ingestion of simple sugars.

How much total energy do we store as carbohydrate?

A common method to express the concentration of carbohydrate stored in the body is in millimoles (mmol). A **millimole** is 1/1000 of a mole, which is the term representing gram molecular weight. In essence, a mole represents the weight in grams of a particular substance such as glucose. The chemical formula for glucose is $C_6H_{12}O_6$, so it contains six parts of carbon and oxygen and twelve parts of hydrogen. The atomic weight of carbon is 12, hydrogen is 1, and oxygen, 16. If you multiply the number of parts by the respective atomic weights of each of the elements for glucose [(6 × 12) + (12 × 1) + (6 × 16)], you would get a total of 180. Thus, one mole of glucose is 180 grams, or about 6 ounces. One millimole is 1/1000 of 180 grams, or 180 milligrams. (See Figure 4.7.)

As an illustration, the normal glucose concentration is about 5 mmol per liter of blood, or 90 mg/100 ml, (90 mg/dL). To calculate, 5 mmol × 180 mg = 900 mg/liter, which is the same as 90 mg/100 ml. The normal individual has about 5 liters of blood. Thus, this individual would have a total of 25 mmol of glucose in the blood, or a total of 4,500 milligrams (25 × 180), or 4.5 grams.

These calculations have been presented here because this is the means whereby concentrations of glucose, glycogen, and other nutrients are expressed in contemporary scientific literature. A knowledge of these mathematical relationships should help you interpret research more effectively. However, because we are using the Calorie as the measure of energy in this book, and because each gram of carbohydrate equals approximately 4 Calories, an estimate of the energy content of the major human energy sources of carbohydrate may be obtained.

The body has three energy sources of carbohydrate—blood glucose, liver glycogen, and muscle glycogen. Initial stores of blood glucose are rather limited, totaling only about 5 grams, or the equivalent of 20 Calories (C). However, blood glucose stores may be replenished from either

Handwritten notes at bottom left: "Bglu – E / glycogen (store) / Fat storage / Excreted in urine"

Handwritten notes at bottom right: "B glu 5gm → 20 cal / Liver glycogen 75-100gm → 300-400cal / Muscle glycogen 360gm → 1440 cal"

Handwritten right margin: "1 gm CHO = 4 Cal / Bglu / glycogen muscle liver"

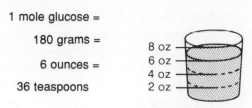

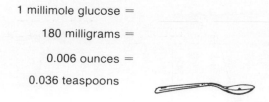

1 mole glucose =

180 grams =

6 ounces =

36 teaspoons

1 millimole glucose =

180 milligrams =

0.006 ounces =

0.036 teaspoons

Figure 4.7 The millimole concept. The concentration of some nutrients in the body is often expressed in millimoles. See text for explanation.

Table 4.6 Approximate carbohydrate stores in the body of a normal, sedentary adult

Source	Amount in grams	Equivalent amount in Calories
Blood glucose	5	20
Liver glycogen	75–100	300–400
Muscle glycogen	300–400	1,200–1,600

liver glycogen or absorption of glucose from the intestine. The liver has the greatest concentration of glycogen in the body. However, because its size is limited, the liver normally contains only about 75–100 g of glycogen, or 300–400 C. One hour of aerobic exercise uses over half of the liver glycogen supply. It is also important to note that the liver glycogen content may be decreased by starvation or increased by a carbohydrate-rich diet. Fifteen hours or more of starvation will deplete the liver glycogen, while certain dietary patterns may nearly double the glycogen content of the liver, a condition that may be useful in certain tasks of physical performance.

The greatest amount of carbohydrate stored in the body is in the form of muscle glycogen. This is because the muscles compose such a large proportion of the body mass as contrasted to the liver. One would expect large differences in total muscle glycogen content between different individuals because of differences in body size. However, for an average-sized, untrained man with about 30 kg of his body weight consisting of muscle tissue, one could expect a total muscle glycogen content of approximately 360 g, or 1,440 C. This would represent a concentration of about 66 mmol, or 12 grams, per kg of muscle tissue. As with liver glycogen, the muscle glycogen stores also may be decreased or increased, with considerable effects on physical performance. For example, a trained endurance athlete may have twice the amount of stored muscle glycogen that an untrained sedentary individual has.

If we calculate the body storage of carbohydrate as blood glucose, liver glycogen, and muscle glycogen, the total is only about 1,800–1,900 C, not an appreciable amount. One full day of starvation could reduce it con-

siderably. Some normal ranges of carbohydrate stores are presented in Table 4.6.

Can the human body make carbohydrates from protein and fat?

Because the carbohydrate stores in the body are rather limited, and because blood glucose is normally essential for optimal functioning of the central nervous system, it is important to be able to produce glucose internally if the stores are depleted by starvation or a zero-carbohydrate diet. This process in the body is called **gluconeogenesis,** meaning the new formation of glucose. A number of different substrates from each of the three energy nutrients may be used and are depicted graphically in Figure 4.8.

Protein may be a significant source of blood glucose. Protein breaks down to amino acids in the body, and certain of these amino acids, notably alanine, may be converted to glucose in the liver. This is referred to as the **glucose-alanine cycle,** which is explained further in Chapter 6. A number of other amino acids also are gluconeogenic. Glucose is essential for the brain and several other tissues. If at least 50–100 grams of carbohydrate are not consumed daily, then the body will produce the glucose it needs, primarily from protein in the body.

Fats in the body break down into fatty acids and glycerol. Although there is no mechanism in human cells to convert the fatty acids to glucose, glycerol may be converted to glucose through the process of gluconeogenesis in the liver.

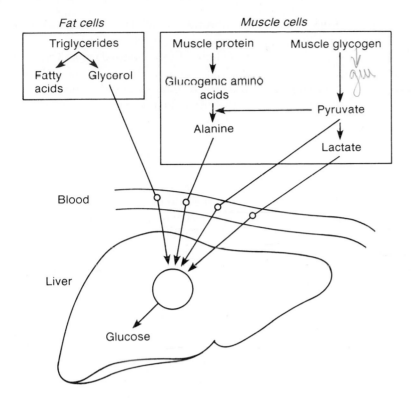

Figure 4.8 Gluconeogenesis. The liver is the major site for gluconeogenesis in the body. The breakdown products of fats, protein, and carbohydrate from other parts of the body may be transported to the liver by the blood for eventual reconversion into glucose. Glycerol, glucogenic amino acids, lactate, and pyruvate may be important sources for the new formation of glucose.

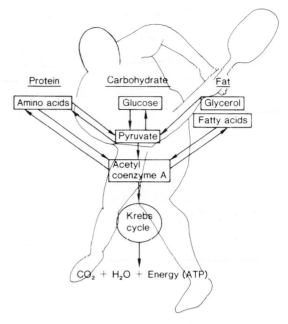

Figure 4.9 Interrelationships among carbohydrate, fat, and protein metabolism in humans. All three nutrients may be utilized for energy, although the major energy sources are carbohydrate and fat. Excess carbohydrate may be converted to fat; the carbohydrate structure also may be used to form protein, but nitrogen must be added. Fat cannot be used to generate carbohydrate to any large extent because acetyl CoA cannot be converted to pyruvate. The glycerol component of fat possibly may form very small amounts of carbohydrate. Fats may serve as a basis for the formation of protein, but again nitrogen must be added. Excess protein cannot be stored in the body but can be converted to either carbohydrate or fat.

In addition, certain by-products of carbohydrate metabolism, notably pyruvate and lactate, may be converted back to glucose in the liver. Figure 4.9 illustrates some of the interrelationships among carbohydrate, fat, and protein in human nutrition.

What are the major functions of carbohydrate in human nutrition?

The major function of carbohydrate in human metabolism is to supply energy. Some body cells, such as the nerve cells in the brain and retina and the red blood cells, are normally totally dependent upon glucose for energy and require a constant source. Through a series of biochemical reactions in the body cells, glucose is oxidized, eventually producing water, carbon dioxide, and energy. As noted in Chapter 3, carbohydrate can be used to produce energy either aerobically or anaerobically. Recall that in the lactic acid system, ATP is produced rapidly via anaerobic glycolysis, but for this system to continue functioning, the end product of glycolysis, pyruvic acid or pyruvate, must be converted into lactic acid. In the oxygen system, aerobic glycolysis predominates and pyruvic acid is converted into

acetyl CoA, which enters into the Krebs cycle and electron transfer system for complete oxidation and the production of relatively large amounts of ATP. For the same amount of carbohydrate, anaerobic metabolism yields only two ATP, whereas aerobic metabolism yields thirty-six to thirty-eight ATP. See Appendix K, Figures K.1 to K.3, for more detail.

Carbohydrates have some functions in the body other than energy production. Monosaccharides can be used to form other smaller carbohydrate molecules such as trioses and pentoses. These substances may combine with other nutrients and form body chemicals essential to life, such as glycolipids or glycoproteins. Glycoproteins are very important components of cell membranes, serving as receptors to help regulate cell function. Ribose is a key pentose (5-carbon sugar) that is a part of a number of indispensable compounds in the body. One of those compounds is RNA, or ribonucleic acid, which plays an important part in anabolic processes in the cells.

Carbohydrates for Exercise

Both hypoglycemia and depleted muscle glycogen may precipitate fatigue, so maintaining optimal levels of blood glucose, liver glycogen, and muscle glycogen is essential in various athletic endeavors, particularly prolonged exercise tasks. In this section we discuss the role of carbohydrate as an energy source during exercise, the effect of training to enhance carbohydrate use for energy when needed, and various methods to provide adequate carbohydrate nutrition to the athlete before, during, and after exercise.

In what types of activities does the body rely heavily on carbohydrate as an energy source?

Carbohydrate supplies approximately 40 percent of the body's energy needs during rest. During very light exercise fat is an important energy source, but as one engages in moderate exercise, carbohydrate use increases to 50 percent or more. When exercise becomes more intense, such as when a person is working at 70–80 percent of capacity, carbohydrate is the preferred fuel. At maximal or supramaximal exercise levels, it is used almost exclusively. Thus, carbohydrate may be the prime energy source for high-intensity anaerobic events lasting for less than one minute and high-intensity aerobic events lasting over an hour or two.

Carbohydrate use, then, is associated with the intensity level of the exercise. The more intense the exercise, the greater the percentage contribution of carbohydrate. Of course, the more intense the exercise, the sooner exhaustion occurs. A fairly well-conditioned person may be able to exercise for many hours at 40–50 percent of VO_2 max, for 1 to 2 hours or so at 70–80 percent of VO_2 max, but only for minutes at maximal or supramaximal levels of VO_2 max. As noted in Chapter 3, the fatigue that occurs in very high-intensity exercise of short duration, such as a minute or two, is probably due to the increased acidity resulting from the rapid production of lactic acid. On the other hand, the fatigue associated with more prolonged exercise may be connected with inadequate supplies of liver and muscle glycogen, both of which may be affected by dietary practices and exercise intensity and duration.

Carbohydrate intake is most important for prolonged endurance events lasting more than 90–120 minutes. Data from such endurance tasks as the Tour de France, the Daedalus project of human-powered flight over 70 miles across the Aegean Sea, the bicycle Race Across America, and the Ironman Triathlon, illustrate the importance of dietary carbohydrate in sustaining high energy output for prolonged periods. Most of the athletes in these events consumed high-caloric diets rich in carbohydrates both before and during competition. A classic example is the ultradistance runner from Greece, Yannis Kouros, who won the Sydney to Melbourne race in Australia, a distance of approximately 600 miles, in 5 days and 5 hours, or about 114 miles of running per day. He consumed up to 13,400 Calories per day, with up to 98 percent being derived from carbohydrates. Data obtained from exercise tasks of lesser magnitude, such as the typical marathon (26.2-mile run), also provide evidence for the importance of carbohydrate as the prime energy fuel as evidenced in recent studies by O'Brien and associates and Tsintzas and colleagues.

Carbohydrate is also an essential energy fuel for prolonged sports involving many intermittent bouts of high-intensity exercise such as soccer, rugby, field hockey, and ice hockey. Athletes in these sports repeatedly use muscle glycogen stored in their fast-twitch muscle fibers, which may lead to a selective depletion in these fibers. In a recent review, Edward Coyle, a renowned researcher in carbohydrate metabolism, noted that muscle glycogen could be depleted in 30–60 minutes of intermittent high-intensity exercise.

The nature of the environment during the event may also influence carbohydrate utilization. Performance at high altitudes and in both warm and very cold environments may increase the utilization of carbohydrate as an energy source. However, relative to exercise in the heat, recent research indicates no adverse effects on the rate of carbohydrate oxidation in subjects who are heat-acclimatized.

Why is carbohydrate an important energy source for exercise?

Carbohydrate is the most important energy food for exercise. Besides being the only food that can be used for anaerobic energy production in the lactic acid system, it is also the most efficient fuel for the oxygen system. If we look at the caloric value of carbohydrate (1 gram = 4 C) and fat (1 gram = 9 C) we might think that fat is a better source of energy. Indeed, this is so if we just look at Calories per gram. However, more oxygen is needed to metabolize the fat, and if we look at how many Calories we get from one liter of oxygen, we will find that carbohydrate yields about 5.05 Calories and fat gives only 4.69. Thus, carbohydrate appears to be a more efficient fuel than fat, by about 7 percent. The metabolic pathways for carbohydrate are also more efficient than those for fat. In essence, carbohydrate is able to produce ATP for muscle contraction up to three times more rapidly than fat.

The primary carbohydrate source of energy for physical performance is muscle glycogen, specifically the glycogen in the muscles that are active. As the muscle glycogen is being used during exercise, blood glucose may enter the muscles and also enter the energy pathways. In turn, the liver will release some of its glucose to help maintain blood glucose levels and prevent hypoglycemia. During moderate exercise, Coyle noted that muscle glycogen and liver glycogen contribute equally to carbohydrate oxidation. At higher intensities, muscle glycogen use increases.

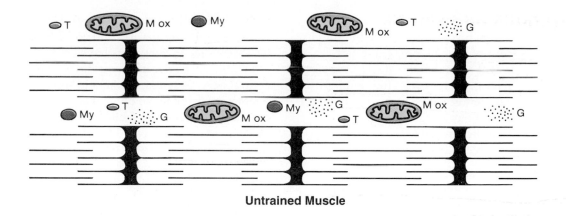

Untrained Muscle

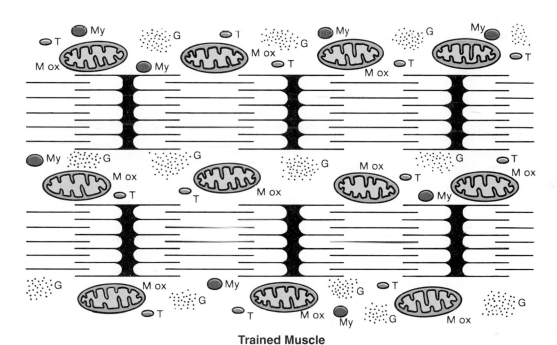

Trained Muscle

Figure 4.10 Some of the effects of aerobic or endurance training upon skeletal muscle. Increases in glycogen (G) and triglyceride (T) provide a greater energy store, while the increase in mitochondria size and number (M), myoglobin content (My), oxidative enzymes (ox), and slow-twitch muscle fiber size facilitates the use of oxygen for production of energy.

Thus, all body stores of carbohydrate—blood glucose, liver glycogen, and muscle glycogen—are important for energy production during various forms of exercise. Proper physical training is essential to optimize carbohydrate utilization during exercise, as is proper carbohydrate nutrition.

What effect does endurance training have on carbohydrate metabolism?

Since carbohydrate is a primary fuel for exercise, as you initiate an endurance exercise program a major proportion of your energy will be derived from your muscle glycogen stores. Exercise itself exerts an insulin-type effect by facilitating the transport of blood glucose into the muscle both during and immediately following the exercise bout.

As you continue your endurance exercise program, such as running or bicycling, your body undergoes several significant changes that have implications for physical performance and the fuels used. Figure 4.10 schematically represents some of these changes at the cellular level. The following have been noted to occur after several months of endurance training:

1. You will increase your VO_2 max through beneficial changes in your cardiovascular system and the oxygen system in your muscle tissues. This will help your body deliver and utilize more oxygen at the muscle tissue, significantly increasing your endurance capacity.

2. Of equal or greater importance, you will be able to work at a greater percentage of your VO_2 max

exercise — an insulin-type effect

without fatigue. At the beginning of your training program you may reach your steady-state threshold at about 50 percent of your VO₂ max and start producing lactic acid more rapidly, which may cause an early onset of fatigue. However, after training you may be able to perform at 70 percent or higher of your VO₂ max without excess lactic acid accumulation. World-class marathoners may operate above 80 percent. You may wish to refer back to Figure 3.14.

3. The enzymes that metabolize carbohydrate in the muscle cells will increase, especially oxidative enzymes associated with the Krebs cycle. This allows your muscles to process carbohydrate more efficiently. All muscle fiber types can increase their oxidative capacity to metabolize carbohydrates during exercise.

4. As we shall see in the next chapter, training also enhances the use of fat during exercise. By doing so, there is less reliance on carbohydrate oxidation during submaximal exercise. Recent research by Friedlander and others reveals that the oxidation of blood glucose decreases during both absolute and relative exercise intensity tasks. These changes may minimize the possibility of hypoglycemia.

5. More glycogen is stored in the muscle. This means you may maintain an optimal speed for a longer time.

What do all these changes mean? You may be able to run a 10-kilometer (6.2 miles) road race at a 7-minute-per-mile pace instead of 8 minutes. You can cruise in high gear for longer periods because you have increased your ability to produce energy from carbohydrates. Also, by reducing your reliance on carbohydrates at lower running speeds, you may compete in more prolonged races, such as marathons, without becoming hypoglycemic.

How is hypoglycemia related to the development of fatigue?

As noted previously, blood glucose is in very short supply, so as it is being used during exercise it must be replenished from liver glycogen stores. A depletion of liver glycogen may lead to hypoglycemia during exercise because gluconeogenesis normally cannot keep pace with glucose utilization by the muscles.

Hypoglycemia is known to impair the functioning of the central nervous system and is often accompanied by acute feelings of dizziness, muscular weakness, and fatigue. The normal blood glucose level usually ranges from 80–100 mg of glucose per 100 ml of blood (4.4–5.5 mmol per liter). As this level gets progressively lower, hypoglycemic symptoms may develop. The point usually used to identify hypoglycemia during research studies with exercise is 45 mg per 100 ml, or 2.5 mmol per liter, although some investigators have used higher levels.

Since hypoglycemia may disrupt functioning of the central nervous system (brain and spinal cord), the body attempts to maintain an optimal blood glucose level. Exercise itself, like insulin, facilitates the transport of blood glucose into the muscle. Thus, insulin levels normally drop during exercise so as to help maintain normal serum glucose. Other hormones—epinephrine (adrenaline), glucagon, and cortisol—also help maintain, and even increase, blood glucose levels during exercise.

Epinephrine is secreted from the adrenal gland during exercise, particularly intense exercise, and stimulates the liver to release glucose; it also accelerates the use of glycogen in the muscle. Glucagon and cortisol levels generally increase during the stress of exercise, cortisol particularly during prolonged exercise. Glucagon is released from the pancreas and generally increases the rate of gluconeogenesis in the liver. Cortisol is secreted from the adrenal gland and facilitates the breakdown and release of amino acids from muscle tissue to provide some substrate to the liver for gluconeogenesis. Blood glucose normally increases during the initial stages of exercise and is normally well maintained by these hormonal mechanisms. A summary of hormonal actions in the regulation of blood glucose is presented in Table 4.7.

Hypoglycemia may be a concern of athletes in several situations. One possibility is a reactive hypoglycemia following the consumption of a high-carbohydrate meal 30–60 minutes or more prior to an athletic event. If hypoglycemia develops just prior to or during the early stages of the event, the effect could impair performance. This possibility will be covered later in this section.

Hypoglycemia may also develop during prolonged exercise tasks, but it may be dependent upon the intensity level of the exercise. In low-intensity exercise, such as 30–50 percent of VO₂ max, the primary fuel is fat, and hence the use of carbohydrate is minimized. Moreover, at this low intensity level, gluconeogenesis can help maintain blood glucose above hypoglycemic levels. However, in exercise tasks above 50–60 percent VO₂ max (or higher percentages in highly-trained individuals), muscle glycogen use increases, more blood glucose is used, and gluconeogenesis is not rapid enough to replace that which is used.

During the early part of prolonged exercise, muscle glycogen is the major source of energy derived from carbohydrate, although some blood glucose is utilized. However, as muscle glycogen levels get low in the latter stages of an endurance task, blood glucose may account for 75–90 percent of the muscular energy from carbohydrate. At this high rate of blood glucose utilization, the liver glycogen stores become rapidly depleted, and thus the blood glucose levels fall toward hypoglycemia.

Table 4.7 Major hormones involved in regulation of blood glucose levels

Hormone	Gland	Stimulus *(Secreted in response to)*	Action
Insulin	Pancreas	Increase in blood glucose	Helps transport glucose into cells; decreases blood glucose levels
Glucagon	Pancreas	Decrease in blood glucose; exercise stress	Promotes gluconeogenesis in liver; helps increase blood glucose levels
Epinephrine	Adrenal	Exercise stress; decrease in blood glucose	Promotes glycogen breakdown and glucose release from the liver; helps increase blood glucose levels
Cortisol	Adrenal	Exercise stress; decrease in blood glucose	Promotes breakdown of protein and resultant gluconeogenesis; helps increase blood glucose levels

Whether hypoglycemia impairs physical performance may depend upon the individual. Some earlier research reported that exercise-induced hypoglycemia led to the expected symptoms, including dizziness and partial blackout. However, more contemporary research from three different laboratories has revealed that a number of subjects may become hypoglycemic during the latter stages of a prolonged exercise task to exhaustion at 60–75 percent of their VO_2 max, and yet are able to continue exercising while hypoglycemic, even at levels as low as 25 mg per 100 ml. It appears that the role hypoglycemia plays in the etiology of fatigue in prolonged exercise has not been totally elucidated, although there appears to be individual susceptibility. Nevertheless, prevention of hypoglycemia is one of the major objectives of carbohydrate consumption during prolonged exercise.

How is low muscle glycogen related to the development of fatigue?

Investigators generally agree that prolonged, moderately high- to high-intensity aerobic exercise is limited by muscle glycogen stores. The depletion of muscle glycogen seems to be a limiting factor when exercising at 65–90 percent of VO_2 max. A number of studies have shown that physical exhaustion was correlated with very low muscle glycogen levels, but others have shown some glycogen remaining even though subjects were exhausted. Costill has indicated that performance would be adversely affected only when muscle glycogen levels went below 40 mmol/kg of muscle tissue. It may be that complete depletion of muscle glycogen is not necessary for performance to suffer, for glycolysis may be impaired with lower glycogen levels or the glycogen in the muscle fiber may be located where it is not readily available for glycolysis.

The fatigue that develops may be related to the depletion of muscle glycogen from specific muscle fiber types. In prolonged exercise at 60–75 percent of VO_2 max, Type I fibers (red, oxidative slow twitch) and Type IIa fibers (red, oxidative-glycolytic fast twitch) are recruited during the early stages of the task, but as muscle glycogen is depleted, the athlete must recruit Type IIb fibers (white, glycolytic fast twitch) to maintain the same pace. However, it takes more mental effort to recruit the Type IIb fibers, which will be more stressful to the athlete. Type IIb fibers also are more likely to produce lactic acid, increasing the acidity, which may increase the perceived stress of the exercise. What probably happens is that as muscle glycogen becomes depleted in the red fiber types, the muscle cell will rely more on fat as the primary energy source. Since fat is a less efficient fuel than carbohydrate, the pace will slow down.

Fatigue in very high-intensity, anaerobic-type exercise generally is attributed to the detrimental effects of the acidity in the muscle cell associated with lactic acid production. Research has now shown that maximal high-intensity exercise, lasting only about 60 seconds, is not impaired by a very low muscle glycogen concentration, approximately 30 mmol/kg muscle. However, with somewhat longer anaerobic tasks, approximating 3 minutes, one laboratory study reported a reduced performance in the time to exhaustion test after 4 days of a low-carbohydrate, high-fat diet when compared to a normal, mixed diet and a high-carbohydrate diet. Although muscle glycogen levels were not measured, a logical assumption is that they were lower on the low-carbohydrate diet.

In addition, field research has suggested that slower overall sprint speed, such as in the latter parts of prolonged athletic contests like soccer and ice hockey, may be due to muscle glycogen depletion. Muscle biopsies of these athletes revealed very low glycogen levels, which were attributed not only to the strenuous exercise in the contest but also to the fact that these athletes were consuming diets low in carbohydrates. Also, as shall be noted below, low muscle glycogen stores may lead to a decrease in exercise intensity during training.

In summary, low levels of glycogen in the white, fast-twitch IIb muscle fibers may limit performance in intermittent, anaerobic-type exercise tasks. Both hypoglycemia and low glycogen in the red muscle fiber types, most likely a combination of the two, may be contributing factors to fatigue in prolonged endurance exercise.

How are low endogenous carbohydrate levels related to the central fatigue hypothesis?

Decreased endogenous carbohydrate stores may possibly cause fatigue by other mechanisms as well. In the latter stages of prolonged exercise bouts, low muscle glycogen, in combination with decreased blood glucose levels, will stimulate gluconeogenesis from protein. In particular, branched-chain amino acids (BCAA) in the muscle will be catabolized to provide substrate for the formation of glucose by the liver. Because BCAA release from the liver may be decreased or uptake by the muscle may increase, blood levels of BCAA decline. The central fatigue hypothesis during prolonged exercise suggests that this decline in blood BCAA may contribute to fatigue. In general, fatigue is hypothesized to occur when BCAA levels drop and the concentration of another amino acid—tryptophan—increases in its free form, or free tryptophan (fTRP). BCAA compete with fTRP for similar receptors that facilitate their entry into the brain, so high BCAA levels prevent brain uptake of fTRP. With an increased fTRP:BCAA ratio, entry of fTRP into the brain cells will be facilitated. Increased brain levels of tryptophan may stimulate the formation of serotonin, a neurotransmitter in the brain that may be related to fatigue sensations. Preventing the decline in the fTRP:BCAA ratio is theorized to prevent the premature development of fatigue, and the use of BCAA supplements in this regard will be covered in Chapter 6. However, carbohydrate supplements may also be helpful, as discussed later in this section.

Will eating carbohydrate immediately before or during an event improve physical performance?

Because hypoglycemia or muscle glycogen depletion may be causes of fatigue during endurance exercise, supplementation with glucose or other forms of carbohydrate before or during exercise may be theorized to delay the onset of fatigue and improve performance. Thousands of studies have been conducted on this topic since carbohydrates were identified as the most efficient energy source for exercise over 70 years ago, and researchers' interest in this topic remains unabated today. In recent years the research designs have usually been highly sophisticated as investigators have attempted to provide specific answers relative to the type, amount, and timing of carbohydrate ingestion before and during performance. Although some problems remain in providing quantitative data, the use of

stable isotopes of ingested carbohydrates (referred to as exogenous carbohydrates in comparison to endogenous stores in the body) as detailed by Wolfe and George has enhanced our understanding of their metabolic fate when ingested prior to or during exercise.

However, the reviewer attempting to synthesize the available research is confronted with a difficult task since the experimental designs varied considerably. The amount and type of carbohydrate ingested, the use of liquid or solid forms, the method of administration (oral ingestion or venous infusion), the time prior to or during the exercise that it was taken, the diet of the subject several days prior to the study, the amount of glycogen in the muscle and liver, the intensity and duration of the exercise, the type of exercise task (running, swimming, cycling, etc.), the fitness level of the subjects, the environmental temperature, and the method used to evaluate blood glucose and muscle glycogen utilization are some of the important differences between studies.

Although the results from all of these studies were not similar, some general consistencies have evolved. The role of carbohydrate supplementation on exercise performance has been the subject of numerous reviews, and a number of contemporary reviews may be found in the reference list at the end of this chapter. Based on these reviews and an overall review of specific studies, the following generalizations appear to be logical. More specific information relative to practical recommendations is provided following this discussion.

Initial Endogenous Stores If the individual has normal liver and muscle glycogen stores, glucose feedings are unnecessary for continuous exercise bouts lasting 60–90 minutes or less. Since the body can store carbohydrate in the muscles and liver, the usefulness of glucose or other carbohydrate intake before or during exercise depends on the adequacy of those supplies already in the muscle and liver to meet energy needs. The muscle and liver glycogen stores should be adequate to meet carbohydrate energy needs. The critical point is to consume substantial amounts of carbohydrates a day or two prior to the event and to decrease the duration and intensity of training to assure ample endogenous glycogen supplies.

The available research has shown that the consumption of glucose, fructose, sucrose, maltodextrin (a glucose polymer), or other carbohydrate combinations immediately prior to events of short or moderate duration has a negligible effect upon performance. Adding a gallon of gas to a full tank will not make a car go faster during a short ride. The same is true of sugar to a muscle already filled with glycogen. On the other hand, if muscle glycogen levels are low and the exercise task is somewhat prolonged, then ingestion of carbohydrate prior to the exercise bout may improve performance. It is important to note, however, that in order to enhance performance, the exogenous carbohydrate source must be able to delay the onset of fatigue that might otherwise occur as a result of premature depletion of endogenous carbohydrate sources.

Exercise Intensity and Duration

The potential beneficial effects of carbohydrate supplementation depend on the interaction of exercise intensity and duration, which of course are interrelated. The shorter the duration, the greater the exercise intensity can be. The following time frames are representative of those that have been studied to evaluate the effects of carbohydrate supplementation.

Very high-intensity exercise for less than 30 minutes Research suggests that carbohydrate supplementation will not enhance performance in high-intensity exercise bouts less than 30 minutes in length. In a recent study, Jenkins and others reported no beneficial effect of carbohydrate ingestion on five sixty-second all-out cycling tests following three days of a very low-carbohydrate diet. Nevertheless, if carbohydrate supplements could ameliorate a muscle or liver glycogen deficiency, performance might improve. For example, Walberg-Rankin reported that carbohydrate supplementation improved high-intensity exercise performance in wrestlers following a drastic weight reduction program with very limited carbohydrate intake. Presumably, the carbohydrate supplement, consumed in a 5-hour period before testing, increased either liver or muscle glycogen levels, enhancing carbohydrate oxidation and subsequent performance.

Very high-intensity resistance exercise training In a recent review, Conley and Stone noted that resistance, or strength, training, may use considerable amounts of muscle glycogen, which can lead to fatigue and strength loss. However, they noted that there are inadequate data to determine whether or not carbohydrate supplements increase performance if consumed before or during training.

High-intensity exercise for 30 to 90 minutes Normally, with adequate muscle and liver glycogen, carbohydrate supplements have not been found to improve exercise performance in this time frame. However, some recent research has suggested that supplementation may benefit well-trained athletes who may be able to exercise at high intensity for about an hour. For example, Jeukendrup and el-Sayed, with their associates, recently reported that cyclists exercising for about an hour at high intensity significantly improved their performance following ingestion of a carbohydrate supplement, as compared to a placebo. Also, Ball and others reported that carbohydrate intake during a simulated time trial improved performance in a sprint at the end of 50 minutes of high-intensity cycling. In such cases, it is possible that the ingested carbohydrates may help provide glucose to the fast-twitch muscle fibers or prevent premature depletion in the slow-twitch fibers.

Intermittent high-intensity exercise for 60 to 90 minutes Research has shown that individuals engaged in endurance-type contests with intermittent bouts of sprinting, such as soccer or ice hockey, may benefit from carbohydrate supplements taken before and during the game. Most of the benefits occurred in the latter stages of the contest. Although some research notes that carbohydrate supplementation in soccer players did not influence tackling, heading, dribbling, or shooting activity, other research reported more goals scored and less conceded during the second half of the game. In ice hockey, carbohydrate supplements improved distance skated, number of shifts skated, and skating speed. In a review, Hawley and others attributed these benefits to a possible sparing of muscle glycogen.

High- to moderate-intensity exercise greater than 90 minutes If the exercise intensity is high enough, research generally supports a beneficial effect of carbohydrate intake on exercise performance tasks greater than 90 minutes, particularly so when the task is more prolonged, such as 2 hours or more.

Timing of Carbohydrate Intake

Athletes may consume diets rich in carbohydrate for several days prior to competition, as discussed later under carbohydrate loading. Most of the studies evaluating the effect of carbohydrate supplements on subsequent exercise performance have used time frames ranging from 4 hours prior to immediately prior to the task, and at various times during the exercise task.

Four hours or less before exercise Carbohydrate intake 60–240 minutes prior to prolonged exercise tasks (longer than 90 minutes) may enhance performance. Research has demonstrated improved performance when adequate carbohydrate was consumed either 1, 3, or 4 hours prior to a prolonged exercise task involving simulated racing conditions during the latter stage. Other research revealed no significant differences in 30-kilometer run performance when equal amounts of carbohydrate were supplemented either 4 hours before or during the run, suggesting the ingested carbohydrate was available for energy production using either strategy.

Less than 1 hour before exercise Individuals who may be prone to reactive hypoglycemia should avoid carbohydrate intake, particularly high-glycemic-index foods, 15–60 minutes prior to performance. Simple sugars ingested within this time frame may actually impair physical performance in such individuals because of the adverse effects of reactive hypoglycemia, such as muscular weakness. Moreover, this same insulin response may speed up muscle glycogen utilization. This may be a disadvantage to the marathoner, whose glycogen levels may be depleted too early in the race. Several earlier studies showed that run time to exhaustion was shorter by about 20–25 percent after athletes consumed 2–3 ounces of glucose within an hour before the endurance test.

However, not all individuals experience reactive hypoglycemia. In a study by John Seifert and others, subjects were given various carbohydrate solutions to raise their insulin levels; when their insulin levels peaked, they undertook an exercise task at 60 percent of VO_2 max for 50 minutes. No hypoglycemia developed, nor were there any adverse sensory or psychological responses.

Other well-controlled studies have reported no adverse effects of glucose, fructose, or maltodextrin ingestion 30–45 minutes prior to prolonged exercise. Compared to placebo conditions with artificially sweetened water, the various carbohydrate solutions elicited no significant differences in muscle glycogen utilization or exercise capacity when subjects were exercising at 55–75 percent of VO_2 max.

For individuals not prone to reactive hypoglycemia, the consumption of carbohydrates within 15–60 minutes prior to performance may confer some benefits. Possible increases in liver and muscle glycogen may offset the reported increase in muscle glycogen utilization.

Immediately before exercise   Carbohydrate intake immediately prior to (within 5–10 minutes) prolonged endurance exercise tasks of 2 hours or more may help delay the development of fatigue and improve performance if the athlete is exercising at a level greater than 50 percent VO_2 max, such as 60–75 percent. The majority of the studies, including controlled laboratory investigations and field research involving different types of endurance athletes, support this point of view. At this level of exercise intensity the insulin response to glucose ingestion is suppressed; in addition, the secretion of epinephrine is increased. These two hormonal responses interact to help maintain or elevate the blood glucose level and prevent the hypoglycemic response that typically may occur in reactive individuals if more time elapses between the ingestion of the carbohydrate and the initiation of exercise.

During exercise   Carbohydrate ingested during prolonged exercise can help maintain blood glucose levels and reduce the psychological perception of effort, as measured by the ratings of perceived exertion, during the latter stages of an endurance task. As the exercise task continues and the muscle glycogen level falls, the amount of energy derived from the ingested carbohydrates increases. Most research supports the benefits of consuming carbohydrates early in and throughout the exercise task, but even a single carbohydrate feeding late in a prolonged exercise bout may help replenish blood glucose levels, increase carbohydrate oxidation, and delay fatigue.

All major investigators who have published extensive reviews, including David Costill, Edward Coyle,

William Sherman, and Mark Hargreaves, conclude that carbohydrate intake during prolonged exercise, when contrasted with placebo conditions, will enhance performance. This general finding is supported by both laboratory and field studies.

Use of the Ingested Carbohydrate   Using labeled carbohydrate sources and analyzing the expired carbon dioxide for radioactivity, investigators have shown that some of the ingested, or exogenous, carbohydrate may be used as an energy source within 5–10 minutes, indicating that it may empty rapidly from the stomach, be absorbed from the small intestine into the blood, and enter into metabolic pathways. Peak use of exogenous carbohydrate appears to occur 75 to 90 minutes after ingestion. A number of studies have shown that the ingested carbohydrate may contribute a significant percentage of the carbohydrate energy source during exercise, ranging from 20–40 percent in some studies, but as much as 60–70 percent during the latter stages of exercise when endogenous liver and muscle glycogen stores become depleted.

Possible Fatigue-Delaying Mechanisms   The precise mechanism whereby glucose ingestion helps delay the onset of fatigue during moderate- to high-intensity exercise (i.e., > 65 percent VO_2 max) has not been totally elucidated, but the available data suggest the delaying effect may be related to the maintenance of higher blood glucose levels, possibly by sparing liver glycogen, and the prevention of hypoglycemia in susceptible individuals; blood glucose would be available to enter the muscle and provide a source of energy for aerobic glycolysis. As noted above, exogenous glucose is used increasingly as the exercise task becomes prolonged. Some research has shown that glucose ingestion could make an endurance task psychologically easier and suggested that the physiological effects of the glucose, either in the brain or in the muscles, reduced the stressful effects of exercise.

Although sparing of muscle glycogen could be another benefit of carbohydrate ingestion before or during moderate- to high-intensity exercise, this does not appear to be the case. David Costill has noted that no data are available to support the concept that carbohydrate intake during exercise reduces the muscle reliance upon muscle glycogen stores. In a unique experiment from the University of Texas, subjects received venous glucose infusions to maintain a hyperglycemic state during 2 hours of exercise at 73 percent of VO_2 max, but the net rate of muscle glycogen utilization was not affected compared to control conditions. Other research has also noted no muscle glycogen sparing effect following carbohydrate supplementation.

On the other hand, Yaspelkis and others, also from the University of Texas, noted that during low-intensity exercise (i.e., < 50 percent VO_2 max) or during low- to moderate-intensity exercise tasks, carbohydrate supplementation during exercise could spare use of muscle glycogen in slow-twitch muscle fibers and enhance performance. They noted that during low-intensity exercise the serum levels of both glucose and insulin were elevated, which could promote muscle use of serum glucose and sparing of muscle glycogen. Bosch and others, as well as Tsintzas and others, recently reported that carbohydrate intake during prolonged exercise at about 70 percent VO_2 max did spare muscle glycogen use, and the Tsintzas group reported the sparing effect occurred in the Type I, slow-twitch muscle fibers.

Nevertheless, Costill notes that understanding of the mechanisms underlying the enhanced utilization of carbohydrate intake during exercise and improved performance is still unclear. For example, relative to the hypothesis regarding the fTRP:BCAA ratio discussed previously, in several recent studies carbohydrate supplementation during exercise has been reported to prevent the decrease in serum BCAA during the later stages of prolonged exercise, possibly by mitigating secretion of cortisol. According to the hypothesis, preventing an increase in the fTRP:BCAA ratio would deter the onset of fatigue.

Conceivably, multiple mechanisms are operating. In all likelihood, one or more of these mechanisms may be functioning in a given athlete during an exercise task that is dependent primarily on carbohydrate metabolism for energy.

Limitations to Prevent Fatigue Although glucose ingestion may help delay fatigue during moderately high-intensity exercise, it cannot totally prevent the onset of fatigue. It appears that blood glucose cannot meet the energy demands of the muscle at this intensity level, and therefore when muscle glycogen stores are reduced to a critical level, fatigue will be evident by a reduced pace. Research suggests that the maximal amount of energy that may be derived from the exogenous carbohydrate is approximately 1 gram per minute, much lower than the energy needs at 65–85 percent of VO_2 max.

Optimal Supplementation Protocol Research by Wright and associates from Ohio State University has indicated that although the intake of carbohydrate either before or during exercise may separately enhance performance, the best effect was observed when carbohydrate was consumed both before and during exercise.

When, how much, and in what form should carbohydrates be consumed before or during exercise?

The most common athletic events or physical performance activities that may benefit from carbohydrate feedings are those associated with long duration (90–120 minutes or more) at moderate to high intensity levels. Marathon running, cross-country skiing, and endurance cycling are common sports of this kind. Other sports that require intermittent bouts of intensive activity over a prolonged period, such as soccer, may also benefit. However, the individual participating in these activities, particularly under warm or hot environmental conditions, also needs to replenish fluid losses incurred through sweating. In such cases, fluid replenishment is more critical than carbohydrate. The topic of fluid replacement during exercise is covered in more detail in Chapter 9, but since carbohydrate is one of the contents in the majority of the sport drinks developed as fluid replacements for athletes, its role is discussed briefly here.

Many studies have been conducted in recent years to determine the best carbohydrate feeding regimen to prevent fatigue during prolonged exercise. A number of different variables have been studied, such as the timing of the feeding and the type, amount, and concentration of carbohydrate.

Again, based on current reviews by the primary investigators regarding carbohydrate supplementation for exercise performance and a careful analysis of individual studies, the following points represent the general conclusions and recommendations for individuals who may be exercising at 60–80 percent of their VO_2 max or greater for 1–2 hours or longer. These points may also be applicable to athletes engaged in intermittent high-intensity exercise sports that last an hour or more. But remember, different individuals may have varied reactions to carbohydrate intake, so athletes should experiment in training before using these recommendations in actual competition.

1. The amount of carbohydrate ingested 4 hours prior to performance should be based upon body weight. Several studies have used 4–5 grams/kg with good results. For an athlete who weighs 60 kg (132 pounds), the recommended amount would be 240–300 grams. The carbohydrates could be consumed in any of several forms, including fluids such as juices or glucose polymer solutions, or solid carbohydrates such as fruits or starches. The fiber content should be minimized to prevent possible intestinal problems during exercise. Keep in mind that 300 grams of carbohydrate is about 1,200 Calories, a somewhat substantial meal. You may consult Appendix F for an expanded list of foods high in carbohydrate, but use the following for a quick estimate of carbohydrate content:

   1 fruit exchange = 15 grams carbohydrate
      1 apple
      1 orange
      1/2 banana
      4 ounces orange juice

1 starch exchange = 15 grams carbohydrate
  1 slice bread
  1/2 cup cereal
  1/4 large bagel
  1/2 cup cooked pasta
  1 small baked potato
Sports drinks: 7–8 ounces = 15 grams carbohydrate
  Gatorade
  Power Ade
  Sport Ade
Sports bars = 20–50 grams carbohydrate
  1 PR Bar
  1 Power Bar
Sports gels = 20–30 grams carbohydrate
  1 Power Gel packet
  1 ReLode packet

The guidelines presented on pages 56–57 relative to precompetition meals provide appropriate guidelines. McDonald's, the fast-food restaurant, developed a menu for athletes with meals containing 60–68 percent of Calories from carbohydrate.

2. If carbohydrate is consumed approximately 1 hour prior to performance, about 1–2 grams/kg (60–120 grams for a 60-kg athlete) may be recommended, for these levels have been shown to enhance performance in several studies. One study using only 12 grams 1 hour prior to performance has shown no beneficial effect. Both glucose polymers and foods with a low glycemic index have been used successfully.

3. If carbohydrates are consumed immediately before exercise, that is, within 10 minutes of the start, about 50–60 grams of a glucose polymer in a 40–50 percent solution has been used effectively in some studies. Dry glucose polymers are available commercially, such as GatorLode (not Gatorade). One teaspoon is 5 grams. To make a 50 percent solution containing 50 grams of the polymer, put 10 level teaspoons of the polymer into 100 milliliters (about 3–4 ounces) of water. To make a 7.5 percent solution containing 15 grams, put 3 teaspoons of the polymer into 200 milliliters (about 7 ounces) of water.

4. During exercise, feedings every 15–30 minutes appear to be a reasonable schedule. Although you may consume considerable quantities of carbohydrate during exercise, your ability to use this exogenous source for energy is limited. The reason is not known, but there may be insufficient absorption or impaired delivery to the active muscles.

Reasonable estimates from the research literature suggest that athletes may use approximately 30–60 grams of ingested carbohydrate per hour, about 0.5–1 gram per minute. Therefore, the athlete should attempt to consume a 5–10 percent solution containing about 15–20 grams of carbohydrate every 15–20 minutes during exercise. Eight ounces (about 240 ml) of a sports drink like Gatorade provides about 14–18 grams of carbohydrate. Consumption of solutions above 10 percent during exercise may delay gastric emptying and cause gastrointestinal distress, but some athletes may tolerate larger concentrations such as 15–20 percent. Ultramarathoners, who may exercise at a relatively low intensity, may tolerate higher concentrations, ranging from 20–50 percent.

Probably the most effective protocol would be to use a high concentration immediately before or during the first 20 minutes of the exercise (about 1 gram/kg body weight), and then use the lower concentrations (about 0.2–0.3 gram/kg body weight) at regular intervals. Moreover, taking a single more concentrated dose, such as 100–200 grams total, in the latter stages of prolonged exercise has also been recommended by some investigators. Because of the nature of their sport, soccer players and other such athletes may need to consume a high concentration before the game and during halftime.

5. A number of different types of carbohydrates have been studied, including glucose, glucose polymers, fructose, and sucrose, both individually and in various combinations, as well as soluble starch (a very long polymer), high-glycemic-index foods like potatoes, and low-glycemic-index foods such as legumes. In general, there appears to be no difference between these different types of carbohydrates as a means to enhance endurance performance when used appropriately. However, there may be some important considerations relative to the use of fructose, glucose polymers, solid foods, and complex carbohydrates.

Fructose has been theorized to be a better source of carbohydrate than glucose because it is absorbed more slowly from the intestine and hence will not create an insulin response and the potential reactive hypoglycemia. Indeed, research has shown that fructose, compared to glucose, may lead to a more stable blood sugar during the early stages of prolonged exercise when ingested 45 minutes prior to the activity, for most ingested fructose is eventually converted to glucose in the liver. However, when fructose is ingested immediately before or during exercise, its effect on the blood sugar and carbohydrate metabolism appears to be little different than that of glucose. Moreover, fructose does not spare the use of muscle glycogen any more or less effectively than glucose. In addition, since fructose is absorbed slowly from the intestinal tract, it can create a significant osmotic effect in the intestines leading to diarrhea and gastrointestinal distress in some individuals. A study from the Exercise Physiology Laboratory at the Quaker Oats Company indicated that a 6 percent solution of fructose, when compared to similar solutions of glucose and sucrose, caused significant gastrointestinal distress and an impairment in exercise performance. The athlete should be cautious in using fructose as the sole source of carbohydrate before or during exercise. Sports drinks containing fructose do so in small concentrations.

Recall that a glucose polymer is a molecular chain of glucose molecules that is shorter than starch but longer than the simple sugars and is derived via a partial hydrolysis of polysaccharides, such as cornstarch. Its major characteristics include a rapid gastric emptying, digestibility, and absorption due to a lesser osmotic effect than simple sugars. A recent meta-analysis (a statistical method comparing the findings of a large number of different studies) revealed that glucose polymer solutions, as compared with simple sugar solutions, caused less inhibition of gastric emptying both at rest and during exercise. Thus, glucose polymers can provide both glucose and fluids rather effectively. Many of the studies cited as showing improvements in performance when carbohydrate was ingested immediately before or during exercise used glucose polymers. Some recent research from South Africa has indicated that glucose polymers, in addition to more rapid gastric emptying, also may be oxidized more readily compared to glucose or sucrose. Although these overall findings suggest that glucose polymers may be the preferable choice, most of the studies that have compared different types of carbohydrates consumed during exercise have reported little or no differences among the types relative to physical performance.

In a recent review, Ellen Coleman noted that solid and liquid forms of carbohydrate were equally effective in maintaining blood glucose levels and enhancing exercise performance. However, subsequent to Coleman's review, Peters and others noted that triathletes who consumed a liquid form of carbohydrates performed better on a 3-hour cycling-running exercise task when compared to both a placebo trial and a trial in which the triathletes consumed isocaloric semi-solid carbohydrate foods (orange juice, white bread, marmalade, and bananas). The authors did note that the athletes may have had a negative perception toward eating solid foods during performance, which could have adversely affected their performance in that trial. Although the effects of consuming equivalent amounts of carbohydrate in either liquid or solid form would appear to be minimal (providing adequate fluid intake in each case), more research is desirable to explore this issue, particularly with ultraendurance performance events where many athletes may consume liquid and solid carbohydrate sources.

In a recent review, Guezennec indicated that a low-glycemic-index meal, such as lentils, consumed prior to prolonged exercise might provide an advantage over a high-glycemic-index meal, such as potatoes. The underlying mechanism might be a slower rate of absorption resulting in a blunted insulin response and maintenance of higher blood glucose levels during prolonged exercise. Guezennec indicated some preliminary research showed improved performance with low-glycemic-index foods, but recommended verification of these findings. Subsequent research has not supported an ergogenic effect. Febbraio and others provided either a low-glycemic-index meal, a high-glycemic-index meal, or a control meal to trained individuals before cycling at 70 percent VO_2 max for 2 hours followed by a 15-minute performance ride. Although the high-glycemic-index food increased blood glucose levels and depressed free fatty acid levels during the early stages, there were no differences later in the exercise task and no effects on the rate of muscle glycogen use or exercise performance.

Along these lines, other investigators have evaluated the effect of various forms of starch on exercise performance. Amylose is a straight-chain starch that is more resistant to digestion compared to amylopectin, a branched-chain starch. The normal ratio of amylose to amylopectin is 1:4 in complex carbohydrates such as potatoes, breads, pasta, rice, and other starchy products. Using a liquid solution of 100 percent amylopectin and one containing 30 percent amylopectin and 70 percent amylose, Goodpaster and others from David Costill's laboratory compared their effect with glucose and a placebo on performance in a 90-minute cycle ride at 66 percent VO_2 max followed by a 30-minute isokinetic cycling task to generate as much work as possible. All carbohydrates elicited similar blood glucose responses, but the glucose and amylopectin solutions allowed the athletes to perform more work than the placebo trial, whereas the amylopectin-amylose solution did not. These investigators noted that amylopectin starch provides an ergogenic effect similar to glucose, but that amylose starch may not. Because amylose starch is resistant to digestion, lesser amounts of carbohydrate may be provided for oxidation.

The potential role of various starches and low-glycemic-index foods is an important consideration for the endurance athlete, and more research is needed to evaluate their effect on prolonged endurance performance. For details of the glycemic index and exercise metabolism, the interested reader is referred to the recent reviews by Walberg-Rankin and Walton and Rhodes.

6. Probably the most important recommendation is for the athlete to experiment with different types and amounts of carbohydrate during training before using them in competition. Just as it is important for you to know your optimal race pace for an endurance event, so too must you know how well you can tolerate different concentrations and types of carbohydrates. For example, a highly concentrated sugar consumed just prior to competition may create an osmotic effect and actually hold excess fluid in the stomach or intestines, which may cause gastrointestinal distress and impaired performance. Just as you train your muscles to learn their capacity, you may also be able to train your digestive system to know its limits. Ron Maughan, an internationally respected authority in sport nutrition, indicated that the optimal strategy relative to carbohydrate utilization is to use your own subjective experience.

What is the importance of carbohydrate replenishment after prolonged exercise?

There are several possible applications of this question. One is the athlete who may be involved in a prolonged exercise bout, have a rest period of 1–4 hours, and then must exercise again, such as athletes who train two or three times daily. Benefits may accrue to anaerobic endurance-, aerobic endurance-, and resistance-trained individuals. A second application is the athlete who trains intensely every day and must have an adequate recovery in the one-day rest interval. A third application, covered in the next section, is the technique of carbohydrate loading.

Several studies have shown that ingesting carbohydrate during the rest interval between two prolonged exercise bouts improves performance in the second bout. This finding is comparable to the beneficial effects of carbohydrate intake during prolonged exercise bouts. The carbohydrate can help restore blood glucose levels but may also be used to resynthesize muscle glycogen. In cases such as this, where the rate of muscle glycogen resynthesis is important, high-glycemic-index foods such as potatoes, bread, glucose, or glucose polymers would be the preferred

source of carbohydrate, for they apparently lead to a faster restoration of muscle glycogen than does a meal rich in low-glycemic-index foods. For repeat prolonged exercise tasks with about a 4-hour interval, a general recommendation is to consume 1 gram of carbohydrate per kilogram body weight immediately after the first event and again 2 hours prior to the second event. Additional carbohydrate may also be consumed immediately before and during the second event.

However, research by Zawadzki and his associates has found that the combination of protein and carbohydrate induced a faster rate of glycogen resynthesis in 4 hours compared to either the carbohydrate or protein given alone. The dosage used was approximately 112 grams of carbohydrate and 41 grams of protein, given immediately after exercise and again 2 hours later. The authors reported significantly higher blood glucose and insulin levels with this treatment, factors that would stimulate glucose uptake by the muscle and activation of glycogen synthase in the muscle to convert the glucose to glycogen.

Some commercial products that combine high amounts of carbohydrate and protein are available. Gator-Pro, for example, contains 59 grams of carbohydrate and 17 grams of protein in an 11-ounce can, but there are also 7 grams of fat. Two cans would provide all of the carbohydrate and most of the protein amounts used in the Zawadzki study. Three Power Bars would contain 120 grams of carbohydrate, 30 grams of protein, and 6 grams of fat. Another approach would be to consume a large bagel, 3 ounces of lean turkey breast, and 24 ounces of Power Ade, which would provide approximately 110 grams of carbohydrate and 33 grams of protein.

Although the combination carbohydrate/protein mixture appears to be the most effective for rapid resynthesis, other protocols may facilitate full replenishment over a 24-hour period. Overall, for athletes who train intensely on a daily basis with either resistive or aerobic exercise that leads to muscle glycogen depletion, approximately 8–10 grams of carbohydrate per kilogram body weight should be consumed daily in order to restore muscle glycogen levels to normal. For an individual who weighs 70 kilograms, this approximates 560–700 grams of carbohydrate, or 2,240–2,800 carbohydrate Calories. This amount of carbohydrate would represent about 65–80 percent of the daily caloric intake of an athlete consuming 3,500 Calories. Athletes involved in ultraendurance events may need 14 grams of carbohydrate/kilogram body weight or more.

To facilitate full glycogen synthesis, research by Blom and Ivy suggests that about 0.7–1.0 grams of high-glycemic-index foods per kilogram body weight should be consumed immediately after the exercise bout, and every 2 hours for the next 4 to 6 hours. Again, for a 70-kg athlete, this would be about 50–70 grams each time. However, several recent studies have noted no difference in

24-hour muscle glycogen resynthesis if the first feeding was not taken until 2 hours after exercise or if the carbohydrate was consumed in four large meals or sixteen smaller ones, as long as the same amount of carbohydrate was consumed. Over the 24-hour period, the rate of muscle glycogen recovery is approximately 5–7 percent per hour. Sports drinks may be a convenient means to consume carbohydrate immediately after exercise. The remaining carbohydrate should be derived from other natural sources in the diet, including both simple carbohydrates in fruits and complex carbohydrates in grains, potatoes, and other foods with adequate dietary fiber and other nutrients. The inclusion of high-glycemic-index foods in the daily diet will help speed resynthesis of muscle glycogen over the 24-hour period, and may be very compatible with the Healthy North American Diet that contains other low-glycemic-index foods.

Will a high-carbohydrate diet enhance my daily exercise training?

Most scientists and sport nutritionists who study carbohydrate metabolism in athletes recommend a high-carbohydrate diet for most athletes, particularly endurance athletes, because success in athletic competition is contingent upon optimal training, and for the endurance athlete, optimal training may be contingent upon adequate nutrition, primarily the ingestion of sufficient carbohydrate every day.

There are some limited data supporting the concept of enhanced training following a high-carbohydrate diet. A number of field and laboratory studies with athletes have attempted to mimic actual sport conditions. For example, one group of soccer players improved performance on an intermittent exercise task designed to mimic physical activity in a game, while another group improved performance in a standardized intermittent running task and a run to exhaustion. In other studies, runners were able to endure longer on a treadmill run to exhaustion, while triathletes experienced a significant improvement in treadmill endurance following 30 minutes of swimming, cycling, and running. In two studies, the psychological status of athletes, as measured by the vigor and fatigue components of the Profile of Mood States (POMS) questionnaire, and their rating of perceived exertion (RPE) during exercise were improved when they switched to higher carbohydrate diets. In general, the normal carbohydrate intake of these athletes was increased from approximately 40–45 percent to 65–70 percent of the daily Calories for varying periods, but usually a week or more.

However, in a comprehensive review of the available research, Sherman and Wimer concluded there is little support for the hypothesis that moderate intake of dietary carbohydrate impairs training or athletic performance. In a subsequent study with his colleagues, Sherman and others concluded that although a high-carbohydrate diet (84 percent carbohydrate) over 7 days helped to maintain muscle glycogen levels in athletes during training, compared to a significant reduction in muscle glycogen while on a moderate-carbohydrate diet (42 percent carbohydrate), neither training capability nor high-intensity exercise performance were impaired with the moderate-carbohydrate diet.

A recent diet that has been advocated for athletes recommends that the daily intake of carbohydrate be restricted to 40 percent of the total caloric intake. Although no research is available to determine whether this approach will help exercise performance, the study by Sherman and others cited above suggests it is possible that 40 percent carbohydrate Calories may be sufficient for some athletes to maintain their training protocol. For an active athlete consuming 4,000 Calories per day, 40 percent carbohydrate would be 1,600 Calories, or 400 grams, which may provide ample amounts to sustain training. Although most endurance athletes need adequate muscle glycogen for training, they normally do not do sufficient exercise to deplete muscle glycogen on a daily basis.

Sherman and Wimer indicate that more research is needed to resolve this issue. Nevertheless, these authors note that because carbohydrate is such an important energy source for many athletic endeavors, and because such a diet does not impair performance, it is prudent to recommend a high-carbohydrate diet for athletes in training. Kuipers also indicates that a high-carbohydrate diet may help prevent symptoms associated with the overtraining syndrome, i.e., fatigue and staleness in training. Some research suggests that carbohydrate intake helps reduce cortisol levels, a hormone that may suppress our immune response. An impaired immune response is one possible factor associated with the overtraining syndrome.

Selecting foods high in carbohydrate content, highlighted earlier in this chapter, provides a sound guide to increase the carbohydrate content of the diet, as do some of the recommendations in the following section regarding carbohydrate loading. Chapter 11 will provide additional information specific to daily caloric intake for planning a diet. Several excellent articles are available that focus on high-carbohydrate diets for the athlete, including those in the references authored by Edward Coyle and Effie Coyle, Linda Houtkooper, and Nancy Clark.

Additionally, as noted above, carbohydrates are often incorporated in liquid solutions for ease of ingestion. Because fluids may be useful to help regulate temperature when exercising under warm environmental conditions, this topic is covered in Chapter 9. Table 9.9 on page 300 provides an overview of carbohydrate and fluid intake before, during, and after exercise.

Carbohydrate Loading

What is carbohydrate, or glycogen, loading?

Because carbohydrate becomes increasingly important as a fuel for muscular exercise as the intensity of the exercise increases, and because the amount of carbohydrate stored in the body is limited, muscle and liver glycogen depletion could be factors that may limit performance capacity in distance events characterized by high levels of energy expenditure for prolonged periods. **Carbohydrate loading,** also called glycogen loading and glycogen supercompensation, is a dietary technique designed to promote a significant increase in the glycogen content in both the liver and the muscles in an attempt to delay the onset of fatigue. It is generally used for 3–7 days in preparation for major athletic competitions.

What type of athlete would benefit from carbohydrate loading?

In general, carbohydrate loading is primarily suited for those individuals who will sustain high levels of continuous energy expenditure for prolonged periods, such as long-distance runners, swimmers, bicyclists, triathletes, cross-country skiers, and similar athletes. In addition, athletes who are involved in prolonged stop-and-go activities, such as soccer, lacrosse, and tournament-play sports like tennis and handball, may benefit. In essence, carbohydrate loading may be effective for athletes engaged in events that use muscle glycogen as the major energy source and that may lead to a depletion of glycogen in the muscle fibers. Bodybuilders have been reported to carbohydrate load in attempts to appear more muscular owing to increased muscle glycogen levels and associated water retention.

Recall from Chapter 3 that humans have several different types of skeletal muscle fibers. In general, the slow-twitch red and fast-twitch red fibers are used mainly during long, continuous activities and are aerobic in nature, whereas the fast-twitch white fibers are used for short, fast activities and are anaerobic in nature. Consider the differences between a distance runner and a soccer player. The former may run at a steady pace for hours, whereas the latter will constantly be changing speeds, with many bouts of full speed interspersed with recovery periods of slower running. Research has shown that glycogen depletion patterns of the two different muscle fiber types are related to the type of exercise. Long, continuous exercise depletes glycogen principally in the slow-twitch red and fast-twitch red fibers, whereas fast, intermittent bouts of exercise with periods of rest, actually a form of interval training, primarily deplete glycogen in the fast-twitch white fibers. However, it should be noted that glycogen depletion may occur in all types of fibers in either prolonged continuous or intermittent exercise and may be quite appreciable, depending upon intensity and duration of the exercise bouts. If carbohydrate loading works for the specific muscle fiber involved, then both types of athletes may benefit. Both should have greater glycogen stores in the latter stages of their respective athletic contests.

How do you carbohydrate load?

As you might suspect, the key to carbohydrate loading is to switch from the normal, balanced diet to one very high in carbohydrate content. The original, classic carbohydrate loading technique, emanating from earlier Scandinavian research, involved a glycogen depletion stage induced by prolonged exercise and a restricted diet. For example, a runner might go for an 18- to 20-mile run to use as much stored glycogen as possible, and then ingest very little carbohydrate in the following 2- to 3-day period. Exercise is continued during this 2- to 3-day period to keep glycogen stores low. Following the depletion stage, the loading stage began. During this phase, carbohydrate may contribute 70 or more percent of the caloric intake. The intensity and duration of exercise during this phase was reduced considerably. The usual case was to rest fully for 2 to 3 days. Thus, the classic carbohydrate loading pattern involved three stages: depletion, carbohydrate deprivation (high-fat/protein diet), and carbohydrate loading. However, this original method may be particularly difficult to tolerate, especially if one tries to exercise at high levels during the depletion phase. The lack of carbohydrate in the diet combined with the exercise bouts may elicit symptoms of hypoglycemia (weakness, lethargy, irritability). Moreover, prolonged exhaustive exercise may lead to muscle trauma, which may actually impair the storage of extra glycogen. This classic, original method is presented in Table 4.8.

Although some early research supported this technique, more recent data suggest that this strict routine may be unnecessary, particularly the total program of depletion. For example, in trained runners, research has shown that simply changing to a very high-carbohydrate diet, combined with 1 or 2 days of rest or reduced activity levels (tapering), will effectively increase muscle and liver glycogen. Well-controlled research by Blom, Costill, and Vollestad noted that exhaustive running is not necessary to achieve muscle glycogen supercompensation. It appears to be important to continue endurance training, or other high-intensity training specific to the sport, during the 7–14 days prior to competition. Such training will serve to maintain adequate levels of glycogen synthase, the enzyme in the muscle that synthesizes glycogen from glucose. Evidence also suggests that if the total carbohydrate content is consumed over the entire week, in contrast to concentrating it in 2–3 days, there will be little difference in the muscle glycogen content between the two techniques.

Table 4.8 Different methods for carbohydrate loading

A recommended method		Original, classic method	
1st day:	depletion exercise (optional)	1st day:	depletion exercise
2nd day:	mixed diet, moderate carbohydrate; tapering exercise	2nd day:	high-protein/fat diet; low carbohydrate; tapering exercise
3rd day:	mixed diet, moderate carbohydrate; tapering exercise	3rd day:	high-protein/fat diet; low carbohydrate; tapering exercise
4th day:	mixed diet, moderate carbohydrate; tapering exercise	4th day:	high-protein/fat diet; low carbohydrate; tapering exercise
5th day:	high-carbohydrate diet; tapering exercise	5th day:	high-carbohydrate diet; tapering exercise
6th day:	high-carbohydrate diet; tapering exercise or rest	6th day:	high-carbohydrate diet; tapering exercise or rest
7th day:	high-carbohydrate diet; tapering exercise or rest	7th day:	high-carbohydrate diet; tapering exercise or rest
8th day:	competition	8th day:	competition
		High-carbohydrate diet: 400–700 g per day depending on body weight; about 70–80 percent of dietary Calories should be carbohydrate.	

Although there may be a number of variations in the carbohydrate loading protocol, a generally recommended format is also presented in Table 4.8. The interested athlete may want to experiment with both techniques, and also make adjustments through experience.

The high-carbohydrate diet should contain about 8–10 grams of carbohydrate per kilogram of body weight, or about 400–700 grams per day, depending on the size of the individual, which is not too different from the generally recommended dietary content of carbohydrate for the endurance athlete in regular training. It is important to note that the athlete should not change his or her diet drastically prior to competition. Consuming a high-carbohydrate diet during training will condition the body to metabolize carbohydrate properly during this loading phase. Table 4.9 represents a general dietary plan for carbohydrate loading. The total caloric value and grams of carbohydrate should be adjusted to individual needs. They are dependent upon the size of the individual and daily energy expenditure in exercise. It is important not to consume excess Calories, for they may be converted into body fat if in excess of the maximal storage capacity of the muscle and liver for glycogen.

Some guidelines for rapid replenishment of glycogen were presented earlier. Because glycogen loading for long-distance events occurs over 2 to 3 days, it would be wise to stress complex carbohydrates in the diet because of their higher nutrient content. However, simple carbohydrates may also be used effectively to increase muscle glycogen stores, as can high-carbohydrate sports drinks such as Gatorlode and Ultra Fuel. Moreover, the diet should also include the daily requirements for protein and fat.

Most prolonged endurance events begin in the morning. The last large meal should be about 15 hours prior to race time, possibly topped off with a simple carbohydrate snack before retiring for the night. Some athletes use a glucose polymer for the last major meal to avoid the presence of intestinal residue the morning of competition. A carbohydrate breakfast such as orange juice, toast, jelly, or other carbohydrates may be eaten 3 to 4 hours prior to competition. This overall dietary regimen should help maximize muscle and liver glycogen stores. The athlete should then follow the guidelines presented previously relative to carbohydrate intake before and during performance.

How do I know if my muscles have increased their glycogen stores?

The most accurate way would be to have a muscle biopsy taken (a needle is inserted into the muscle and a small portion is extracted and analyzed), but this is not very practical. However, keeping an accurate record of your body weight, which should be recorded every morning as you arise and after you urinate, may help you determine the answer to this question. Approximately 3 grams of water are bound to each gram of stored glycogen. If your

Table 4.9 Daily food plan for carbohydrate loading

Dietary sources of fats, proteins, and carbohydrates	Amount and Calories	Grams of carbohydrate, protein, and fat
Meat, fish, poultry, eggs, cheese, select low-fat items	6–8 oz Calories: 330–440	0 grams carbohydrate* 42–56 grams protein 18–24 grams fat
Breads, cereals, and grain products	10–20 servings Calories: 800–1,600	150–300 grams carbohydrate 24–60 grams protein
Vegetables, high Calorie (such as corn)	4 servings Calories: 280	60 grams carbohydrate 8 grams protein
Fruits	4 servings Calories: 240	60 grams carbohydrate
Fats and oils	2–4 teaspoons Calories: 90–180	10–20 grams fat
Milk, skim	2 servings Calories: 180	24 grams carbohydrate 16 grams protein
Desserts, like pie	2 servings Calories: 700	102 grams carbohydrate 6 grams protein 30 grams fat
Beverages, naturally sweetened	8–24 ounces Calories: 80–240	20–60 grams carbohydrate
Water	8 or more servings Calories: 0	
TOTAL KCAL	2,700–3,860	

TOTAL GRAMS AND APPROXIMATE % OF DIETARY CALORIES

Carbohydrate	416–606	65%
Protein	96–146	15%
Fat	58–74	20%

Consult Table 4.2 for specific high-carbohydrate foods in each of the food sources.

*Beans are listed in the meat group because of their high protein content; however, they are also low in fat and high in carbohydrates, so they are an excellent selection from this food group. Substitution of beans for meat will increase the total grams of carbohydrate and the percentage of dietary Calories from carbohydrate.

Including high-carbohydrate drinks, such as glucose polymers, can add significant amounts of carbohydrate to the diet and may substitute for other foods, such as desserts.

Source: Adapted from M. Forgac, "Carbohydrate Loading: A Review" in *Journal of the American Dietetic Association* 75:42–5, 1979.

body stores an additional 300–400 grams of glycogen, along with 900–1,200 grams of water, your body weight will increase about 1,200–1,600 grams, or 2.5–3.5 pounds above your normal training weight during the loading phase. The weight gain would be greater with additional glycogen storage. This is indicative that the carbohydrate loading has been effective, since rapid weight gains from one day to another are usually due to changes in body water content.

Bodybuilders may use carbohydrate loading because the increased muscle water content may hypertrophy the muscles, leading to a more muscular, aesthetic appearance in competition. However, Horowitz and others reported no increase in the girths of seven different muscle groups following a carbohydrate loading regimen in resistance-trained bodybuilders.

Will carbohydrate loading increase muscle glycogen concentration?

Most, but not all, studies show that an appropriate carbohydrate loading protocol, compared to normal or low dietary carbohydrate intake, will substantially increase muscle glycogen levels, at least in males. Research by

Tarnopolsky and others indicates that female endurance athletes did not increase muscle glycogen levels following accepted carbohydrate loading procedures, while male endurance athletes did, possibly because the female athletes consumed lower absolute amounts of carbohydrate or relied more on fat as an energy source which may not have created a stimulus to store more glycogen. These investigators recommend more research to confirm their findings.

Glycogen content in the muscle has been reported to increase about two to three times beyond normal and liver glycogen content nearly doubled following a carbohydrate loading regimen, and this increase may last at least 3 days in a rested athlete. However, it may be important to taper and rest about 2 days prior to the event because Fogelholm and others reported no increase in muscle glycogen following the classic loading protocol if athletes continued to train 45–60 minutes per day, even though the training was easy. This finding merits confirmation, as other studies have shown muscle glycogen supercompensation when individuals tapered, although most studies use at least 1 day of rest before the competitive exercise test.

Hargreaves and others note that the increased muscle glycogen may be used more readily in exercise tasks approximating 65–70 percent VO_2 max, which might be a reasonable pace for an average runner competing in a marathon. If muscle glycogen were used more rapidly during the early stages of a marathon, theoretically carbohydrate loading would provide no advantage during the latter stages of the race. However, Bosch and others note that although carbohydrate loading may reduce the relative contribution of blood glucose to overall carbohydrate oxidation, the improved performance may be attributed to the initially greater amount of muscle glycogen.

Will carbohydrate loading improve exercise performance?

Although athletes in most sports may benefit from an increased carbohydrate content in the diet, the full procedure of carbohydrate loading is not necessary for the vast majority of athletes.

In general, carbohydrate loading has not been found to enhance performance in single high-intensity exercise tasks ranging up to 30 minutes or so. For example, Vandenberghe and others found no effect of muscle glycogen levels (manipulated by carbohydrate loading) on muscle glycolytic rate during very high intensity exercise (125 percent VO_2 max) or on all-out performance at this exercise intensity, a time approximating 3 minutes. Various other studies have reported that carbohydrate loading does not increase the speed of runners in events ranging from 10 kilometers to the half-marathon. However, Pizza and others, using an exercise task consisting of a 15-minute submaximal run followed by a run to exhaustion at 100 percent VO_2 max reported an increase in performance associated with carbohydrate loading. The run to

exhaustion approximated 5 minutes. In general, this finding is an exception to the rule, but additional research is warranted.

Carbohydrate loading may benefit athletes involved in prolonged intermittent high-intensity exercise tasks. Most recently, Akermark and others, using elite Swedish ice hockey players on two competitive teams as subjects, reported that the team that carbohydrate loaded between two games had higher muscle glycogen levels, which were associated with improvement in distance skated, number of shifts skated, and skating speed in the second game.

Carbohydrate loading has been studied most extensively as a means to improve performance in more prolonged aerobic endurance exercise tasks. In general, the results are supportive of an ergogenic effect. Laboratory studies have shown that exercise time to exhaustion is closely associated with the amount of muscle glycogen available or the amount of carbohydrate in the diet. When endurance performance is compared after subjects have been on either a high-fat/high-protein diet, a mixed, balanced diet, or a high-carbohydrate diet for 4–7 days, performance on the high-fat/high-protein diet is worse than on the other two. However, research findings comparing a mixed, balanced diet with a high-carbohydrate diet have been equivocal, with some results favoring the high-carbohydrate diet and others revealing no difference between the two. Unfortunately, the performance tests in many of these studies may not have been long enough for the individual to derive the full benefit from carbohydrate loading; they lasted less than 2 hours.

One of the most supportive studies was conducted by Clyde Williams in England. Male and female runners performed a 30-kilometer (18.6 miles) run on a treadmill and then were divided into two groups, one used a carbohydrate loading technique for a week while the other group maintained their normal carbohydrate intake. Although there were no significant differences between the groups for overall performance time in the 30 kilometers, the carbohydrate-loading group ran the last 5 kilometers significantly faster compared to their initial trial.

A recent study by Rauch and others compared the effects of a 3-day carbohydrate loading protocol (10 grams carbohydrate per kilogram body weight per day, versus a normal mixed diet at 6 grams per kilogram) on performance in a 3-hour cycling task. Endurance-trained cyclists rode 2 hours at 75 percent VO_2 max, interspersed with five 60-second sprints every 20 minutes, and then completed a 60-minute performance ride. The carbohydrate loading regimen significantly increased the distance covered in the performance ride.

Moreover, several field studies with runners and cross-country skiers have shown improved performances with carbohydrate loading. In general, carbohydrate loading, in contrast to a mixed diet, did not enable these athletes to go faster during the early stages of their events, but the high glycogen levels enabled them to perform longer at a given speed. The end result was an overall faster time. Failure to carbohydrate load has also been identified as one of the factors contributing to collapse of runners in an ultramarathon. In a recent update, Hawley and others concluded that carbohydrate loading would postpone fatigue in endurance events lasting over 90 minutes, and may improve endurance performance in events where a set distance is covered as fast as possible.

Although carbohydrate loading appears to be an effective technique to enhance performance in prolonged aerobic endurance events, research suggests the most effective protocol is to carbohydrate load and use carbohydrate supplements during the event. Kang and others recently noted this method can exert an additional ergogenic effect by preventing a decline in blood glucose levels and maintaining carbohydrate metabolism during the later stages of prolonged aerobic exercise.

Are there any possible detrimental effects relative to carbohydrate loading?

From a performance standpoint, the extra body weight associated with the increased water content may be a disadvantage. In activities where moving the body weight is important, extra energy will be required to lift the extra 2–3 pounds of body water. However, in most performance events for which carbohydrate loading is advocated, the benefits from the energy aspects of the increased glycogen should more than offset the additional water weight. Moreover, if the individual is performing in a hot environment, the extra water could be available as a source of sweat and may be helpful in controlling body temperature during exercise in the heat. Although one study suggested that the water stored with glycogen did not confer any advantage in regulation of body temperature while exercising in heat, the duration of the exercise, only 45 minutes, would not be sufficient to benefit from the increased water levels. Another study conducted in South Africa revealed no beneficial or detrimental effects of carbohydrate loading on body temperature during 2.5 hours of exercise in a moderate environment (70° Fahrenheit; 21° Celsius). However, performance in longer exercise tasks with greater levels of water losses might be benefited.

From a health standpoint there may be some potential hazards to individuals with certain conditions. Although diabetics have been known to carbohydrate load, they should consult their physicians prior to using the technique. Individuals with high blood-lipid or cholesterol levels should avoid the high-fat/high-protein diet phase of the depletion stage if, for some reason, they prefer the original, classic method of carbohydrate loading. Blood serum lipids and cholesterol have been reported to rise significantly during this phase. In addition, these individuals should eat mostly complex carbohydrates during the loading phase because an increased intake of simple carbohydrates may raise blood-lipid levels. Furthermore, hypoglycemia may occur during the high-fat/high-protein phase.

Several laboratory studies and one case study have reported electrocardiographic (ECG) abnormalities in individuals who used the classic carbohydrate loading technique. Although no cause and effect relationship was determined, these investigators speculated that hypoglycemia or glucose intolerance may be involved. On the other hand, other well-controlled research with marathoners and typical joggers revealed no ECG changes following the classic method of carbohydrate loading.

Several investigators theorized that carbohydrate loading could possibly lead to destruction of muscle fibers by excessive glycogen storage, but no data were presented to support their contentions.

Other potential problems with the high-carbohydrate phase are diarrhea, nausea, and cramping, particularly when the diet is changed drastically or large amounts of simple carbohydrates are consumed. Individuals who wish to carbohydrate load should experiment with such diets during their training and not just before competition.

In general, however, the recommended carbohydrate loading technique presented in Table 4.8, which at the most is only a 7-day dietary regimen, poses no significant health hazards to the normally healthy individual.

Carbohydrates: Ergogenic Aspects

Throughout this chapter you have learned that carbohydrate intake, in a variety of ways, may be used to enhance physical performance. Truly, carbohydrates represent one of our most important ergogenic nutrients. You have also learned that certain forms of carbohydrate, such as fructose, possess the potential to impair performance in some individuals if consumed in excess. Such an effect may be ergolytic, the opposite of ergogenic. In this brief section we shall look at several forms of carbohydrate that might possess either ergogenic or ergolytic properties, including honey, alcohol (a by-product of carbohydrate fermentation), and metabolic by-products of glycolysis.

Is honey more effective than glucose or other carbohydrates?

One of the main foods of athletes over the years has been honey. In a best-seller entitled *Folk Medicine*, Jarvis suggested that honey gives quick energy release and enables athletes who expend energy heavily to recuperate rapidly from exertion. Although he claimed that honey was an excellent source of potassium, iron, calcium, and a host of other nutrients, the amounts are actually so small that honey is not considered to be a good nutrient source other than for its carbohydrate content, 40 percent of which is fructose.

One of the main advocates for honey as an ergogenic aid is Percival, who published his experiences with honey relative to athletic nutrition in the *American Bee Journal*—the reader may perceive the implications. Without reporting any experimental design or quantified results, Percival reported that athletes participating in endurance tests, such as distance running and repeated 50-yard sprints and 100-yard swims, performed better when fed 2 tablespoons of honey 30 minutes prior to testing. Performance also suffered when the honey was withdrawn. Percival concluded that, without reservation, honey is an ideal energy and fatigue-recovery fuel. Unfortunately, no research specifically concerned with the effect of honey upon physical performance has been uncovered, so the lack of experimental data makes it difficult to accept Percival's conclusions. However, the role of honey may be similar to that of glucose and fructose discussed earlier in this chapter. Since it tastes good, it may be a good source of carbohydrate to incorporate into the diet. On the other hand, the high fructose content may cause gastrointestinal problems in some individuals, so experimentation with its use in training is important.

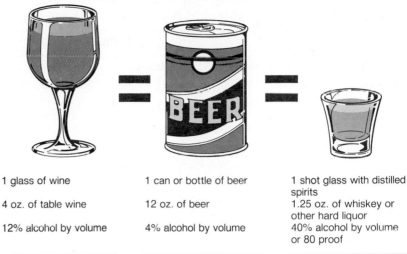

1 glass of wine	1 can or bottle of beer	1 shot glass with distilled spirits
4 oz. of table wine	12 oz. of beer	1.25 oz. of whiskey or other hard liquor
12% alcohol by volume	4% alcohol by volume	40% alcohol by volume or 80 proof
4 x 0.12 = 0.48 oz. of ethyl alcohol per serving	12 x 0.04 = 0.48 oz. of ethyl alcohol per serving	1.25 x 0.40 = 0.50 oz. of ethyl alcohol per serving

Figure 4.11 Alcohol equivalencies and drinking.

Is alcohol an effective ergogenic aid?

The alcohol produced for human consumption is ethyl alcohol, or **ethanol.** It is a transparent, colorless liquid derived from the fermentation of sugars in fruits, vegetables, and grains. Although classified legally as a drug, alcohol is a component of many common beverages served throughout the world. In the United States, alcohol is consumed mainly as a natural ingredient of beer, wine, and liquors. Although the alcohol content may vary in different types, in general, beer is about 4–5 percent alcohol, wine is about 12–14 percent alcohol, and typical bar liquor (whiskey, rum, gin, vodka) is about 40–45 percent alcohol. The term **proof** is a measure of the alcohol content in a beverage and is double the percentage; an 86-proof bottle of whiskey is 43 percent alcohol, while a 150-proof bottle of Caribbean rum is 75 percent alcohol (Figure 4.11).

One drink of alcohol is the equivalent of one-half ounce of pure ethyl alcohol or the equivalent of about 13–14 grams of alcohol. The following amounts of beer, wine, and liquor contain approximately equal amounts of alcohol and are classified as one drink:

12 ounces (one bottle) of beer

4 ounces (one wine glass) of wine

1.25 ounces (one jigger or shot glass) of liquor

Technically, alcohol may be classified as a food because it provides energy, one of the major functions of food. Alcohol contains about 7 Calories per gram, almost twice the value of an equal amount of carbohydrate or protein. Beer and wine also contain some carbohydrate, a source of additional Calories. In general, a bottle of regular beer has about 150 Calories, while a 4-ounce glass

of wine or a shot glass of liquor contains about 100 Calories. Table 4.10 provides an approximate analysis of the caloric content of common alcoholic beverages and nonalcoholic beer.

In general, the Calories found in beer, wine, and liquor are empty Calories. Although wine and beer contain trace amounts of protein, vitamins, and minerals, liquor is void of any nutrient value. Alcohol may have a certain value to us as a social beverage, but its value as a food and source of nutrients is virtually nil.

About 20 percent of the alcohol ingested may be absorbed by the stomach; the remainder passes on to the intestine for absorption. The absorption is rapid, particularly if the digestive tract is empty. The alcohol enters the blood and is distributed to the various tissues, being diluted by the water content of the body. A small portion of the alcohol, about 3–10 percent, is excreted from the body through the breath, urine, or sweat, but the majority is metabolized by the liver, the organ that metabolizes other drugs. As the blood circulates, the liver of an average adult male will metabolize about one-third ounce (8–10 grams) of alcohol per hour, or somewhat less than the amount of alcohol in one drink.

Although alcohol is derived from the fermentation of carbohydrates, it is metabolized in the body like fat. The liver helps convert the metabolic by-products of alcohol into fatty acids, which may be stored in the liver or transported into the blood. Several other compounds, such as lactate, acetate, and acetaldehyde, may also be released into the blood. These products may eventually be utilized for energy and converted into carbon dioxide and water. A schematic of alcohol metabolism is presented in Figure 4.12.

As noted above, the liver of a 150-pound male can metabolize only about one-third ounce of alcohol, or less

Table 4.10 Caloric content of typical alcoholic beverages

| Beverage | Amount | Carbohydrate | | Alcohol | | Total |
		Grams	Calories	Grams	Calories	Calories
Beer, regular	12 ounces	13	52	13	91	150
Beer, light	12 ounces	7	28	11	77	109
Beer, nonalcoholic	12 ounces	12	48	1	7	55
Beer, alcohol-free	12 ounces	12	48	0	0	48
Wine, table	4 ounces	4	16	12	84	100
Liquor, 80 proof	1.25 ounces	0	0	14	98	100

The small discrepancies in the calculation of total Calories for beer and liquor may be attributed to a small protein content in beer and trace amounts of carbohydrate in liquor.

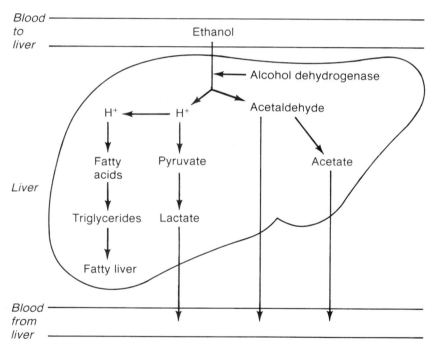

Figure 4.12 Simplified metabolic pathways of ethanol (alcohol) in the liver. Hydrogen ions are removed from ethanol as it is converted to acetaldehyde, which may be released into the blood for transport to other tissues. The excess hydrogen ions may combine with fatty acids to form triglycerides or with pyruvate to form lactate. Excessive accumulation of triglycerides may lead to the development of a fatty liver and eventually to cirrhosis.

than one drink, per hour. The rate is lower in smaller individuals and higher in larger individuals. Thus, consumption of alcohol at a rate greater than one drink per hour will result in an accumulation of alcohol in the blood; this is measured as the **blood alcohol content (BAC)** in grams per 100 milliliters of blood. For the average male, one drink will result in a BAC of about 0.025; four drinks in an hour would lead to a BAC of approximately 0.10.

For over a century, athletes have consumed alcohol just prior to or during competition in attempts to improve performance. Alcohol has been alleged to alter energy metabolism, improve physiological processes, or modify psychological factors so as to benefit the athlete. Let us look at the available research to evaluate the truth of these allegations.

Although alcohol contains a relatively large number of Calories and its metabolic pathways in the body are short, the available evidence suggests that it is not utilized to any significant extent during exercise. First, the major sources of energy for exercise are carbohydrates and fats, which are in ample supply in most individuals. Alcohol may help form fats, but there is no evidence that it can substitute for other fat sources in the body. Even if it could, this would be of no benefit because the body has more than enough fat to supply energy during prolonged exercise. Second, the by-products of alcohol metabolism that are released by the liver into the blood may enter the skeletal muscles but appear to be of little importance to exercising muscle. Third, even if the energy from alcohol could be used, it would represent an uneconomical source. The amount of oxygen needed to release the Calories from alcohol is greater than for an equivalent amount of carbohydrate and fat. And lastly, the rate at which the liver metabolizes alcohol limits its use as an energy source during exercise, particularly in an individual working at a high level of intensity. In summary, these four factors suggest alcohol is not a key energy source during exercise, and even if it were, it would not offer any advantages over natural supplies of carbohydrate and fat. Recent research with carbon labeling revealed alcohol did not significantly modify endogenous carbohydrate and fat utilization during exercise.

Research also supports the finding that alcohol in small amounts (one to two drinks) neither improves nor deteriorates physiological processes associated with maximal aerobic exercise, including VO_2 max and maximal heart rate; neither does it affect other indicators of maximal aerobic performance such as exercise tests to exhaustion. Moreover, tests of anaerobic performance such as strength and local muscular endurance also are not affected.

However, a few studies have reported some potential adverse effects of consuming alcohol during exercise. Most of the studies alluded to above were conducted on males. A recent study reported some adverse acute effects of moderate alcohol consumption on cardiovascular and metabolic responses in females. In a submaximal cycling exercise task for 30 minutes, ingestion of alcohol increased the heart rate, oxygen consumption, blood pressure, and blood lactate, which the investigators indicated were negative effects. Moreover, some recent research reported a significant decrease in aerobic endurance when alcohol was ingested before and during a treadmill run at about 80–85 percent VO_2 max, which may have been associated with an impaired glucose metabolism. Alcohol also reduces gluconeogenesis by the liver and glucose uptake by the legs during the latter stages of exercise. In prolonged exercise, such as marathons, these effects could lead to an earlier onset of hypoglycemia or muscle glycogen depletion and a subsequent decrease in performance. Moreover, some studies have reported reduced absorption of vitamin B_1 associated with moderate intakes of alcohol. Theoretically, this could impair physical performance of an endurance nature because vitamin B_1 is involved in the aerobic metabolism of carbohydrate. Additional research is merited to document any adverse effects of alcohol on cardiovascular or metabolic processes during exercise.

Alcohol also has been used as an ergogenic aid for its psychological effects. It is a narcotic, a depressant, that affects the brain. As a depressant, alcohol would not be advocated as a means to improve performance; however, some have contended that increased feelings of self-confidence, reduced anxiety levels, and a perceived decrease in sensitivity to pain may offset any depressant effects and possibly benefit performance. Moreover, alcohol in small doses may exert a paradoxical stimulation effect. Parts of the brain that normally inhibit behavior may be depressed by alcohol, leading to a transitory sensation of excitement.

Although these effects may occur, research does not support the use of alcohol in sports involving psychological processes such as perceptual-motor abilities. Perceptual-motor activities involve the perception of a stimulus, integration of this stimulus by the brain, and an appropriate motor response (movement). The evidence overwhelmingly supports the conclusion that alcohol adversely affects psychomotor performance skills, such as reaction time, balance, hand/eye coordination, and visual perception, that are important in events with rapidly changing stimuli such as tennis.

In one form of athletic competition, such as marksmanship in riflery, pistol shooting, dart throwing, and archery, alcohol may be used to decrease muscle tremor and thereby improve accuracy for competition. Although research generally is not supportive of an improved performance, a recent study with archers revealed a tendency toward reduced tremor with low blood alcohol levels, resulting in a smoother release. However, no actual performance data were revealed. Throwing accuracy improved in darts at a BAC of 0.02, but was impaired at a BAC of 0.05. This area of study merits additional research.

Only a limited number of studies have been conducted relative to the effect of social drinking upon physical performance, but there is rather general agreement that light social drinking will not impair performance on the following day. Tests of reaction time, strength, power, and cardiovascular performance were not adversely affected following the consumption of one drink the night before. On the other hand, heavy drinking may impair performance on the following day owing to hangover effects, involuntary eye movement, or dehydration.

The use of alcohol by Olympic athletes had been banned previously by the IOC, but because wine and beer are commonly consumed as a part of many traditional European meals it was removed from the banned list prior to the 1972 Olympics. However, individual sports federations within the IOC still may consider alcohol use during competition as grounds for disqualification. At the present time, only the sports that involve shooting competition ban the use of alcohol.

Do the metabolic by-products of carbohydrate exert an ergogenic effect?

Recall that the primary mechanism in the transformation of muscle glycogen into energy is glycolysis. The end product during aerobic metabolism is normally pyruvate. However, glycolysis leading to the formation of pyruvate involves production of a number of metabolic by-products in a chain of about a dozen sequential steps, each step being controlled by an enzyme. (See Appendix K.) One theory of fatigue is that if one of these steps is blocked by inactivation of an enzyme, glycolysis may not continue at an optimal rate since a necessary metabolic by-product may be in short supply. This blocked step could represent a weak link in the chain, reducing the rate at which ATP could be produced. Thus, a few investigators have studied the effects of several of these metabolic by-products during exercise for their possible bioenergetic effects, which could possess ergogenic potential. The metabolic by-product lactate has also been studied as a possible ergogenic aid.

Fructose 1,6-diphosphate (FDP) FDP is a natural metabolic by-product of glycolysis. It has been shown to play an important function in the regulation of glycogen metabolism. Some research has shown that the infusion of exogenous FDP helped prevent glycogen breakdown and stimulate glycogen synthesis in individuals who suffered heart attacks. If such an effect could be produced in healthy individuals, endurance performance might be enhanced. Thus, Myers and his associates infused FDP into physically trained subjects to study the metabolic response to exercise during 1 hour at 70 percent of VO_2 max. However, what may have been effective in diseased individuals with poor metabolic status was not shown to be effective in healthy individuals during exercise. The investigators noted no beneficial effects of FDP upon a wide variety of physiological, metabolic, or hormonal responses during this exercise task.

Dihydroxyacetone and Pyruvate (DHAP) DHAP is a combination of two three-carbon metabolic by-products of glycolysis—dihydroxyacetone and pyruvate. Previous studies with animals have shown that DHAP increases muscle glycogen content, so Ronald Stanko and his associates at the University of Pittsburgh investigated the potential ergogenic effect of DHAP in humans. Two studies were conducted, both using untrained males as subjects. The dosage of DHAP in both studies was 100 grams per day for 7 days; DHAP was prepared in a 3:1 ratio of dihydroxyacetone (75 g) to sodium pyruvate (25 g) and administered either in Jello or artificially sweetened fluids. The placebo in both studies was 100 grams of Polycose, a carbohydrate. The DHAP or Polycose was substituted for a portion of the carbohydrate in the diet. Both studies were well designed, using a double-blind, placebo, repeated-measures crossover approach. In the first study, the diet was standardized at 55 percent carbohydrate of the daily caloric intake. The criterion test was an arm ergometer exercise task to exhaustion at 60 percent VO_2 peak following a week of supplementation. DHAP significantly increased endurance time, attributed primarily to an increased muscle glycogen concentration and increased extraction of blood glucose, both factors providing more glucose to the exercising muscle. In the second experiment, subjects consumed a high-carbohydrate diet (70 percent of the daily caloric intake). The criterion test was a cycle ergometer exercise task to exhaustion at 70 percent VO_2 peak. DHAP improved performance in an identical fashion to the first study, the effect being attributed to an increased blood glucose extraction by the exercising muscle. The results of these two well-controlled studies indicate an ergogenic effect of DHAP with untrained subjects, but confirming data are needed with well-trained athletes.

Lactate Salts As noted previously, lactic acid is a metabolic by-product of anaerobic glycolysis. We also indicated that although lactic acid is often associated with fatigue, it is the hydrogen ion release that increases the acidity and impairs performance, not the lactate itself. Lactate is actually a small metabolite of glucose; its formula is $C_3H_5O_3$, about half of that of glucose, $C_6H_{12}O_6$. Thus, lactate still possesses considerable energy, and researchers in California have developed a product called polylactate, a combination of lactate and an amino acid. In a study presented at a regional meeting of the American College of Sports Medicine, Larsen and his associates investigated the effect of polylactate upon physiological and psychological responses to a 3-hour bicycle ergometer exercise task at 50 percent of VO_2 max. Compared to a sweetened placebo, they reported that polylactate can help maintain blood glucose, reduce perceived exertion, and enhance blood buffering capacity (lower blood acidity). No performance data were presented. On the basis of these findings, it would appear polylactate is comparable to other carbohydrate supplements, although the potential effect of the improved blood buffering capacity would appear to have some ergogenic potential. However, Fred Brouns and his colleagues at Maastricht in the Netherlands reported that 3 weeks of supplementation with oral lactate salts did not influence the removal of lactate during and following exercise, suggesting no value to lactate supplementation in this regard.

Unfortunately, there are few data available regarding the ergogenic effect of these carbohydrate by-products.

Dietary Carbohydrates: Health Implications

Although improving, the diet of the typical American still appears to be unbalanced. In general, we consume too many Calories, too much fat and refined sugar products, and not enough complex carbohydrates. Such a diet may pose several health problems. As we shall see in Chapter 5, excessive consumption of dietary fat appears to be of major concern relative to the development of several chronic diseases and, as is discussed in Chapter 10, a significant contributor to the development of obesity. On the other hand, nutritional objectives in *Healthy People 2000* recommend that consuming more carbohydrates, particularly complex carbohydrate and fiber-containing foods, while moderating intake of refined sugars and alcohol (a by-product of carbohydrate fermentation) may produce some significant health benefits.

How do refined sugars affect my health?

If you consume the typical American diet, approximately 18–20 percent of your daily caloric intake is derived from simple carbohydrates including natural sugars found in milk and fruit, and refined sugars such as ordinary table sugar and the high-fructose corn syrup added to numerous processed foods; over half of our simple carbohydrate intake is from refined sugar. Over the years, dietary intake of refined sugar has been alleged to contribute to a wide variety of health problems, particularly psychological afflictions such as hyperactivity, premenstrual syndrome (PMS), and even mental illness.

Carbohydrate intake, particularly sugars such as sucrose, has been studied for its effect on mood and behavior. As discussed previously, increases in the fTRP:BCAA ratio facilitates the entry of tryptophan into the brain, possibly stimulating the formation of the neurotransmitter serotonin, which may affect mood states and behavior. A diet high in carbohydrates may stimulate a release of insulin, which not only moves glucose into the body cells, but amino acids as well, particularly the BCAA into muscle cells. Thus, high-glycemic-index foods may increase the fTRP:BCAA ratio and affect mood. Serotonin formation in the brain may induce relaxation and sleepiness, and may function somewhat as an antidepressant. In certain syndromes such as PMS and seasonal affective disorder (SAD), carbohydrate cravings for sweet, starchy foods may develop, which may be related to the effect on serotonin production and possible antidepressant effects. Paradoxically, hyperactivity has been theorized to result from excess sucrose intake in children, but a review by Gans indicates there are few scientific data to support this relationship.

Refined sugar has also been alleged to contribute to other health problems as well, including obesity, diabetes, and cardiovascular disease. Although the role carbohydrates, including refined sugars, may play in the development of these health problems is still under investigation, The National Research Council, in its major treatise on diet and health, stated there is minimal evidence linking refined sugar intake per se to these specific health problems. However, as we shall see in Chapter 10, high-sugar foods are often high in fat as well, and may be linked to the development of obesity.

At the present time, scientific data support a relationship between refined sugar intake and only one health problem, dental caries. Even with dental caries, tooth decay is not necessarily a matter of how much sugar one eats, but in what form and how often. Sticky, chewy, sugary foods eaten often between meals increase the risk of developing dental caries. Starchy foods that adhere to teeth, like bread, are also cariogenic. To prevent caries, brush and floss your teeth.

Nevertheless, many health organizations around the world have recommended a reduced intake of refined sugars, generally to amounts less than 10 percent of the daily caloric intake. Because refined sugar contains no nutrients, but only Calories, its intake should be limited in any well-balanced diet. Suggestions to decrease sugar intake were presented in Chapter 2. To reiterate some of these points:

Read food labels and select foods low in sugar.

Know the different ways in which sugar may appear on a food label. Sugar is sugar. There is no additional nutritional value of "natural" sugars compared to ordinary table sugar (sucrose).

Reduce the sugar in foods prepared at home.

Use less sugar at the table.

Eat more fruits for a naturally-occurring source of sugar.

Decrease intake of soft drinks with sugar.

Use other sweeteners, such as cinnamon, nutmeg, ginger, or artificial sweeteners.

Are artificial sweeteners safe?

A number of artificial sweeteners have been produced over the years, but currently only three are approved for use in the United States. Saccharin, 300 times as sweet as sucrose, is a noncaloric derivative of coal tar. Aspartame, 180 times as sweet as sucrose, is derived from two amino acids (aspartic acid and phenylalanine) and contains 4 Calories per gram. Acesulfame K, 200 times as sweet as sucrose, is a naturally-occurring potassium salt.

Saccharin in extremely large doses has been shown to cause urinary bladder cancer in laboratory animals, and according to the Delaney clause, it should be banned as an additive to food products. However, the United States Congress passed a law exempting saccharin from the Delaney clause, and its use continues. Epidemiological data with humans have not shown any relationship between urinary bladder cancer and saccharin at levels normally consumed by the general population, so it is assumed to be safe. Nevertheless, products containing saccharin have warnings on the label indicating that they may be hazardous to your health. The safety of aspartame, also known as Equal or NutraSweet, has been questioned because some reports have associated it with headaches, dizziness, or fatigue in some individuals, which may have been an allergic reaction; more recent reports have associated it with brain tumors. However, following a detailed analysis of the scientific evidence, the Food and Drug Administration and other federal health agencies consider aspartame to confer no significant health risks, with the exception of individuals who have phenylketonuria (PKU), a rare genetic disease that limits the ability to metabolize phenylalanine. Such individuals are aware of their condition, and products containing aspartame must carry a warning on the label that the product contains phenylalanine. Acesulfame K (Sunette, Sweet One) is considered safe and needs no warning on the label.

Artificial sweeteners may be effective in weight-control programs, and their role will be discussed in Chapter 11.

Why are complex carbohydrates thought to be beneficial to my health?

To increase consumption of total carbohydrate in the diet while reducing the consumption of refined sugars, one must increase the consumption of complex carbohydrates. A diet rich in complex carbohydrates may also reduce the percentage contribution from fats, which may confer significant health benefits as noted in the next chapter. Complex carbohydrates are found primarily in starchy vegetables and whole grains, but small amounts are also found in fruits. As noted in Chapter 2 relative to the vegetarian diet, these foods contain a number of healthful nutrients, such as protein, essential fats, minerals, antioxidant vitamins, and various phytochemicals. They also contain one of the most important health-related nutrients, dietary fiber.

Why should I eat foods rich in dietary fiber?

Americans do not consume enough dietary fiber. There is considerable epidemiological evidence, and some experimental evidence, to support the value of adding dietary fiber to the diet as a sound preventative measure against many chronic diseases. For example, epidemiological studies with vegetarians, who consume diets high in complex carbohydrates and fiber, have shown lower levels of obesity and many other chronic diseases. Exactly how dietary fiber may be protective is not known, but several mechanisms have been proposed that may help in the prevention of certain forms of cancer, coronary heart disease, obesity, diabetes, hypertension, and various disorders of the gastrointestinal tract.

Fiber may add bulk to the contents of the large intestine, stimulating peristalsis and speeding up the transit time of food through the intestines. The increased bulk may dilute any possible cancer-causing agents (carcinogens) that might attack cell walls, while faster transit diminishes the time carcinogens may have to act. Epidemiological studies have shown that populations with high-fiber diets have lower incidence of colon and rectal cancer. Increased bulk and peristalsis also decreases the incidence rate of diverticulosis, an inflammatory disorder in the large intestine that may cause rupture, leading to serious complications.

Fiber, particularly gummy forms of soluble fiber like beta-glucans in oats, may bind with various substances in the gastrointestinal tract. Soluble fiber may bind with carcinogens so that they are excreted by the bowel, again reducing the risk of colorectal cancer. Soluble fiber may also bind with and lead to the excretion of bile salts, which contain cholesterol; normally bile salts are reabsorbed into the body, but excretion of bile salts, along with their cholesterol content, may help reduce serum cholesterol levels. This effect may decrease the risk of coronary heart disease because high serum cholesterol levels increase the risk of atherosclerosis, a major cause of heart disease.

Fiber slows down gastric (stomach) emptying and thereby slows glucose absorption in the small intestine. This effect may lead to better control of blood sugar and may also lengthen the sensation of fullness or satiety, which may be important to individuals on weight-loss diets. Thus, high-fiber diets may be useful in the prevention or treatment of obesity. Some recent research with women has indicated that diets with low cereal fiber and high-glycemic-index foods increase the risk of diabetes, so theoretically increases in dietary fiber may be protective.

Some soluble fibers may be fermented in the large intestine to form short-chain fatty acids (SCFA). SCFA may confer several benefits: they may be absorbed and transported to the liver where they may suppress cholesterol synthesis, possibly helping to decrease serum cholesterol levels and the risk of coronary heart disease.

Fiber may reduce circulating levels of estrogen in the body. In a recent review, Stoll identified several mechanisms whereby dietary fiber could reduce estrogen levels, including a reduction of enterohepatic recirculation of estrogens and reduced production of biologically active forms of estrogens produced by body fat. Stoll noted that if these and other proposed mechanisms could synergistically reduce circulating estrogens, the risk of breast cancer in women could be reduced.

High-fiber diets may even complement a diet that is low in fat and cholesterol to help protect against coronary heart disease. A meta-analysis of experimental studies has reported reduced blood cholesterol levels after a diet high in soluble fibers such as oat bran, even when consumed as part of a low-saturated fat/low-cholesterol diet. But even with diets higher in fat and saturated fat, recent research by Rimm and his associates indicated that a high-fiber diet could reduce the risks associated with a high-fat diet. Nevertheless, the best strategy is to reduce fat and increase fiber, a combination that will enhance overall healthful effects.

Although this area is still under investigation, several hypotheses link potential health benefits to the specific type of fiber consumed. Foods that are rich in the water-insoluble type of fiber, such as whole wheat products, wheat bran cereals, brown rice, and lentils, are more likely to increase the fecal bulk, maximizing the dilutant effect and speed of transit through the colon, and hence helping prevent diseases of the large intestine and rectum. Foods richer in water-soluble fiber, such as apples, bananas, citrus fruits, carrots, and oats, have more of a binding effect and are theorized to be more likely to reduce serum cholesterol. However, as a leading investigator on the health effects of dietary fiber, Joanne Slavin notes it is difficult to generalize as to the physiological effects of fiber based on its classification as either water soluble or insoluble. For example, Slavin notes that rice bran, which is devoid of soluble fiber, has been shown to reduce serum cholesterol, and SCFA generated from fermentation of soluble fibers may help prevent colon cancer. Recent research has also supported the effect of insoluble fiber to reduce the risk of heart disease. A balanced intake of both soluble and insoluble dietary fiber appears to be the best approach.

The National Research Council has cautioned that data relative to a protective effect of fiber per se against the development of certain chronic diseases are inconclusive at present. Nevertheless, the council recognizes the value of the epidemiological data supportive of a protective effect of a diet high in whole-grain products, legumes, fruits, and vegetables. Its current recommendation is to obtain approximately 20–35 grams of dietary fiber through the consumption of natural, wholesome foods, not fiber supplements. It is important to recognize that the health benefits attributed to fiber may be associated with the form in which the fiber is consumed—as part of a whole, natural food containing other potential health-promoting nutrients such as vitamins, rather than by consumption of a purified supplement form.

Obtaining 20–35 grams of fiber daily is not difficult, but you have to eat more whole grains, fruits, vegetables, and legumes. The following general equivalencies may help you reach this goal:

3 fruits	=	6 grams fiber
3 vegetables	=	9 grams fiber
3 slices of whole-grain bread	=	6 grams fiber
1/2 cup beans	=	7 grams fiber
1 serving bran cereal	=	9 grams fiber
Total	=	37 grams fiber

According to one physician, a good way to see if you are eating enough fiber is to observe the buoyancy of your stool in the toilet. It should float, or at least appear flaky and break apart. If it sinks or does not break apart, you are not eating enough fiber.

There appear to be few or no health disadvantages to a high-fiber diet. As we shall see in Chapter 8, there has been some concern that high-fiber diets could lead to increased losses of certain minerals, such as iron and zinc, but research has shown that such concerns are generally unwarranted if one follows the recommendations just given.

What is lactose intolerance?

About one in nine Americans may develop gastrointestinal distress when they consume dairy products containing substantial amounts of lactose, particularly milk. Such individuals lack the enzyme lactase and hence cannot metabolize lactose in the digestive tract. The most common symptoms of **lactose intolerance** are gas, bloating, abdominal pain, and diarrhea, although headache and fatigue may also occur.

Individuals may be diagnosed as being lactose intolerant through a lactose tolerance test administered by a physician. One physician suggests, however, that a self-detection technique may be an effective approach. If you experience problems such as gas and diarrhea after consuming milk, abstain from all dairy products for 2 weeks and then evaluate the results. If the symptoms resolve, and then reoccur when you resume dairy food consumption, you may need to reduce the amount of lactose in your diet. Unfortunately, usually this means a reduced intake of dairy foods, which are considered to be the main dietary source of not only lactose, but calcium as well.

In order to obtain adequate calcium intake, the lactose-intolerant individual may use several strategies. In some cases, milk may be consumed in small amounts, such as one-half cup, without triggering adverse effects, for the intestinal tract may be able to process smaller amounts. Consuming small amounts of milk over the course of the day may provide significant amounts of calcium. Reduced-lactose milk is available, as are enzyme supplements, such as Lactaid, to help prevent indigestion. Other dairy products which have been fermented, such as yogurt, may be tolerated and provide a good calcium source. Cheese may also be a good source of calcium, although it is high in fat. Dark-green leafy vegetables, tofu, sardines, and salmon are all nondairy sources of calcium. Additionally, calcium supplements may be useful.

What effect can drinking alcohol have upon my health?

Consumption of alcoholic beverages is a popular pastime worldwide. People drink mainly for social reasons, but when and how much they drink may have a significant impact on their health and the health of others. Although many of the effects of alcohol may negatively affect health status, some effects may be positive.

Negative Effects Alcohol affects all cells in the body, and many of these effects may have significant health implications. Drinking alcoholic beverages, particularly in large amounts, is associated with over 100,000 deaths per year.

Direct toxic effects Alcohol has a direct toxic effect on the intestinal walls; it tends to impair the absorption of vitamins such as thiamin (B$_1$). Individuals who drink alcohol also have a higher incidence rate of pharyngeal and esophageal cancer, which may possibly be associated with the direct effect of alcohol as it contacts these tissues during ingestion. Combining alcohol with certain medication such as aspirin or nonsteroidal anti-inflammatory agents (ibuprofen) may promote gastrointestinal bleeding. Drinking alcohol may also aggravate certain health conditions, such as peptic ulcers.

Liver function The liver is the only organ in the body that metabolizes alcohol, and alcohol may affect liver function in several ways. It may interfere with the metabolism of other drugs, increasing the effect of some and lessening the effects of others. Even with a balanced diet high in protein, consuming six drinks a day for less than a month has been shown to cause significant accumulation of fat in the liver. If continued over years, the liver cells degenerate. Eventually the damaged liver cells are replaced by non-functioning scar tissue, a condition known as **cirrhosis.** As liver function deteriorates, fat, carbohydrate, and protein metabolism are not regulated properly; this has possible pathological consequences for other body organs such as the kidney, pancreas, and heart.

Mental processes Following absorption, the most immediate effects of alcohol are on the brain; often these effects are paradoxical. Although alcohol is a depressant, a small amount often exerts a stimulating effect because it may release some of the normal inhibitory control mechanisms in the brain. For the most part, however, alcohol acts as a depressant, and its effects on the brain are dose-dependent. The effects occur in a hierarchical fashion related to the development of the brain. In general, alcohol first affects the higher brain centers. With increasing dosages, lower levels of brain function become depressed with subsequent disturbance of normal functions. This hierarchy of brain functions, from higher levels to lower levels, and some of the functions affected by alcohol may be generalized as follows:

Thinking and reasoning—Judgment

Perceptual-motor responses—Reaction time

Fine motor coordination—Muscles of speech

Gross motor coordination—Walking

Visual processes—Double vision

Alertness—Sleep, coma

Respiratory control—Respiratory failure, death

An overview of the effects of increasing blood alcohol content on mental and physical functions is presented in Table 4.11.

Table 4.11	Typical effects of increasing blood alcohol content	
Number of drinks* consumed in 2 hours	Blood** alcohol content	Typical effects
2–3	.02–.04	Reduced tension, relaxed feeling, relief from daily stress
4–5	.06–.09	Legally drunk in some states, impaired judgment, a high feeling, impaired fine motor ability and coordination
6–8	.11–.16	Legally drunk in all states, slurred speech, impaired gross motor coordination, staggering gait
9–12	.18–.25	Loss of control of voluntary activity, erratic behavior, impaired vision
13–18	.27–.39	Stuporous, total loss of coordination
19 and above	> .40	Coma, depression of respiratory centers, death

*One drink = 12 ounces regular beer
4 ounces wine
1.25 ounces liquor

**BAC based on body weight of 160 pounds (72.6 KG). The BAC will increase proportionally for individuals weighing less (such as a 120-pound female) and will decrease proportionally for individuals weighing more (such as a 200-pound football player). For example, four to five drinks in 2 hours could lead to a BAC of 0.08–0.12 in a 120-pound individual.

If you want to avoid mental impairment associated with alcohol, abstinence is the simplest approach. For those who do drink, abstinence is advised under certain conditions. The acute effects of excessive alcohol consumption include impairment of both motor coordination and judgment—two factors that are extremely important in the safe operation of an automobile. At the least, being arrested for drunk driving may have serious social and personal consequences. At the worst, alcohol is involved as a cause of nearly one-half of all automobile fatalities—20,000 deaths per year in the United States alone. As the saying goes, "Don't drink and drive!"

Alcohol usage also is correlated highly with aggressive tendencies. Laboratory studies have indicated aggressive behavior is directly related to the quantity of alcohol consumed. Alcohol abuse is associated with sexual abuse, homicide, and suicide.

Most of these adverse effects are associated with excessive alcohol intake, particularly as practiced in binge drinking. Recent surveys indicate that almost half of college students binge, and one of the most significant factors underlying alcohol-related behavior problems is the amount of alcohol consumed; the greater the amount of alcohol consumed, the more serious the problem.

DNA damage Laboratory research has shown that in vitro (that is, in a test tube) alcohol and acetaldehyde cause changes in DNA (the genetic material in body cells) comparable to changes elicited by carcinogens. This DNA damage may occur at an alcohol concentration equivalent to one to two drinks. In those who drink, this finding could be related to the increased risk of certain forms of cancer, including pharyngeal and esophageal cancer as mentioned above, and also breast and colon cancer.

One of the most debated issues is the risk of breast cancer. Possible mechanisms have been identified; in addition to potential DNA damage, alcohol ingestion may also increase estrogen levels, a factor that increases breast cancer risk. Research associating increased incidence of breast cancer with alcohol consumption is epidemiological in nature. Several reviews have concluded that there is a significant relationship between alcohol intake and breast cancer, even in moderate amounts, but these reviews did not infer causality. In a more recent detailed review, Roth and others indicated the association between moderate alcohol intake and breast cancer was weak and does not support a causal relationship. Hopefully, similar detailed studies in the near future may help resolve this controversy.

Women who drink should abstain during pregnancy because alcohol may affect DNA in the embryo and fetus. The term **fetal alcohol syndrome (FAS)** refers to the effects upon the development of a fetus if a mother consumes alcohol while pregnant. The child may experience retardation in growth and mental development as well as facial birth defects (Figure 4.13). **Fetal alcohol effects (FAE)** may be observed in children when full-blown FAS is not present. Children with FAE are easily distracted and have poor attention spans. Both FAS and FAE are associated with learning disorders in children. No "safe" amount of alcohol during pregnancy has been determined. Thus, the safest approach is abstinence.

Obesity Alcohol is a significant source of Calories, about 7 per gram, somewhat comparable to the caloric content of fat. Recent research has indicated that if small amounts of alcohol (5 percent of daily caloric intake) are inter-

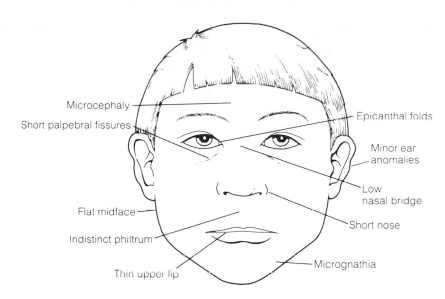

Figure 4.13 Common facial characteristics of children with fetal alcohol syndrome (FAS). Features labeled on the left are seen frequently; those on the right are less specific to this syndrome.

changed for an equivalent caloric intake from carbohydrates, there is no effect on daily energy expenditure. In other words, alcohol Calories themselves will not increase body fat as long as total daily caloric intake matches daily caloric expenditure. Actually, one study indicates alcohol may slightly increase the resting metabolic rate of female social drinkers. However, Angelo Tremblay, an esteemed scientist in weight control, and his colleagues recently found that alcohol has no inhibitory effect on food intake and its energy content, and when consumed in conjunction with a high-fat diet promotes overfeeding, a primary determinant of obesity.

Excessive drinking and alcoholism Heavy alcohol consumption aggravates most of the health problems mentioned above and may lead to addiction. Research has shown that three or more drinks per day increase the risk of developing high blood pressure and may increase blood lipid levels. These conditions are associated with cardiovascular disease, and heavy alcohol consumption is linked to sudden death from heart failure and stroke.

Alcohol abuse is the major drug problem in the United States, posing a problem for one in seven males and one in sixteen females, or about one out of every ten drinkers. Excessive intake of alcohol may lead to a disorder known as **alcoholism,** a condition whose etiology is unknown but probably is related to a variety of physiological, psychological, and sociological factors. The National Council on Alcoholism suggests that there is no pat definition for alcoholism; it may be evidenced by a variety of behaviors. The number of behaviors exhibited by the drinker may be related to various stages in the progression toward alcoholism. Appendix D, a questionnaire developed by the National Council on Alcoholism, provides for an assessment of these behaviors.

Positive Effects On the positive side, most recent epidemiological research has shown that moderate consumption of alcohol (one to three beers or glasses of wine per day) is associated with lessened mortality, primarily because of a reduced rate of coronary heart disease (CHD) in men, but some data supports favorable effects for women as well. The mechanism is not known, but several have been proposed based on epidemiological and experimental studies.

One theory suggests small amounts of alcohol induce a relaxation effect, which may reduce emotional stress, a risk factor associated with CHD.

Another theory has focused upon the effect of alcohol to raise levels of HDL cholesterol, the form of cholesterol that protects against the development of CHD (see discussion on pages 162–163). A significant number of studies have supported this effect, although the mechanisms have not been determined. Some studies have shown an increase in one form of cholesterol, HDL_2, which is believed to be protective. Other studies note an increase in HDL_3, which may also elicit a protective effect. Gaziano and others noted alcohol may reduce the risk of heart disease by raising the levels of both HDL_2 and HDL_3.

Another theory suggests alcohol decreases platelet aggregability (clotting ability) by increasing the activity of a clot-dissolving enzyme in the blood. In addition, certain alcoholic beverages may augment this effect. Red wine contains flavonoids (as does purple grape juice) which may slow the activity of platelets.

Other mechanisms may be operating as well. Alcohol may increase tissue response to insulin, possibly diminishing the role insulin levels play in increasing blood pressure and triglycerides, potential risk factors for CHD.

Although these factors may be important, some investigators contend that individuals who drink moderately may practice other life-style behaviors that reduce the risk for CHD. For example, a recent study from the University of Virginia reported that, contrary to expectations, runners drink more alcohol than non-exercisers. However, those with a history of drinking problems actually drank less. Additionally, a South Carolina research survey found that moderate, and even heavy, drinkers who do not smoke were more likely than nondrinkers to report engaging in regular leisure time physical activity. As noted in Chapter 1, exercise itself may reduce the risk of CHD.

Because of the potential for abuse, addiction, and all types of injuries, abstinence from alcohol or prudent consumption is generally recommended by health authorities. As noted above, abstinence is the best policy for pregnant women or if you plan to operate a motor vehicle. Health professionals, however, generally support the view that alcohol consumed in moderation, along with a balanced diet, should not pose any health problem to the average healthy individual. The definition of moderation has varied, but ranges from no more than 1 to 2 drinks per day, for women, and 1 to 3 drinks per day for men. Nevertheless, although there are actually some possible health benefits associated with alcohol consumption in moderation, health authorities caution that these potential benefits are not sufficient cause to start drinking if you currently abstain. You should consult with your physician if you are considering drinking for its possible health benefits.

References

Books

Hunt, S., and Groff, J. 1990. *Advanced Nutrition and Human Metabolism.* St. Paul, MN: West Publishing Company.

Jarvis, D. 1958. *Folk Medicine.* New York: Holt.

Jeukendrup, A. 1997. *Aspects of Carbohydrate and Fat Metabolism During Exercise.* Haarlem, Netherlands: De Vrieseborch.

National Research Council. 1989. *Diet and Health: Implications for Reducing Chronic Disease Risk.* Washington, DC: National Academy Press.

U.S. Department of Health and Human Services Public Health Service. 1991. *Healthy People 2000: National Health Promotion and Disease Prevention Objectives.* Washington, DC: Government Printing Office.

Wolinsky, I., and Hickson, J. 1993. *Nutrition in Exercise and Sport.* Boca Raton, FL: CRC Press.

Reviews

Anderson, O. 1997. Fat vs. carbohydrate: Which source of energy fuels finer running? *Running Research News* 13(3):1, 4–10.

Applegate, E. 1991. Nutritional considerations for ultraendurance performance. *International Journal of Sports Nutrition* 1:118–26.

Bennett, B., and Dotson, C. 1990. Effects of carbohydrate solutions on gastric emptying: A meta-analytic investigation. *Medicine and Science in Exercise and Sport* 22:S21.

Bennett, W., and Cerda, J. 1996. Benefits of dietary fiber. Myth or medicine? *Postgraduate Medicine* 99:153–72.

Clark, N. 1995. Energy bars: Are these fast fuelers for you? *Physician and Sportsmedicine* 23(9): 7–8.

Coate, D. 1993. Moderate drinking and coronary heart disease mortality: Evidence from NHANES I and the NHANES I follow-up. *American Journal of Public Health* 83:888–90.

Coggan, A. 1997. Symposium: Metabolic adaptations to endurance training: Recent advances. *Medicine and Science in Sports and Exercise* 29:620–76.

Coggan, A., and Swanson, S. 1992. Nutritional manipulations before and during endurance exercise: Effects on performance. *Medicine and Science in Sports and Exercise* 24 (No. 9 Supplement):S331–S335.

Coleman, E. 1994. Update on carbohydrate: Solid versus liquid. *International Journal of Sport Nutrition* 4:80–88.

Conley, M., and Stone, M. 1996. Carbohydrate ingestion/supplementation for resistance exercise and training. *Sports Medicine* 21:7–17.

Consumers Union. 1995. Fiber bounces back. *Consumer Reports on Health* 7:25–28.

Consumers Union. 1996. Alcohol: Spirit of health? *Consumer Reports on Health* 8:37–40.

Costill, D. 1988. Carbohydrates for exercise: Dietary demands for optimal performance. *International Journal of Sports Medicine* 9:1–18.

Coyle, E. 1991. Timing and method of increased carbohydrate intake to cope with heavy training, competition and recovery. *Journal of Sport Sciences* 9:29–52.

Coyle, E. 1992. Carbohydrate supplementation during exercise. *Journal of Nutrition* 122:788–95.

Coyle, E. 1993. Effects of diet on intermittent high intensity exercise. In *Intermittent High Intensity Exercise,* ed. D. MacLeod, et al. London: E. and F. N. Spon.

Coyle, E. 1995. Substrate utilization during exercise in active people. *American Journal of Clinical Nutrition* 61 (Supplement): 968S–979S.

Coyle, E., and Coyle, E. 1993. Carbohydrates that speed recovery from training. *Physician and Sportsmedicine* 21 (February): 111–23.

Coyle, E., and Montain, S. 1992. Carbohydrate and fluid ingestion during exercise: Are there trade-offs? *Medicine and Science in Sports and Exercise* 24:671–78.

Davis, J. M. 1996. Carbohydrates, branched-chain amino acids and endurance: The central fatigue hypothesis. *Sports Science Exchange* 9 (2): 1–6.

Food and Drug Administration. 1996. FDA statement on aspartame. *FDA Talk Paper* T96–75, November 18.

Gans, D. 1991. Sucrose and unusual childhood behavior. *Nutrition Today* 26 (May/June): 8–14.

Gibbons, B. 1992. Alcohol: The legal drug. *National Geographic* 181:3–35.

Greenhaff, P., et al. 1993. Carbohydrate metabolism. In *Principles of Exercise Biochemistry,* ed. J. Poortmans. Basel, Switzerland: Karger.

Guezennec, C. 1995. Oxidation rates, complex carbohydrates and exercise. *Sports Medicine* 19:365–372.

Hargreaves, M. 1996. Carbohydrates and exercise performance. *Nutrition Reviews* 54: S136–S139.

Hawley, J., and Hopkins, W. 1995. Aerobic glycolytic and aerobic lipolytic power systems. *Sports Medicine* 19:240–250.

Hawley, J., et al. 1997. Carbohydrate-loading and exercise performance: An update. *Sports Medicine* 24:73–81.

Hawley, J., et al. 1994. Carbohydrate, fluid, and electrolyte requirements of the soccer player: A review. *International Journal of Sport Nutrition* 4:221–236.

Hawley, J., et al. 1992. Oxidation of carbohydrate ingested during prolonged endurance exercise. *Sports Medicine* 14: 27–42.

Holloszy, J., and Kohrt, W. 1996. Regulation of carbohydrate and fat metabolism during and after exercise. *Annual Reviews of Nutrition* 16:121–38.

Houtkooper, L. 1992. Food selection for endurance sports. *Medicine and Science in Sports and Exercise* 24: S349–S359.

Howe, G., et al. 1992. Dietary intake of fiber and decreased risk of cancers of the colon and rectum: Evidence from the combined analysis of 13 case-control studies. *Journal of the National Cancer Institute* 84:1887–96.

International Life Science Institute. 1995. Complex carbohydrates: The science and the label. *Nutrition Reviews* 53:186–93.

Ivy, J. 1991. Muscle glycogen synthesis before and after exercise. *Sports Medicine* 11:6–19.

Klatsky, A., et al. 1992. Alcohol and mortality. *Annals of Internal Medicine* 117:646–53.

Kuipers, H. 1996. How much is too much? Performance aspects of overtraining. *Research Quarterly for Exercise and Sport* 67 (Supplement): S65–S69.

Kune, G., and Vitetta, L. 1992. Alcohol consumption and the etiology of colorectal cancer: A review of the scientific evidence from 1957 to 1991. *Nutrition and Cancer* 18:97–111.

Liebman, M., and Wilkenson, J. 1993. Carbohydrate metabolism and exercise. In *Nutrition in Exercise and Sport,* eds. I. Wolinsky and J. Hickson. Boca Raton, FL: CRC Press.

Lindeman, A. 1992. Eating for endurance or ultraendurance. *Physician and Sportsmedicine* 20 (March): 87–104.

Maughan, R. 1991. Carbohydrate-electrolyte solutions during prolonged exercise. In *Perspectives in Exercise Science and Sports Medicine. Ergogenics: The Enhancement of Sports Performance,* eds. D. Lamb and M. H. Williams. Indianapolis, IN: Benchmark.

Maughan, R., et al. 1997. Diet composition and the performance of high-intensity exercise. *Journal of Sports Sciences* 15:265–75.

Miller, G. 1993. Carbohydrates in ultra-endurance exercise and athletic performance. In *Nutrition in Exercise and Sport,* eds. I. Wolinsky and J. Hickson. Boca Raton, FL: CRC Press.

Mufti, S. 1992. Alcohol acts to promote incidence of tumors. *Cancer Detection and Prevention* 16:157–62.

National Diary Council. 1997. Dairy food sensitivity: Facts and fallacies. *Dairy Council Digest* 68 (3): 13–18.

Newsholme, E. 1993. Basic aspects of metabolic regulation and their application to provision of energy in exercise. In *Principles of Exercise Biochemistry,* ed. J. Poortmans. Basel, Switzerland: Karger.

Newsholme, E. 1993. Application of knowledge of metabolic integration to the problem of metabolic limitations in sprints, middle distance and marathon running. In *Principles of Exercise Biochemistry,* ed. J. Poortmans. Basel, Switzerland: Karger.

O'Brien, C. 1993. Alcohol and sport. *Sports Medicine* 15:71–77.

Pascoe, D., and Gladden, L. 1996. Muscle glycogen resynthesis after short term, high intensity exercise and resistance exercise. *Sports Medicine* 21:98–118.

Percival, L. 1955. Experience with honey in athletic nutrition. *American Bee Journal* 95:390–93.

Ripsin, C., et al. 1992. Oat products and lipid lowering: A meta-analysis. *Journal of the American Medical Association* 267:3317–25.

Rose, D. 1990. Dietary fiber and breast cancer. *Nutrition and Cancer* 13:1–8.

Roth, H., et al. 1994. Alcoholic beverages and breast cancer: Some observations on published case-control studies. *Journal of Clinical Epidemiology* 47:207–16.

Schneeman, B., and Tietgen, J. 1994. Dietary fiber. In *Modern Nutrition in Health and Disease,* eds. M. Shils, et al. Philadelphia: Lea and Febiger.

Sherman, W. 1991. Carbohydrate meals before and after exercise. In *Perspectives in Exercise Science and Sports Medicine. Ergogenics: The Enhancement of Sports Performance,* eds. D. Lamb and M. H. Williams. Indianapolis, IN: Benchmark.

Sherman, W., and Wimer, G. 1991. Insufficient dietary carbohydrate during training: Does it impair athletic performance? *International Journal of Sports Nutrition* 1:28–44.

Short, S. 1993. Surveys of dietary intake and nutrition knowledge of athletes and their coaches. In *Nutrition in Exercise and Sport,* eds. I. Wolinsky and J. Hickson. Boca Raton, FL: CRC Press.

Singh, A., et al. 1994. Dietary requirements for ultra-endurance exercise. *Sports Medicine* 18:301–8.

Slavin, J. 1994. Whole grains and health: Separating the wheat from the chaff. *Nutrition Today* 29 (4): 6–11.

Slavin, J. 1992. Dietary fiber and cancer update. *Contemporary Nutrition* 17(8): 1–2.

Slavin, J. 1990. Dietary fiber: Mechanisms or magic on disease prevention? *Nutrition Today* (November/December) 25: 9–13.

Steinmetz, G. 1992. Fetal alcohol syndrome: The preventable tragedy. *National Geographic* 181:36–39.

Stoll, B. 1996. Can supplementary dietary fibre suppress breast cancer growth? *British Journal of Cancer* 73:557–59.

Suh, I., et al. 1992. Alcohol use and mortality from coronary heart disease: The role of high-density lipoprotein cholesterol. *Annals of Internal Medicine* 116:881–87.

Walberg-Rankin, J. 1997. Glycemic index and exercise metabolism. *Sports Science Exchange* 10(1): 1–7.

Walberg-Rankin, J. 1995. Dietary carbohydrate as an ergogenic aid for prolonged and brief competitions in sport. *International Journal of Sport Nutrition* 5:S13–S28.

Walsh, J. 1996. Sugar found innocent of charges but what it does to diets is criminal. *Environmental Nutrition* 19 (11): 1, 6.

Walton, P., and Rhodes, E. 1997. Glycaemic index and optimal performance. *Sports Medicine* 23:164–72.

Williams, M. 1992. Alcohol and sports performance. *Sports Science Exchange* 4(40):1–4.

Wolfe, R., and George, S. 1993. Stable isotopic tracers as metabolic probes in exercise. *Exercise and Sports Science Reviews* 21:1–31.

Specific Studies

Akermark, C., et al. 1996. Diet and muscle glycogen concentration in relation to physical performance in Swedish elite ice hockey players. *International Journal of Sport Nutrition* 6:272–84.

Ball, T., et al. 1995. Periodic carbohydrate replacement during 50 min of high intensity cycling improves subsequent sprint performance. *International Journal of Sport Nutrition* 5:151–58.

Bangsbo, J. 1992. The effect of carbohydrate diet on intermittent exercise performance. *International Journal of Sports Medicine* 13:152–57.

Barrett, D., et al. 1995. The association between alcohol use and health behaviors related to the risk of cardiovascular disease: The South Carolina Cardiovascular Disease Prevention Project. *Journal of Studies on Alcohol* 56:9–15.

Below, P., et al. 1995. Fluid and carbohydrate ingestion independently improve performance during 1 h of intense exercise. *Medicine and Science in Sports and Exercise* 27:200–10.

Bianchi, C., et al. 1993. Alcohol consumption and the risk of acute myocardial infarction in women. *Journal of Epidemiology and Community Health* 47:308–11.

Blair, S., et al. 1980. Blood lipid and ECG response to carbohydrate loading. *Physician and Sports Medicine* 8:69–75.

Blom, T., et al. 1987. The effects of different post-exercise sugar diets on the rate of muscle glycogen resynthesis. *Medicine and Science in Sports and Exercise* 19:491–96.

Borg, G., et al. 1990. Effect of alcohol on perceived exertion in relation to heart rate and blood lactate. *European Journal of Applied Physiology* 60:382–84.

Bosch, A., et al. 1994. Influence of carbohydrate ingestion on fuel substrate turnover and oxidation during prolonged exercise. *Journal of Applied Physiology* 76:2364–72.

Brouns, F., et al. 1995. Chronic oral lactate supplementation does not affect lactate disappearance from blood after exercise. *International Journal of Sport Nutrition* 5:117–24.

Burke, L., et al. 1993. Muscle glycogen storage after prolonged exercise: Effect of the glycemic index of carbohydrate feedings. *Journal of Applied Physiology* 75:1019–23.

Burke, L., et al. 1996. Muscle glycogen storage after prolonged exercise: Effect of the frequency of carbohydrate feedings. *American Journal of Clinical Nutrition* 64:115–19.

Carey, K., and Correia, C. 1997. Drinking motives predict alcohol-related problems in college students. *Journal of Studies on Alcohol* 58:100–105.

Chryssanthopoulos, C., et al. 1994. Comparison between carbohydrate feedings before and during exercise on running performance during a 30-km treadmill time trial. *International Journal of Sport Nutrition* 4:374–86.

Chryssanthopoulos, C., et al. 1994. The influence of pre-exercise glucose ingestion on endurance running capacity. *British Journal of Sports Medicine* 28:105–9.

Clark, N., et al. 1992. Feeding the ultraendurance athlete: Practical tips and a case study. *Journal of the American Dietetic Association* 92:1258–62.

Davis, J., et al. 1992. The effects of carbohydrate feedings on plasma free tryptophan and branched-chain amino acids during prolonged cycling. *European Journal of Applied Physiology* 65 (6): 513–19.

Derman, K., et al. 1996. Fuel kinetics during intense running and cycling when fed carbohydrate. *European Journal of Applied Physiology* 74:36–43.

el-Sayed, M., et al. 1997. Carbohydrate ingestion improves performance during a 1 h simulated cycling trial. *Journal of Sports Sciences* 15:223–30.

el-Sayed, M. 1995. Effects of carbohydrate feeding before and during prolonged exercise on subsequent maximal exercise performance capacity. *International Journal of Sport Nutrition* 5:215–24.

Essen, B. 1978. Glycogen depletion of different fiber types in human skeletal muscle during intermittent and continuous exercise. *Acta Physiologica Scandinavica* 103:446–55.

Fallowfield, J., et al. 1995. The influence of ingesting a carbohydrate-electrolyte beverage during 4 hours of recovery on subsequent endurance capacity. *International Journal of Sport Nutrition* 5:285–89.

Febbraio, M., et al. 1996. Effect of CHO ingestion on exercise metabolism and performance in different ambient temperatures. *Medicine and Science in Sports and Exercise* 28:1380–87.

Febbraio, M., and Stewart, K. 1996. CHO feeding before prolonged exercise: Effect of glycemic index on muscle glycogenolysis and exercise performance. *Journal of Applied Physiology* 81:1115–20.

Fogelholm, M., et al. 1991. Carbohydrate loading in practice: High muscle glycogen concentration is not certain. *British Journal of Sports Medicine* 25:41–44.

Fraenkel-Conrat, H., and Singer, B. 1988. Nucleoside adducts are formed by cooperative reactions of acetaldehyde and alcohols: Possible mechanism for the role of alcohol in carcinogenesis. *Proceedings of the National Academy of Sciences* 85:3758–61.

Friedlander, A., et al. 1997. Training-induced alterations of glucose flux in men. *Journal of Applied Physiology* 82:1360–69.

Gaziano, J., et al. 1993. Moderate alcohol intake, increased levels of high-density lipoprotein and its subfractions, and decreased risk of myocardial infarction. *New England Journal of Medicine* 329:1829–34.

Goforth, H., et al. 1997. Persistence of supercompensated muscle glycogen in trained subjects after carbohydrate loading. *Journal of Applied Physiology* 82:342–47.

Goodpaster, B., et al. 1996. The effects of pre-exercise starch ingestion on endurance performance. *International Journal of Sports Medicine* 17:366–72.

Gutgesell, M., et al. 1996. Reported alcohol use and behavior in long-distance runners. *Medicine and Science in Sports and Exercise* 28:1063–70.

Hargreaves, M., et al. 1995. Influence of muscle glycogen on glycogenolysis and glucose uptake during exercise in humans. *Journal of Applied Physiology* 78:288–92.

Hawley, J., et al. 1991. High rates of exogenous carbohydrate oxidation from starch ingested during prolonged exercise. *Journal of Applied Physiology* 71:1801–06.

Horowitz, J., et al. 1989. Effects of carbohydrate loading and exercise on muscle girth. *Medicine and Science in Sports and Exercise* 21:S58.

Ivy, J., et al. 1988. Muscle glycogen synthesis after exercise: effect of time of carbohydrate ingestion. *Journal of Applied Physiology* 64:1480–85.

Jandrain, B., et al. 1993. Fructose utilization during exercise in man: Rapid conversion of ingested fructose to circulating glucose. *Journal of Applied Physiology* 74:2146–54.

Jarvis, J., et al. 1992. The effect of food matrix on carbohydrate utilization during moderate exercise. *Medicine and Science in Sports and Exercise* 24:320–26.

Jenkins, D., et al. 1994. The influence of dietary carbohydrate and pre-exercise glucose consumption on supramaximal intermittent exercise performance. *British Journal of Sports Medicine* 28:171–76.

Jeukendrup, A., et al. 1997. Carbohydrate-electrolyte feedings improve 1 h time trial cycling performance. *International Journal of Sports Medicine.* 18:125–29.

Jozsi, A., et al. 1996. The influence of starch structure on glycogen resynthesis and subsequent cycling performance. *International Journal of Sports Medicine* 17:373–78.

Kang, J., et al. 1996. Effect of carbohydrate substrate availability on ratings of perceived exertion during prolonged exercise of moderate intensity. *Perceptual and Motor Skills* 82:495–506.

Kang, J., et al. 1995. Effect of carbohydrate ingestion subsequent to carbohydrate supercompensation on endurance performance. *International Journal of Sport Nutrition* 5:329–43.

Keith, R., et al. 1991. Alterations in dietary carbohydrate, protein, and fat intake and mood state in trained female cyclists. *Medicine and Science in Sports and Exercise* 23:212–16.

Kendrick, Z., et al. 1993. Effect of ethanol on metabolic responses to treadmill running in well-trained men. *Journal of Clinical Pharmacology* 33:136–39.

Klesges, R., et al. 1994. Effects of alcohol intake on resting energy expenditure in young women social drinkers. *American Journal of Clinical Nutrition* 59:805–9.

Lamb, D., et al. 1991. Muscle glycogen loading with a liquid carbohydrate supplement. *International Journal of Sport Nutrition* 1:52–60.

Lamb, D., et al. 1990. Dietary carbohydrate and intensity of interval swim training. *American Journal of Clinical Nutrition* 52:1058–63.

Larsen, J., et al. 1988. Effects of ingesting polylactate during prolonged cycling. Paper presented at Southwest Regional Meeting of the American College of Sports Medicine, Las Vegas, NV. December 1988.

Liu, S., et al. 1997. Prevalence of alcohol-impaired driving. *Journal of the American Medical Association* 277:122–25.

Macfarlane, G., et al. 1996. The influence of alcohol consumption on worldwide trends in mortality from upper aerodigestive tract cancers in men. *Journal of Epidemiology and Community Health* 50:636–39.

Madsen, K., et al. 1996. Effects of glucose, glucose plus branched-chain amino acids, or placebo on bike performance over 100 km. *Journal of Applied Physiology* 81:2644–50.

Marmy-Conus, N., et al. 1996. Preexercise glucose ingestion and glucose kinetics during exercise. *Journal of Applied Physiology* 81:853–57.

Mason, W., et al. 1993. Carbohydrate ingestion during exercise: Liquid vs solid feedings. *Medicine and Science in Sports and Exercise* 25:966–69.

Massicotte, D., et al. 1992. Metabolic availability of oral glucose during exercise: A reassessment. *Metabolism* 12: 1284–90.

McConell, G., et al. 1996. Effect of timing of carbohydrate ingestion on endurance exercise performance. *Medicine and Science in Sports and Exercise* 28:1311–20.

Millard-Stafford, M., et al. 1992. Carbohydrate-electrolyte replacement improves distance running performance in the heat. *Medicine and Science in Sports and Exercise* 24:934–40.

Murray, R., et al. 1989. The effects of glucose, fructose, and sucrose ingestion during exercise. *Medicine and Science in Sports and Exercise* 21:275–82.

Myers, J., et al. 1990. Effect of fructose 1,6-diphosphate infusion on the hormonal response to exercise. *Medicine and Science in Sports and Exercise* 22:102–5.

Niekamp, R., and Baer, J. 1995. In-season dietary adequacy of trained male cross-country runners. *International Journal of Sport Nutrition* 5:45–55.

Nishibata, I., et al. 1993. Glucose ingestion before and during exercise does not enhance performance of daily repeated endurance exercise. *European Journal of Applied Physiology* 66:65–69.

O'Brien, M., et al. 1993. Carbohydrate dependence during marathon running. *Medicine and Science in Sports and Exercise* 25:1009–17.

Okano, G., et al. 1996. Effect of 4 h preexercise high carbohydrate and high fat meal ingestion on endurance performance and metabolism. *International Journal of Sports Medicine* 17:530–34.

Parkin, J., et al. 1997. Muscle glycogen storage following prolonged exercise: Effect of timing of ingestion of high glycemic index food. *Medicine and Science in Sports and Exercise* 29:220–24.

Peronnet, F., et al. 1992. Exogenous substrate oxidation during exercise: Studies using isotopic labelling. *International Journal of Sports Medicine* 13 (Supplement 1): S123–S125.

Peters, H., et al. 1995. Exercise performance as a function of semi-solid and liquid carbohydrate feedings during prolonged exercise. *International Journal of Sports Medicine* 16:105–13.

Pitsiladis, Y., et al. 1996. Effects of alterations in dietary carbohydrate intake on running performance during a 10 km treadmill time trial. *British Journal of Sports Medicine* 30:226–31.

Pizza, F., et al. 1995. A carbohydrate loading regimen improves high intensity, short duration exercise performance. *International Journal of Sport Nutrition* 5:110–16.

Rauch, L., et al. 1995. The effects of carbohydrate loading on muscle glycogen content and cycling performance. *International Journal of Sport Nutrition* 5:25–36.

Rehrer, N., et al. 1992. Gastric emptying, absorption, and carbohydrate oxidation during prolonged exercise. *Journal of Applied Physiology* 72:468–75.

Reilly, T., and Scott, J. 1993. Effects of elevating blood alcohol levels on tasks related to dart throwing. *Perceptual and Motor Skills* 77:25–26.

Rimm, E., et al. 1996. Vegetable, fruit, and cereal fiber intake and risk of coronary heart disease among men. *Journal of the American Medical Association* 275:47–51.

Rumpler, W., et al. 1996. Energy value of moderate alcohol consumption by humans. *American Journal of Clinical Nutrition* 64:108–14.

Salmeron, J., et al. 1997. Dietary fiber, glycemic load, and risk of non-insulin-dependent diabetes mellitus in women. *Journal of the American Medical Association* 277:472–77.

Saris, W. 1989. Study of food intake and energy expenditure during extreme sustained exercise. The Tour de France. *International Journal of Sports Medicine* 10:S26–S31.

Seifert, J., et al. 1994. Glycemic and insulinemic response to preexercise carbohydrate feedings. *International Journal of Sport Nutrition* 4:46–53.

Sherman, W., et al. 1993. Dietary carbohydrate, muscle glycogen, and exercise performance during 7 d of training. *American Journal of Clinical Nutrition* 57:27–31.

Snyder, A., et al. 1993. Carbohydrate consumption prior to repeated bouts of high-intensity exercise. *European Journal of Applied Physiology* 66:141–45.

Spohr, H., et al. 1993. Prenatal alcohol exposure and long-term developmental consequences. *Lancet* 341:907–10.

Stanko, R., et al. 1990. Enhanced leg exercise endurance with a high-carbohydrate diet and dihydroxyacetone and pyruvate. *Journal of Applied Physiology* 69:1651–56.

Stanko, R., et al. 1990. Enhancement of arm exercise endurance capacity with dihydroxyacetone and pyruvate. *Journal of Applied Physiology* 68:119–24.

Suter, P., et al. 1992. The effect of ethanol on fat storage in healthy subjects. *New England Journal of Medicine* 326:983–87.

Tarnopolsky, M., et al. 1995. Carbohydrate loading and metabolism during exercise in men and women. *Journal of Applied Physiology* 78:1360–68.

Taylor, S., and Chermack, S. 1993. Alcohol, drugs, and human physical aggression. *Journal of Studies on Alcohol Supplement* 11:78–88.

Thomas, D., et al. 1991. Carbohydrate feeding before exercise: Effect of glycemic index. *International Journal of Sports Medicine* 12:180–86.

Tremblay, A., et al. 1995. Alcohol and a high-fat diet: A combination favoring overfeeding. *American Journal of Clinical Nutrition* 62:639–44.

Tsintzas, O., et al. 1996. influence of carbohydrate supplementation early in exercise on endurance running capacity. *Medicine and Science in Sports and Exercise* 28:1373–79.

Tsintzas, O., et al. 1996. Carbohydrate ingestion and single muscle fiber glycogen metabolism during prolonged running in men. *Journal of Applied Physiology* 81:801–9.

Tsintzas, O., et al. 1995. Influence of carbohydrate-electrolyte drinks on marathon running performance. *European Journal of Applied Physiology* 70:154–60.

Vandenberghe, K., et al. 1995. No effect of glycogen level on glycogen metabolism during high intensity exercise. *Medicine and Science in Sports and Exercise* 27:1278–83.

Van Horn, L., et al. 1991. Effects on serum lipids of adding instant oats to usual American diets. *American Journal of Public Health* 81:183–88.

Vollestad, N., et al. 1984. Muscle glycogen depletion patterns in type I and subgroups of type II fibers during prolonged severe exercise in man. *Acta Physiologica Scandinavica* 122:433–41.

Wagenmakers, A., et al. 1991. Carbohydrate supplementation, glycogen depletion, and amino acid metabolism during exercise. *American Journal of Physiology* 260:E883–E890.

Walberg-Rankin, J., et al. 1996. Effect of weight loss and refeeding diet composition on anaerobic performance in wrestlers. *Medicine and Science in Sports and Exercise* 28:1292–99.

Wang, M., et al. 1995. The acute effect of moderate alcohol consumption on cardiovascular responses in women. *Journal of Studies on Alcohol* 56:16–20.

Wannamethee, G., and Shaper, A. 1992. Alcohol and sudden cardiac death. *British Heart Journal* 68:443–48.

Wechsler, H., et al. 1994. Health and behavioral consequences of binge drinking in college. *Journal of the American Medical Association* 272:1672–77.

Williams, C., et al. 1992. The effect of a high carbohydrate diet on running performance during a 30-km treadmill time trial. *European Journal of Applied Physiology* 65:18–24.

Wright, D., et al. 1991. Carbohydrate feedings before, during, or in combination improve cycling endurance performance. *Journal of Applied Physiology* 71:1082–88.

Yaspelkis, B., et al. 1993. Carbohydrate metabolism during exercise in hot and thermoneutral environments. *International Journal of Sports Medicine* 14:13–19.

Yaspelkis, B., et al. 1993. Carbohydrate supplementation spares muscle glycogen during variable-intensity exercise. *Journal of Applied Physiology* 75:1477–85.

Zachwieja, J., et al. 1991. Influence of muscle glycogen depletion on the rate of resynthesis. *Medicine and Science in Sports and Exercise* 23:44–48.

Zawadzki, B., et al. 1992. Carbohydrate-protein complex increases the rate of muscle glycogen storage after exercise. *Journal of Applied Physiology* 72:1854–59.

Zeederberg, C., et al. 1996. The effect of carbohydrate ingestion on the motor skill proficiency of soccer players. *International Journal of Sport Nutrition* 6:348–55.

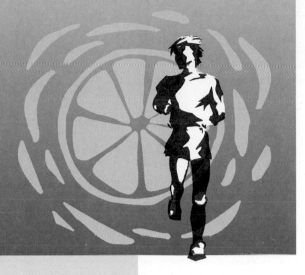

Fat: An Important Energy Source During Exercise

CHAPTER 5

KEY CONCEPTS

- The three major lipids in human nutrition are triglycerides, cholesterol, and phospholipids.

- The fat content of foods varies considerably, but generally the fruit, vegetable, and starch food exchanges are good sources of unsaturated fats and are low in total fat, whereas the meat and milk food exchanges have a high total fat and saturated fat content.

- Although some fat is essential in the diet as a source of essential fatty acids and the fat-soluble vitamins, these nutrients may be obtained from polyunsaturated fats.

- Cholesterol is a nonfat substance vital to human metabolism, and although it may be obtained in the diet only from animal foods, the body can produce its own supply from other dietary nutrients such as saturated fats.

- Dietary lipids may be utilized as an energy source, stored in the adipose tissue, or used as part of body-cell structure. By-products of fat metabolism, eicosanoids, may act as local hormones and affect a variety of physiological functions.

- Fats are transported in the blood primarily as lipoproteins, but plasma free fatty acids from adipose tissue are a major source of energy during lower intensity exercise.

- One of the major functions of fat is to provide energy. Although fat may be an important energy source for low- to moderate-intensity exercise, it is not the optimal energy source during high-intensity aerobic or anaerobic exercise.

- Fat loading, wheat germ oil, lecithin, carnitine, omega-3 fatty acids, and fasting do not appear to be effective ergogenic aids; additional research is needed with medium-chain triglycerides.

- Research suggests that caffeine may improve performance in a variety of athletic endeavors. Some evidence indicates that caffeine may be beneficial in prolonged endurance events, possibly through a glycogen-sparing effect, and also in short-term aerobic exercise tasks, possibly through a psychological effect.

- Low-density forms of lipoproteins (LDL) may predispose certain individuals to coronary heart disease whereas high-density forms (HDL) may be protective.

- Diets high in saturated fats and cholesterol may increase the risk of coronary heart disease, so the recommended dietary intake of total fat is 30 percent or less of the total caloric intake with saturated fats at less than 10 percent of the total. The recommended cholesterol intake is less than 300 milligrams per day, or 100 milligrams per 1,000 Calories.

- In general, a low-fat diet is recommended for both health and physical performance. One should consume less high-fat meat and dairy products and more fruits, vegetables, whole-grain products, dietary fiber, lean meats, and skim milk.

KEY TERMS

alpha-linolenic acid
angina
apolipoprotein
arteriosclerosis
atherosclerosis
beta-oxidation
caffeine
carnitine
cholesterol
chylomicron
coronary artery disease (CAD)
coronary heart disease (CHD)
coronary occlusion
coronary thrombosis
eicosanoids
ester
fatty acids
fat loading
fat substitutes
glycerol
hidden fat
HDL (high-density lipoproteins)
ischemia
ketones
LDL (low-density lipoproteins)
lecithin
linoleic acid
lipids
lipoprotein
lipoprotein (a)
medium-chain triglycerides (MCTs)
monounsaturated fatty acid
myocardial infarct
omega-3 fatty acids

INTRODUCTION

From a health standpoint dietary fat is the nutrient of greatest concern to a variety of health organizations, such as the American Heart Association and the American Cancer Society, for excessive consumption of certain types of fat has been associated with the development of a host of pathological conditions, including coronary heart disease, cancer, and obesity. Thus, one of the major recommendations advocated in *Healthy People 2000* for a healthier diet is to reduce the amount of dietary fat intake to a reasonable level. Part of the rationale for this recommendation and some general guidelines for implementing it are presented in this chapter, but additional information may also be found in Chapters 2 and 11.

We need some fat in our diet. Despite its potential health hazards, dietary fat contains several essential nutrients that serve a variety of important functions in human nutrition. For the endurance athlete, one of the most important functions of fat is to provide energy during exercise, and researchers have explored a variety of techniques in attempts to improve endurance performance by increasing the ability of the muscle to use fat as a fuel.

To clarify the role of dietary fat in health and its possible relevance to sports, this chapter presents information on the basic nature of dietary fats and the associated compound cholesterol, the metabolic fate and physiological functions of fats and cholesterol in the body, the role of fat as an energy source during exercise, the use of various dietary practices or ergogenic aids to improve fat metabolism and endurance performance, and possible health problems associated with excessive dietary fat.

Dietary Fats

What are the different types of dietary fats?

What we commonly call fat in our diet actually consists of several substances classified as lipids. **Lipids** represent a class of organic substances that are insoluble in water but soluble in certain solvents like alcohol or ether. The three major lipids of importance to humans are triglycerides, cholesterol, and phospholipids. All three have major functions in the body.

What are triglycerides?

The **triglycerides,** also known as the true fats or the neutral fats, are the principal form in which fats are eaten and stored in the human body. Triglycerides are composed of two different compounds—fatty acids and glycerol. When an acid (fatty acid) and an alcohol (glycerol) combine, an **ester** is formed, the process being known as esterification. (Three fatty acids are attached to each glycerol molecule.) Figure 5.1 is a diagram of a triglyceride.

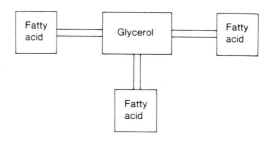

Figure 5.1 Structure of a triglyceride. Three fatty acids combine with glycerol to form a triglyceride.

Fatty acids, one of the components of fat, are chains of carbon, oxygen, and hydrogen atoms that vary in length and in the degree of saturation of carbon with hydrogen. Short-chain fatty acids contain fewer than six carbons, medium-chain fatty acids have six to twelve carbons, long-chain fatty acids have fourteen or more carbons. A **saturated fatty acid** contains a full quota of hydrogenated ions so that all of its chemical bonds are full. Unsaturated fatty acids may absorb more hydrogen because they have some unfilled bonds, or double bonds. These latter fatty acids may be classified as **monounsaturated,** having a single double bond and capable of absorbing two hydrogen ions, and **polyunsaturated,** having two or more double bonds and capable of absorbing four or more hydrogen ions. At room temperature, saturated fats are usually solid, while unsaturated fats are usually liquid. **Partially hydrogenated fats** or oils have been treated by a process that adds hydrogen to some of the unfilled bonds, thereby hardening the fat or oil. In essence, the fat becomes more saturated. During the hydrogenation process, the normal position of hydrogen ions at the double bond known as *cis*, or same side, may be partly transposed so that hydrogen ions are on opposite sides of the double bond, resulting in a **trans fatty acid. Omega-3 fatty acids** are a special class of polyunsaturated fatty acids found mainly in fish oils. Figure 5.2 represents the structural difference between a saturated, a monounsaturated, an unsaturated (cis and trans), and an omega-3 fatty acid. The health implications of these different types of fats are discussed later in this chapter. In general though, excess intake of saturated and trans fatty acids is associated with increased health risks, whereas adequate intake of monounsaturated, polyunsaturated, and omega-3 fatty acids may be associated with neutral or some beneficial health effects. Bell and others noted recently that food technology is evolving to create structured triglycerides that may possess health benefits.

Glycerol is an alcohol, a clear, colorless syrupy liquid. It is obtained in the diet as part of triglycerides, but it also may be produced in the body as a by-product of carbohydrate metabolism. On the other hand, glycerol can be converted back to carbohydrate in the process of gluconeogenesis in the liver.

What are some common foods high in fat content?

The fat content in foods can vary from 100 percent, as found in most cooking oils, to minor trace amounts, less than 5–10 percent, as found in most fruits and vegetables. Some foods obviously have a high-fat content: butter, oils, shortening, mayonnaise, margarine, and the visible fat on meat. However, in other foods the fat content may be high but not as obvious. This is known as **hidden fat.** For example, whole milk, cheese, nuts, desserts, crackers, potato chips, and a wide variety of commercially prepared foods may contain considerable amounts of fat. For example, a 5-ounce baked potato contains 145 Calories with about 3 percent fat, while a 5-ounce serving of potato chips contains 795 Calories, over 60 percent of them from fat. Figure 5.3 presents some examples of hidden fat.

In general, animal foods found in the meat and milk groups are high in fat, particularly saturated fat. However, careful selection

and preparation of foods in these groups will considerably reduce fat content. The percentage of fat in meats may vary considerably. In the meat group, beef and pork products usually contain considerable amounts of fat, up to 70 percent fat Calories. However, the meat industry is responding to dietary modifications by many Americans

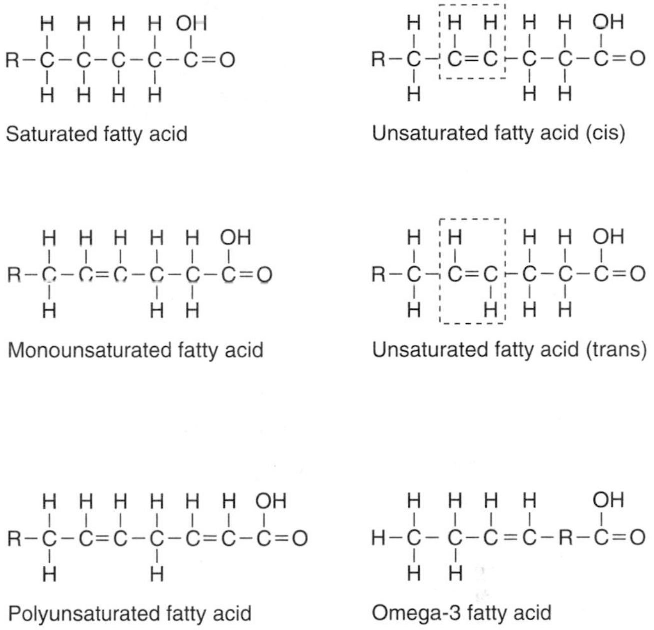

Figure 5.2 Structural differences between saturated, monounsaturated, and polyunsaturated fatty acids (including the cis and trans forms) and the omega-3 fatty acid. Note there is a single double bond between carbon atoms in the monounsaturated fatty acid and two or more in the polyunsaturated fatty acid. In the omega-3 fatty acid, the double bond is located three carbons from the last, or omega, carbon. The R represents the radical, or the presence of many more C—H bonds. In the trans configuration, one of the hydrogen ions is moved to the opposite side.

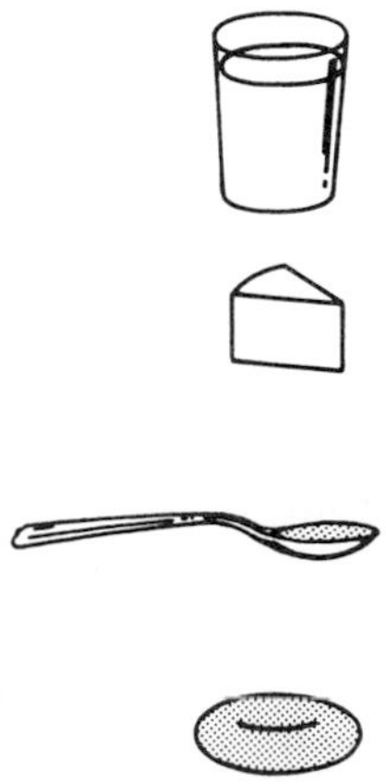

	Calories	Grams of fat	Percentage fat Calories
8 ounces whole milk	150	8	48%
1 ounce cheddar cheese	115	9	70%
1 tablespoon peanut butter	95	8	76%
1 doughnut	100	5	45%

Figure 5.3 Hidden fat. Many of the foods we consume may contain significant amounts of Calories in the form of hidden fat.

Table 5.1 — Approximate percentage of fatty acids in common fats and oils*

Oil/fat	Saturated fat	Monounsaturated fat	Polyunsaturated fat
Beef fat (tallow)	50+	43	4
Butterfat	62+	30	4
Chicken fat	30	46	22
Cocoa butter (chocolate)	60+	33	3
Coconut oil	87+	6	2
Canola oil (rapeseed oil)	6	62+	30
Corn oil	13	25	60+
Cottonseed oil	26	18	53+
Margarine (soft tub)	21	48	31
Olive oil	14	74+	9
Palm kernel oil	84+	12	2
Palm oil	50+	38	10
Peanut oil	17	48	33
Pork fat (lard)	40	47	12
Safflower oil	9	12	78+
Shortening (animal)	44	48	5
Shortening (vegetable)	26	43	25
Soybean oil	15	24	58+
Sunflower oil	11	20	66+
Tuna fat	27	26	37
Wheat germ oil	20	16	64+

*May not total 100 percent owing to the presence of other fatty substances
+ = high-content source

and is making low-fat red meats available to consumers. For example, 3 ounces of beef eye of round or pork tenderloin contain about 140 Calories, 4 grams of total fat, and 1.5 grams of saturated fat; both cuts of meat contain fewer than 30 percent of their Calories as fat. Poultry and fish have much lower levels of fat. Trimming the fat from meats or removing the skin from poultry drastically reduces the fat content. Some fish, such as flounder and tuna, are remarkably low in fat while others, such as salmon and mackerel, are higher in total fat content but contain greater amounts of omega-3 fatty acids. In the milk group, whole milk contains about 8 grams of fat per cup; skim milk contains about 0.5–1.0 grams, which is much less than whole milk.

Small amounts of trans fatty acids are found naturally in beef, butter, and milk, but deep-fried foods and commercially prepared products, particularly stick margarine and snack foods such as chips, cakes, and cookies, may contain substantial amounts.

Most plant foods, such as vegetables, fruits, beans, and natural whole-grain products, generally are low in fat content, and the fat they do contain is mostly unsaturated. On the other hand, some plant foods, such as nuts, seeds, and avocados, are very high in fat, but again primarily unsaturated fats. However, coconuts and palm kernels are extremely high in both total and saturated fats.

Since later in this chapter we discuss some health implications relating to the types of fats we eat, Table 5.1 presents an approximate percentage of the amount of saturated, monounsaturated, and polyunsaturated fatty acids found in some common oils and fats. Several high-content sources for each of the three types of fatty acids are noted.

Table 5.2 Calculation of the percentage of Calories in foods that are derived from fat

Method A. Data from food label

Amount per serving
Calories = 90

Calories from fat = 30

To calculate percentage of food Calories that consists of fat, simply divide the Calories from fat by the Calories per serving and multiply by 100 to express as a percent.

$$30/90 = 0.33 \qquad 0.33 \times 100 = 33 \text{ percent fat Calories}$$

Method B. Data from food composition table

Amount per serving
Calories = 90

Total fat, grams = 8

Saturated fat, grams = 3

To calculate percentage of food Calories that consists of total fat or saturated fat, use the caloric value for fat of 1 gram = 9 Calories.

Total fat = 8 grams

Total fat calories = 8 grams × 9 Calories/gram = 72 Calories

Use the same procedure as in Method A.

$$72/90 = 0.80 \qquad 0.80 \times 100 = 80 \text{ percent fat Calories}$$

Saturated fat = 3 grams

Saturated fat Calories = 3 grams × 9 Calories/gram = 27 Calories

$$27/90 = 0.30 \qquad 0.30 \times 100 = 30 \text{ percent saturated fat Calories}$$

How do I calculate the percentage of fat Calories in a food?

It is important to realize that a product advertised as 95 percent fat free (or only 5 percent fat) may contain a considerably higher percentage of its Calories as fat: The advertised percentage refers to the weight of the product, not its caloric content. The product may contain a considerable amount of water, which contains no Calories. Thus, luncheon meat advertised as 95 percent fat free may actually contain more than 40 percent of its Calories from fat depending upon the water weight. Foods with a high water content contain even higher percentages of fat Calories. A striking example is whole milk, which is only 3.5 percent fat by weight; however, one glass of milk contains about 150 Calories and 8 grams of fat, which accounts for 48 percent of the caloric content (8 × 9 = 72; 72/150 = 48). Even low-fat milk (2 percent fat) contains about 37 percent fat Calories.

If you want to calculate the percentage of fat calories in most foods you eat, you can get the information you need from the food label, which will include the total Calories and the Calories from fat; additional mandatory information is the total fat and saturated fat content. The label optionally may list the Calories from saturated fat and the amounts of polyunsaturated and monounsaturated fat. If you do not have a food label, then you will need to know the Calories and grams of fat for the food. Both of these values can be obtained from a food composition table found in most basic nutrition texts. Table 5.2 presents the methods for calculating the percent of fat Calories and percent of saturated fat Calories from either a food label or food composition table. Table 5.3 represents the percentage of food energy that is derived from fat in some common foods; the percentages are indicated for both total fat and saturated fat. Additional information is presented in Chapter 11, where the focus is on reducing high-fat foods in the diet as a means to Calorie control.

What are fat substitutes?

Fat substitutes, or fat replacers, are supposedly designed to provide the taste and texture of fats, but without the Calories (9 Calories per gram), saturated fat, or cholesterol.

Table 5.3 Percentage of total fat Calories and saturated fat Calories in some common foods*

Food	% Calories total fat	% Calories saturated fat	Food	% Calories total fat	% Calories saturated fat
Meat group			*Vegetables*		
Bacon	80	30	Asparagus	8	2
Beef, lean and fat (untrimmed)	70	32	Beans, green	7	1.5
			Broccoli	12	1.5
Beef, lean only (trimmed)	35	15	Carrots	4	< 1
Hamburger, regular	62	29	Potatoes	1	< 1
			Fruits		
Chicken, breast (with skin)	35	11	Apples	5	< 1
Chicken, breast (without skin)	19	5	Bananas	5	2
			Oranges	4	< 1
Luncheon meat (bologna)	82	35	*Starches/Breads/Cereals*		
Salmon	37	7	Bread		
Flounder, tuna	8	2	White	12	2
Egg, white and yolk	67	22	Whole wheat	12	2
			Crackers	30	12
Egg, white	0	0	Doughnuts	43	7
Milk group			Macaroni	5	< 1
Milk, whole	45	28	Macaroni and cheese	46	20
Milk, skim	5	2.5	Oatmeal	13	2
Cheese, cheddar	74	47	Pancakes, wheat	30	7
Cheese, mozzarella, part skim	56	35	Spaghetti	5	< 1
			Fats and oils		
Ice cream	49	28	Butter	99	62
Ice milk	31	18	Lard	99	40
Yogurt, partially skim milk	29	14	Margarine	99	21
			Oil, corn	100	13
Dried beans and nuts			Oil, coconut	100	87
Beans, dry, navy	4	< 1	Salad dressings		
Beans, navy, canned with pork	28	12	French	95	15
			French, special dietary low fat	14	< 1
Peanuts	77	17			
Peanut butter	76	19			

< 1 = less than 1 percent
*Percentages may vary. See food labels for specific information when available.

They are found in many normally high-fat products, such as ice cream, that are marketed as fat free. Fat substitutes may be manufactured from carbohydrate, protein, or fats. Although a number of fat substitutes are under development, the following are commonly used.

Some carbohydrates, such as starches and gums, provide thickness and structure and are useful as fat substitutes. Guar gum, gum arabic, and cellulose gel are examples. Oatrim, made from oats, is being used to replace fat in milk. Depending on the form used, the caloric content may range from 0–4 Calories per gram. These substances are generally recognized as safe and have been approved by the Food and Drug Administration (FDA).

Simplesse is manufactured from milk or egg protein by a microparticulation process so that it has the taste and texture of fat. The caloric value of Simplesse is only 1.3 Calories per gram. The use of Simplesse has been approved by the FDA.

Salatrim, which is an acronym for short- and long-chain fatty acid triglyceride molecule, is a modified fat containing only 5 Calories per gram. Olestra is an ester of sucrose with long-chain fatty acids, a structure that cannot be absorbed by the gastrointestinal tract and therefore supplies no Calories to the body. Although Olestra has been approved by the FDA, its use may interfere with the absorption of several fat-soluble vitamins and beta-carotene, and may cause intestinal cramps and loose stools in some individuals.

The use of fat substitutes to help decrease dietary fat intake is covered later in this chapter, and their use in weight-control programs is detailed in Chapter 11.

What is cholesterol?

Cholesterol is one of the lipids known as sterols. It is not a fat, but it is a fat-like pearly substance found in animal tissues. Cholesterol is not an essential nutrient for it is manufactured naturally in the liver of animals from fatty acids and from the breakdown products of carbohydrate and protein—glucose and amino acids.

What foods contain cholesterol?

Cholesterol is found only in animal products and is not found in fruits, vegetables, nuts, grains, or other nonanimal foods. Table 5.4 presents some foods from the meat and milk groups with the cholesterol content in milligrams. Several foods from the bread/cereal group are also included, indicating that the preparation of some bread/cereal products may add cholesterol by including some animal product containing cholesterol, mainly eggs. (See Figure 5.4.)

What are phospholipids?

Chemically, **phospholipids** are somewhat comparable to triglycerides. They have a glycerol base, one or two attached fatty acids, and an additional structure that con-

Table 5.4 Cholesterol content, in milligrams, for some common foods	Amount	Cholesterol
Meat group		
Beef, pork, ham	1 oz	25
Poultry	1 oz	23
Fish	1 oz	21
Shrimp	1 oz	45
Lobster	1 oz	25
Eggs	1	220
Liver	1 oz	120
Milk group		
Milk, whole	1 cup	27
Milk, 2%	1 cup	15
Milk, skim	1 cup	7
Butter	1 tsp	12
Margarine	1 tsp	0
Cream cheese	1 tbsp	18
Ice milk	1 cup	10
Ice cream	1 cup	85
Bread/Cereal group		
Bread	1 slice	0
Biscuit	1	17
Pancake	1	40
Sweet roll	1	25
French toast	1 slice	130
Doughnut	1	28
Cereal, cooked	1 cup	0
Fruits, vegetables, grains, and nuts have no cholesterol.		

tains a phosphate group. One of the most common phospholipids is lecithin, whose structure is depicted as a simple diagram in Figure 5.5. Phospholipids are not essential nutrients as the body can make them from triglycerides. As discussed later in this chapter, lecithin has been studied as a potential ergogenic aid.

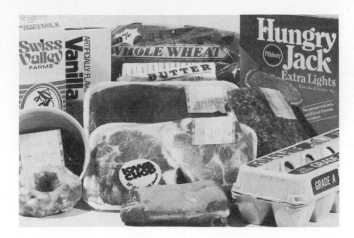

Figure 5.4 Foods high in cholesterol. Eggs added to flour in some products in manufacturing or preparation (for example, bread and pancake mix) will increase cholesterol content.

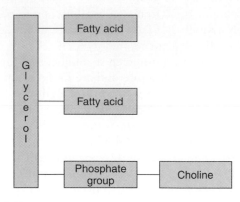

Figure 5.5 Simplified diagram of the phospholipid lecithin.

What foods contain phospholipids?

Egg yolks provide substantial amounts of lecithin, and other good sources include liver, wheat germ, and peanuts. However, lecithin may be degraded in the digestive tract to smaller constituents. Your body can make all of the phospholipids it needs. Because dietary phospholipids are not associated with any health risks, there is little concern with dietary intake.

How much fat and cholesterol do we need in the diet?

Dietary fat is essential to human metabolism for it provides us with a source of essential fatty acids and a means whereby fat-soluble vitamins are taken into the body. Most fatty acids may be synthesized in the body, but according to the National Research Council, **linoleic acid,** an essential polyunsaturated fatty acid, must be supplied in the diet because the body can not produce it from other fatty acids. **Alpha-linolenic acid,** an omega-3 fatty acid, is also considered to be an essential fatty acid. Research is continuing to determine whether other fatty acids must also be obtained through the diet. As shall be noted later, certain types of fatty acids may confer some health benefits.

Although no specific RDA has been established for the total amount of fat, the National Research Council recommends a minimum daily adequate amount of 3–6 grams of linoleic acid. Since almost all foods have some fat, sufficient amounts of this essential fatty acid are found in the average diet. Even on a vegetarian diet of fruits, vegetables, beans, and grain products, about 5–10 percent of your total Calories would be derived from fat and would provide an ample supply of linoleic acid. Approximately 15 grams of fat from vegetable sources would provide 5 grams of linoleic acid, so 1 tablespoon of a high-polyunsaturated fat, about 15 grams, would provide 5 grams of linoleic acid, within the minimum daily adequate amount recommended by the NRC.

Although the situation is improving, many Americans still eat too much fat. In the 1970s, the average American derived about 40 percent of dietary Calories from fat and about 15 percent from saturated fat, but the most recent data indicate those percentages have dropped to 33 and 12, respectively. Nevertheless, these values are still considered to be excessive and conducive to certain chronic diseases. The goals of the Healthy North American Diet are to reduce overall fat consumption to less than 30 percent of dietary Calories, with less than 10 percent from saturated fats, about 10–15 percent from monounsaturated fats, and no more than 10 percent from polyunsaturated fats. Some nutritionists also recommend that the consumption of omega-3 fatty acids, as a form of polyunsaturated fats, be increased through an increased intake of high-fat fishes like salmon. However, these goals are for adults, not for young children, particularly infants and children under 2 years of age, who need adequate energy and nutrients found in fat to support growth and development.

Cholesterol is vital to human physiology in a variety of ways, so the body needs an adequate supply. Because cholesterol may be manufactured in the body from either fats, carbohydrate, or protein, however, there is apparently little need for us to obtain large amounts, if any, in the foods we eat. Also, because a positive relationship has been established between high blood cholesterol levels and coronary heart disease, reduction of dietary cholesterol has been advocated by a number of health-related associations. The goal of the Healthy North American Diet is to reduce the average American intake of 400–500 milligrams or more of cholesterol per day to less than 300 milligrams, or about 100 milligrams of cholesterol for every 1,000 Calories you eat. Table 5.5 indicates the grams of fat and saturated fat and milligrams of cholesterol that

Table 5.5 Daily allowance for grams of fat and saturated fat, and milligrams of cholesterol*				
Total Calories	**Fat Calories**	**Grams of fat**	**Grams of saturated fat**	**mg of cholesterol**
1,000	300	33	11	100
1,500	450	50	16	150
2,000	600	66	22	200
2,500	750	83	27	250
3,000	900	100	33	300

*Based upon a diet containing 30 percent of Calories as fat with 100 milligrams of cholesterol per 1,000 Calories.

may be consumed daily on a diet containing 30 percent of the Calories as fat and less than 300 milligrams of cholesterol. For the 30 percent recommendation, a very simple method to determine the grams of total fat you may consume on a given caloric diet is to simply drop the zero from the daily caloric total and divide by 3. For example,

2,100 Calorie diet

2,100 = 210

210/3 = 70 grams total fat

For lower percentages of fat Calories, say 20 percent, simply multiply the daily caloric intake by the percentage desired and divide by 9 to get the grams of fat allowed per day. For example, 20 percent of 2,500 Calories would permit 500 Calories from fat, or about 55 grams per day.

As we shall see later in this chapter and in Chapter 11, excessive consumption of dietary fat and cholesterol may be linked to a variety of chronic diseases, including heart disease and obesity. In certain individuals with blood lipid abnormalities, the recommended reduction in dietary fats and cholesterol is even greater than the Healthy North American Diet, with the total dietary Calories from fat being 20 percent or lower in some diet plans, as in the Ornish and Pritikin diet plans.

Recent dietary surveys also indicate that many athletes still consume substantial amounts of fat, ranging from 35–45 percent of the daily caloric intake. High-fat diets may be deleterious to physical performance in several ways. The fat may displace carbohydrate in the diet, may lead to excessive caloric intake and body weight, and may cause gastrointestinal distress if consumed as part of a pregame meal. All of these factors could possibly impair physical performance.

Metabolism and Function

In this section we briefly cover the digestion of dietary lipids, their metabolic disposal in the body, interactions with carbohydrate and protein, the major functions of fats in the body, and energy stores of fat.

How does dietary fat get into the body?

The major dietary sources of lipids are the triglycerides, comprising about 95 percent, while the other 5 percent consists mainly of sterols and phospholipids. Most of the dietary triglycerides contain long-chain fatty acids (14 or more carbons). Lipids are insoluble in water, and therefore their digestion and absorption is somewhat more complicated than that of carbohydrates. As lipids enter the small intestine, they stimulate hormonal secretion by the intestines that culminates in the secretion of bile from the gallbladder and lipases from the pancreas into the intestinal lumen. The bile salts serve as emulsifiers, breaking up the lipid droplets into smaller segments that may be hydrolyzed by the lipid enzymes, pancreatic lipases, and cholesterases. In essence, lipids are hydrolyzed into free fatty acids (FFA), glycerol, cholesterol, and phospholipids, which through an intricate process are then absorbed into the cells of the intestinal mucosa. Here they are combined into a fat droplet called a **chylomicron,** which contains a large amount of triglyceride and smaller amounts of cholesterol, phospholipids, and protein. The chylomicron is one form of a **lipoprotein,** which, by its name, you can see is composed of lipids and protein. A diagram of a lipoprotein is presented in Figure 5.6. The chylomicron then leaves the intestinal cell and is absorbed by the lacteal in the villi, where it is eventually transported in the lymphatic system to the blood. A schematic of this process is presented in Figure 5.7.

Medium-chain triglycerides (MCTs) release fatty acids with shorter carbon chain lengths (6–12 carbons), enabling them to be absorbed directly into the blood without being converted into chylomicrons. They are transported directly to the liver. Because of this rapid processing, MCTs have been theorized to possess ergogenic potential, and their efficacy in this regard will be discussed in a later section.

What happens to the lipid once it gets in the body?

The digestion of lipids into chylomicrons is slow, and the absorption after a high-fat meal can last several hours. As the chylomicron circulates in the blood, it reacts with

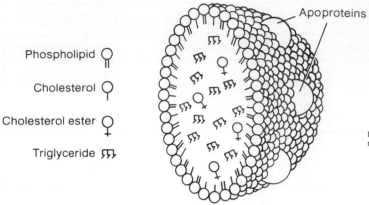

Phospholipid

Cholesterol

Cholesterol ester

Triglyceride

Figure 5.6 Schematic of a lipoprotein. Lipoproteins contain a core of triglycerides and cholesterol esters surrounded by a coat of apoproteins, cholesterol, and phospholipids. The proportion of protein, cholesterol, triglycerides, and phospholipids varies between the different types of lipoproteins.

various cells in the body, particularly cells in the muscle and adipose tissues. Specific proteins in the outer coat of lipoproteins are known as apolipoproteins. **Apolipoproteins** enable the various lipoproteins to react with specific receptors in cells throughout the body. The apolipoproteins in the chylomicron interact with an enzyme, lipoprotein lipase, which is produced in the muscle and adipose cells and released to the capillary blood vessels surrounding the cells. The lipoprotein lipase releases fatty acids and glycerol from the chylomicron. The fatty acids are absorbed into the cells while the glycerol is transported primarily to the liver for conversion to glucose. The remains of the chylomicron, the chylomicron remnant, are transported to the liver for disposal.

In the muscle, the fatty acids may either be used as a source of energy or may combine with newly generated glycerol, which is derived as a metabolic by-product of glycolysis, leading to the formation and storage of muscle triglycerides. In the adipose cell, most of the fatty acids combine with glycerol and are stored as adipose cell triglycerides.

The key organ in the body for the metabolism of most nutrients is the liver. It is a clearinghouse in human metabolism. As blood passes through the liver, its cells take the basic nutrients and convert them into other forms. As mentioned in Chapter 4, the liver is able to manufacture glucose from a variety of other nutrients, including glycerol. Pertinent to our discussion here is its role in lipid metabolism. As noted above, glycerol and chylomicron remnants, including phospholipids, are transported to the liver, as are the MCTs directly from the intestinal tract. Adipose cells are metabolically active in the sense that they are constantly releasing fatty acids for use by the body, including the liver. The major role of the liver is to combine these various components (fatty acids, glycerol, cholesterol, and phospholipids), along with protein, into various forms of lipoproteins.

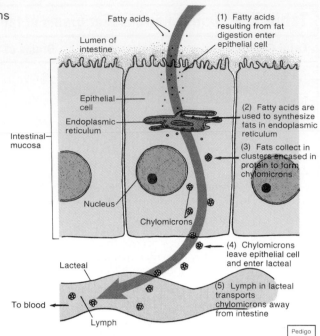

Figure 5.7 The absorption of lipids. In the lumen of the intestine, several lipases, assisted by bile salts, digest lipids to various forms of fatty acids, phospholipids, cholesterol, and glycerol, which are absorbed by an intricate process into the epithelial cells of the intestinal mucosa. Here they are combined with protein to form chylomicrons, a form of lipoprotein, which are transported out of the cell and into the lacteal, where the lymph eventually carries them to the blood.

What are the different types of lipoproteins?

After the chylomicrons have been cleared from the blood, which may take several hours, lipoproteins constitute approximately 95 percent of the serum lipids. The metabolism of lipoproteins is complex, for they are constantly being synthesized and catabolized by the liver and other body tissues. As a result, there is an exchange of protein and lipid components among the different classes of lipoproteins, which can lead to the conversion of one form into another.

The classification of lipoproteins may be determined by several methods. One of the methods is by the type of apolipoprotein present and its functions. Lipoproteins have a number of different apoproteins, which enable them to react with different tissues. The letters A, B, C, D, and E, including subdivisions such as A-I and A-II are common designations. The second method, most popularly known, is based on the density of the lipoprotein particle. Designations range from high to very low density.

The chylomicron is one form of lipoprotein, but because it is relatively short-lived, it is not considered a major lipoprotein. For our purposes in this book, the major classifications of lipoproteins along with their suggested composition and function are listed next; a graphical depiction is presented in Figure 5.8. However, it should

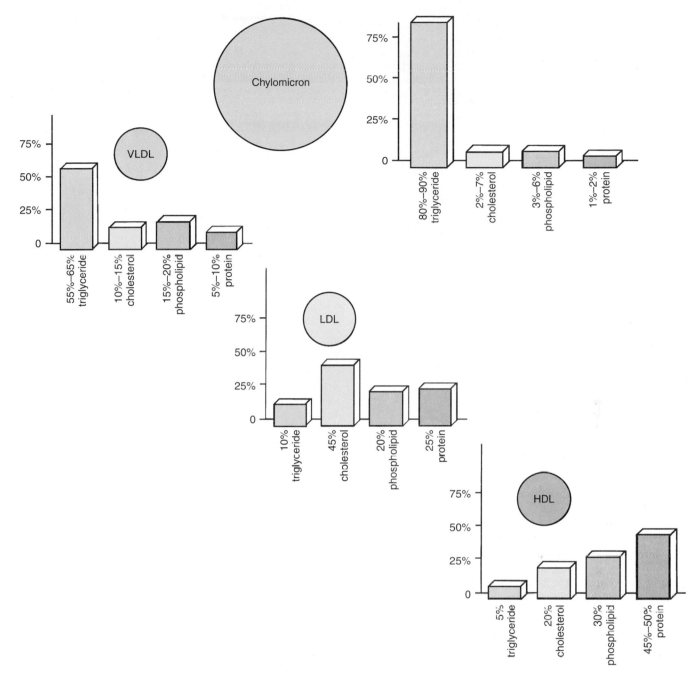

Figure 5.8 The approximate content of four different types of lipoproteins.

From G. M. Wardlow and P. M. Insel, *Perspectives in Nutrition*. St. Louis: Mosby, 1996. 3rd Edition.

be noted that a wide variety of lipoproteins exist based upon their specific lipid and protein content. Additionally, their metabolism and complete functions have not been totally elucidated.

VLDL (very low-density lipoproteins). **VLDL** consist primarily of triglycerides from endogenous sources, whereas chylomicrons contain triglycerides from exogenous sources, that is, the diet. These triglycerides are transported to the tissues to

provide fatty acids and glycerol. The loss of triglycerides to the tissues will increase VLDL's density to a form called IDL (intermediate-density lipoprotein), which is between VLDL and LDL. Apoprotein B is the major apoprotein associated with both VLDL and IDL.

LDL (low-density lipoproteins). **LDL** contain a high proportion of cholesterol and phospholipids, but little triglycerides. LDL are formed after the VLDL

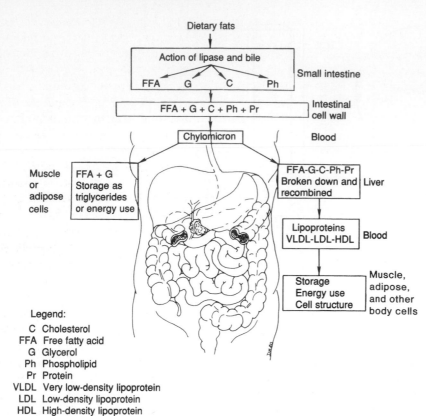

Dietary fats

Action of lipase and bile — Small intestine

FFA   G   C   Ph

FFA + G + C + Ph + Pr — Intestinal cell wall

Chylomicron — Blood

Muscle or adipose cells

FFA + G
Storage as triglycerides or energy use

FFA-G-C-Ph-Pr
Broken down and recombined — Liver

Lipoproteins
VLDL-LDL-HDL — Blood

Storage
Energy use
Cell structure

Muscle, adipose, and other body cells

Legend:
C   Cholesterol
FFA Free fatty acid
G   Glycerol
Ph Phospholipid
Pr Protein
VLDL Very low-density lipoprotein
LDL Low-density lipoprotein
HDL High-density lipoprotein

Figure 5.9 Simplified diagram of fat metabolism. After digestion, most of the fats are carried in the blood as chylomicrons. Through the metabolic processes in the body, fat may be utilized as a major source of energy, used to help develop cell structure, or stored as a future energy source.

and IDL release their stores of triglycerides. Recently, a new LDL, small or dense LDL, has been uncovered. Apolipoprotein B is the major apolipoprotein associated with LDL.

HDL (high-density lipoproteins). **HDL** contain a high proportion of protein (about 45–50 percent), moderate amounts of cholesterol and phospholipids, and very little triglycerides. Several subclasses of HDL have been identified, most notably HDL_2 and HDL_3. Apolipoprotein A is the major apolipoprotein associated with HDL.

Lipoprotein (a). **Lipoprotein (a)** is very similar to the LDL, being in the upper LDL density range. The principal apolipoprotein associated with lipoprotein (a) is apolipoprotein (a).

A simplified schematic of fat metabolism is presented in Figure 5.9.

Can the body make fat from protein and carbohydrate?

You may recall that glycogen is made up of many individual glucose molecules and is a glucose polymer. In essence, fatty acids are polymers of acetyl CoA, the primary substrate for the Krebs cycle.

As noted in Figure 4.9, the amino acids of protein may be converted to acetyl CoA, which can then be converted into fat. Carbohydrates also may be converted to fat

via acetyl CoA. It is important to understand that the body will take excess amounts of both these nutrients and convert them to fat when caloric expenditure is less than caloric intake. Thus, in general, it is not necessarily what you eat, but rather how much, that determines whether or not you gain body fat. However, as discussed in Chapters 10 and 11, there is some evidence to suggest that dietary fat may be stored as body fat more readily than carbohydrate or protein, and thus may be a factor in the development of obesity.

It is important to note that although carbohydrates and protein may be converted to fat (primarily fatty acids), fatty acids cannot be converted to carbohydrate or protein. If excess nitrogen is available from protein, it may combine with metabolic by-products of fatty acids to form nonessential amino acids—but fatty acids cannot be converted into protein without this excess nitrogen.

What are the major functions of the body lipids?

The body lipids are derived from the dietary lipids and other carbon sources, namely carbohydrate and protein, but with the exception of linoleic fatty acid and several of the omega-3 fatty acids, all lipids essential to human metabolism may be produced by the liver. The body lipids serve a variety of functions, including all three purposes of food: they form body structures, help regulate metabolism, and provide a source of energy.

Structure   The structure of virtually all cell membranes, including the nerve membranes, consists partly of lipids, notably cholesterol and phospholipids. The structural fat deposits in the adipose tissues are used as insulators to conserve body heat and shock absorbers to protect various organs.

Metabolic Regulation   Cholesterol is a component of several hormones, such as testosterone and estrogen, which have diverse effects in the regulation of human metabolism. The majority of cholesterol in the body is used by the liver to produce bile salts, essential for the digestion of fats. Phospholipids are also instrumental for blood clotting.

Some derivatives of specific fatty acids formed by oxidation have some potent biologic functions in the body. These derivatives—prostaglandins, prostacyclins, thromboxanes, and leukotrienes—are collectively known as **eicosanoids.** These eicosanoids possess hormone-like properties that influence a number of physiological functions, including several that may have implications for health or physical performance. Several important eicosanoids are derived from omega-3 fatty acids, and the theorized health and performance implications will be discussed in later sections of this chapter.

Energy Source   In general, the function of the majority of the body lipids, the triglycerides, is to provide energy to drive metabolic processes. The majority of the triglycerides in the body are stored in the adipose tissue. They break down to free fatty acids (FFA) and glycerol, which are released into the blood, with the FFA being transported to the tissues and the glycerol going to the liver. In the tissues, the FFA are reduced to acetyl CoA and enter the Krebs cycle to produce energy via the oxygen system. The glycerol is used by the liver to form other lipids or glucose.

During rest, nearly 60 percent of the energy supply is provided by the metabolism of fats when the individual consumes a mixed diet. Most of the energy provided is presented to body cells as fatty acids, but some energy may be provided by ketones. As the liver metabolizes fatty acid, substances known as ketoacids, or **ketones,** are produced from excess acetyl CoA, diffuse from the liver into the blood, and are transported to the body tissues where they can eventually be used as a source of energy. The major ketones are acetoacetic acid, beta-hydroxybutyric acid, and acetone. These ketones usually are produced in small amounts, but when the use of fatty acids as an energy source is high (such as with fasting, high-fat diets, and diabetes) ketone levels in the blood will increase. Ketones are an important energy source during fasting or starvation. However, excessive accumulation may lead to acidosis (ketosis) in the blood, a condition which may cause coma and death, such as in uncontrolled diabetes.

How much total energy is stored in the body as fat?

The greatest amount of energy stored in the body is fat in the form of triglycerides. Fat is a very efficient, compact means to store energy for several reasons. First, fat has 9 Calories per gram, more than twice the value of carbohydrate and protein. Also, there is very little water in body fat compared to the 3–4 grams of water stored with each gram of carbohydrate or protein. In essence, body fat is about 5–6 times as efficient an energy store as carbohydrate and protein. If the average 154-pound man had to carry all the potential energy of his fat stores as carbohydrate, he would weigh nearly 300 pounds.

Most of the triglycerides are stored in the adipose tissues, approximately 80,000–100,000 Calories of energy in the average adult male with normal body fat. The triglycerides within and between the muscle cells may provide approximately 2,500–2,800 Calories, while those in the blood provide only about 70–80 Calories. The free fatty acids (FFA) in the blood total about 7–8 Calories. The liver also contains an appreciable store of triglycerides. Thus, you can see that the human body contains a huge reservoir of energy Calories in the form of fat.

Fats and Exercise

Are fats used as an energy source during exercise?

The two major energy sources for the production of ATP during exercise are carbohydrates in the form of muscle glycogen and fats in the form of fatty acids. In steady-state exercise, both can be converted to acetyl CoA for subsequent oxidation in the citric acid cycle. In general, a mixture of both fuel sources is used during exercise, although the quantitative values may vary depending on a variety of factors, including the intensity and duration of the exercise bout, the diet, and the training status of the individual.

The fatty acids used by the muscle cells during exercise may be derived from a variety of sources, including the plasma triglycerides in the chylomicrons and VLDL but Martin indicates they may provide only about 10 percent of fat energy. The two major sources are the plasma FFA and the muscle triglycerides. The plasma FFA are in very short supply, so they must be replenished by the vast stores of triglycerides in the adipose tissue. An enzyme in the adipose cells, known as hormone-sensitive lipase (HSL), catabolizes the intracellular triglycerides to FFA and glycerol. The FFA are released into the blood, bound to the protein albumin as a carrier, and transported to the muscle cells or other cells where they are transported into the cell and metabolized for energy. Intracellularly, an enzyme complex using a carrier called **carnitine** is necessary to transport the fatty acid into the mitochondria. The muscle triglycerides may also be metabolized to fatty acids and glycerol by an enzyme similar to HSL, and the fatty acids may be processed into the mitochondria. (See Figure 5.10.)

During rest, most of the fat energy needs of the body are met by the supply of plasma FFA to the cells. Fatty acids are constantly being mobilized from the adipose tissues to replenish the plasma FFA. Most of the FFA released during rest, about 70 percent, are actually re-esterified back into triglycerides, the remainder being delivered to the body cells for energy.

During exercise, only about 25 percent of these FFA are re-esterified, so this alone provides a substantial increase in FFA delivery to the muscle cells. Additionally, hormones that activate HSL, such as epinephrine, are secreted during exercise, stimulating the breakdown of adipose cell triglycerides and the release of FFA into the blood for transport and entrance to the muscle cell. Epinephrine also stimulates intramuscular lipases to catabolize muscle triglycerides into FFA. These fatty acids then enter the mitochondria and are degraded to acetyl CoA. The metabolism of long-chain FFA into acetyl CoA (a 2-carbon molecule) in the cell is known as **beta-oxidation,** for the beta carbon is the second carbon on the long chain.

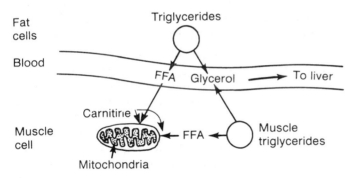

Figure 5.10 Fat as an energy source during exercise. Free fatty acids (FFA) are an important energy source during endurance exercise. They may be released by the adipose tissue triglycerides and travel by the blood to the muscle cells, and also may be derived from the muscle cell triglycerides. Carnitine is needed to transport the FFA into the mitochondria. The glycerol that is released from the triglycerides may be transported to the liver for gluconeogenesis. (See Appendix K, Figure K.4, for more details.)

Recent reviews by Coyle and Martin have noted that during mild exercise at about 25 percent of VO_2 max, 20 percent or less of the total energy cost is derived from carbohydrate while the other 80 percent or more comes from fat. The plasma FFA provided by the adipose tissue appear to be the major source of fat energy during mild exercise, but their percentage use decreases and that of muscle triglycerides increases as the exercise intensity increases up to about 65 percent VO_2 max. At this point, fats and carbohydrates appear to contribute equally to the energy expenditure, and the plasma FFA and muscle triglycerides contribute equally to the energy derived from fats. However, Coyle and others indicated that carbohydrate ingestion within an hour of moderate exercise will inhibit long-chain fatty acid oxidation. At high intensity exercise levels, about 85 percent VO_2 max, the percentage contribution from fats (mostly muscle triglycerides) diminishes to 25 percent or less as muscle glycogen becomes the preferential energy source. These findings have been documented using substrate tracer methodology, particularly in an excellent study by Romijn and others. A summary of fat utilization during exercise is presented in Table 5.6.

One of the key factors that determines which body fuel is used during exercise is the exercise intensity. As noted in previous chapters, carbohydrate is the preferred energy source during high-intensity exercise, such as 65–70 percent of VO_2 max and above. It appears that there is a metabolic limit in the ability to generate ATP from FFA, so that FFA alone could not sustain exercise at this intensity. Although fatty acids do provide some of the energy in intense exercise, their contribution diminishes as the exercise intensity increases above 60–70 percent VO_2 max. George Brooks refers to the increasing use of carbohydrate and the decreasing use of fat as the "crossover" effect. There may be various factors that limit the role of FFA as the major energy source during high-intensity exercise, including the following:

Inadequate rate of release from the adipose cells

Inadequate transport capacity by albumin

Inadequate uptake by the muscle cell

Inadequate use in the cell

Table 5.6 Fat energy sources during exercise	
Plasma chylomicrons	Not a major source
Plasma VLDL	Not a major source
Plasma FFA	Major source; replenished by adipose cell release of FFA; Used in exercise at low to moderate intensity, i.e., 25–65 percent VO_2 max; Use decreases as exercise intensity increases toward 65 percent VO_2 max
Muscle FFA	Major source; released from intramuscular triglycerides; Low use during mild exercise; Used increasingly as exercise intensity increases toward 65 percent VO_2 max
Note: With high-intensity exercise, 65 percent VO_2 max or higher, total fat oxidation falls.	

Although the limiting factor is not known, Hodgetts and others suggested it may be due to inadequate release of FFA from the adipose tissues. A possible mechanism is the suggestion that increased serum lactic acid levels, which may occur in high-intensity exercise, may block the release of FFA from the adipose tissues. Possible limitations may also occur within the muscle, such as a decreased ability to transport the FFA into the mitochondria.

As noted in previous chapters, the amount of energy that may be obtained from muscle and liver glycogen is rather limited. Hence, within about an hour or so of high-intensity exercise, glycogen stores approach very low levels and the body shifts to an increasing usage of FFA, leading to a decrease in the intensity of the exercise. In cases such as prolonged endurance tasks like ultramarathons, FFA may provide nearly 90 percent of the energy in the latter stages of the event.

Although ketones may be utilized by the muscle, they do not appear to contribute significantly to energy production during exercise.

Do women use fats more efficiently during exercise than men?

Women possess a greater percentage of body fat than men, and several writers for popular runners' magazines have suggested that women could process this fat more efficiently and thus be more effective in ultramarathon events. Several previous studies have reported that when men and women are matched for their aerobic capacity, the utilization of fat as an energy source during prolonged exercise is similar. However, in a recent study regarding the effect of carbohydrate loading on energy substrate use and exercise performance in similarly trained male and female endurance athletes, Tarnopolsky and others, using the respiratory exchange ratio to evaluate energy substrate utilization, reported that women oxidized significantly more fat and less carbohydrate than men when exercising at 75 percent VO_2 max. However, the men improved their performance in the exercise task following carbohydrate loading but the women did not.

The investigators suggested that estrogen may influence energy substrate use during exercise, favoring fat use in women. However, this issue is still controversial and merits additional research.

What effect does exercise training have on fat metabolism during exercise?

A number of studies have shown that trained athletes use more fat than untrained athletes during a standardized exercise task. For example, if you ran an 8-minute mile both before and after a 2-month endurance training program, you would use the same amount of caloric energy each time. However, after training, more of that energy would be derived from fat. Hence, training helps you become a better fat burner, so to speak, which may help spare some of the glycogen in your muscles.

Although all of the exact mechanisms have not been identified, several factors may be involved. Some research indicates that exercise training increases the sensitivity of the adipose cells to epinephrine, possibly enhancing HSL activity to facilitate the release of FFA into the blood during exercise. Training also increases the muscle triglyceride content—possibly due to an enhanced insulin sensitivity—which regulates movement of FFA into cells. Additionally, the trained individual may use ketones as an energy source more effectively. Exercise training also leads to improved enzyme functions and other changes in the muscle cells, such as enhanced carnitine activity. These changes make muscle cells more efficient in taking up serum FFA and processing fatty acids from both the muscle triglycerides and serum FFA for ATP production. According to Martin, the increased content and use of muscle triglycerides may be the primary mechanism underlying the greater capacity of trained muscle to oxidize fatty acids during exercise. Increased utilization of fat during exercise is one of the major effects of training experienced by the endurance athlete.

Although carbohydrate becomes more important as an energy source during high-intensity exercise, Eric Newsholme noted that highly trained endurance athletes may be able to use fats more efficiently at exercise intensity levels greater than 50 percent VO_2 max, and in a recent review Pendergast and his associates concluded that fat, particularly intramuscular fat, plays an important role in metabolism at exercise intensities as high as 80 percent of VO_2 max or more in trained endurance athletes. In this regard, Dr. David Costill has noted that some highly-trained runners could derive as much as 75 percent of their energy from fat even when they were running at about 70 percent of their VO_2 max. The ability to derive a substantial proportion of the energy demands of intensive exercise from fatty acids is extremely important for athletes such as marathoners who may be able to save some of their muscle glycogen for utilization in the latter stages of the race. The mixture of fatty acids and glycogen for energy will enable them to sustain their pace, whereas the total depletion of muscle glycogen and subsequent reliance on fatty acids as the sole energy supply would force them to slow down. Thus, it is important for the endurance athlete to become a better "fat burner," and a variety of ergogenic aids have been proposed to enhance this effect.

Fats: Ergogenic Aspects

Because exercise training leads to an increased utilization of fatty acids as an energy source and improved performance in endurance events (theoretically by sparing muscle glycogen), a variety of dietary practices, dietary supplements, and pharmacological agents have been employed in attempts to facilitate this metabolic process during exercise. Dietary strategies have been used to increase the concentration of muscle triglycerides or serum level of FFA. Such strategies include high-fat diets, fasting, and even infusion of lipids into the bloodstream. Dietary supplements and drugs have been used to either increase the supply of oxidizable fats or the rate of fat metabolism. Dietary supplements include medium-chain triglycerides, wheat germ oil, lecithin, glycerol, and carnitine, while the main drug used is caffeine.

What is fat loading?

Dietary strategies designed to increase the supply or metabolism of fat as an energy source during exercise may be referred to as **fat loading.** Because the rate at which FFA are oxidized in the muscle is dependent in part upon their concentration in the blood plasma, several different dietary techniques have been tried in attempts to increase plasma FFA levels. Additionally, these dietary strategies have been used to enhance metabolism of fats in the muscle, including the endogenous muscle triglycerides.

The acute effects of high-fat meals and the chronic effects of high-fat diets have been studied in attempts to enhance exercise performance. There appear to be no benefits associated with consumption of a high-fat meal several hours prior to performance. For example, comparing the effects of a high-fat (61 percent fat Calories) versus a low-fat (10 percent fat Calories) meal consumed 4 hours prior to performance, Okano and others reported no significant differences between the treatments on performance in a ride to exhaustion at 80 percent VO_2 max following 2 hours of riding at 60 percent VO_2 max. A high-fat dietary strategy does not appear to enhance performance, and, in fact, may actually impair performance if it contributes to gastrointestinal distress because of the delayed gastric emptying associated with fats. Research has shown that consuming a high-fat diet for 1 or 2 days, another acute approach, may actually impair performance in high-intensity exercise tasks.

When an individual is placed on a chronic low-carbohydrate and high-fat diet for several weeks, the body adjusts its metabolism to use fats more efficiently. Studies conducted in the 1980s have shown that although this diet strategy may improve the use of fats during submaximal exercise at about 60–65 percent VO_2 max, endurance performance was not improved. However, in a recent review, Pendergast and others hypothesized that increased dietary fat, while maintaining normal muscle glycogen levels, may increase VO_2 max and muscle triglyceride levels, which may result in improved endurance exercise performance. Several studies support this hypothesis. For example, Muoio and others manipulated the percentage of fat Calories in the diet of six highly-trained runners from a normal level of 24 percent up to 38 percent on a high-fat diet and down to 15 percent on a high-carbohydrate diet. Each diet was consumed for approximately 1 week. In a treadmill run to exhaustion, the runners performed better following the week of the high-fat diet. However, the authors acknowledged limitations to the experimental design in this prototype study, such as no random assignment of the three diet conditions, and they recommended additional research. They also noted it would not be prudent to advise fat intake in excess of 30 percent of total Calories. In another study using a crossover experimental protocol, Lambert and others placed athletes on a high-fat diet (70 percent fat Calories) or low-fat diet (12 percent fat Calories) for 2 weeks, testing the effects on three performance tests done in consecutive order with 30 minutes rest between each. The three exercise tests included a Wingate high-power test, a high-intensity test to exhaustion at 90 percent VO_2 max, and a moderate-intensity test to exhaustion at 60 percent VO_2 max. Although there were no significant effects between the two diets for performance in the first two exercise tests, the cyclists rode significantly longer on the moderate-intensity test following adaptation to the high-fat diet. The investigators noted that adaptation to the high-fat diet decreased the reliance on carbohydrate as an energy source during exercise, and thus suggested the improved performance was due to muscle-glycogen sparing. Although an interesting study that merits confirmation, the exercise protocol used does not appear to have any application to contemporary sport events. The interested reader is referred to the recent review by Lambert and others.

A diet plan advertised to burn more fat or burn fat faster has been popularized in the best-selling book *The Zone*, by Barry Sears. The 40:30:30 diet consists of a set ratio of Calories from carbohydrate (40 percent), fat (30 percent), and protein (30 percent). Although this is not considered to be a high-fat diet, it may be regarded to be a low-carbohydrate, high-protein diet as the nutrient ratios 40:30:30 vary from those normally recommended, i.e., 58:30:12. More is said about the high protein content in the next chapter. The book is targeted primarily at those who desire to lose body fat for health or appearance, and reviewers suggest it may be effective because the diet plan is actually low in Calories, which is the key point of a diet to lose weight. Nonetheless, this diet plan has also been marketed to athletes as a means to optimize performance, partly because of the nature of the fats recommended in this diet plan.

Sears suggests that certain fats may be of value to athletes. Some companies manufacture food products based on the 40:30:30 ratio and target them at the sports nutrition market. Several reports in swimming magazines indicated that such a diet was instrumental in the success of the Stanford University swim team, but the data presented were anecdotal rather than scientific. Part of the theory underlying the application of this diet to sport performance may be eicosanoid-generating fatty acids, particularly the omega-3 fatty acids, discussed later in this chapter.

The "zone" diet has been criticized by health writers, such as Bonnie Liebman, and sport nutritionists, like Ellen Coleman. Both note numerous flaws in the diet plan, and Coleman indicates the diet may actually impair training and subsequent performance if it contains inadequate carbohydrate. However, this diet plan may provide adequate carbohydrate for training provided the athlete consumes adequate Calories. For example, an endurance athlete who consumes 3,000 Calories per day during training would derive 1,200 Calories from carbohydrate ($0.40 \times 3,000$), which is 300 grams of carbohydrate. For a 60-kilogram athlete, this amounts to 5 grams per kilogram body weight, which although not the recommended amount for endurance athletes, has been shown to be sufficient to sustain training on a daily basis, although training may appear more stressful psychologically. Nevertheless, there are no reputable scientific data showing that the 40:30:30 diet plan enhances athletic performance. Although some fat is essential in the diet, a high-carbohydrate diet is recommended for most athletes, particularly those involved in prolonged exercise training.

In summary, in a recent major review, Sherman and Leenders noted that although the hypothesis that "fat loading" may increase fat oxidation, decrease carbohydrate utilization, and enhance performance is intriguing, the current scientific literature is not supportive. Additional well-controlled research is merited.

Will fasting help improve my performance?

Sherman and Leenders indicate that fasting for 24 hours may increase the plasma FFA availability. Unfortunately, endurance exercise performance is usually impaired because fasting reduces muscle glycogen stores or induces hypoglycemia. The effect of fasting on physical performance when athletes attempt to lose body weight for sport competition is covered in Chapter 10.

Can the use of medium-chain triglycerides improve endurance performance?

Medium-chain triglycerides (MCTs) have been suggested to be ergogenic, possibly because they are water soluble and can be absorbed by the portal circulation and delivered directly to the liver instead of via the chylomicron route in the lymph. MCTs have been marketed commercially, one brand being CapTri®. CapTri® has been advertised to increase energy levels, extend endurance, promote muscularity, enhance fat metabolism, and lower body fat. Research has shown that MCTs do not inhibit gastric emptying as common fat does and may be absorbed rapidly in the small intestine. Also, Massicotte and his associates reported exogenous MCTs are oxidized at a rate comparable to exogenous glucose, being oxidized within the first 30 minutes of exercise.

Earlier research has not supported an ergogenic effect of MCT supplementation. High-fat meals using MCTs have been given to subjects 1–4 hours prior to exercise performance. The usual dose was about 25–45 grams, or about 225–400 Calories. Although high-fat meals may lead to a greater oxidation of fats, they have not been shown to improve performance. Moreover, in one study comparing equivalent caloric intakes of either fat or carbohydrate ingested 1 hour prior to a 2-hour endurance task at 67 percent of VO_2 max, more endogenous carbohydrate was used following the fat diet. Furthermore, high-fat meals caused gastric distress in some subjects.

More recently, Van Zyl and others suggested that not enough MCTs were used in previous studies. Using endurance-trained cyclists, they compared the effects of three supplements on an endurance performance task consisting of a 2-hour ride at 60 percent VO_2 max followed by a 40-kilometer performance ride. The three supplements, consumed throughout the performance task, were carbohydrate only, MCTs only, and carbohydrate with MCTs; the MCT dose was about 86 grams. Compared to the carbohydrate supplement, the MCT supplement actually impaired 40-kilometer performance, whereas the combination carbohydrate-MCT supplement improved performance. These investigators suggested that the carbohydrate-MCT supplement improved performance in the 40-kilometer performance ride by decreasing oxidation of muscle glycogen during the preliminary submaximal 2-hour ride, thus sparing the glycogen for the more intense exercise task. However, in several studies with his University of Maastricht colleagues in the Netherlands, Jeukendrup investigated similar supplementation protocols and reported very little contribution of ingested MCTs to energy metabolism during exercise. Using a protocol comparable to the Van Zyl research group, but also incorporating a placebo trial and using a 15-minute cycle performance task instead of a 40-kilometer ride, Jeukendrup and colleagues also found that MCT supplementation impaired performance and attributed the impairment to gastrointestinal distress. However, in contrast to the Van Zyl study, they reported no significant differences between the other trials, suggesting the carbohydrate-MCT combination was not an effective ergogenic.

Whether or not the appropriate dosage and timing of MCT supplementation enhances prolonged endurance exercise performance is presently uncertain. In the most recent review, Berning notes that while some of the research is promising, more scientific research is needed to evaluate the ergogenic potential of MCT supplementation.

Will infusion of fats into the bloodstream improve fat oxidation and performance?

As discussed previously, the digestion and absorption of ingested fats is a rather slow process. Most ingested fats are absorbed slowly into the lymph and then are processed into the blood. One technique that has been used to increase serum levels of FFA is the infusion, not ingestion, of a fat emulsion, such as Intralipid. Hargreaves and others have shown that this technique may rapidly increase plasma FFA, leading to a decrease in glucose uptake and an increase in ketone uptake by leg muscles exercising for 1 hour at 80 percent of maximal work capacity. However, Intralipid had no effect on leg uptake of plasma FFA or on muscle glycogen utilization. No performance data were reported. Intralipid had been used by one national team in the Tour de France, but the entire team withdrew from the race allegedly due to adverse reactions.

Is the glycerol portion of triglycerides an effective ergogenic aid?

As you may recall, glycerol is one of the by-products of triglyceride breakdown. Because glycerol may be converted to glucose in the liver, researchers theorized that it could be an efficient energy source during exercise. However, in well-controlled research, glycerol feedings did not prevent either hypoglycemia or muscle glycogen depletion patterns in several prolonged exercise tasks. Apparently the rate at which the human liver converts glycerol to glucose is not rapid enough to be an effective energy source during strenuous prolonged exercise. However, as noted in Chapter 9, glycerol may be used to increase body water stores, including plasma volume, prior to exercise, which may improve cardiovascular functions and help regulate body temperature more effectively, possible ergogenic effects.

Do wheat germ oil supplements enhance athletic performance?

One of the most enduring yet controversial ergogenic foods on the market is wheat germ oil, which has been advertised to improve endurance, stamina, and vigor. **Wheat germ oil** is extracted from the embryo of wheat; it is high in linoleic fatty acid, vitamin E, and octacosanol, a solid white alcohol that has been theorized to be the ergogenic ingredient. It is interesting to note that a product called Octacol 4 was endorsed by one of the best marathoners in the United States.

Several theories have been advanced about the beneficial physiological effects of wheat germ oil supplements for athletes, such as enhanced glycogen metabolism and increased oxygen uptake. The principal investigator, who studied wheat germ oil for nearly 20 years, stated that the supplements were to be taken in conjunction with training and were beneficial primarily for endurance. However, the research literature does not provide the necessary objective data to actually pinpoint the exact metabolic role of the wheat germ oil or octacosonal in humans that would improve endurance performance. Moreover, a thorough analysis of approximately thirty-five studies has not supported the contention that wheat germ oil is an effective ergogenic aid. This evidence was used successfully by the Federal Trade Commission to ban advertising claims that wheat germ oil could improve endurance, stamina, and vigor.

How effective are lecithin or choline supplements?

Lecithin is a phospholipid that occurs naturally in a variety of foods, such as beans, eggs, and wheat germ. Because it is an important component of many types of human body tissues, contains choline needed for the synthesis of acetylcholine (an important neurotransmitter), and contains phosphorus, it has been theorized to be ergogenic in nature. Several German studies conducted over 50 years ago reported increases in power and strength following several days of supplementation with 22–83 milligrams of lecithin. However, these early studies have been discredited because of poor experimental design. In a study with better experimental design, Staton reported that 30 grams of lecithin supplementation daily for 2 weeks had no effect upon grip strength.

Although lecithin does not appear to be an effective ergogenic aid, several of its constituents have been theorized to enhance exercise performance. Choline, an amine, is discussed in Chapter 6, and the mineral phosphate salts are covered in Chapter 8.

Why are omega-3 fatty acids suggested to be ergogenic, and do they work?

Omega-3 fatty acids are theorized to be ergogenic, not because of their energy content, but because they may elicit favorable physiological effects relative to several types of physical performance. One theory is based on the finding that omega-3 fatty acids may be incorporated into the membrane of the red blood cell (RBC), making the RBC less viscous and less resistant to flow. Another theory is based on the role of certain by-products—the eicosanoids mentioned previously—whose production in the body cells is related to omega-3 fatty acid metabolism. In particular, two specific forms of the eicosanoids, prostaglandin E_1 (PGE_1) and prostaglandin I_2 (PGI_2), may elicit a vasodilation effect on the blood vessels and may stimulate the release of human growth hormone. Theoretically, the less viscous RBC and the vasodilative effect should enhance blood flow, facilitating the delivery of blood and oxygen to the muscles during exercise, benefitting the endurance athlete. Additionally, the increased secretion of human growth hormone might stimulate muscle growth and benefit the strength/power athlete and may also facilitate recovery from intense exercise bouts.

Several food bars marketed for athletes, such as the Bio/Syn energy bar, are a blend of vegetable and fish oils that contain a mixture of fatty acids, including omega-3 fatty acids, along with carbohydrate and protein.

Unfortunately, although the ergogenic potential of omega-3 fatty acids is an interesting hypothesis, there are few supportive scientific data. Bucci, in his book discussing nutritional ergogenic aids, cites several studies with Eico-max®, a commercially available blend of fish oils and vegetable oils. The studies were conducted with university football teams and focused on measures of strength and speed, possibly testing the potential anabolic effect of omega-3 fatty acids via stimulated release of human growth hormone. In one of the studies, there was no control group. Bucci notes that both studies reported improved performance with the use of Eicomax®, however, perusal of the cited references reveals that these studies have not appeared in the scientifically reviewed literature, but were published in the training manual of the company that produces Eicomax®. If indeed these are valid findings, they need to be published in the scientific literature and confirmed.

Using a more sophisticated experimental design, Brilla and Landerholm studied the effect of fish oil supplements containing 4 grams per day of omega-3 fatty acids, either separately or in combination with an aerobic exercise training program, on aerobic fitness as measured by a test of VO_2 max. They reported that although exercise training increased VO_2 max, the omega-3 fatty acids yielded no ergogenic effect when taken without exercise training, nor did they have any additive effect with training. Raastad and others also reported that daily supplementation of 2.6 grams omega-3 fatty acids for 10 weeks did not improve maximal aerobic power or running performance in well-trained male soccer players.

At the present time, there do not appear to be sufficient data to support an ergogenic effect of omega-3 fatty acids.

Can carnitine supplements enhance fat metabolism and physical performance?

Carnitine is a water-soluble, vitamin-like compound that facilitates the transport of long-chain fatty acids into the mitochondria. There are basically two forms of carnitine, L-carnitine and D-carnitine, but other forms are available, such as L-propionylcarnitine. L-carnitine is the physiologically active form in the body, so in the following discussion, carnitine will refer mostly to L-carnitine, but in some studies L-propionylcarnitine has been used.

Carnitine was discovered in 1905 and was considered to be an essential vitamin at one time. Although Broquist has indicated that carnitine is an extremely important catalyst for metabolic reactions in the muscle, carnitine is not an essential dietary nutrient because it may be formed in the liver from other nutrients—principally two amino acids, lysine and methionine. Also, carnitine is found in substantial amounts in animal foods, particularly meats, with much lesser amounts in plant foods. For example, for similar weights, beef has about 300 times as much carnitine as bread; 3 ounces of beef contains about 60 mg of carnitine. There is no RDA for carnitine. Most individuals consume enough carnitine in the daily diet, and the body also has an effective conservation system. The typical non-vegetarian diet provides about 100–300 milligrams per day. Although deficiencies are very rare, vegetarians have been reported to have lower plasma levels of carnitine compared to individuals on a mixed diet.

Carnitine supplementation has been theorized to enhance physical performance because of several of its metabolic functions in the muscle cell. Approximately 90 percent of the body supply of carnitine is located in the muscle tissues. Theoretically, supplemental carnitine might facilitate the transport of fatty acids into the mitochondria for oxidation, which would be an important consideration if the oxidation of fatty acids was limited by their transport into the mitochondria. Recent research has reported an increase in respiratory chain enzymes in the mitochondria of long-distance runners following carnitine supplementation. Combining these two potential effects, carnitine would theoretically be beneficial for athletes in very prolonged endurance events by increasing the utilization of fatty acids during exercise and sparing the use of muscle glycogen. This is the primary theory underlying carnitine supplementation for endurance athletes.

Carnitine plays other metabolic roles that have been theorized to be ergogenic. Wagenmakers notes that carnitine may facilitate the oxidation of pyruvate, which may possibly enhance the utilization of glucose and reduce the production of lactic acid during exercise, factors that may enhance performance in short-term maximal or supramaximal exercise, such as in a 400-meter or 800-meter run. Wagenmakers also notes that carnitine may increase blood flow both at rest and during exercise, which may enhance delivery of both oxygen and energy substrate to the muscle during exercise, a theoretical ergogenic effect independent of the role of carnitine in the muscle cells. Conversely, Wagenmakers notes that carnitine may expedite the oxidation of branched-chain amino acids (BCAA), leading to a series of biochemical reactions that could lead to premature fatigue, an ergolytic rather than ergogenic effect.

Carnitine supplementation, particularly L-propionylcarnitine, has been used effectively to improve exercise capability in patients with serious diseases. After carnitine supplementation for several weeks, patients with peripheral vascular disease increased their walking distance before experiencing pain. Several studies have also reported improved exercise capacity in patients with heart disease following carnitine supplementation.

Although these are logical theories and interesting medical applications, the available scientific evidence is somewhat equivocal, and in general does not appear to support an ergogenic effect of carnitine supplementation. Major reviews regarding the effect of carnitine supplementation on physical performance have been published in recent years, and the following are the key points regarding the ergogenic effects of carnitine supplementation emanating from these reviews.

1. Supplementation will increase plasma levels of carnitine, but much of this will be excreted by the kidneys. However, muscle levels may be slightly greater during training if carnitine supplements are taken. Doses of 2 grams per day for 4 weeks or more may be needed to increase muscle carnitine levels. Such doses may help prevent carnitine losses during strenuous training.

2. Acute supplementation does not appear to enhance performance. Although not studied extensively, Colombani and others, in a well-designed, double-blind, placebo, crossover study, reported no significant effect on performance in either a marathon or a 20-kilometer run after supplements of 2 grams of carnitine 2 hours before the events. Such short-term supplementation may not be adequate to increase muscle levels of carnitine.

3. Chronic supplementation, with as much as 6 grams per day for 7 days, has no effect on lactic acid accumulation during high-intensity anaerobic exercise, nor does it increase performance in such exercise tasks. For example, Trappe and others reported no effect of carnitine supplementation on performance in five repeat 100-yard swims with a 2 minute recovery.

4. The effect of chronic carnitine supplementation on VO_2 max is equivocal, but most reviewers believe it has no significant effect. The effects of carnitine supplementation on aerobic endurance performance has not been studied extensively, but those data that are available, such as the effect on a 70-minute cycling task and a 5-kilometer run, have shown no beneficial effect. There are no scientific data showing a beneficial effect of chronic carnitine supplementation on very prolonged aerobic endurance tasks, such as a marathon.

5. The primary theory underlying carnitine supplementation is enhanced fat utilization. However, recent research by Decombaz and colleagues and Vukovich and colleagues reported no effect of chronic carnitine supplementation on fat oxidation or muscle glycogen sparing under exercise conditions maximizing fatty acid oxidation.

6. D-carnitine may be toxic, as it can deplete L-carnitine, leading to a carnitine deficiency. L-carnitine appears to be a safe supplement, but some reviewers recommend no more than 2–5 grams per day, possibly for only one month at a time.

For a detailed review of carnitine metabolism and its potential ergogenic effect, the interested reader is referred to the excellent critiques by Bucci, Clarkson, Leibovitz and Mueller, Wagenmakers, and most recently, Heinonen. Although interpretation of the scientific data regarding the ergogenic value of carnitine supplementation may vary somewhat, most believe scientific data are lacking to support a beneficial effect. However, most also agree that additional research is warranted.

Does caffeine improve exercise performance?

Caffeine is a naturally occurring compound in many of the foods and beverages that we consume every day, such as coffee, tea, colas, caffeinated waters and juices, and chocolate. It is also found in various dietary supplements, such as kola nuts and guarana, and even some over-the-counter stimulant supplements targeted to athletes. Yet caffeine is legally classified as a drug and has some powerful physiological effects on the human body. A normal therapeutic dose of caffeine may range from 100–300 milligrams. Some approximate amounts in the beverages we consume are 100–150 mg in a cup of perked coffee, 20–50 mg in a cup of tea, 35–55 mg in a can of cola, and 55–110 mg in a can of high-caffeine soda. Unfortunately, most of these products do not list the caffeine content on the label. Various stimulant tablets, such as Vivarin, contain about 200 milligrams per tablet.

Caffeine is a central nervous system stimulant that will enhance psychological processes. These psychological processes may underlie some of the ergogenic effects of caffeine supplementation.

Caffeine also has profound effects on metabolic processes. Caffeine stimulates heart function, blood circulation, and release of epinephrine (adrenaline) from the adrenal gland. Epinephrine, also a stimulant, augments these effects and also, in conjunction with caffeine, stimulates a wide variety of tissues. Together they potentiate muscle contraction, raise the rate of muscle and liver glycogen breakdown, increase release of FFA from adipose tissue, and increase use of muscle triglycerides. One of the most observed effects at rest is an increase in blood levels of FFA. These varied physiological responses are mediated by the action of caffeine, or epinephrine, to enhance appropriate intracellular functions in specific cells; functions such as increased calcium release to excite muscle contraction or elevated enzymic activity to release FFA from adipose tissue cells. Caffeine is degraded rapidly in the liver to dimethylxanthines, metabolites which may also affect metabolism favorably.

Because some of these physiological effects could be theorized to improve physical performance, the International Olympic Committee (IOC) banned the use of caffeine as a drug prior to the 1972 Olympics. However, because caffeine is a natural ingredient in some beverages that athletes consume, the IOC removed it from the doping list from 1972–1982. The use of large amounts of caffeine was again banned for the 1984 Olympic games, probably because some recent research had suggested that caffeine could artificially improve performance. Olympic athletes are permitted to consume small amounts of caffeine, but the use of large doses, such as the equivalent of 5–6 cups of strong coffee or only 4 Vivarin tablets in a short time, is grounds for disqualification. About 800 mg of caffeine consumed in 2–3 hours would exceed the legal limit, which is 12 micrograms of caffeine per milliliter of urine. In a 70-kilogram (154-pound) male, the consumption of 100 milligrams would lead to the excretion of approximately 1.5 micrograms/milliliter. The excretion rate would be more or less depending upon body weight.

Caffeine has been studied for its possible ergogenic effects for nearly 100 years. Early research focused on improvements in strength, power, and psychomotor parameters such as reaction time. However, since research by Costill's laboratory in the late 1970s suggested caffeine could increase endurance, many researchers have investigated the effects of caffeine on fat metabolism as a means to enhance performance of endurance athletes, such as marathoners, primarily because of caffeine's potential to spare the use of muscle glycogen. In recent years, increased research attention has also refocused on the ergogenic potential of caffeine in tasks of higher exercise intensity and shorter duration.

Literally hundreds of studies have been conducted to test the ergogenic effectiveness of caffeine. Considerable differences exist in the experimental designs of caffeine studies in such aspects as caffeine dosage (3–15 mg per kg body weight), the type of exercise task (power, strength, reaction time, short-term endurance, prolonged endurance), the intensity of the exercise (submaximal exercise, maximal exercise), the training status of the subject (trained, untrained), the pre-exercise diet (high-carbohydrate, mixed), the subjects' caffeine status (user, abstainer), and individual variability (reactor, nonreactor). These differences complicate interpretation of the results.

Several reviews regarding the effect of caffeine on physical performance have been published recently, and the interested reader is referred to the articles by Dodd and others, Graham and Spriet, Spriet, and J. Williams. Based on these reviews and an independent analysis of key studies, the following points represent a general summary of the available research.

1. Caffeine can increase alertness, which may improve simple reaction time. Doses of 200 milligrams have been effective, particularly when subjects are mentally fatigued. Larger doses, above 400 milligrams, may increase nervousness and anxiousness, and thus may adversely affect performance in events characterized by fine motor skills and control of hand steadiness, such as pistol shooting.

2. The vast majority of earlier studies revealed that caffeine did not improve performance in events characterized by strength, speed, power, or local muscular endurance, nor in endurance events lasting less than 30 minutes, and this is the general conclusion of the review by Williams, which focuses on high-intensity exercise performance. More recent studies are inconsistent. Several support this general conclusion; however, other recent well-designed, double-blind, placebo, crossover studies have shown caffeine-induced improvement in several high-intensity exercise tasks. For example, Anselme and others reported significant improvements in maximal power (watts) production in 6 seconds; Collomp and others reported faster 100-meter swim times in highly-trained swimmers; Wiles and others noted significantly faster run times for 1,500 meters, particularly increased speed in the latter part of the race, in trained middle-distance runners; MacIntosh and Wright found significantly faster times in a 1,500-meter swim; Jackman and others reported increased time to exhaustion when exercising at 100 percent VO_2 max, a time approaching 5 minutes.

The enhanced performance noted in these exercise tasks may be attributed to psychological factors. In support of this point, Cole and others recently had subjects perform cycling tasks at several set ratings of perceived exertion (RPE), which is a scale representing how psychologically stressful the exercise appeared to be. In the three levels of RPE used, the subjects produced more work following caffeine ingestion as compared to the placebo. Although the subjects perceived the work tasks to be identical by the RPE scale, they actually generated more work with caffeine.

3. It is well established that caffeine may raise serum FFA levels at rest just before exercise, but there appears to be some controversy regarding serum FFA levels during exercise when trials with and without caffeine are compared. A number of studies that involved subjects who consumed caffeine beverages regularly and who also used a small dose of caffeine (5 mg/kg) have reported no significant differences between caffeine and placebo trials. The most likely reason is that exercise itself, as a stressor, stimulates epinephrine release and raises FFA levels comparable to the small dose. However, other studies that have involved subjects who were not regular caffeine users or who abstained from caffeine use for 4–7 days and which also employed large doses of caffeine (15 mg/kg) have noted significantly higher levels of FFA during exercise compared to placebo trials. Bucci reported fifteen studies in which caffeine increased FFA over the effect of exercise alone. Whether or not there are changes in plasma FFA may be irrelevant, for as Tarnopolsky notes, plasma concentrations do not provide us with appropriate information regarding

the flux of the FFA, that is, the rate at which it appears in the blood from the adipose tissue and the rate of entry into the muscle cell.

4. Even though caffeine may elevate FFA during exercise, whether the use of fat as an energy source is increased during exercise is debatable. Several reviewers have noted an inconsistency in the results when the respiratory quotient (RQ) was used to assess fuel utilization; the RQ may serve as a general guide to the percentage use of carbohydrate and fat during submaximal, mild- to moderate-intensity exercise. Although the data are inconsistent, the current belief is that caffeine will enhance the metabolism of FFA, either the FFA delivered in the plasma or the FFA derived from the intramuscular stores of triglycerides. In research done nearly 20 years ago, Essig noted that caffeine elicited an increased utilization of muscle triglycerides during exercise.

5. Current data suggest that caffeine ingestion prior to exercise will induce a glycogen-sparing effect. In all studies that have taken muscle biopsies, caffeine has been shown to exert a glycogen-sparing effect. Recent well-designed studies headed by Lawrence Spriet and Terry Graham from Canada show clearly that caffeine will spare the use of muscle glycogen during the first 15 minutes of exercise, supporting the research findings of Essig years ago. This glycogen-sparing will allow the subject to perform longer because of higher concentrations of muscle glycogen late in the exercise task. In the study by Spriet and others, no crossover design was used, for all subjects received the placebo first and then 1 week later, the caffeine. Muscle biopsies were taken at the point of exhaustion in the placebo trial. During the caffeine trial, the subjects were stopped for a muscle biopsy at the exact same time they reached exhaustion in the placebo trial; they were still performing but were stopped for the biopsy and then continued cycling. The muscle glycogen was higher in the caffeine trial compared to the placebo trial, strong evidence of a glycogen-sparing effect that allowed the athletes to continue to cycle.

6. As the duration of the endurance event increases to an hour or more, the research indicates, although not uniformly so, that caffeine may enhance performance. In many studies with improved performance, the psychological effect of caffeine was hypothesized as the cause. A number of studies have shown that caffeine may exert a stimulating effect on psychological processes, such as alertness and mood, which may diminish the perception of effort during exercise and thereby improve performance.

Several recent well-designed studies have shown significant increases in epinephrine levels during exercise following caffeine ingestion, both in elite and recreational athletes. Epinephrine responses to caffeine ingestion may be greater in nonusers versus habitual caffeine users. Epinephrine may exert a stimulating psychological effect, or it may promote glycogen-sparing. Although epinephrine release during exercise normally stimulates muscle glycogen catabolism, researchers suggest that caffeine may interfere with this effect within the cell, and the overall effect is enhanced fat oxidation and muscle-glycogen sparing, as noted above. Whatever the effect, recent studies by Graham and Spriet, Spriet and others, and French and others have shown remarkable improvements in performance with caffeine. For example, Graham and Spriet used elite distance runners as subjects and found that caffeine improved mean run time to exhaustion at 85 percent of VO_2 max from 49.2 minutes following the placebo to 71.0 minutes after caffeine (9 mg/kg body weight), a 44 percent improvement. Performance on a comparable cycling test to exhaustion revealed similar results. In most studies, the caffeine was taken 1 hour prior to performance, but French and others found that caffeine was effective even if taken immediately before the performance task.

7. Previous research has shown that carbohydrate loading and having a high-carbohydrate breakfast prior to competition may negate the metabolic effects of caffeine. High-carbohydrate levels stimulate insulin release, which appears to block the effect of caffeine in raising FFA levels. However, given the conflicting data as to whether or not plasma FFA accurately reflect the FFA flux, this observation may not be too meaningful. Moreover, the subjects in the study by Graham and Spriet did load with carbohydrates for several days prior to the exercise task, both in the placebo and caffeine trials, and it did not appear to affect the ergogenic effect of caffeine adversely.

8. One possible factor determining whether caffeine is an effective ergogenic aid is the caffeine status of the subjects. In many of the studies that report an ergogenic effect, subjects abstained from caffeine use for 2–4 days prior to the experiment; they became caffeine-free for several days to possibly heighten the caffeine effect when taken. This abstention period was based on some research reporting no effects of caffeine on epinephrine or FFA levels if subjects abstained for less than 1 day. Other research documented a decreased sensitivity to caffeine following 6 weeks of increased caffeine ingestion; that is, the epinephrine level was

decreased during exercise following this period of increased caffeine intake. However, in a recent review, Graham and Spriet suggest that caffeine withdrawal may have little effect on actual performance, and that subjects may consume caffeine products up to the day of the event.

9. Caffeine is a diuretic and also stimulates metabolism. Theoretically, increased water losses and an elevated metabolism before competition could impair exercise performance under warm, humid environmental conditions, possibly because of retarded sweat losses and excessive increases in body temperature. However, research has shown no changes in sweat loss, plasma volume, or body temperature following caffeine ingestion. Moreover, Cohen and others reported that caffeine ingestion did not impair performance in a 13.1-mile (21.1 km) half-marathon run outdoors under hot, humid conditions. Although running performance was not impaired by caffeine, nor was it improved. Wemple and others also found that drinking caffeinated sports drinks during exercise does not increase urine production.

10. Caffeine use has provided ergogenic effects when given in the range of very low doses (3 mg/kg) to very high doses (15 mg/kg). However, it should be noted that the maximal dose recommended without exceeding the IOC legal limit approximates 8–10 mg/kg body weight. For a 70-kg athlete, this would be 560–700 milligrams, about 4–6 cups of coffee or 3 Vivarin tablets. However, because there may be individual differences in caffeine clearance rates in the body, some researchers recommend the dose be limited to 7 mg/kg or less to avoid a positive drug test for excess caffeine use.

11. In general, studies have not reported a decrease in performance following caffeine ingestion. However, it should be noted that individuals vary in their responses to any drug. For example, in several of the studies the investigators reported that some subjects had adverse reactions to the caffeine and thus had an impaired performance.

12. If you are considering using caffeine as a potential ergogenic aid, it is wise to experiment with its use in training prior to use in competition. You might start by drinking 1–2 cups of coffee about an hour prior to some of your workouts. For example, if you are a distance runner, do your long runs periodically with and without the coffee or other caffeine source, and judge for yourself if it works for you. To make it a more valid case study, have someone randomly give you regular or decaffeinated coffee before the runs, but without informing you which type you are drinking until you have done each several times. Try this procedure also after abstaining from caffeine for 4–5 days. Keep a record of your feelings and times after the runs so you can compare differences.

Caffeine appears to be an effective ergogenic aid in doses that are both safe and legal. However, some athletes believe taking caffeine may be considered unethical because it is an artificial means to enhance performance. Given its safety and legality, the decision to use caffeine as a performance-enhancer rests with the ethical standards of the individual athlete.

Dietary Fats and Cholesterol: Health Implications

In Chapter 2, a number of dietary fat-reduction strategies were presented to reduce the consumption of total fat, saturated fat, and cholesterol, deriving most of the dietary fat from monounsaturated fats and polyunsaturated fats, including the omega-3 fatty acids. Such dietary changes are theorized to reduce the prevalence of certain chronic diseases and health problems, including obesity and the associated incidence of breast cancer and diabetes; cancer of the colon, rectum, and prostate; and risk factors associated with several cardiovascular diseases. Although the relationship between various forms of dietary fats and the development of chronic diseases is becoming clearer, there is still need for considerable research because the etiology of most chronic diseases is complex, involving multiple risk factors, only one of them being the composition of the diet. Remember, if you want to optimize your health, eliminating or reducing as many risk factors as possible is the best approach.

Researchers are attempting to unravel the specific mechanisms underlying the complex role of dietary fat in the etiology of various chronic diseases. One possibility, to be discussed in Chapter 10, is the role of total dietary fat intake in the development of obesity. For example, the role of dietary fat in the etiology of breast cancer is controversial. While some studies report an increased risk of breast cancer with increased dietary fat intake, a recent review by Hunter and others revealed no increased risk, and one recent study from Italy actually revealed a decreased risk of breast cancer with increased fat intake, an effect the authors attributed to the associated higher intake of vegetables. However, women who are obese appear to be more likely to develop breast cancer because excess body fat may lead to increased serum levels of estrogen, which is associated with an increased incidence of breast cancer. Obesity itself is also a risk factor for other forms of cancer, diabetes, hypertension, and cardiovascular disease. Another possibility is that specific dietary fats may elicit biochemical reactions in the body that may either promote or deter risk factors associated with chronic diseases. For example, saturated fats may lead to increased serum levels of cholesterol, whereas monounsaturated fats may decrease them. It is also possible that diets high in

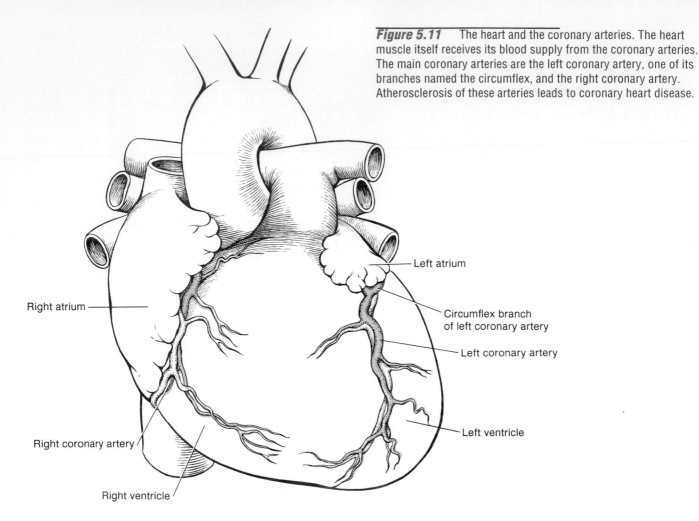

Figure 5.11 The heart and the coronary arteries. The heart muscle itself receives its blood supply from the coronary arteries. The main coronary arteries are the left coronary artery, one of its branches named the circumflex, and the right coronary artery. Atherosclerosis of these arteries leads to coronary heart disease.

Left atrium

Circumflex branch of left coronary artery

Left coronary artery

Left ventricle

Right atrium

Right coronary artery

Right ventricle

fat are low in complex carbohydrates, fruits and vegetables, thus diminishing dietary fiber and other nutrients regarded to be healthful.

Because the available evidence relating dietary lipids to cardiovascular diseases is so compelling, we shall treat this subject in some detail. However, note that the dietary and exercise recommendations advanced later in this chapter for the prevention of cardiovascular disease may also help prevent other chronic diseases, such as obesity and certain forms of cancer.

How does cardiovascular disease develop?

Nearly one out of every two deaths in the United States is due to diseases of the heart and blood vessels. Each year, approximately one million Americans die from some form of cardiovascular disease, including coronary heart disease, stroke, hypertensive disease, rheumatic heart disease, and congenital heart disease.

Coronary heart disease is the major disease of the cardiovascular system; of the million deaths noted previously, it is responsible for over half. Although the total percentage of deaths due to coronary heart disease has been declining in recent years, it is still an epidemic and the number one cause of death among Americans.

Coronary heart disease (CHD) is also known as **coronary artery disease (CAD)** because obstruction of the blood flow in the coronary arteries is responsible for the pathological effects of the disease. The coronary arteries are illustrated in Figure 5.11. The major manifestation of CHD is a heart attack, which results from a stoppage of blood flow to parts of the heart muscle. A decreased blood supply, known as **ischemia,** will deprive the heart of needed oxygen. In some individuals, ischemia results in **angina,** a sharp pain in the chest, jaw, or along the inside of the arm indicative of a mild heart attack. Other terms often associated with a heart attack include **coronary thrombosis,** a blockage of a blood vessel by a clot (thrombus), **coronary occlusion,** which simply means blockage, and **myocardial infarct,** death of heart cells that do not get enough oxygen due to the blocked coronary artery. The major cause of blocked arteries is atherosclerosis.

Arteriosclerosis is a term applied to a number of different pathological conditions wherein the arterial walls thicken and lose their elasticity. It is often defined as hardening of the arteries. **Atherosclerosis,** one form of arte-

Figure 5.12 The developmental process of atherosclerosis and thrombosis. Deposits of cholesterol and other debris (plaque) accumulate in the inner lining of the artery, leading to a decrease or cessation of blood flow to the tissues. Atherosclerosis in the coronary arteries is a major cause of heart disease.

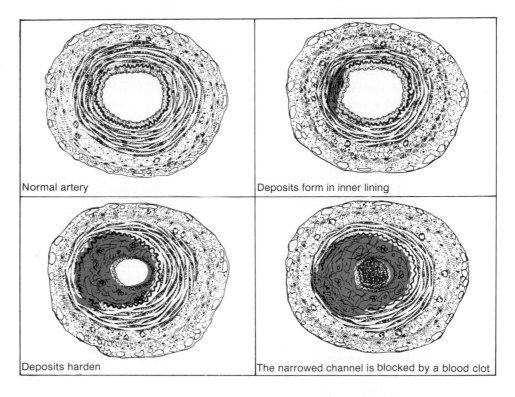

Normal artery

Deposits form in inner lining

Deposits harden

The narrowed channel is blocked by a blood clot

Figure 5.13 An enlargement of atherosclerotic plaque. Oxidized LDL cholesterol, macrophages, foam cells, fibrous material, and other debris collect beneath the endothelial cells lining the coronary artery. The site of the plaque may be initiated by some form of injury to the cell lining, possibly an ulceration as shown.

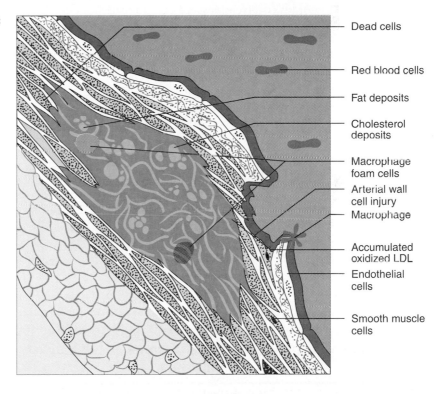

Dead cells

Red blood cells

Fat deposits

Cholesterol deposits

Macrophage foam cells

Arterial wall cell injury

Macrophage

Accumulated oxidized LDL

Endothelial cells

Smooth muscle cells

riosclerosis, is characterized by deposits of fat, oxidized LDL cholesterol, macrophages (white blood cells that oxidize LDL cholesterol), foam cells, cellular debris, calcium, and fibrin on the inner linings of the arterial wall. These deposits, known as **plaque,** result in a narrowing of the blood channel, making it easier for blood clots to form and eventually resulting in complete blockage of blood flow to vital tissues such as the heart or the brain. Figure 5.12 illustrates the gradual, progressive narrowing of the arterial channel. Figure 5.13 presents a schematic of the content of arterial plaque.

Atherosclerosis is a slow, progressive disease that begins in childhood and usually manifests itself later in life. Because of its prevalence in industrialized society, scientists throughout the world have been conducting intensive research to identify the cause or causes of atherosclerosis and coronary heart disease. The actual cause has not yet been completely identified, but considerable evidence has identified factors that may predispose an individual.

As noted previously, a risk factor represents a statistical relationship between two items such as high serum cholesterol and heart attack. This does not mean that a cause and effect relationship exists, although such a relationship is often strongly supported by the available evidence. The three principal risk factors associated with CHD are high blood pressure, high serum cholesterol levels, and cigarette smoking. Several major professional and governmental health organizations also believe that physical inactivity is a fourth principal risk factor. Other interacting risk factors are heredity, diabetes, diet, obesity, age, gender, stress, and several others. A guide to assessing your risk factor profile is presented in Appendix H.

How do the different forms of serum lipids affect the development of atherosclerosis?

In atherosclerosis, the plaque that develops in the arterial walls is composed partly of fats and cholesterol. Hence, high levels of blood lipids (triglycerides and cholesterol) are associated with increased plaque formation. However, as you recall, triglycerides and cholesterol may be transported in the blood in a variety of ways but primarily as constituents of lipoproteins. Considerable research has been devoted to identifying those specific lipoproteins and other lipid components that may predispose to CHD, and although there is some debate about the meaningfulness of specific serum lipid profiles, some theories prevail.

The major villain appears to be serum cholesterol, as depicted in Figure 5.14. Total cholesterol, expressed in milligrams per 100 milliliters of blood, is a significant risk factor. As noted in Table 5.7, a cholesterol level below 200 is considered to be desirable, between 200 and 239 is borderline-high, and above 240 is high. However, you should be aware that there is a rather large standard error

of measurement involved in some tests of cholesterol, being on the order of 30 milligrams. What this means is that if your blood cholesterol is reported as 220 (borderline-high), it may be possible that you actually have a cholesterol level of 190 (desirable) or 250 (high) if you vary, respectively, one standard error below or above your actual measurement of 220. For this reason, it may be a good idea to have a second test completed if you are concerned with your total cholesterol level.

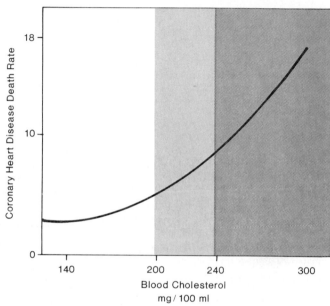

Figure 5.14 A desirable blood cholesterol is below 200 milligrams per deciliter (mg/dl). The rise of coronary heart disease fatalities increases progressively in individuals with borderline-high (200–240 mg/dl) and high blood cholesterol (> 240 mg/dl).

Source: U.S. Department of Health and Human Services, Public Health Service, National Institutes of Health, "So you have high blood cholesterol . . . ," in *NIH Publication No. 8972922*, 1989, U.S. Government Printing Office, Washington, DC.

Table 5.7	Recommended cholesterol and triglyceride levels* of the National Cholesterol Education Program sponsored by the National Heart, Lung, and Blood Institute			
	Total cholesterol classification	**LDL cholesterol classification**	**Serum triglyceride classification**	**HDL cholesterol classification**
Desirable	< 200	< 130	< 250	> 60
Borderline/high risk	200–239	130–159	250–400	—
High risk	> 240	> 160	> 400	< 35

*Levels expressed in mg/dl

The form by which cholesterol is transported in your blood may also be related to the development of atherosclerosis. In general, high levels of low-density lipoproteins (LDL) are associated with atherosclerosis. A current theory suggests various forms of LDL, such as small, dense LDL and the variant lipoprotein (a), may be more prone to oxidation by macrophages at an injured site in the arterial epithelium, leading to an influx into the cell wall and the formation of plaque. The presence of oxygen free radicals has been suggested to accelerate this process. Other mechanisms, such as increased clotting ability, may be operative. As noted in Table 5.7, LDL levels less than 130 are desirable, while those above 160 pose a high risk. Although not normally listed in risk factor tables, lipoprotein (a) values greater than 25–30 milligrams per deciliter of blood are associated with increased risk of CHD.

Conversely, high levels of high-density lipoproteins (HDL), particularly the subfraction HDL_2 and HDL with apolipoprotein A-I, appear to be protective against the development of atherosclerosis, although research is continuing to explore other relationships. Levels of 60 milligrams or more of HDL appear desirable, but because HDL varies daily, several measurements over time may be required to obtain an accurate reading. Research suggests that HDL interacts with the arterial epithelium, acting as a scavenger by picking up cholesterol from the arterial wall and transporting it to the liver for removal from the body, known as reverse cholesterol transport. HDL may also inhibit LDL oxidation and platelet aggregation.

Recent research by Stampfer and his colleagues suggests that increased levels of serum triglycerides is an independent risk factor for CHD. Also, they are often associated with increased levels of LDL and decreased levels of HDL. A summary of serum lipid factors associated with increased risk of atherosclerosis is presented in Table 5.8, representing new guidelines from the National Cholesterol Education Program.

If your total blood cholesterol is borderline or high, a determination of the LDL and HDL levels may be desirable, for they provide additional information relative to your risk. Based on epidemiological data, several ratios have been developed to assess risk of CHD, with the lower the ratio, the lower the risk.

One common comparison is the ratio of total cholesterol (TC) to the HDL level, or TC/HDL. A ratio of about 4.5 is associated with an average risk for CHD. For example, an individual with a total cholesterol of 200 and an HDL of 60 would have a ratio of 3.33 (200/60), or a lower risk, while someone with the same total cholesterol but an HDL of 20 would have a much higher risk with a ratio of 10 (200/20).

Another comparison is the ratio of LDL to HDL, or LDL/HDL. An LDL to HDL ratio of about 3.5 is considered to be an average risk for CHD. Thus, a ratio of 140/60, or 2.3, would be a much lower risk than 140/20, or 7.0.

Table 5.8 Serum lipid factors associated with increased risk of atherosclerosis

High levels of total cholesterol

High levels of LDL cholesterol

High levels of dense form of LDL cholesterol

High levels of abnormal apolipoprotein, apolipoprotein (a)

High levels of triglycerides

Low levels of HDL cholesterol

Low levels of HDL_2 cholesterol

Low levels of apolipoprotein A-I

Can I reduce my serum lipid levels and possibly reverse atherosclerosis?

Certain forms of hypercholesteremia are genetic in nature and for some individuals, drug therapy may be required to reduce serum lipid levels. Some drugs stimulate liver degradation and excretion of cholesterol, while others may bind with bile salts in the intestines so that they are not reabsorbed; because bile salts are derived from cholesterol, it is effectively excreted from the body.

However, a Positive Health Life-Style may not only help to prevent the development of atherosclerosis, but may also lead to regression of coronary artery blockage. In a recent review, Greg Brown and others noted that the available data support the hypothesis that lowering of serum lipids may lead to the regression of atherosclerotic lesions and elicit improved clinical effects. For those who are interested in preventing the development of atherosclerosis or reversing its progress, an appropriate diet and exercise program are two key elements of the Positive Health Life-Style that are recommended by health professionals. Both factors may not only have favorable effects on serum lipid levels, but other risk factors for CHD as well, such as obesity and hypertension.

What should I eat to modify my serum lipid profile favorably?

The National Cholesterol Education Program (NCEP) was developed with the general goal of reducing the prevalence of high serum cholesterol in the United States. One of the first steps is to identify those individuals with high serum cholesterol by various simplified screening techniques, such as the measurement of total cholesterol by small samples of blood obtained through fingertip capillary blood. If this measure is borderline-high (200–239 mg/dl) or high (> 240 mg/dl), venous blood samples may be taken

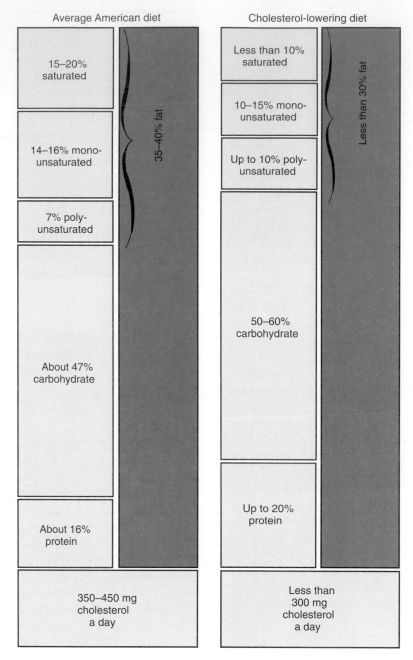

Figure 5.15 Comparison of the composition of the average American diet to the National Cholesterol Education Program Step 1 cholesterol-lowering diet.

Source: U.S. Department of Health and Human Services.

to determine LDL and HDL levels. If high serum cholesterol levels are detected, dietary modifications and other appropriate life-style changes may be recommended.

Figure 5.15 illustrates the composition of the average American diet and the Step 1 diet of the NCEP. Although the differences between the two diets appear to be small, such changes may reduce serum lipids. A sensible plan to reduce serum lipid levels is presented in Figure 5.16, and representative results are shown in Figure 5.17. If the original dietary plan is not effective after several months, the Step 2 NCEP diet may be recommended, which is essentially the same as the Step 1 diet but with less than 7 percent of the dietary Calories from saturated fat and less than 200 milligrams of cholesterol per day.

Several health organizations, including the American Heart Association, the National Institutes of Health, and the National Heart, Lung, and Blood Institute have recommended a number of dietary guidelines that have been shown to lower serum cholesterol or serum triglycerides.

Measuring your progress: A sensible plan

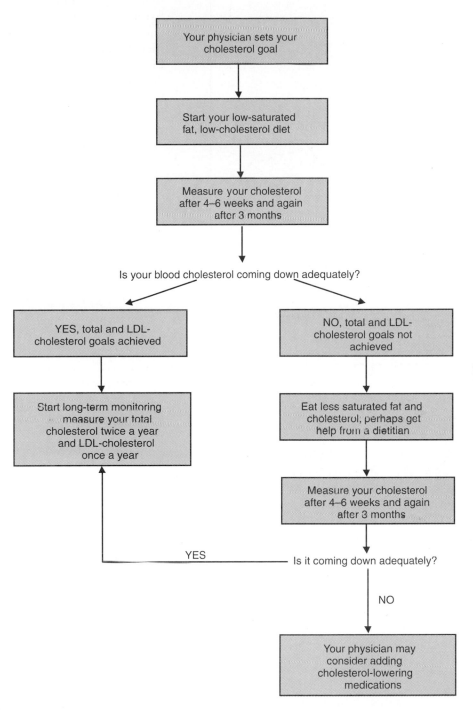

Figure 5.16 A sensible plan to monitor the effects of a cholesterol-lowering diet. The initial diet plan may involve the National Cholesterol Education Program Step 1 diet, but if unsuccessful, the Step 2 diet may be implemented. In individuals highly resistant to dietary modifications, drug therapy may be prescribed.

Source: U.S. Department of Health and Human Services.

Based on the available scientific evidence, the following guidelines appear to be prudent. Although these guidelines have been developed to help individuals reduce high serum lipid profiles, they will also help to maintain normal levels and thus may be regarded as preventive medicine. As you may note, these recommendations are extensions of some guidelines for the Healthy North American Diet.

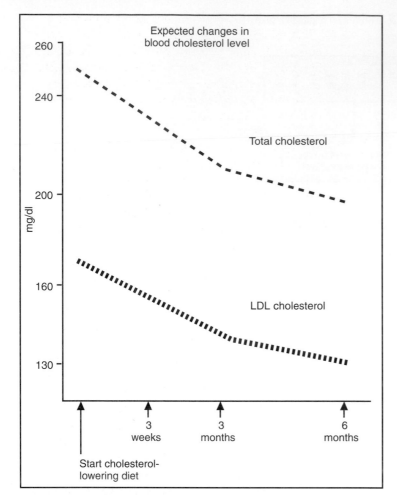

Figure 5.17 Representative expected changes in total serum cholesterol and LDL cholesterol associated with appropriate dietary modifications, such as switching from the typical American diet to the Step 1 diet of the National Cholesterol Education Program (NCEP).

Source: U.S. Department of Health and Human Services.

1. Adjust caloric intake to achieve and maintain ideal body weight. One of the most common causes of high triglyceride levels is too much body fat. In many cases, simply losing body weight or reducing caloric intake will reduce these levels.

2. Reduce the total amount of fats in the diet. As mentioned previously, less than 30 percent of dietary Calories should be derived from fat. Reducing the total amount of fat will usually reduce the amount of Calories also, but nutrient content will actually improve. Reducing total fat intake to 20 percent or even 10 percent of total daily Calories will reduce total and LDL cholesterol even more. However, the carbohydrate Calories that replace the fat Calories should *not* be derived from refined carbohydrates, but rather from complex carbohydrates containing dietary fiber.

3. Reduce the amount of saturated fat to less than 10 percent of dietary Calories. Saturated fats, particularly lauric, myristic, and palmitic fatty acids, have been shown to increase blood cholesterol levels, particularly LDL cholesterol associated with development of atherosclerosis. Saturated fats may also increase blood clotting, another risk factor for CHD. In two recent meta-analyses, Howell and others found that consumption of saturated fatty acids was the major dietary determinant of plasma cholesterol response to diet, while Clarke and others indicated that reducing the intake of saturated fat produced the most significant benefits regarding the prevention of CHD.

4. Reduce the consumption of hydrogenated or partially hydrogenated vegetable oils. They not only become more saturated, but contain a greater proportion of trans unsaturated fatty acids. Research has indicated that trans fatty acids may have an adverse effect on serum lipid levels and increase the risk of CHD; trans fatty acids may increase serum levels of LDL cholesterol and lipoprotein (a) and decrease levels of HDL cholesterol and apolipoprotein A-I. Although some reviewers contend that the adverse effects of trans fatty acids are somewhat less than those associated with saturated fatty acids, the Consumers Union recently cited research indicating that they may be as bad, or even worse. At the present time, the amount of trans present in foods is not indicated on food labels, so you need to look for the terms "hydrogenated" and "partially hydrogenated." Some trans fatty acids appear naturally in meat, but processed foods that contain substantial amounts of trans fatty acids include margarine; vegetable shortening; white bread; packaged goods such as cookies, crackers, potato chips, and cakes; and fried fast foods such as french fries. The major component of each of these foods that adds trans fatty acids is usually partially hydrogenated vegetable oils. Using olive oil or diet and whipped margarine may help reduce one of the major sources of dietary trans fatty acids. Fat-free margarines contain no trans fatty acids.

5. Substitute polyunsaturated and monounsaturated fats for saturated fats. Consume 10 percent or less of the total dietary Calories from polyunsaturated fats and 10–15 percent from monounsaturated fats.

   When substituted for saturated fats, polyunsaturated fatty acids have been reported to reduce total serum cholesterol levels, including LDL cholesterol; however, some research has shown they may also reduce HDL cholesterol levels. Additionally, high amounts of linoleic acid, a polyunsaturated fatty acid, in the diet have been associated with the development of cancer of the colon; thus, try to limit the daily intake of polyunsaturated fats to 10 percent of the total Calories, or less. Researchers theorize that the double bonds in these fatty acids are easily oxidized and may produce carcinogenic free radicals. Fortunately, natural vegetable foods that are high in polyunsaturated fatty acids are also high in certain vitamins that have antioxidant properties and help counteract the oxidation of these bonds. Vegetable foods with polyunsaturated fatty acids also contain alpha-linolenic acid and various phytochemicals that are thought to prevent the development of cancer.

Monounsaturated fats appear to be just as effective as polyunsaturated fats in reducing total and LDL cholesterol without lowering HDL cholesterol. Olive and canola oil are particularly high in monounsaturated fatty acids. Earlier research, primarily with hypercholesteremic individuals, suggested that polyunsaturated fats would also lower HDL cholesterol, an undesirable effect, while monounsaturated fats would not. However, Dreon and others recently noted no HDL-lowering effect of a polyunsaturated fat-enriched diet, when compared with a monounsaturated fat-enriched diet, in healthy individuals on a low-fat diet. With respect to plasma HDL cholesterol levels, these investigators concluded that there is no apparent advantage in using predominantly monounsaturated rather than polyunsaturated fats if subjects are on the generally recommended healthy diet, which is reduced in fat.

The overall general recommendation is to consume more or less equal proportions of saturated, monounsaturated, and polyunsaturated fatty acids, possibly with a slightly higher proportion of monounsaturated fats and a lower proportion of saturated fats. In a recent poll of over 30 nutrition experts conducted by the Consumers Union, although the majority agreed that dietary fat should constitute 30 percent of daily Calories or lower, about a dozen experts indicated the 30 percent limit could be higher if more healthful fats were chosen, such as in the Mediterranean diet rich in monounsaturated fats (olive oil) and polyunsaturated fats (fish, nuts).

6. Consume foods rich in omega-3 fatty acids, a special form of polyunsaturated fatty acids. The main omega-3 fatty acid in plants is alpha-linolenic acid. Fish oils are the primary source of two other omega-3 fatty acids, EPA (eicosapentaenoic acid) and DHA (docosahexaenoic acid). Relative to health effects, EPA and DHA are considered to be more important than alpha-linolenic acid; although EPA and DHA may be formed in the body from alpha-linolenic acid, this process appears to be limited so the most concentrated source of EPA and DHA in the diet is fish oil.

As mentioned earlier, omega-3 fatty acids have been theorized to be ergogenic in nature because of the production of specific eicosanoids. Omega-3 fatty acids are also being studied for their potential health benefits, which also may be related to specific eicosanoids that are produced. Although the health-related role of omega-3 fatty acids and eicosanoids is complex and has not been totally determined, here is a simple summarization. The cell membrane contains a variety of molecular compounds, including phospholipids and their associated fatty acids. When the diet is high in linoleic acid, one of the main fatty acids in the phospholipids is arachidonic acid, which produces one form of eicosanoids when it is metabolized. When the diet is high in fish oils, EPA and DHA become the major source of eicosanoids, which are different in nature compared to those derived from arachidonic acid. In essence, the different forms of eicosanoids, functioning as local hormones, elicit characteristic effects, and those effects associated with omega-3 fatty acid-derived eicosanoids appear to provide some health benefits.

Epidemiological research has suggested populations that consume diets rich in fish products have a lower incidence rate of coronary heart disease, and experimental research has suggested a number of possible mechanisms underlying this relationship. Omega-3 fatty acids may reduce serum triglycerides and may increase HDL cholesterol, although they appear to have no effect on total serum cholesterol. Eicosanoids derived from omega-3 fatty acids may also decrease platelet aggregation and stickiness, possibly helping to prevent clot formation. They may also improve vascular tone and decrease blood viscosity. Collectively, all of these effects could help prevent CHD. Just as there are good and bad forms of cholesterol, there may be good and bad forms of eicosanoids, at least as related to cardiovascular health. Additionally, eicosanoids derived from omega-3 fatty acids may exert beneficial effects on the immune system, possibly helping to inhibit tumor growth associated with cancer.

Fish such as salmon, sardines, mackerel, and tuna, as well as wheat germ oil, canola oil, and common varieties of beans, have substantial amounts of omega-3 fatty acids. Some scientists suggest 1–2 servings of fish per week may provide some beneficial effects. Although the American Heart Association does recommend an increased consumption of fish, it does not recommend the use of commercial fish oil supplements, because their long-term effectiveness and safety have not been established. They are high in Calories in the dosages recommended, and they may have adverse effects in some individuals, such as prolonged bleeding time. Continued research with fish oil supplements should help to resolve this issue in the future.

Whether or not omega-3 fatty acids may protect you against CHD or other diseases may be dependent on your genetics. Some individuals may benefit, others may not, and supplements may actually be harmful to some. The interested reader is referred to the review by Berdanier. But for now, a diet low in saturated fatty acids and high in natural plant and fish sources of omega-3 fatty acids is highly recommended.

7. Decrease the amount of dietary cholesterol. Even though only about 35–40 percent of dietary cholesterol is absorbed, blood serum levels go up with increasing amounts in the diet. This is particularly true for cholesterol responders, those individuals with a genetic predisposition whose body production of cholesterol does not automatically decrease when the dietary intake increases. The average U.S. daily intake is approximately 400–500 milligrams or more. It is recommended that this amount be reduced to 300 milligrams per day or less, or 100 milligrams per 1,000 Calories consumed. The most significant dietary reductions should be saturated fat.

8. If you consume foods with artificial fats, do so in moderation. The American Dietetic Association (ADA) notes that fat substitutes possess the potential to reduce the intake of dietary fat, citing opinions that they may be able to reduce current dietary fat intake to 30 percent or less of the daily Calories. However, the ADA also notes that fat substitutes should be used in the context of the Healthy North American Diet and should not be used to displace healthful foods. Some fat is needed in the diet to provide the essential fatty acids and fat-soluble vitamins, and this fat should be obtained easily through natural, wholesome foods such as whole grains, fruits, and vegetables.

In a review article, David Mela indicates fat substitutes appear to pose little risk to the consumer, and although there are potential health benefits associated with their incorporation into a healthy diet, few data are available to indicate they possess any health benefits. One possible health benefit may

be their application in weight-loss programs, and this topic will be covered in Chapter 11.

9. Reduce intake of refined sugars and increase consumption of foods high in complex carbohydrates and dietary fiber. Table sugar provokes higher triglyceride concentrations more than complex carbohydrates with fiber do. Again, the value of complex carbohydrates in the diet is stressed, particularly high-fiber foods, as a means to help reduce serum cholesterol. Recent research has suggested that without adequate amounts of dietary fiber, a diet low in saturated fats and cholesterol has only modest effects on lowering CHD risk. Thus, replace high-fat foods with high-fiber foods. Increased consumption of fruits and vegetables is recommended as well, for they may provide substantial amounts of the antioxidant vitamins (C, E, and beta-carotene) that may help to prevent undesired oxidations in the body. Guidelines presented in the preceding chapter are helpful to increase carbohydrate intake, and the role of antioxidant vitamins will be discussed in Chapter 7.

10. Nibble food throughout the day. Interestingly, David Jenkins showed a significant reduction in serum LDL cholesterol if subjects consumed their daily Calories, actually the same food, throughout the day rather than in three concentrated meals at breakfast, lunch, and dinner.

In simple practical terms, what do all of these recommendations mean? You should not eliminate all fat from your diet, but simply reduce the amount of fat that you eat. In essence, eat less butter, fatty meats, organ foods such as liver and kidney, egg yolks, whole milk, cheeses, ice cream, gravies, creamed foods, high-fat desserts, and refined sugar. Eat more lean meats, fish, poultry, egg whites, skim and low-fat milk products, fruits and vegetables, beans, and whole-grain products, or the Healthy North American Diet. Table 5.9 provides some specifics.

Can exercise training also elicit favorable changes in the serum lipid profile?

Physical inactivity, or lack of exercise, has been identified as one of the risk factors associated with an increased incidence of atherosclerosis and cardiovascular disease. Hence, exercise programs stressing aerobic endurance-type activities have been advocated as a means of reducing the incidence levels of these conditions, possibly via direct beneficial effects on the heart or blood vessels. However, the precise mechanism whereby exercise may help reduce the morbidity and mortality of CAD has not been identified. Therefore, many authorities believe that the beneficial effect may not be due to exercise itself, but rather the possible associated effects such as reductions in body fat and blood pressure. Although some investigators believe endurance exercise may have a preventive function independent of these associated effects, it also exerts a significant beneficial influence on the serum lipid profile, which, like blood pressure, is one of the major risk factors. An acute exercise session, such as a five-mile run, may elicit a temporary decrease in serum triglycerides and increase in HDL cholesterol, but our concern here is with the more permanent effects associated with a habitual endurance exercise training program.

Literally hundreds of epidemiological and experimental studies have been conducted in the past decade to address the question posed above. Space does not permit a detailed analysis of each, but major reviews of the worldwide literature have been reported by prominent authorities such as Stefanik and Wood from the internationally renowned Stanford University research group. These reviews have noted a rather consistent pattern relating exercise and blood lipids. In general, increased levels of exercise are associated with lower plasma levels of triglycerides and LDL, and higher levels of HDL. Research has also indicated that the individuals at greatest risk, those with a total cholesterol over 240, may experience the greatest benefit. Recent research has shown, however, that neither an acute bout of exercise nor chronic low-intensity or high-intensity exercise has any effect on lipoprotein (a). This risk factor apparently is not influenced by exercise.

To bring about significant changes in the serum lipid profile, endurance exercise equivalent to running 10–15 miles per week, about an additional 1,000 Calories of energy expenditure, appears to be a reasonable estimate of a weekly threshold level. This level must be held for a prolonged period, possibly 3–9 months, before benefits may be noted. Additional caloric expenditure per week may elicit further improvements; lifetime aerobic exercise appears to be the key, but moderately intense leisure-time activity, such as brisk walking, may also elicit beneficial effects.

However, in women, excessive exercise that causes amenorrhea may reverse these benefits. The effects of exercise-induced amenorrhea will be discussed further in Chapters 8 and 10, but it appears that the lower levels of estrogen associated with this condition may lead to lower levels of HDL cholesterol.

Although the precise biochemical mechanisms underlying the beneficial effects of exercise on serum lipids have not been identified, researchers have found that in physically trained males and females, activity levels of several enzymes, such as hepatic lipase and lipoprotein lipase, are modified in such a way as to promote a more rapid catabolism of triglycerides and a greater production of HDL. Exercise may also favorably modify the serum lipid levels by helping the individual lose body fat or influencing changes in other aspects of his or her life-style, such as diet.

Research has revealed that the beneficial effects of exercise training are additive to a diet modified in fat content, such as substitution of polyunsaturated omega-3 fatty acids for saturated fat. Moreover, a low-fat diet will reduce total cholesterol and LDL cholesterol but may also decrease HDL cholesterol. Exercise may prevent or attenuate the decrease in HDL cholesterol. Thus, the combination of both dietary modifications and exercise is the recommended approach to modify favorably serum lipid levels.

Recent research also reveals that highly-trained endurance runners who increase their dietary fat to about 40 percent of daily caloric intake for 4 weeks do not experience any adverse effects in their blood lipid profiles. Although this type of diet is not recommended on a long-term basis, this study by Leddy and others illustrates some of the protective effects of exercise training on serum lipid changes associated with short-term increases in dietary fat.

Does drinking coffee, tea, or other caffeinated beverages pose any significant health risk?

This is one of the most hotly debated questions over the past quarter century. In the early 1970s and 1980s a number of epidemiological studies linked coffee or caffeine consumption with the development of a variety of health problems, including heart disease and associated risk factors such as high serum cholesterol and high blood pressure; pancreatic cancer; fibrocystic breast disease; osteoporosis; and pregnancy-related problems such as infertility, miscarriages, low birth weight, and birth defects. Conversely, other epidemiological studies have shown no relationship between coffee or caffeine consumption and these health problems. Investigators have looked at a variety of factors, including different sources of caffeine such as coffee versus tea, regular versus decaffeinated coffee, and even the method of preparing coffee, such as filtered versus boiled.

Many of the earlier reported adverse findings associated with caffeine consumption were derived from rather small epidemiological studies or from animal research using rather high doses of caffeine. However, more contemporary, larger epidemiological studies have been conducted, and two recent reviews have evaluated these reports and summarized the effect of caffeine on a variety of health problems. The following represent the key points presented in the reviews by Lamarine, The Consumers Union and by the Association of Women's Health, Obstetric and Neonatal Nurses, as well as other independent sources.

Cardiovascular Disease and Associated Risk Factors
Caffeine is a stimulant that may affect heart function. In some individuals it may cause a slight arrhythmia, or irregular heart beat. Caffeine may also acutely increase blood pressure in individuals who are caffeine-sensitive and also in individuals who are under stress. However, these reactions are relatively rare. Individuals

Table 5.9 Food selections to decrease total dietary fat, saturated fat, and cholesterol

	Choose	Go easy on	Decrease
Meat, poultry, fish and shellfish (up to 6 ounces a day)	Lean cuts of meat with fat trimmed, like: beef—round, sirloin, chuck, loin lamb—leg, arm, loin, rib pork—tenderloin, leg (fresh), shoulder (arm or picnic) veal—all trimmed cuts except ground poultry without skin fish, shellfish		"Prime" grade fatty cuts of meat like: beef—corned beef brisket, regular ground, short ribs pork—spareribs, blade roll Goose, domestic duck Organ meats like: liver, kidney, sweetbreads, brain Sausage, bacon, frankfurters, regular luncheon meats Caviar, roe
Dairy products (2 servings a day; 3 servings for women who are pregnant or breast-feeding)	Skim milk, 1% milk, low-fat buttermilk, low-fat evaporated or nonfat milk Low-fat yogurt and low-fat frozen yogurt Low-fat soft cheeses, like: cottage, farmer, pot Cheese labeled no more than 2 to 6 grams of fat an ounce	2% milk Part-skim ricotta Part-skim or imitation hard cheeses, like: part-skim mozzarella "Light" cream cheese "Light" sour cream	Whole milk, like: regular, evaporated, condensed Cream, half-and-half, most nondairy creamers and products, real or nondairy whipped cream Cream cheese, sour cream, ice cream, custard-style yogurt Whole-milk ricotta High-fat cheeses, like: Neufchatel, Brie, Swiss, American, mozzarella, feta, cheddar, Muenster
Eggs (no more than 3 egg yolks a week)	Egg whites Cholesterol-free egg substitutes		Egg yolks
Fats and oils (up to 6 to 8 teaspoons a day)	Unsaturated vegetable oils, like: corn, olive, peanut, rapeseed (canola oil), safflower, sesame, soybean Margarine or shortening made with unsaturated fats listed above: liquid, tub, stick Diet mayonnaise, salad dressings made with unsaturated fats listed above Low-fat dressings	Nuts and seeds Avocados and olives	Butter, coconut oil, palm kernel oil, palm oil, lard, bacon fat Margarine or shortening made with saturated fats listed above Dressings made with egg yolk
Breads, cereals, pasta, rice, dried peas and beans (6 to 11 servings a day)	Breads, like: white, whole wheat, pumpernickel, and rye breads; sandwich buns; dinner rolls; bagels; English muffins; rice cakes Low-fat crackers, like: matzo, pita; bread sticks, rye krisp, saltines, zwieback Hot cereals, most cold dry cereals Pasta, like: plain noodles, spaghetti, macaroni Any grain rice Dried peas and beans, like: split peas, black-eyed peas, chickpeas, kidney beans, navy beans, lentils, soybeans, soybean curd (tofu)	Store-bought pancakes, waffles, biscuits, muffins, cornbread	Croissants, butter rolls, sweet rolls, Danish pastry, doughnuts Most snack crackers, like: cheese crackers, butter crackers, those made with saturated fats Granola-type cereals made with saturated fats Pasta and rice prepared with cream, butter, or cheese sauces; egg noodles

Fruits and vegetables (2 to 4 servings of fruit and 3 to 5 servings of vegetables)	Fresh, frozen, canned, or dried fruits and vegetables		Vegetables prepared in butter, cream, or sauce
Sweets and snacks (avoid too many sweets)	Low-fat frozen desserts, like: sherbet, sorbet, Italian ice, frozen yogurt, popsicles Low-fat cakes, like: angel food cake Low-fat cookies, like: fig bars, gingersnaps Low-fat candy, like: jelly beans, hard candy Low-fat snacks, like: plain popcorn, pretzels Nonfat beverages, like: carbonated drinks, juices, tea, coffee	Frozen desserts, like: ice milk Homemade cakes, cookies, and pies using unsaturated oils sparingly Fruit crisps and cobblers Potato and corn chips prepared with unsaturated vegetable oil	High-fat frozen desserts, like: ice cream, frozen tofu High-fat cakes, like: most store-bought, pound, and frosted cake Store-bought pies, most store-bought cookies Most candy, like: chocolate bars Potato and corn chips prepared with saturated fat Buttered popcorn High-fat beverages, like: frappes, milkshakes, floats, eggnogs
Label ingredients (To avoid much fat, saturated fat, or cholesterol, go easy on products that list first any fat, oil, or ingredients higher in saturated fat or cholesterol. Choose more often those products that contain ingredients lower in fat, saturated fat, and cholesterol.)	Ingredients lower in saturated fat or cholesterol: Carob, cocoa Oils, like: corn, cottonseed, olive, safflower, sesame, soybean, sunflower Nonfat dry milk, nonfat dry milk solids, skim milk		Ingredients higher in saturated fat or cholesterol: Chocolate Animal fat, like: bacon, beef, ham, lamb, meat, pork, chicken or turkey fats, butter, lard Coconut, coconut oil, palm-kernel or palm oil Cream Egg and egg-yolk solids Hardened fat or oil Hydrogeneated vegetable oil Shortening or vegetable shortening, unspecified vegetable oil (could be coconut, palm-kernel, palm)

Source: Adapted from "Report of the Expert Panel of Detection, Evaluation, and Treatment of High Blood Cholesterol in Adults." National Heart, Lung, and Blood Institutes of Health.

who may experience arrhythmias, who are under stress, or who are hypertensive should consult their physicians regarding the use of caffeine.

Several recent reviews have investigated the relationship between coffee consumption and serum lipid levels, noting an inconsistency in the results of most studies. Some studies have shown that both caffeinated and decaffeinated coffee may raise serum cholesterol, but others have reported no effects. In some cases where the cholesterol levels rose, the authors noted the increases were of little clinical significance. Increased serum cholesterol levels have been associated with the method of preparation, particularly boiling coffee as practiced in Scandinavia and other parts of the world. Several cholesterol-raising substances (cafestol and kahweol) have been found in the oil droplets formed in the boiling process. These substances are removed when coffee is filtered, the major means of coffee preparation used in the United States and Canada.

Based on contemporary research, the office of the U.S. Surgeon General reported that evidence of the relationship between coffee and heart disease was too weak to warrant recommending a reduction of coffee consumption, and the American Heart Association stated that moderate coffee consumption does not appear to be harmful to the heart.

Cancer The American Cancer Society, after reviewing the available scientific evidence, indicated there is no known association between the consumption of coffee, tea, or other caffeinated beverages and the development of any type of cancer.

Fibrocystic Breast Disease Fibrocystic breast disease involves the development of benign fibrous lumps in the breast tissue that might develop tenderness or become painful. Although an earlier anecdotal report suggested an association with caffeine intake, a major study by the National Cancer Institute (NCI) revealed no evidence supporting such an association. Both the NCI and a health committee of the American Medical Association stated there is no association between caffeine intake and fibrocystic breast disease.

Osteoporosis Factors underlying the development of osteoporosis are discussed in detail in Chapter 8. Essentially, calcium loss may lead to osteoporosis. For now, we may note that caffeine tends to accelerate the use of calcium from bones and lead to its excretion in the urine. However, the amount is very small, approximating only 5 milligrams of calcium loss for every cup of coffee. Using 2 tablespoons of milk in the coffee would replace the amount of lost calcium. In a recent report, the National Institutes of Health indicated caffeine use does not cause significant losses of calcium. However, drinking milk or eating calcium-rich foods is highly recommended if you drink caffeinated beverages.

Pregnancy-Related Health Problems Animal research has suggested that very high doses of caffeine, administered directly into the stomach via tubes, could impair fertility or interfere with fetal development, causing detrimental pregnancy consequences such as miscarriage, low birth weight, or birth defects. However, other animal research, administering caffeine in fluids as normally consumed by humans, did not produce such effects. Moreover, several major human epidemiological studies have not provided any evidence showing an association between moderate caffeine consumption and adverse effects on pregnancy outcome. Nevertheless, because of the earlier research findings with animals, the Food and Drug Administration and the American Dietetic Association recommend that pregnant women consider abstaining from caffeine use, or if they do drink caffeine beverages to do so in moderation.

Weight Control Caffeine use may stimulate metabolism, increasing the resting metabolic rate about 10 percent for several hours, an effect which theoretically could facilitate weight loss. However, although caffeine was once one of the main ingredients in over-the-counter weight-loss products, its use in this regard has been banned because it does not provide any long-term benefits. Proper weight-control procedures are discussed in Chapters 10 and 11.

Sleeplessness Caffeine use, particularly before retiring for the night, may delay the onset of sleep because of its stimulant effects.

Gastric Distress Some individuals experience stomach irritation due to increased secretion of gastric acids following ingestion of caffeinated beverages. In such cases, individuals should consult their physician or avoid caffeine.

Caffeine Naivete Abstainers or those who consume little caffeine may experience nervousness, irritability, headaches, or insomnia with moderate doses, although long-term consumption of coffee leads to development of tolerance and reduction of these "coffee nerves" symptoms.

Caffeine Dependence Although not classified as an addictive drug, some individuals may develop caffeine dependence, often referred to as caffeinism; caffeine dependence is listed in the *Diagnostic and Statistical Manual of Mental Disorders* published by the American Psychiatric Association. Caffeine-dependent individuals may experience various symptoms upon caffeine withdrawal, including headaches and nervousness. However, caffeine dependence is not considered a serious form of drug abuse.

Death Although rare, death may result from overdoses of caffeine-containing diet or stimulant pills. Individuals who take several different over-the-counter dietary supplements may be taking substantial amounts of caffeine along with other drugs. Such combinations, in excess, may be fatal.

In general though, most professional health organizations note that caffeine is regarded to be a safe drug. If you are healthy and are not on medications, several cups of coffee or caffeinated beverages should pose no health problems. Where moderation is recommended, the dosage is the equivalent of less than 300 milligrams of caffeine per day, or about 2–3 cups of coffee. And we are talking 6-ounce cups of coffee or so, not the supersize 20-ounce cups or higher from local convenience stores.

Caffeine may actually confer some possible health benefits. Caffeine increases alertness, promotes clearer thinking, and diminishes drowsiness, all factors that may contribute to safer automobile operation under certain conditions.

Can very low serum cholesterol levels affect health?

Although most of the focus of this chapter has been on prevention of high levels of serum cholesterol, there has been some recent concern relative to very low levels, those below 160 mg/dl. In 1990, the National Heart, Lung, and Blood Institute held a conference on the association of low cholesterol levels to mortality, and based on a review of nineteen studies, indicated that there was an increase in all cause mortality in individuals who had serum cholesterol levels lower than 160 mg/dl, as compared to those with levels of 160 to 199 mg/dl. There was no increased risk of CHD and a slight increased risk of various forms of cancer associated with low cholesterol levels, but there were major increases in risk for digestive diseases and traumatic death, such as suicide, homicide, and accidental death. Other reports indicate increased mortality due to hemorrhagic stroke, infectious diseases, and alcohol dependence syndrome. An interesting perspective on health benefits and risks of lowering serum cholesterol is presented by Allred.

There may be some cause and effect relationships because very low cholesterol levels may interfere with the production of cellular constituents that help prevent disease. Low serum cholesterol may lead to inadequate amounts of serotonin in the brain, a neurotransmitter that may induce relaxation effects. Decreased serotonin may lead to depression or aggressive behavior. Additionally, low serum cholesterol may prolong bleeding time, which may lead to prolonged hemorrhage. However, a Consumers Union report questions whether or not there is a cause and effect relationship, suggesting low serum cholesterol is the result of illness, not the cause of it. A number of disease conditions, particularly of the liver and pancreas, as well as alcoholism, may depress serum cholesterol levels. As is well known, alcoholism is associated with a variety of digestive disorders and increased incidence rates of violent deaths, i.e., suicide, homicide, and accidental death.

In a recent study, Harris reported that those with low cholesterol levels comprised two distinct groups of people, healthy and unhealthy. In this study, most of the adverse health effects of low serum cholesterol were seen in the elderly, those aged 65 and above. However, older individuals with low cholesterol levels who were physically active, i.e., healthy, had no significant increased mortality rates compared to individuals with higher serum cholesterol levels. Harris concluded low serum cholesterol is not associated with increased mortality in individuals who are classified as healthy. If you are young and healthy, the current advice is not to worry about low serum cholesterol.

This issue is currently being debated, but most authorities suggest that it is still beneficial to reduce serum cholesterol to 200 mg/dl or below, for the health benefits relative to CHD may be substantial. On the other hand, for individuals who have a serum cholesterol between 160–199 mg/dl, aggressive techniques to reduce it even further may not be advisable, for the available data do not appear to support an additional protective effect against CHD with levels lower than 160 mg/dl, and based on the observational data available, there may be some associated health risks with very low levels. Additionally, for those with serum cholesterol levels lower than 160 mg/dl, authorities do not recommend attempts to raise it higher, such as by consumption of high-fat diets.

References

Books

Bucci, L. 1993. *Nutrients as Ergogenic Aids for Sports and Exercise.* Boca Raton, FL: CRC Press.

Byrne, K. 1991. *Understanding and Managing Cholesterol: A Guide for Wellness Professionals.* Champaign, IL: Human Kinetics.

Cureton, T. 1972. *The Physiological Effects of Wheat Germ Oil on Humans in Exercise.* Springfield, IL: C C Thomas.

Jeukendrup, A. 1997. *Aspects of Carbohydrate and Fat Metabolism During Exercise.* Haarlem: De Vriesborch.

Lee, R., and Nieman, D. 1993. *Nutritional Assessment.* Madison, WI: Brown and Benchmark.

National Research Council. 1989. *Recommended Dietary Allowances.* Washington, DC: National Academy Press.

National Research Council. 1989. *Diet and Health: Implications for Reducing Chronic Disease Risk.* Washington, DC: National Academy Press.

Sears, B. 1993. *Essential Fatty Acids, Eicosanoids, and Dietary Endocrinology.* Marblehead, MA: Eicotec Foods.

Spiller, G. 1997. Caffeine. Boca Raton, FL: CRC Press.

U.S. Department of Health and Human Services Public Health Service. 1992. *So You Have High Blood Cholesterol . . .* Bethesda, MD: National Institute of Health.

U.S. Department of Health and Human Services Public Health Service. 1992. *Eating to Lower Your High Blood Cholesterol.* Bethesda, MD: National Institutes of Health.

U.S. Department of Health and Human Services Public Health Service. 1991. *Healthy People 2000: National Health Promotion and Disease Prevention Objectives.* Washington, DC: U.S. Government Printing Office.

U.S. Department of Health and Human Services Public Health Service. 1990. *National Cholesterol Education Program Report of the Expert Panel on Population Strategies for Blood Cholesterol Reduction.* Bethesda, MD: National Institutes of Health.

Wolinsky, I., and Hickson, J. 1994. *Nutrition in Exercise and Sport.* Boca Raton, FL: CRC Press.

Reviews

Allred, J. 1993. Lowering serum cholesterol: Who benefits? *Journal of Nutrition* 123:1453–59.

American Academy of Pediatrics. 1992. Statement on cholesterol. *Pediatrics* 90:469–73.

American Dietetic Association. 1991. Position of the American Dietetic Association: Fat replacements. *Journal of the American Dietetic Association* 91:1285–88.

American Heart Association. 1993. Rationale of the diet-heart statement of the American Heart Association. *Circulation* 88:3008–29.

American Heart Association. 1996. Dietary guidelines for healthy American adults. *Circulation* 94:1795–1800.

Assmann, G., et al. 1993. High density lipoproteins, reverse transport of cholesterol, and coronary artery disease: Insights from mutations. *Circulation* 87:III-28–III-34.

Association of Women's Health, Obstetric and Neonatal Nurses. 1994. Caffeine and women's health. Washington, DC: International Food Information Council Foundation.

Badimon, J., et al. 1993. Coronary atherosclerosis: A multifactorial disease. *Circulation* 87:II-3–II-5.

Bang, O. 1990. Dietary fish oils in the prevention and management of cardiovascular and other diseases. *Comprehensive Therapy* 16:31–35.

Bell, S., et al. 1997. The new dietary fats in health and disease. *Journal of the American Diebetic Association.* 97:280–86.

Berdanier, C. 1994. *W*-3 fatty acids: A panacea. *Nutrition Today* 29 (4): 28–32.

Berning, J. 1996. The role of medium-chain triglycerides in exercise. *International Journal of Sport Nutrition* 6:121–33.

Bjorntorp, P. 1991. Importance of fat as a support nutrient for energy: Metabolism of athletes. *Journal of Sports Sciences* 9: 71–76.

Blair, S. 1994. Physical activity, fitness, and coronary heart disease. In *Physical Activity, Fitness, and Health,* eds. C. Bouchard, et al. Champaign, IL: Human Kinetics.

Breslow, J. 1993. Genetics of lipoprotein disorders. *Circulation* 87:III-16–III-21.

Brooks, G. 1997. Importance of the "crossover" concept in exercise metabolism. *Clinical and Experimental Pharmacology and Physiology* 24:889–95.

Broquist, H. 1994. Carnitine. In *Modern Nutrition in Health and Disease,* eds. M. Shils, et al. Philadelphia: Lea and Febiger.

Brown, G., et al. 1993. Lipid lowering and plaque regression: New insights into prevention of plaque disruption and clinical events in coronary disease. *Circulation* 87:1781–89.

Bulow, J. 1993. Lipid mobilization and utilization. In *Principles of Exercise Biochemistry,* ed. J. Poortmans. Basel, Switzerland: Karger.

Charnock, J., et al. 1992. Dietary modulation of lipid metabolism and mechanical performance of the heart. *Molecular and Cellular Biochemistry* 116:19–25.

Clarke, R., et al. 1997. Dietary lipids and blood cholesterol: Quantitative meta-analysis of metabolic ward studies. *British Medical Journal* 314:112–17.

Clarkson, P. 1992. Nutritional ergogenic aids: Carnitine. *International Journal of Sports Nutrition* 2:185–90.

Colditz, G. 1993. Epidemiology of breast cancer. Findings from the nurses' health study. *Cancer* 71(4):1480–89.

Coleman, E. 1997. Carbohydrate unloading: A reality check. *Physician and Sportsmedicine* 25(2): 97–98.

Coniglio, J. 1992. How does fish oil lower plasma triglycerides? *Nutrition Reviews* 50:195–206.

Consumers Union. 1997. How little fat should we really eat? *Consumer Reports on Health* 9:114–6.

Consumers Union. 1997. The facts about fats. *Consumer Reports on Health* 9:25–28.

Consumers Union. 1997. What caffeine can do for you—and to you. *Consumers Reports on Health* 9:97–101.

Consumers Union. 1995. Cutting cholesterol: More vital than ever. *Consumer Reports on Health* 7:13–14.

Consumers Union. 1992. Is reducing your cholesterol harmful? *Consumer Reports on Health* 4:81–83.

Coyle, E. 1995. Fat metabolism during exercise. *Sports Science Exchange* 8 (6):1–6.

Dattilo, A. 1992. Dietary fat and its relationship to body weight. *Nutrition Today* 27 (January/February):13–19.

Dodd, S., et al. 1993. Caffeine and exercise performance. An update. *Sports Medicine* 15:14–23.

Feldman, E. 1994. Nutrition and diet in the management of hyperlipidemia and atherosclerosis. In *Modern Nutrition in Health and Disease,* eds. M. Shils, et al. Philadelphia: Lea and Febiger.

Franklin, B., and Kahn, J. 1996. Delayed progression or regression of coronary atherosclerosis with intensive risk factor modification. *Sports Medicine* 22:306–20.

Graham, T., and Spriet, L. 1996. Caffeine and exercise performance. *Sports Science Exchange* 9 (1): 1–5.

Guezennec, C. 1992. Role of lipids on endurance capacity in man. *International Journal of Sports Medicine* 13(1): S114–S118.

Hansen, H. 1994. New biological and clinical roles for the *n*-6 and *n*-3 fatty acids. *Nutrition Reviews* 52:162–67.

Hawley, J., and Hopkins, W. 1995. Aerobic glycolytic and aerobic lipolytic power systems. *Sports Medicine* 19:240–50.

Heinonen, O. 1996. Carnitine and physical exercise. *Sports Medicine* 22:109–32.

Holloszy, J. 1990. Utilization of fatty acids during exercise. In *Biochemistry of Exercise VII,* eds. A. Taylor, et al. Champaign, IL: Human Kinetics.

Howell, W., et al. 1997. Plasma lipid and lipoprotein responses to dietary fat and cholesterol: A meta-analysis. *American Journal of Clinical Nutrition* 65:1747–64.

Hunter, D., et al. 1996. Cohort studies of fat intake and the risk of breast cancer: A pooled analysis. *New England Journal of Medicine* 334:356–61.

Jarvis, J., and Miller, G. 1996. Fat in infants' diets. *Nutrition Today* 31 (5):182–91.

Jonnalagadda, S., et al. 1996. Effects of individual fatty acids on chronic diseases. *Nutrition Today* 31:90–106.

Kiens, B. 1997. Effect of endurance training on fatty acid metabolism: Local adaptations. *Medicine and Science in Sports and Exercise* 29:640–45.

Kris-Etherton, P., and Nicolosi, R. 1995. Trans fatty acids and coronary heart disease risk. Washington, DC: International Life Sciences Institute.

Kromhout, D. 1992. Dietary fats: Long-term implications for health. *Nutrition Reviews* 50 (II): 49–53.

Lamarine, R. 1994. Selected health and behavioral effects related to the use of caffeine. *Journal of Community Health* 19:449–66.

Lambert, E., et al. 1997. Nutritional strategies for promoting fat utilization and delaying the onset of fatigue during prolonged exercise. *Journal of Sports Sciences* 15:315–24.

Lawn, R. 1992. Lipoprotein (a) in heart disease. *Scientific American* 266 (June): 54–60.

Leibel, R. 1992. Fat as fuel and metabolic signal. *Nutrition Reviews* 50:12–16.

Leibovitz, B., and Mueller, J. 1993. Carnitine. *Journal of Optimal Nutrition* 2:90–109.

Lichtenstein, A. 1995. Trans fatty acids and hydrogenated fat: What do we know? *Nutrition Today* 30:102–6.

Liebman, B. 1996. Carbo-phobia: Zoning out on the new diet books. *Nutrition Action Healthletter* 23 (6):3–5.

Lifshitz, F., and Tarim, O. 1996. Considerations about dietary fat restrictions for children. *Journal of Nutrition* 126:1031S–1041S.

Linscheer, W., and Vergroesen, A. 1994. Lipids. In *Modern Nutrition in Health and Disease,* eds. M. Shils, et al. Philadelphia: Lea and Febiger.

Mackinnon, L., et al. 1997. Effects of physical activity and diet on lipoprotein (a). *Medicine and Science in Sports and Exercise* 29:1429–36.

Martin, W. 1997. Effect of endurance training on fatty acid metabolism during whole body exercise. *Medicine and Science in Sports and Exercise* 29:635–39.

Martin, W. 1996. Effects of acute and chronic exercise on fat metabolism. *Exercise and Sport Sciences Reviews* 24:203–31.

Marwick, C. 1990. International conference gives boost in including omega fatty acids in diet. *Journal of the American Medical Association* 263:3153–54.

Mela, D. 1992. Nutritional implications of fat substitutes. *Journal of the American Dietetic Association* 92:472–76.

Miller, G., and Groziak, S. 1996. Impact of fat substitutes on fat intake. *Lipids* 31 (Supplement): S293–S296.

Montgomery, A. 1988. Cholesterol tests: How accurate are they? *Nutrition Action Health Letter* 15:1, 4–7, May.

Moore, S. 1994. Physical activity, fitness, and atherosclerosis. In *Physical Activity, Fitness, and Health,* eds. C. Bouchard, et al. Champaign, IL: Human Kinetics.

Murray, T., et al. 1994. Putative effects of diet and exercise on lipids and lipoproteins. In *Nutrition in Exercise and Sport,* eds. I. Wolinsky and J. Hickson. Boca Raton, FL: CRC Press.

National Dairy Council. 1996. Fear of fat. *Dairy Council Digest* 67:25–30.

National Institutes of Health. 1992. Triglyceride, high density lipoprotein, and coronary heart disease. *Consensus Statement* 10 (2): 1–28, February.

Nestel, P. 1993. Contribution of fats and fatty acids to performance of the elite athlete. In *Nutrition and Fitness for Athletes,* eds. A. Simopoulos and K. Pavlou. Basel, Switzerland: Karger.

Newsholme, E. 1993. Basic aspects of metabolic regulation and their application to provision of energy in exercise. In *Principles of Exercise Biochemistry,* ed. J. Poortmans. Basel, Switzerland: Karger.

Newsholme, E. 1993. Application of knowledge of metabolic integration to the problem of metabolic limitations in sprints, middle distance and marathon running. In *Principles of Exercise Biochemistry,* ed. J. Poortmans. Basel, Switzerland: Karger.

Pendergast, D., et al. 1996. The role of dietary fat on performance, metabolism, and health. *American Journal of Sports Medicine* 24:S53–S58.

Reed, D. 1993. Which risk factors are associated with atherosclerosis? *Circulation* 87: Supplement II:II-54–II-55.

Rose, D., and Connolly, J. 1992. Dietary fat, fatty acids and prostate cancer. *Lipids* 27:798–803.

Schardt, D., and Schmidt, S. 1996. Caffeine: The inside scoop. *Nutrition Action Healthletter* 23 (10): 1, 4–7.

Schwartz, C., et al. 1993. A modern view of atherogenesis. *American Journal of Cardiology* 71:9B–14B.

Sherman, W. M., and Leenders, N. 1995. Fat loading: The next magic bullet. *International Journal of Sport Nutrition* 5:S1–S12.

Spriet, L. 1995. Caffeine and performance. *International Journal of Sport Nutrition* 5:S84–S99.

Stefanik, M., and Wood, P. 1994. Physical activity, lipid and lipoprotein metabolism, and lipid transport. In *Physical Activity, Fitness, and Health,* eds. C. Bouchard, et al. Champaign, IL: Human Kinetics.

Swinburn, B., and Ravussin, E. 1993. Energy balance or fat balance. *American Journal of Clinical Nutrition* 57: Supplement, 766S–771S.

Tarnopolsky, M. 1993. Protein, caffeine, and sports. *Physician and Sportsmedicine* 21 (March): 137–49.

Uauy-Dagach, R., and Valenzuela, A. 1992. Marine oils as a source of omega-3 fatty acids in the diet: How to optimize the health benefits. *Progress in Food and Nutrition Science* 16:199–243.

von Duvillard, S. 1997. Symposium: Lipids and lipoproteins in diet and exercise. Introduction. *Medicine and Science in Sports and Exercise* 29:1414–15.

Wagenmakers, A. 1991. L-carnitine supplementation and performance in man. *Medicine and Sport Science: Advances in Nutrition and Top Sport* 32:110–27.

Wallingford, J., and Yetley, E. 1991. Development of the health claims regulations: The case of omega-3 fatty acids and heart disease. *Nutrition Reviews* 49:323–29.

Whitten, P. 1993. Stanford's secret weapon: New nutrition program lifts Cardinal swimmers to record-breaking year. *Swimming World and Junior Swimmer* 34 (March/April): 28–33.

Williams, C. 1995. Macronutrients and performance. *Journal of Sports Sciences* 13:S1–S10.

Williams, J. 1991. Caffeine, neuromuscular function and high-intensity exercise performance. *Journal of Sports Medicine and Physical Fitness* 31:481–89.

Wolf, G. 1996. High-fat, high-cholesterol diet raises plasma HDL cholesterol: Studies on the mechanism of this effect. *Nutrition Reviews* 54:34–37.

Wolfe, R., and George, S. 1993. Stable isotopic tracer as metabolic probes in exercise. *Exercise and Sport Science Reviews* 21:1–31.

Wooten, M., et al. 1996. Trans: The phantom fat. *Nutrition Action Healthletter* 23 (7): 1, 10–13.

Wynder, E., et al. 1992. Breast cancer—The optimal diet. *Advances in Experimental Medicine and Biology* 322:143–53.

Zlotkin, S. 1996. A review of the Canadian "Nutrition Recommendations Update: Dietary Fat and Children" *Journal of Nutrition* 126:1022S–1027S.

Specific Studies

Anselme, F., et al. 1992. Caffeine increases maximal anaerobic power and blood lactate concentration. *European Journal of Applied Physiology* 65:188–91.

Ascherio, A., et al. 1996. Dietary fat and risk of coronary heart disease in men: Cohort follow-up study in the United States. *British Medical Journal* 313:84–90.

Ascherio, A., et al. 1995. Dietary intake of marine n-3 fatty acids, fish intake, and the risk of coronary disease among men. *New England Journal of Medicine* 332:977–82.

Bangsbo, J., et al. 1992. Acute and habitual caffeine ingestion and metabolic responses to steady-state exercise. *Journal of Applied Physiology* 72:1297–1303.

Beckers, E., et al. 1992. Gastric emptying of carbohydrate-medium-chain triglyceride suspensions at rest. *International Journal of Sports Medicine* 13:581–84.

Bonaa, K., et al. 1992. Habitual fish consumption, plasma phospholipid fatty acids, and serum lipids: The Tromso study. *American Journal of Clinical Nutrition* 55:1126–34.

Brevetti, G., et al. 1992. Superiority of L-proprionylcarnitine vs L-carnitine in improving walking capacity in patients with peripheral vascular disease: An acute, intravenous, double-blind, cross-over study. *European Heart Journal* 13:251–55.

Brilla, L., and Landerholm, T. 1990. Effect of fish oil supplementation and exercise on serum lipids and aerobic fitness. *The Journal of Sports Medicine and Physical Fitness* 30:173–80.

Cohen, B., et al. 1996. Effects of caffeine ingestion on endurance racing in heat and humidity. *European Journal of Applied Physiology* 73:358–63.

Cole, K., et al. 1996. Effect of caffeine ingestion on perception of effort and subsequent work production. *International Journal of Sport Nutrition* 6:14–23.

Collomp, K., et al. 1992. Effects of caffeine ingestion on sprint performance in trained and untrained swimmers. *European Journal of Applied Physiology* 64:377–80.

Collomp, K., et al. 1991. Effects of caffeine ingestion on performance and metabolism during the Wingate test. *International Journal of Sports Medicine* 12:439–43.

Colombani, P., et al. 1996. Effects of L-carnitine supplementation on physical performance and energy metabolism of endurance-trained athletes: A double-blind crossover field study. *European Journal of Applied Physiology* 73:434–39.

Corti, M., et al. HDL cholesterol predicts coronary heart disease mortality in older persons. *Journal of the American Medical Association* 274:539–44.

Costill, D., et al. 1978. Effects of caffeine ingestion on metabolism and exercise performance. *Medicine and Science in Sports* 10:155–58.

Coyle, E., et al. 1997. Fatty acid oxidation is directly regulated by carbohydrate metabolism during exercise. *American Journal of Physiology* 273:E268–75.

Daviglus, M., et al. 1997. Fish consumption and the 30-year risk of fatal myocardial infarction. *New England Journal of Medicine* 336:1046–53.

Decombaz, J., et al. 1993. Effect of L-carnitine on submaximal exercise metabolism after depletion of muscle glycogen. *Medicine and Science in Sports and Exercise* 25:733–40.

Dreon, D., et al. 1990. The effects of polyunsaturated fat vs monounsaturated fat on plasma lipoproteins. *Journal of the American Medical Association* 263:2462–66.

Durstine, J., et al. 1996. Effect of a single session of exercise on lipoprotein (a). *Medicine and Science in Sports and Exercise* 28:1277–81.

Esrey, K., et al. 1996. Relationship between dietary intake and coronary heart disease mortality: Lipid research clinics prevalence follow-up study. *Journal of Clinical Epidemiology* 49:211–16.

Essig, D., et al. 1980. Muscle glycogen and triglyceride use during leg cycling following caffeine ingestion. *Medicine and Science in Sports and Exercise* 12:109.

Franceschi, S., et al. 1996. Intake of macronutrients and risk of breast cancer. *Lancet* 347:1351–56.

French, C., et al. 1991. Caffeine ingestion during exercise to exhaustion in elite distance runners. *The Journal of Sports Medicine and Physical Fitness* 31:425–32.

Graham, T., and Spriet, L. 1991. Performance and metabolic responses to a high caffeine dose during prolonged exercise. *Journal of Applied Physiology* 71:2292–98.

Halle, M., et al. 1996. Lipoprotein (a) in endurance athletes, power athletes, and sedentary controls. *Medicine and Science in Sports and Exercise* 28:962–64.

Hansen, J., et al. 1993. Inhibition of exercise-induced shortening of bleeding time by fish oil in familial hypercholesterolemia (type IIa). *Arteriosclerosis and Thrombosis* 13:98–104.

Hardman, A., and Hudson, A. 1994. Brisk walking and serum lipid and lipoprotein variables in previously sedentary women: Effect of 12 weeks of regular brisk walking followed by 12 weeks of detraining. *British Journal of Sports Medicine* 28:261–66.

Hargreaves, M., et al. 1991. Effect of increased plasma free fatty acid concentrations on muscle metabolism in exercising men. *Journal of Applied Physiology* 70:194–201.

Harris, T., et al. 1992. The low cholesterol-mortality association in a national cohort. *Journal of Clinical Epidemiology* 45:595–601.

Hodgetts, V., et al. 1991. Factors controlling fat mobilization from human subcutaneous adipose tissue during exercise. *Journal of Applied Physiology* 71:445–51.

Hubinger, L., and Mackinnon, L. 1992. The acute effect of 30 min of moderate exercise on high density lipoprotein cholesterol in untrained middle-aged men. *European Journal of Applied Physiology* 65:555–60.

Hurley, B., et al. 1986. Muscle triglyceride utilization during exercise: Effect of training. *Journal of Applied Physiology* 60:562–67.

Ivy, J., et al. 1980. Contribution of medium and long chain triglyceride intake to energy metabolism during prolonged exercise. *International Journal of Sports Medicine* 1:15–20.

Jackman, M., et al. 1996. Metabolic catecholamine, and endurance responses to caffeine during intense exercise. *Journal of Applied Physiology* 81:1658–63.

Jenkins, D., et al. 1989. Nibbling versus gorging: Metabolic advantages of increased meal frequency. *New England Journal of Medicine* 321:929–34.

Jeukendrup, A., et al. 1996. Effect of endogenous carbohydrate availability on oral medium-chain triglyceride oxidation during prolonged exercise. *Journal of Applied Physiology* 80:949–54.

Jeukendrup, A., et al. 1996. Effects of carbohydrate (CHO) and fat supplementation on CHO metabolism during prolonged exercise. *Metabolism* 45:915–21.

Lambert, E., et al. 1994. Enhanced endurance in trained cyclists during moderate intensity exercise following 2 weeks adaptation to a high fat diet. *European Journal of Applied Physiology* 69:287–93.

Leddy, J., et al. 1997. Effect of a high or a low fat diet on cardiovascular risk factors in male and female runners. *Medicine and Science in Sports and Exercise* 29:17–25.

MacIntosh, B., and Wright, B. 1995. Caffeine ingestion and performance of a 1,500-metre swim. *Canadian Journal of Applied Physiology* 20:168–77.

Massicotte, D., et al. 1992. Oxidation of exogenous medium-chain free fatty acids during prolonged exercise: Comparison with glucose. *Journal of Applied Physiology* 73:1334–39.

Morgan, R., et al. 1993. Plasma cholesterol and depressive symptoms in older men. *Lancet* 341(8837):75–79.

Morgan, S., et al. 1997. A low-fat diet supplemented with monounsaturated fat results in less HDL-C lowering than a very-low-fat diet. *Journal of the American Dietetic Association* 97:151–56.

Muoio, D., et al. 1994. Effect of dietary fat on metabolic adjustments to maximal VO_2 and endurance in runners. *Medicine and Science in Sports and Exercise* 26:81–88.

Nagel, D., et al. 1989. Effects of an ultra-long distance (1000 km) race on lipid metabolism. *European Journal of Applied Physiology* 59:16–20.

Nordoy, A., et al. 1993. Individual effects of dietary saturated fatty acids and fish oil on plasma lipids and lipoproteins in normal men. *American Journal of Clinical Nutrition* 57:634–39.

Okano, G., et al. 1996. Effect of 4 h preexercise high carbohydrate and high fat meal ingestion on endurance performance and metabolism. *International Journal of Sports Medicine* 17:530–34.

Ornish, D., et al. 1990. Can lifestyle changes reverse coronary heart disease? The lifestyle heart trial. *Lancet* 336:129–33.

Oster, G., and Thompson, D. 1996. Estimated effects of reducing dietary saturated fat intake on the incidence and costs of coronary heart disease in the United States. *Journal of the American Medical Association* 96:127–31.

Poehlman, E., et al. 1994. Effects of endurance training on total fat oxidation in elderly persons. *Journal of Applied Physiology* 76:2281–87.

Raastad, T., et al. Omega-3 fatty acid supplementation does not improve maximal aerobic power, anaerobic threshold and running performance in well-trained soccer players. *Scandinavian Journal of Medicine and Science in Sports* 7:25–31.

Romijn, J., et al. 1993. Regulation of endogenous fat and carbohydrate metabolism in relation to exercise intensity and duration. *American Journal of Physiology* 265:E380–E391.

Sasaki, S., et al. 1993. An ecological study of the relationship between dietary fat intake and breast cancer mortality. *Preventive Medicine* 22:187–202.

Smith-Schneider, L., et al. 1992. Dietary fat reduction strategies. *Journal of the American Dietetic Association* 92:34–38.

Spriet, D., et al. 1992. Caffeine ingestion and muscle metabolism during prolonged exercise in humans. *American Journal of Physiology* 262:E891–E898.

Stampfer, M., et al. 1996. A prospective study of triglyceride level, low-density lipoprotein particle diameter, and risk of myocardial infarction. *Journal of the American Medical Association* 276:882–88.

Starling, R., et al. 1997. Effects of diet on muscle triglyceride and endurance performance. *Journal of Applied Physiology* 82:1185–89.

Staton, W. 1951. The influence of soya lecithin on muscular strength. *Research Quarterly* 22:201–207.

Tarnopolsky, M., et al. 1995. Carbohydrate loading and metabolism during exercise in men and women. *Journal of Applied Physiology* 68:302–8.

Tarnopolsky, M., et al. 1989. Physiological responses to caffeine during endurance running in habitual caffeine users. *Medicine and Science in Sports and Exercise* 21:418–24.

Trappe, S., et al. 1994. The effect of L-carnitine supplementation on performance during interval swimming. *International Journal of Sports Medicine* 15:181–85.

Van Soeren, M., et al. 1993. Caffeine metabolism and epinephrine responses during exercise in users and nonusers. *Journal of Applied Physiology* 75:805–12.

Van Zyl, C., et al. 1996. Effects of medium-chain triglyceride ingestion on fuel metabolism and cycling performance. *Journal of Applied Physiology* 80:2217–25.

Venkatraman, J., et al. 1997. Influence of the level of dietary lipid intake and maximal exercise on the immune status in runners. *Medicine and Science in Sports and Exercise* 29:333–44.

Visich, P., et al. 1996. Effects of exercise with varying energy expenditure on high-density lipoprotein-cholesterol. *European Journal of Applied Physiology* 72:242–48.

Vukovich, M., et al. 1994. Carnitine supplementation: Effect on muscle carnitine and glycogen content during exercise. *Medicine and Science in Sports and Exercise* 26:1122–29.

Watts, G., et al. 1996. Dietary fatty acids and progression of coronary artery disease in men. *American Journal of Clinical Nutrition* 64:202–9.

Wemple, R., et al. 1997. Caffeine vs caffeine-free sports drinks: Effect on urine production at rest and during prolonged exercise. *International Journal of Sports Medicine* 18:40–46.

Wiles, J., et al. 1992. Effect of caffeinated coffee on running speed, respiratory factors, blood lactate and perceived exertion during 1500-meter treadmill running. *British Journal of Sports Medicine* 26:116–20.

Williams, J., et al. 1988. Caffeine, maximal power output, and fatigue. *British Journal of Sports Medicine* 22:132–34.

Wood, P., et al. 1993. Effect of butter, mono- and polyunsaturated fatty acid-enriched butter, trans fatty acid margarine, and zero trans fatty acid margarine on serum lipids and lipoproteins in healthy men. *Journal of Lipid Research* 34:1–10.

Wyss, V., et al. 1990. Effects of L-carnitine administration on VO_2 max and the aerobic anaerobic threshold in normoxia and acute hypoxia. *European Journal of Applied Physiology* 60:1–6.

CHAPTER 6

Protein: The Tissue Builder

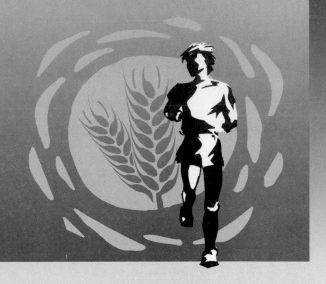

KEY TERMS

alanine
alpha-ketoacid
amino acids
ammonia
choline
complete proteins
creatine
deamination
essential (indispensable)
  amino acids
glucogenic amino acids
HMB
human growth hormone
  (HGH)
incomplete proteins
inosine
ketogenic amino acids
legumes
limiting amino acid
nitrogen balance
nonessential (dispensable)
  amino acids
protein-sparing effect
proteinuria
purines
sports anemia
urea

KEY CONCEPTS

• Protein contains nitrogen, an element essential to the formation of twenty different amino acids, the building blocks of all body cells.

• Essential, or indispensable, amino acids cannot be adequately synthesized in the body and thus must be obtained through dietary protein, whereas nonessential, or dispensable, amino acids may be synthesized in the body. However, all twenty amino acids are necessary for protein formation in the body.

• The human body needs a balanced mixture of essential amino acids, and although animal protein provides all of the essential amino acids in the proper blend, a combination of certain plant proteins, such as grains and legumes, will satisfy this dietary requirement.

• The RDA for protein is based upon the body weight of the individual, and the amount needed per unit body weight is greater during childhood and adolescence than during adulthood. The adult RDA is 0.8 grams of protein per kilogram body weight, or 0.36 grams per pound body weight.

• Dietary protein should comprise approximately 12 percent of the daily caloric intake, and although animal foods in the meat and milk groups have a high protein content, they also may be high in fat. Increasing the proportion of dietary protein intake from plant sources is recommended.

• The major function of dietary protein is to build and repair tissues and to synthesize hormones, enzymes, and other body compounds, but it also may be used as a significant source of energy under certain conditions.

• During exercise, particularly with low carbohydrate stores in the body, muscle protein may supply nearly 5–10 percent of the energy Calories.

• Although protein catabolism may occur during exercise, protein synthesis predominates in the recovery period. The type of protein synthesized is specific to the type of exercise program, such as weight training or aerobic endurance.

• Several recognized authorities have recommended a protein intake of 1.6–1.8 grams per kilogram body weight per day for athletes attempting to gain weight, and about 1.2–1.6 grams per kilogram body weight per day for endurance athletes.

• Although some athletes may benefit from additional protein in the diet, they do not need expensive commercial protein supplements; instead they should obtain the extra protein they need through the increased caloric intake associated with exercise.

• Although several interesting hypotheses have been proposed, amino acid supplements are not currently considered to be effective as a means to improve physical performance; additional research is needed because valid data are sparse.

- Research suggests creatine may be an effective ergogenic aid, particularly for repetitive short-duration, high-intensity exercise tasks. Research findings are equivocal regarding the ergogenic effect of other protein-related supplements, such as choline and HMB. Additional research is needed to document an ergogenic effect of creatine in actual sport competition and to help resolve the ambiguity with other related supplements.
- Dietary deficiencies, as well as dietary excesses, of protein and amino acids may interfere with optimal physiological efficiency, which may lead to impairment of physical performance or health status.

INTRODUCTION

Protein is one of our most essential nutrients. It has a wide variety of physiological functions that are essential to optimal physical performance. For example, protein forms the structural basis of muscle tissue, is the major component of most enzymes in the muscle, and can serve as a source of energy during exercise. Because protein is so important to the development and function of muscle tissue, and because most feats of human physical performance involve strenuous muscular activity in one form or another, it is no wonder that protein has persisted throughout the years as the food of the athlete. Indeed, surveys have revealed that many high school and college athletes believe that athletic performance is improved by a high-protein diet. A best-selling diet book suggests protein is the key macronutrient for the athlete, and for health as well.

Companies that market nutritional supplements for athletes have capitalized on this belief. Probably the athletic groups most susceptible to the lure of protein supplements are bodybuilders and strength-type athletes, such as weight lifters and football players. Numerous high-protein products have been developed for these athletes in attempts to exploit the protein-muscle strength relationship. In recent years, specific amino acids have been theorized to maximize muscle mass and strength gains and have been advertised extensively in magazines for bodybuilders. Some advertisements even suggest that certain amino acid mixtures have an effect similar to drugs such as anabolic steroids, which have been used to stimulate muscle development.

Protein supplements are marketed for other types of athletes as well. Although protein is not regarded as a major energy source during exercise, research has suggested that endurance athletes may use some specific amino acids for energy production under certain conditions. It was not long after publication of these findings that a "new protein discovery" designed to replace these amino acids was advertised in magazines for runners. More recently, specific amino acids have been theorized to delay the onset of fatigue during prolonged exercise through their effect on neurotransmitters in the brain.

There is no doubt that an adequate amount of dietary protein and related essential amino acids is required by all individuals. However, the advertisements directed toward athletes imply that additional protein, usually in the form of protein or amino acid supplements, is necessary for optimal performance. Although most investigators who study protein metabolism during exercise suggest athletes may need to increase their protein intake, the usual recommendation is to increase the intake of natural protein sources.

Other dietary supplements related to protein or amino acids, such as amines or various metabolic by-products, have become increasingly popular in recent years. One of the current hot sellers is creatine, but other supplements such as inosine and choline are available. In most cases these dietary supplements have been marketed to strength-trained athletes as a means to foster muscle growth and strength development, but some are intended for use by athletes involved in other sports, such as aerobic endurance events.

Does the physically active individual need more protein or related dietary supplements in the diet? The information presented in this chapter should provide a general answer to this question. Topics to be covered include dietary needs and sources of protein; metabolic fates and functions in the body; the effects of exercise on protein metabolism and dietary requirements; the ergogenic potential of protein, amino acids, or other related supplements; and health aspects of dietary protein.

Dietary Protein

What is protein?

Protein is a complex chemical structure containing carbon, hydrogen, and oxygen—just as carbohydrates and fats do. Protein has one other essential element—nitrogen, which constitutes about 16 percent of most dietary protein. These four elements are combined into a number of different structures called **amino acids,** each one possessing an amino group (NH_2) and an acid group (COOH), with the remainder being different combinations of carbon, hydrogen, oxygen, and in some cases sulfur. There are twenty amino acids, all of which can be combined in a variety of ways to form the proteins necessary for the structure and functions of the human body. Figure 6.1 depicts the formula of **alanine,** an amino acid discussed later.

Proteins are created when two amino acids link and form a peptide bond; hence, a dipeptide is formed. As more amino acids are added, a polypeptide is formed. Most proteins are polypeptides, combining up to 300 amino acids. Figure 6.2 depicts the building of a protein.

Protein is contained in both animal and plant foods. Humans obtain their supply of amino acids from these two general sources.

Is there a difference between animal and plant protein?

To answer this question, let us first look at a basic difference between two groups of amino acids. Humans can synthesize some amino acids in their bodies but cannot synthesize others. The nine amino acids that cannot be manufactured in the body are called **essential,** or **indispensable, amino acids** and must be supplied in the diet. Those that may be formed in the body are called **nonessential,** or **dispensable, amino acids.** Although nutrition scientists prefer the terms indispensable and dispensable, this text uses the terms essential and nonessential because they are most commonly used.

It should be noted that all twenty amino acids are necessary for protein synthesis in the body and must be present simultaneously for optimal maintenance of body growth and function. The use of the terms essential and indispensable in relation to amino acids is to distinguish those that must be obtained in the diet. Table 6.1 presents the dietary essential and nonessential amino acids.

All natural, unprocessed animal and plant foods contain all twenty amino acids. However, the amount of each amino acid in specific foods varies. Over the years a number of different techniques have been used, usually with animals, to assess the quality of protein in selected foods. We need not go into a detailed discussion of all techniques to evaluate protein quality, but essentially they focus on the concept of **nitrogen balance,** the ability of the body to retain nitrogen. In essence, nitrogen balance is protein balance. In positive nitrogen balance the body is retaining protein to adequately support growth and development, while in negative nitrogen balance the body is losing protein, with possible impairment in growth and development. The quality of the protein in foods we eat may affect nitrogen balance.

In general, those foods that contain an adequate content of all nine essential amino acids to support both life and growth are known as **complete proteins,** or high-quality proteins, while those that have a deficiency of one or more essential amino acids and are unable to support life or growth are called **incomplete proteins,** or low-quality proteins. The essential amino acid that is in short supply in a particular food is labeled the **limiting amino acid.**

The proteins ingested as animal products are generally regarded to be of a higher quality than those found in plants. This is not to say that an amino acid found in a plant is inferior to the same amino acid found in an animal. They are the same. When we look at the distribution of all the

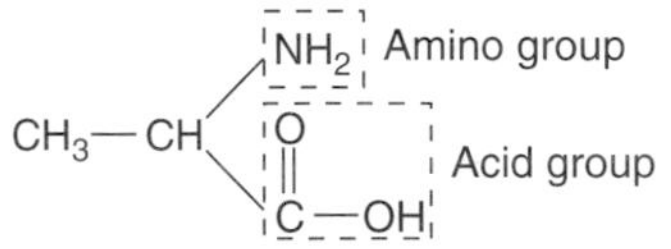

Figure 6.1 The chemical structure of alanine, an amino acid. The amino group (NH_2) contains nitrogen, while the acid group is represented by COOH.

Table 6.1   The dietary amino acids

Essential amino acids	Nonessential amino acids
Histidine	Alanine
Isoleucine*	Arginine
Leucine*	Asparagine
Lysine	Aspartic acid
Methionine	Cysteine
Phenylalanine	Glutamic acid
Threonine	Glutamine
Tryptophan	Glycine
Valine*	Proline
	Serine
	Tyrosine

*Branched-chain amino acids

AA	Amino acid
AA–AA	Dipeptide
AA–AA–AA	Tripeptide
AA–AA–AA–AA–AA–AA– . . . –AA	Polypeptide (50–100 AA)
AA–AA–AA–AA–AA–AA–AA–AA–AA–AA–AA– . . . . –AA	Protein (> 100 AA)

Figure 6.2 Formation of peptides and polypeptides from amino acids, with eventual formation of proteins.

amino acids in the two food sources, however, we can then see two major reasons why animal protein is called a high-quality protein, whereas plant protein is of lower quality.

First, animal protein is a complete protein because it contains all the essential amino acids. Second, it contains the essential amino acids in larger amounts and in the proper proportion. As noted above, all twenty amino acids must be present simultaneously for the body to synthesize them into necessary body proteins. If one amino acid is in short supply, protein construction may be blocked. Having the proper amount of animal protein in the diet is a good way to ensure receiving a balanced supply of amino acids.

Although plant proteins are regarded as being of lower quality than animal proteins, they still may provide you with all the protein and amino acids you need for optimal growth and development. However, proteins usually exist in smaller concentrations in plant foods. For example, 2 ounces of fish contain about 14 grams of protein, while 2 ounces of cooked macaroni only have 2 grams; 2 ounces of beans, which are generally regarded to be good sources of protein, have only 5 grams. In addition, most plant proteins have insufficient amounts of one or more of the essential amino acids, i.e., limiting amino acids. Grain products are usually deficient in lysine, whereas legumes are low in methionine. An exception to this generality is the protein isolated from soybeans, which is comparable to animal protein. As noted in Chapter 2, if plant foods are eaten in proper combinations over the course of the day, the individual may receive a balanced supply of amino acids. Some populations receive most of their protein from plant sources.

What are some common foods that are good sources of protein?

Animal foods in the milk and meat groups generally have substantial amounts of high-quality protein. One glass of milk or its equivalent contains about 7–8 grams of protein, as does 1 ounce of meat, fish, or poultry. **Legumes,** such as dry beans (black, garbanzo, great northern, kidney, lima, navy, pinto, soybeans), lentils, and peas (black-eyed, split), are relatively good sources of protein. Legumes also are high in carbohydrate and for this reason are currently classified as a starch food exchange. However, because of their relatively high protein content, legumes may be included within the meat exchange list. One-half cup contains about 7–9 grams of protein. Nuts contain fair amounts of protein but are high in fat. Fruits, vegetables, and grain products all have some protein, but the content varies; generally speaking, the protein content is low, ranging from less than 1 gram to about 3 grams of protein per serving, although some products may contain more, such as protein-enriched pasta (e.g., Superoni). Some sports drinks and sports bars contain significant amounts of protein.

Table 6.2 and Figures 6.3 and 6.4 present some common foods in each of several food groups, with the number

Table 6.2 Protein content in some common foods

Food	Amount	Protein (grams)
Milk list		
Milk, whole	1 c	8
Milk, skim	1 c	8
Cheese, cheddar	1 oz	7
Yogurt	1 c	8
Meat list		
Beef, lean	1 oz	8
Chicken breast	1 oz	8
Luncheon meat	1 oz	5
Fish	1 oz	7
Eggs	1	6
Navy beans, cooked*	1/2 c	7
Peanuts, roasted	1/2 c	18
Peanut butter	1 tbsp	4
Vegetable list		
Broccoli	1/2 c	2
Carrots	1	1
Fruit list		
Banana	1	1
Orange	1	1
Pear	1	1
Starch list		
Bread, wheat	1 slice	3
Bran flakes	1 c	4
Doughnuts	1	1
Macaroni	1/2 c	3
Macaroni and cheese	1/2 c	9
Peas, green	1/2 c	4
Potato, baked	1	3
Sports drinks and bars		
GatorPro	11 oz	17
Power Bar	1	10

Protein (grams) may vary slightly from the food exchange lists because these data were derived from food analyses reported by the United States Department of Agriculture.

*Found in both the meat and meat substitutes and starch lists in Appendix F.

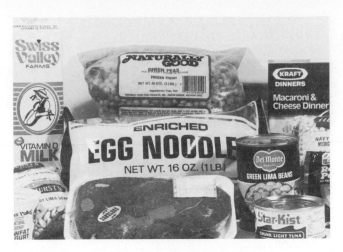

Figure 6.3 Foods high in protein include meats, milk, and plants such as legumes.

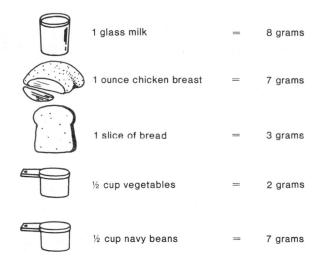

1 glass milk	=	8 grams
1 ounce chicken breast	=	7 grams
1 slice of bread	=	3 grams
½ cup vegetables	=	2 grams
½ cup navy beans	=	7 grams

Figure 6.4 Protein in food.

of grams of protein in each. Notice the effect combination-type foods have on protein content: for example, macaroni and cheese versus plain macaroni. Most food labels today will list the grams of protein per serving.

How much dietary protein do I need?

Humans actually do not need protein per se, but rather an adequate amount of nitrogen and essential amino acids. However, because all nine essential amino acids and almost all dietary nitrogen are derived from dietary protein, it serves as the basis for our daily requirements.

In the United States, the recommended dietary intake of protein is based upon the RDA. The amount of protein necessary in the diet varies in different stages of the life cycle. During the early years of life, children manufacture protein tissue during rapid growth stages, with the rate of growth (and thus the protein needs) varying from infancy through late adolescence. In young adulthood, the protein requirement stabilizes. Throughout the life cycle, however, the protein requirement established in the RDA is based upon the body weight of the individual. As a person passes from infancy to adulthood, the protein RDA per unit body weight decreases.

Table 6.3 presents the amount of protein needed per kilogram or per pound of body weight for different age groups. A variety of scientific techniques have been used over the years to determine human protein needs, and more recent research has reaffirmed these estimates for adults and children. The values in this table are dependent upon adequate daily energy intake (i.e., Calories), for a low-energy diet will increase protein needs. To calculate your requirement, simply determine your body weight in kilograms or pounds and multiply by the appropriate figure for your age group. Recall that one kilogram is equal to 2.2 pounds. As an example, compute the protein requirement for a 154-pound, or 70-kg, average 23-year-old male:

$$0.36 \text{ g protein/pound} \times 154 \text{ pounds} = 55.4 \text{ or } 56 \text{ g protein/day}$$

$$0.8 \text{ g protein/kg} \times 70 \text{ kg} = 56 \text{ g protein/day}$$

However, the minimum necessary intake of protein is much less than the RDA. If all proteins were the same quality as egg protein, then the RDA would be approximately 0.34 g protein/kg body weight per day. Allowances are made in the RDA for the fact that individual protein needs vary, that the biologic quality of all dietary protein is not as good as egg protein, and that the efficiency of utilization decreases at higher dietary protein-intake levels. Hence, the RDA is adjusted upward to account for these factors.

The RDA for protein, as noted above, is based upon body weight of the individual at different ages. If you would take the recommended energy intake in Calories for each age group, say 2,200 C for the average adult female, and calculate the percentage of this value that the RDA for protein supplies, the values are less than 10 percent for each age group. Mathematically, 56 grams of protein, at 4 Calories per gram, total 224 Calories, which is about 10 percent of 2,200. This value is slightly lower than the generally recommended dietary protein content, that is, about 12–15 percent of daily caloric intake.

Table 6.3	Grams of protein needed per kilogram or per pound body weight during the life cycle		
Age in years	**Grams/kg body weight**	**Grams/ pound body weight**
0.0–0.5	2.2	1.00
0.5–1.0	1.6	.71
1–3	1.2	.56
4–6	1.2	.56
7–14	1.0	.45
15–18	0.9	.41
19 and up	0.8	.36

Table 6.4	Estimated RDA for the essential amino acids in an adult male (70 kg)	
	RDA (mg/kg)	**Total mg**
Histidine	8–12	560–840
Isoleucine	10	700
Leucine	14	980
Lysine	12	840
Methionine plus cysteine	13	910
Phenylalanine plus tyrosine	14	980
Threonine	7	490
Tryptophan	3.5	245
Valine	10	700
Total		6,405–6,685

How much of the essential amino acids do I need?

For the average adult, about 10–15 percent of the total protein requirement should consist of the essential amino acids; this amounts to a little over 6 grams. Table 6.4 lists the estimated RDA for these nine amino acids for an adult male. Phenylalanine is an essential amino acid, whereas tyrosine is normally listed as a nonessential amino acid. Both are of similar chemical structure so that when substantial quantities of tyrosine are contained in the diet, the need for phenylalanine will decrease somewhat. The same holds true for the essential sulfur-containing amino acid methionine and its chemically related counterpart, cysteine. Although some nutrition scientists have suggested that the RDA for essential amino acids are too low and have recommended an intake about twice as high, individuals who obtain the RDA for protein should have no problem obtaining even these higher recommended values.

Fortunately we do not need to memorize these amino acids and check our food products to see if they are present. A few general rules can help ensure that we receive a balanced supply in our diet.

What are some dietary guidelines to ensure adequate protein intake?

To answer in one sentence: Eat a wide variety of animal and plant foods. The high-quality, complete proteins are obtained primarily from animal foods. Meat, fish, eggs, poultry, milk, and cheese contain the type and amount of the essential amino acids necessary for maintaining life and promoting growth and development. They are high-nutrient-density foods. Because animal protein is of high quality, you do not need as much of it to satisfy your RDA. For example, although the average male needs about 56 grams of protein per day, he only needs 45 grams if it is animal protein. One glass of milk, with 8 grams of protein, will provide almost 20 percent of his protein RDA. Two glasses of milk, one egg, and 3 ounces of lean meat, fish, or poultry will provide 100 percent of his RDA. In addition, a substantial proportion of daily vitamin and mineral needs will also be supplied in these foods. As noted in Chapter 5, selection of low-fat foods will enhance the nutrient density by reducing Calories.

Plant foods also may provide good sources of protein. Grain products such as wheat, rice, and corn, as well as soybeans, peas, beans, and nuts, have a substantial protein content. However, most plant foods contain incomplete proteins because they lack a sufficient quantity of some essential amino acids. For this reason, the protein RDA for the average adult male is 65 grams per day when plant proteins are the primary source. However, if certain plant foods are eaten over the course of a day, such as grains and legumes, they may supply all the essential amino acids necessary for human nutrition and be as complete a protein as animal protein.

Some recent research has suggested that if the daily dietary protein is obtained through a mixture of animal and plant foods in a ratio of 30:70, that is 30 percent of the protein from animal foods and 70 from plant foods, the protein quality would be similar to the use of animal foods alone. Mixing animal and plant foods in the same meal is common, and is also healthful and nutritious. Animal foods provide excellent sources of essential minerals, such as iron, zinc, and calcium, while plant foods provide carbohydrate, dietary fiber, and various phytochemicals.

Metabolism and Function

What happens to protein in the human body?

Dietary protein consists of long, complex chains of amino acids. In the digestive process, enzymes (proteases) in the stomach and small intestine break the complex protein down into polypeptides and then into individual amino acids. The amino acids are absorbed through the wall of the small intestine, pass into the blood, and then to the liver via the portal vein. The digestion of protein takes several hours, but once the amino acids enter the blood they are cleared within 5–10 minutes. There is a constant interchange of amino acids among the blood, the liver, and the body tissues. The liver is a critical center in amino acid metabolism. It is continually synthesizing a balanced amino acid mixture for the diverse protein requirements of the body. These amino acids are secreted into the blood and carried as free amino acids or as plasma proteins such as albumin.

The most important metabolic fate of the amino acids is the formation of specific proteins, including the structural proteins such as muscle tissue and the functional proteins such as enzymes. Body cells obtain amino acids from the blood, and the genetic apparatus in the cell nucleus directs the synthesis of proteins specific to the cell needs. The body cells may also use some of the nitrogen from the amino acids to form non-protein nitrogen compounds, such as creatine. For example, the muscle cells will form contractile proteins as well as the enzymes and creatine phosphate necessary for energy production. The body cells will use only the amount of amino acids necessary to meet their protein needs. They cannot store excess amino acids to any significant amount, although the protein formed may be catabolized to release amino acids back to the blood.

Because the human body does not have a mechanism to store excess nitrogen, it cannot store amino acids per se. Through the process of **deamination** the amino group (NH_2) containing the nitrogen is removed from the amino acid, leaving a substrate known as an **alpha-ketoacid.** The excess nitrogen must be excreted from the body. In essence, the liver forms **ammonia** (NH_3) from the excess nitrogen; the ammonia is converted into **urea,** which passes into the blood and is eventually eliminated by the kidneys into the urine.

The alpha-ketoacid that is released may have several fates. For one, it can recombine with another amino group and be reconstituted to an amino acid. It also may be channeled into the metabolic pathways of carbohydrate and fat. The liver is the main organ where this conversion occurs. In essence, some of the amino acids are said to be **glucogenic amino acids,** that is, glucose forming. At various stages of the energy transformations within the liver, the glucogenic amino acids may be converted to glucose. This process is called gluconeogenesis. The **ketogenic amino acids** are metabolized in the liver to acetyl CoA, which may be used for energy production via the Krebs cycle or converted to fat. The glucose and fat produced may be transported to other parts of the body to be used. Thus, although excess protein cannot be stored as amino acids in the body, the energy content is not wasted, for it is converted to either carbohydrate or fat.

Figure 6.5 presents a summary of the fates of protein in human metabolism. See also Appendix K, figure K.5.

Can protein be formed from carbohydrates and fats?

Yes, but with some major limitations. Protein has one essential element, nitrogen, which is not possessed by either carbohydrate or fat. However, if the body has an

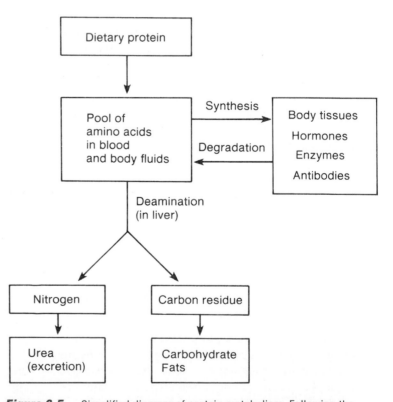

Figure 6.5 Simplified diagram of protein metabolism. Following the digestion of dietary proteins, one of the major functions of the amino acids is the sythesis of body tissues, enzymes, hormones, and antibodies. However, protein also is constantly being degraded by the liver. The excess nitrogen is excreted as urea while the carbon residue may be converted into carbohydrate or fat.

excess of amino acids, the liver may be able to use the nitrogen-containing amino groups from these excess amino acids and combine them with alpha-ketoacids derived from either carbohydrate or fat metabolism. A key alpha-ketoacid from carbohydrate is pyruvic acid, while fat yields acetoacetic acid. The net result is the formation in the body of some of the nonessential amino acids using carbohydrates and fats as part of the building materials. Keep in mind that nitrogen must be present for this to occur, and its source is through dietary protein.

What are the major functions of protein in human nutrition?

Dietary protein may be utilized to serve all three major functions of food. Through the action of the individual amino acids, protein serves as the structural basis for the vast majority of body tissues, is essential for regulating metabolism, and can be used as an energy source. In one way or another protein is involved in almost all body functions. Its individual roles are beyond the scope of this text, so the following discussion represents just some of its major functions of importance to health and fitness. Table 6.5 highlights the major functions of protein in the body.

Protein is the main nutrient used in the formation of all body tissues. This role is extremely important in periods of rapid growth, such as childhood and adolescence. Athletes who attempt to gain muscle tissue also need an adequate dietary supply of protein to create a positive energy balance. Certain amino acids, such as the branched-chain amino acids (BCAA) leucine, isoleucine, and valine, constitute a significant amount of muscle tissue.

Protein is critical in the regulation of human metabolism. It is used in the formation of almost all enzymes, many hormones, and other compounds that control body functions. Insulin, hemoglobin, and the oxidative enzymes

in the mitochondria are all proteins that have important roles in regulating metabolism during exercise. Other metabolic roles of protein include the maintenance of water balance and acid-base balance, regulation of the blood clotting process, prevention of infection, and development of immunity to disease. Proteins also serve as carriers for nutrients in the blood, such as the free fatty acids (FFA) and the lipoproteins, and help transport nutrients into the body cells.

Although protein is not a major energy source for humans at rest, it can serve such a function under several conditions. In nutritional balance, the priority use of dietary protein is to promote synthesis of body proteins essential for optimal structure and function. However, as noted above, excess dietary protein may be converted to carbohydrate or fat and then enter metabolic pathways for energy production or storage. On the other hand, during periods of starvation or semistarvation, adequate amounts of dietary or endogenous carbohydrates and dietary fats may not be available. Both dietary protein and the body protein stores are used for energy purposes in such a situation, because energy production takes precedence over tissue building in metabolism. Hence, if the active individual desires to maintain lean body mass, it is essential to have not only adequate protein intake but also sufficient carbohydrate Calories in the diet to provide a **protein-sparing effect.** In other words, carbohydrate Calories will be used for energy production, thus sparing utilization of protein as an energy source and allowing it to be used for its more important metabolic functions.

Although body proteins are composed of all twenty amino acids, individual amino acids may have important specific effects in the body. For example, the amino acid glycine is a neurotransmitter substance, tryptophan and tyrosine are important for the formation of several chemical transmitters in the brain, while the branched-chain

---

Table 6.5 Summary of the functions of proteins and amino acids in human metabolism

1. Structural function	Form vital constituents of all cells in the body, such as contractile muscle proteins
2. Transport function	Transport various substances in the blood, such as the lipoproteins for conveying triglycerides
3. Enzyme function	Form almost all enzymes in the body to regulate numerous diverse physiological processes
4. Hormone and neurotransmitter function	Form various hormones, such as insulin; form various neurotransmitters, or neuropeptides, that function in the central nervous system, such as serotonin
5. Immune function	Form key components of the immune system, such as antibodies
6. Acid-base balance function	Buffer acid and alkaline substances in the blood to maintain optimal pH
7. Fluid balance function	Exert osmotic pressure to maintain optimal fluid balance in body tissues, particularly the blood
8. Energy function	Provide source of energy to the Krebs cycle when deaminated; excess protein may be converted to glucose or fat for subsequent energy production
9. Movement function	Provide movement when structural muscle proteins use energy to contract

amino acids (leucine, isoleucine, and valine) are major components of muscle tissue that may provide a source of energy.

Because of the diverse roles of protein and amino acids in the body, athletes have used protein supplements for years in attempts to improve performance. Amino acid supplements have only recently been introduced for this purpose. The effectiveness of such supplements is evaluated in later sections.

Proteins and Exercise

Are proteins used for energy during exercise?

Protein generally has not been regarded as an important source of energy during exercise because, as noted in the previous two chapters, carbohydrate and fats serve this purpose quite well. Research has now shown, however, that protein may be a significant source of energy during exercise under certain conditions.

Scientists have used a variety of techniques to study protein metabolism during exercise. Because urea is a by-product of protein metabolism, its concentration in the urine, blood, and sweat has been analyzed. Also, the presence in the urine of a marker for muscle protein breakdown known as 3-methylhistidine, a modified amino acid, has been studied to evaluate protein catabolism. The nitrogen balance technique consists of precisely measuring nitrogen intake and excretion to determine whether the individual is in positive or negative protein balance. Finally, labeled isotopes of amino acids have been ingested or injected to study their metabolic fate during exercise. However, even with such techniques Michael Rennie and his colleagues, in a recent review, noted that we still have limited knowledge regarding the effects of exercise on nitrogen metabolism in humans.

Nevertheless, using these techniques, most investigators in this area, most recently including Gail Butterfield, William Evans, Peter Lemon, Jacques Poortmans, Mark Tarnopolsky, and Robert Wolfe, have reported that the available data appear to support an increased use of protein, or amino acids, as an energy source during exercise. However, questions still remain concerning the specific protein sources and their proportionate contribution. In the majority of exercise tasks, including strenuous weight training, protein appears to be a relatively minor source of energy and accounts for less than 5 percent of the total energy cost of the activity. As Poortmans has noted, protein may be used to produce significant amounts of ATP in the muscle, but the rate of production is much slower than with carbohydrate and fat, the preferred fuels. On the other hand, Lemon has reported that in the latter stage of prolonged endurance exercise, protein could contribute up to 15 percent of the total energy cost. In this regard, prolonged exercise may be comparable to a state of starvation. As the endurance athlete depletes the endogenous carbohydrate stores, the body catabolizes some of its protein for energy or eventual conversion to glucose. Protein catabolism has been shown to increase significantly even when muscle glycogen is depleted by only about 33–55 percent.

In general, a brief session of exercise lowers the rate of protein synthesis and speeds protein breakdown. The exact mechanisms of protein metabolism during exercise have not been determined, though several mechanisms have been proposed. Parkhouse has reported that exercise, particularly exercise to exhaustion, activates specific proteolytic enzymes in the muscle that degrade the myofibrillar protein. Fitts and Metzger found elevated levels of proteolytic enzymes in fatigued muscle. A number of amino acids released by muscle tissue breakdown could enter the energy pathways, but the major research effort has focused on the fate of leucine, one of the branched-chain amino acids in the muscle. The oxidation of leucine has been shown to increase during exercise. In essence, the by-products of leucine catabolism eventually combine with pyruvate in the muscle cell and are converted to alanine and an alpha-ketoacid. The alpha-ketoacid may enter the Krebs cycle and be used for energy production. The alanine is released into the bloodstream and transported to the liver where it is converted into glucose. The glucose may then be released into the blood to be used by the central nervous system and may eventually find its way to the contracting muscle to be used as an energy source. Alanine appears to be an important means of transporting the amino group to the liver for excretion as urea. This overall process involving gluconeogenesis, known as the glucose-alanine cycle, is depicted graphically in Figure 6.6. Some investigators have noted that during the latter part of endurance exercise, the blood levels of alanine increase, presumably because more is released from the muscle. However, the estimated glucose production approximates only 4 grams per hour, which might be important in mild-intensity exercise but is possibly insignificant during high-intensity exercise when carbohydrate use may approximate 3 grams per minute. Additionally, several investigators have reported an increased release of branched-chain amino acids (BCAA) from the liver during endurance exercise, with subsequent uptake by the muscle cells.

Thus, protein (amino acids) can be utilized during exercise to provide energy directly in the muscle and via glucose produced in the liver, particularly when the body stores of glycogen and glucose are low. A low-carbohydrate diet will facilitate this process. On the other hand, adequate carbohydrate intake before and during prolonged exercise will help reduce the use of body protein for this purpose, because the presence of adequate muscle glycogen appears to inhibit enzymes that catabolize muscle protein. Scientists from the University of Maastricht in the Netherlands recently noted that high-carbohydrate diets may have a protein-sparing effect for endurance athletes.

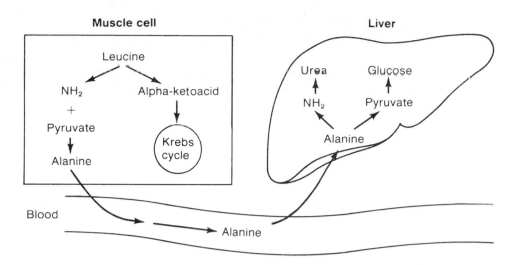

Figure 6.6 Glucose-alanine cycle. Alanine may be produced in the muscle tissue from the breakdown of other amino acids, most notably leucine. The alanine is then released into the blood and travels to the liver for eventual conversion to glucose through the process of gluconeogenesis. (See Appendix K, Figure K.5, for other amino acids that may enter energy pathways.)

Although the available evidence suggests that metabolism of protein and its use as an energy source are increased during exercise, the magnitude of its contribution may depend on a variety of factors, such as the intensity and duration of exercise and the availability of other fuels, such as glycogen, in the muscle. This topic is the subject of continuing research.

Does exercise increase protein losses in other ways?

Exercise has been shown to increase protein losses from the body in several other ways. For one, exercise causes an elevated level of protein in the urine, a condition known as **proteinuria.** This condition has been observed following competition in a wide variety of sports, including running, football, basketball, and handball. Research suggests that the greater the intensity of the exercise, the greater the loss of protein in the urine. Poortmans indicated there may be a decreased reabsorption of protein in the kidney tubules during intense exercise. However, the total amount of protein lost in this manner appears to be rather negligible, amounting to less than 3 grams per day.

Protein also may be lost in the sweat. Several investigators have reported the presence of both amino acids and proteins in exercise-induced sweat. Again, the losses are relatively minor, on the order of 1 gram per liter of sweat in adult males. This avenue could account for 2–4 grams of protein in an endurance athlete training in a warm environment.

What effect does exercise training have upon protein metabolism?

This question may be addressed from several perspectives. First, how does training influence protein metabolism during exercise? And second, what happens during the recovery period between training bouts?

As for the first part of this question, you may recall from previous chapters that there is substantial research to support the conclusion that aerobic endurance training improves the ability of the muscle cell to use both carbohydrate and fat as energy sources during exercise. Although extensive evidence is not available, in a recent review, Graham and others noted that following endurance training the muscles appear to develop the potential for increased capacity for oxidation of leucine and the other branched-chain amino acids. Thus, endurance training may increase the capacity of the muscle to derive energy from protein in a fashion similar to the increased utilization of fat, another possible means to spare the use of carbohydrates such as blood glucose and muscle glycogen. Additionally, when exercising at a standardized work load before and after training, training may also decrease the production or accumulation of ammonia, a nitrogen by-product of protein catabolism. Extrapolating from animal research, some investigators theorize that instead of forming ammonia, the nitrogen is incorporated into other amino acids, such as alanine, for transportation from the muscle to the liver.

In general, these changes in protein metabolism through training would appear to be contrary to preservation of body protein stores, but they may represent another means whereby the body adapts to endurance training in an attempt to preserve carbohydrate as an energy source when endogenous supplies are decreased. Another possibility is to prevent fatigue associated with ammonia. Although no underlying mechanism has been identified, increasing levels of ammonia in the body have been associated with fatigue, somewhat comparable to the accumulation of lactic acid. One theory is that increased ammonia levels in the muscle may impair oxidative processes, thus decreasing energy production, while another theory suggests increased plasma ammonia may impair brain functions and induce central fatigue. Because ammonia is formed in the muscle from the amino group, removal of the amino group by alanine or another amino acid, glutamine, may help decrease the production of ammonia and delay the onset of fatigue. Thus, increased production of alanine theoretically could be a beneficial effect of training.

Regarding the second part of this question, although protein catabolism may occur during exercise, even following training, the recovery period is marked by an increase in protein synthesis. Numerous studies have found that after resistance or endurance exercise, protein balance is maintained or becomes positive. Trained individuals, during rest, have been shown to experience a preferential oxidation of fat and a sparing of protein, as measured by leucine metabolism and the respiratory quotient. The exercise task apparently stimulates the DNA in the muscle cell nucleus to increase the synthesis of protein, and the type of protein that is synthesized is specific to the type of exercise. Aerobic exercise stimulates synthesis of mitochondria and oxidative enzymes, which are composed of protein and are necessary for energy production in the oxygen system. Resistance training promotes synthesis of the contractile muscle proteins. These adaptations to training are the key factors in improving performance.

The effect of training in producing a positive nitrogen balance or a positive protein balance during the recovery period depends on an adequate dietary supply of protein and Calories.

Do individuals in strenuous physical training, including the developing adolescent athlete, need more protein in the diet?

There appears to be a difference of opinion about the answer to this question. For example, the National Research Council, in its 1989 RDA, states there is little evidence that muscular activity increases the need for protein, except for the small amounts needed for the development of muscle during physical conditioning. The council further suggests that in view of the margin of safety in the RDA, no increment is needed during training. One investigator even contends that because exercise training increases the ability of the body to retain protein in the recovery period, athletes in training may need less protein than sedentary individuals if they consume enough Calories to maintain body weight.

On the other hand, many investigators who have studied the protein needs of athletes have recommended that athletes' protein requirements may be increased during periods of heavy physical training. Because weight lifters and bodybuilders are attempting to increase lean muscle mass and strength, the extra protein is recommended to maximize muscle protein synthesis. Additional dietary protein also has been recommended for endurance athletes who may utilize protein as an energy source during exercise, and who also need to synthesize oxidative enzymes and mitochondria. Others have suggested that protein supplementation is particularly important during the early stages of training to help prevent sports anemia. The recommended range of protein varies with the type of athlete, but recent recommendations, based on reputable research, range from 1.2–1.8 grams per kilogram body weight.

The following is a brief summary of the available research relative to the protein needs of, and the effect of protein supplementation upon, athletes involved in either strength-type or endurance-type activities, including the special condition of sports anemia.

Strength-Type Activities   Individuals involved in these activities include weight lifters, bodybuilders, and football players. They are usually interested in increasing muscle mass and decreasing body fat, as well as improving strength and power. It is unlikely that such athletes use considerable amounts of protein for energy during training. Tarnopolsky and his associates recently reported that 1 hour of circuit weight lifting did not affect leucine turnover for several hours afterwards, but Pivarnik and others did note increased urinary levels of 3-methylhistidine in untrained subjects after the third day of training, suggesting the skeletal muscle was being degraded through strength-building exercises.

Several studies have attempted to determine the protein requirement for maintaining nitrogen balance during weight lifting. Greg Paul conducted a thorough review of the available literature and reported values of 0.82–1.94 grams of protein per kilogram body weight per day. More recent research by Tarnopolsky suggests a value near the RDA is sufficient to maintain nitrogen balance. In the Pivarnik study, there was no indication that the reported breakdown of muscle tissue increased protein requirements, and one of the coinvestigators, James Hickson, was cited as indicating that the RDA was sufficient. These findings may be appropriate for maintaining nitrogen balance but possibly not for creating a positive nitrogen balance, hopefully as muscle mass.

Unfortunately there is very little scientific information about the specific protein requirements for the development of lean muscle mass in weight-training programs. Protein balance is usually positive during these programs, and research studies have suggested that weight lifters could retain between 7 and 28 grams of protein per day. Although it might be assumed this protein would be assimilated as muscle tissue, this has not been determined. A number of respected investigators have recommended that weight lifters and other athletes training to increase muscle mass and strength, particularly the developing adolescent athlete and those in the early stages of training, consume more protein. Peter Lemon, in a 1996 review, recommended between 1.7 and 1.8 grams of protein per kilogram body weight per day, whereas Mark Tarnopolsky in 1993 recommended between 1.2 and 1.76 grams of protein per kilogram body weight. Gail Butterfield recommended a value of twice the RDA plus an additional 200 Calories per day. These general recommendations are for athletes and others involved in strenuous resistance training.

Both laboratory and field studies have been conducted to investigate the effect of additional dietary protein upon body weight and composition during physical training. Although the field studies with athletes such as football players were relatively uncontrolled in regard to diet and amount of exercise, most of them reported that increased protein in the form of dietary supplements led to increases in body weight. However, most of these field studies did not evaluate body composition or the changes in lean body tissue such as muscle versus body-fat changes. Several better-controlled laboratory studies have compared the effect of normal protein intake, about 0.8–1.4 grams per kilogram, to higher levels, such as 1.6–2.8 grams per kilogram, on body composition changes during a weight-training program. In general, these studies revealed that although protein balance could be maintained or even be positive with the consumption of a normal amount of protein, the body protein balance was even more positive with the larger amounts. The additional body weight also appears to be in the form of lean body mass. However, in a recent well-designed study using nuclear magnetic resonance to measure leg muscle, Weideman and others reported no significant increase in leg muscle hypertrophy following 13 weeks of weight training with 2.94 grams of protein per kilogram per day, nor did Lemon and others find increased muscle mass when subjects consumed 2.62 grams of protein per kilogram per day, as compared to 1.35 grams per kilogram.

Another important consideration in weight-gaining programs is sufficient dietary energy in the form of carbohydrate or fat. This topic is covered in Chapter 12.

Although available research suggests that the effects of increased protein intake appear to be beneficial relative to body protein balance during training, the effect upon actual physical performance is very questionable. Field studies that reported increased strength levels following protein supplementation were poorly designed. For example, one study used a milk-protein supplement with elite weight lifters, increasing their daily protein intake from a normal 2.5 grams to 3.5 grams per kilogram body weight. The investigators noted significant gains in both lean body mass and strength following a period of several months when the athletes consumed the supplement, compared to a decrease in these variables after the athletes had consumed a placebo for several months. Although this may appear to be a well-designed study, the protein supplement was given during two periods when the athletes were peaking for world championship competition, while the placebo was given during a period of apparently less intensive training between competitions. Thus the effects could be due to the more intensive training presumed to occur in the peak training periods. Several other well-

designed studies have not revealed any beneficial effects of protein supplementation upon physical performance. In the Weideman study cited above, 2.94 grams of protein/kg/day did not increase strength. Lemon and others reported that increasing dietary protein intake from 1.35 to 2.62 grams per kilogram body weight also had no effect on strength gains during the early stages of training.

Endurance-Type Activities   As noted previously, the use of protein as an energy source may increase during prolonged endurance exercise, although the precise source of the protein thus utilized has not been identified. Hickson and Wolinsky, in a recent review, noted that whatever the source of the protein catabolized during exercise, skeletal muscle tissue or otherwise, the fact that protein catabolism occurs suggests that protein needs may be increased with endurance-building activities. Current research appears to support this point of view. Paul reviewed a number of studies involving endurance athletes and found that 0.97–1.37 grams of protein per kilogram per day were needed to attain nitrogen balance. Other investigators have reported similar findings or recommendations. Lemon recently reported values of 1.2–1.4 grams per kilogram per day; Tarnopolsky suggested 1.2–1.6 grams; Butterfield concluded from her review that 1.26 grams were necessary; and Poortmans recommended 1.2 grams. Individual endurance athletes can vary greatly in their ability to retain dietary protein, possibly owing to such factors as total energy intake, particularly carbohydrate, and protein quality. In particular, female endurance athletes may need higher values since their energy intakes are usually lower. Athletes attempting to lose body weight for competition may also need more protein. Some investigators suggest a greater safety margin when establishing dietary protein recommendations for endurance athletes, possibly up to 1.8–2.0 grams of protein per kilogram per day.

Few data are available regarding the effect of high-protein diets upon endurance performance. One early study did note that low protein intake, only 4 grams per day, did not lower maximal endurance capacity over a 10-day period, but energy intake was adequate. Sharp and his colleagues investigated the effect of a protein supplement (0.8 g/kg/day) during 8 weeks of combined aerobic and anaerobic training on a bicycle ergometer. Although the protein supplement did not increase VO_2 max or mean power output, the subjects were able to generate more work output at the anaerobic (lactate) threshold. These investigators also reported favorable effects of protein supplementation upon anabolic hormones, particularly testosterone, and such an effect could benefit performance. On the other hand, Bigard and others reported that although at moderate altitude VO_2 max was unaffected, bicycle ergometer endurance time was impaired significantly on an isocaloric diet when protein intake was increased from 12 percent to 20 percent of daily caloric intake and carbohydrate intake was correspondingly decreased.

Most recently, the 40:30:30 "zone diet" alluded to in Chapter 5 may be considered to be a high-protein diet because 30 percent of the daily Calories are derived from protein; 40 percent are derived from carbohydrate and 30 percent from fat. Although such a diet could be palatable to an athlete, there are no scientific data to suggest it improves performance compared to diets higher in carbohydrate and balanced in fat and protein. In a recent review of functional foods in sport edited by Brouns, John Hawley, an expert on sport nutrition from South Africa, criticized the "zone diet" book, noting that the claims of improved sport performance are based on anecdotal reports and selectively-quoted research, not sound scientific evidence. Hawley contends that the book is confusing and contradictory.

However, for weight-restricted athletes attempting to lose body fat or maintain a low body weight for sports competition, some investigators recommend increased protein intake. With a 1,500 Calorie diet, a 30 percent protein allotment would be 450 Calories, or approximately 112 grams of protein. For a lean athlete, this amount of protein may help insure protein adequacy and may fall in the range of recommended protein intake.

Intermittent High-Intensity Activities   Very little research has been conducted relative to the protein requirements of athletes involved in sports or activities characterized by prolonged, intermittent high-intensity exercise, such as soccer, field or ice hockey, lacrosse, and basketball. However, in a recent review, Lemon indicated such activities represent a balance of strength/power and endurance activities, and recommended a protein intake ranging from 1.4–1.7 grams per kilogram body weight. This value is in accord with those recommended for strength-trained and endurance-trained individuals.

Sports Anemia   Some investigators have suggested that additional protein be taken during the early stages of an endurance training program to prevent the development of a condition labeled as **sports anemia.** Sports anemia is thought to occur as the body adapts to the exercise in the early stages of the program and uses protein to synthesize myoglobin, mitochondria, and other muscle protein compounds essential for oxygen utilization at the expense of hemoglobin. Thus there is a transitory decline in the serum hemoglobin levels resulting in the appearance of anemia.

Most of the early research relative to protein requirements to prevent sports anemia was conducted in Japan. These studies suggested that 1.5–2.0 grams of protein per kilogram body weight were needed daily for the first month of training to prevent this condition. On the other hand, a more recent report from Japan, although noting the development of sports anemia in individuals with low protein intake (0.5 grams per kilogram), also stated that normal protein intake of 1.25 grams per kilogram would prevent its development. Other research has suggested that sports anemia is not caused by a loss of hemoglobin but rather by an expansion of the plasma, which simply dilutes the hemoglobin concentration and gives the appearance of anemia. Moreover, sports anemia has not been shown to occur in all subjects initiating a strenuous training program, particularly in those on a balanced diet. Sports anemia also has been associated with iron nutrition and is discussed further in Chapter 8.

What are some general recommendations relative to dietary protein intake for athletes?

Although the available research does not provide us with any definitive data about exact protein requirements during training, it does suggest that athletes need at least the RDA of approximately 0.8–1.0 grams per kilogram body weight and possibly more to maintain or increase protein balance. The following mathematical presentations are possible scenarios for various athletes who may wish to maintain or increase protein balance. The protein needs are based upon the RDA, a rough estimate of the amount of protein used during strenuous exercise, and additional protein needs for the individual who wants to gain weight.

Let us look first at the young athlete who wants to gain body weight, preferably in the form of muscle tissue, through a weight-training program. The protein RDA for an adolescent male is 1.0 grams per kilogram. At moderate activity levels, the average 70-kg adolescent male would be in protein balance with 70 g daily. However, according to the suggested upper recommendation of about 1.8 grams per kilogram, he would need about 126 g daily if involved in a strenuous training program. Is this a reasonable amount?

One pound of muscle tissue is equal to 454 grams, and its composition is approximately 70 percent water, 7 percent lipids, and 22 percent muscle tissue. Hence, 1 pound of muscle contains about 100 grams of protein ($454 \times .22$). If the desired weight gain is 1 pound of lean body mass per week, a reasonable goal, then this young male would need an additional 14 grams of protein per day (100 grams/7 days) to supply the amount in 1 pound of muscle tissue. A gain of 2 pounds per week, although probably more difficult to accomplish, would require 28 additional grams of protein per day. Let us be liberal and estimate an additional 22 grams of protein per day to cover losses due to exercise. In summary, assuming that a portion of these protein needs are not covered by the safety margin incorporated in the RDA, this young athlete would need approximately 120 grams of protein per day (70 + 28 + 22) to gain 2 pounds of lean body tissue per week, or about 1.7 grams of protein per kilogram body weight. This value falls within the recommended range.

Endurance athletes are not necessarily interested in gaining weight, but they may need to replenish the protein that may serve as an energy source during training. Running 10 miles per day would expend approximately 1,000

Calories. If 10 percent of this energy cost, or 100 Calories, was derived from protein, then approximately 25 grams of protein (100 Calories/4 Calories per gram of protein) would need to be replaced. With a liberal estimated additional loss of 10 grams of protein in the urine and sweat, the total daily protein requirement for a 70-kg male, again assuming that these additional needs are not accounted for by the safety margin in the RDA, would be 105 grams (70 + 25 + 10), or 1.5 g/kg. Again, this value falls within the recommended range.

These protein needs could be satisfied easily by small adjustments to the normal diet already being consumed in the United States. For example, the average caloric intake for a moderately active young male averages 2,500–3,000 C. This caloric intake may be increased through physical training as more Calories are expended. Thus, caloric intake would be increased to approximately 3,500–4,000 C. It is important to note that adequate energy intake, primarily in the form of carbohydrates, will improve protein balance. In essence, an increased energy intake appears to decrease protein requirements somewhat.

If the protein content of the dietary Calories averaged 12 percent, which represents the approximate intake in the United States, then the intake of protein would approximate 1.5–1.7 grams per kilogram, which parallels the amounts estimated in the examples cited above. Increasing the protein content to 15 percent would provide a value of 1.9–2.1 grams per kilogram body weight.

These values approach the higher amounts recommended by some investigators for individuals in training. The calculations are presented in Table 6.6.

Dietary surveys of athletes have revealed that many strength-type athletes, such as football players, are currently consuming about 2 grams of protein per kilogram per day. Grandjean recently reported an intake of 1.4–3.0 grams of protein per kilogram body weight in elite male athletes, and 1.0–2.0 grams in elite female athletes. On the other hand, athletes such as wrestlers and gymnasts, who are in greater need of protein because of low caloric intake, have been reported to consume less than their RDA. In female athletes, low dietary protein intake has been associated with amenorrhea, a topic discussed further in Chapters 8 and 10.

It is important for the athlete to obtain adequate protein nutrition. Wise selection of high-quality protein foods will provide adequate amounts through a balanced diet to meet bodily needs during the early and continued stages of training. It is not difficult to increase the protein content of the diet. For example, 8 ounces of roasted, skinless chicken breast and two glasses of skim milk, a total of less than 600 Calories, will provide over 70 grams of high-quality protein, the RDA for our typical 70-kg adolescent and more than half of the 125 grams that may be recommended for such an athlete attempting to gain muscle mass. Perusal of Table 6.2 and Appendix F will help you select

Table 6.6	Calculation of grams protein/kilogram body weight	
Body weight: 70 kg		
One gram protein = 4 Calories		
Daily caloric intake:	3,500–4,000	3,500–4,000
Percent protein:	15	12
Calories in protein:	525–600	420–480
Grams of protein:	131–150	105–120
Grams protein/kg:	1.9–2.1	1.5–1.7

high-protein foods. Additional points on this subject are covered in Chapter 12 under the topic of gaining weight.

The importance of carbohydrate in the diet of the athlete or physically active individual, particularly those involved in endurance exercise, should also be reiterated, for adequate dietary carbohydrate will decrease the oxidation of amino acids and the formation of ammonia. Besides its efficiency as a metabolic fuel during exercise, carbohydrate also provides a potent protein-sparing effect. As discussed in Chapter 2, dietary carbohydrate is stressed in the precompetition meal, particularly when consumed within an hour of competition, and protein intake should be limited. A recent study by Wiles and others noted an increased oxygen consumption during various exercise intensities (an indicator of impaired efficiency), particularly the more intense levels, when protein was consumed 1 hour prior to the exercise task, and ratings of perceived exertion were also higher with the protein diet. The protein meal content was 0.4 grams per kilogram body weight. However, no adverse effects were noticed when the same protein intake was consumed 3 hours prior to the exercise task. These findings suggest protein intake should be restricted in any precompetition feedings within an hour of exercise, particularly intense exercise near 100 percent VO_2 max.

Other investigators have studied the effect of protein supplementation upon possible muscle damage during training, but the results are contradictory. One study reported that 15 grams of protein consumed immediately after exercise enhanced muscle repair, as measured by changes in enzyme status associated with muscle damage. Conversely, another study, using 37.5 grams of protein, showed no facilitation in recovery from muscle damage, as measured by a strength test.

More recently, Zawadzki and others reported that adding protein to a carbohydrate supplement increased the rate of muscle glycogen synthesis during the recovery period immediately following exercise when compared to the carbohydrate supplement alone; approximately 40 grams of protein were added to 112 grams of carbohydrate. The authors noted increased levels of insulin with the

Table 6.7 Recommended protein intakes in grams per kilogram body weight for sedentary and physically active individuals

	Grams of protein/kg body weight
Sedentary	0.8
Strength-trained, maintenance	1.2–1.4
Strength-trained, gain muscle mass	1.6–1.8
Endurance-trained	1.2–1.4
Weight-restricted	1.4–1.8

The values presented represent a synthesis of those recommended by leading researchers involved in protein metabolism and exercise. Teenagers should add 10 percent to the calculated values.

To calculate body weight in kilograms, simply multiply your weight in pounds by 0.454. Then, multiply your weight in kilograms by the appropriate value in the grams per kilogram body weight column to determine the range of grams of protein intake per day. Teenagers should increase this amount by 10 percent.

protein/carbohydrate mixture, which would speed muscle glycogen resynthesis. Similar findings were reported by Chandler and others following a weight-training workout, and the authors suggested a carbohydrate-protein supplement after weight-training exercise may elicit hormonal responses during recovery that may be favorable to muscle growth. However, no performance data were reported in these studies. It is clear that additional research is necessary before we can make any sound conclusions about the effect of protein supplementation on exercise performance.

It is becoming increasingly clear that athletes involved in intense resistance or aerobic endurance training need more protein in the diet. Table 6.7 presents a summary of the recommended daily protein intakes for sedentary and physically active individuals. Whether or not certain diet strategies, such as high protein intake immediately before or after strenuous exercise, cause any beneficial or detrimental effect is less certain and merits additional research.

Protein: Ergogenic Aspects

Given the potential importance of protein to optimal physical performance, a wide variety of ergogenic aids associated with protein nutrition have been used in attempts to enhance performance, such as special protein foods, amino acids, and by-products of protein metabolism.

Are special protein supplements necessary?

As already discussed, the available research data suggest that athletes involved in weight training to gain weight or in strenuous endurance exercise may need somewhat more than the RDA for protein to maintain or increase protein balance, particularly if energy intake (Calories) is not adequate to meet daily energy expenditure. However, as also noted, the ability of protein supplementation to improve physical performance above and beyond the effects of the training program itself is obscure.

To provide additional protein to the diet, investigators have used powdered protein sources, canned liquid meals high in protein and energy, or special foods and concoctions high in protein content. However, the protein content is actually derived from natural protein, such as milk, egg, or soy protein. As Bucci has indicated, supplements of intact proteins, such as the proteins found in these products, offer no advantages over protein found in other food sources, since these supplements are in fact derived from natural foods. In addition, many of these protein supplements are expensive when compared to natural protein that may be obtained easily in high-protein foods such as powdered milk, skim milk, eggs, and chicken. Blending powdered milk into a glass of skim milk, with some vanilla or other flavoring, will provide substantial amounts of high-quality protein—your own personal protein supplement. Some comparative costs for different sources of protein are presented in Table 6.8.

Nevertheless, commercial supplements may be a convenient means for some busy athletes to secure additional protein in the diet. Many of these products contain high-quality protein, such as milk or egg protein; provide a balanced mixture of protein, carbohydrate, and fat for additional Calories; and may also contain supplemental vitamins and minerals. Although these products do not contain all of the nutrients of natural foods, they may be useful adjuncts to a balanced diet. Certain brands have been available for years, such as Nutrament, but several companies have recently marketed products specifically for physically active individuals, such as Nitrofuel by Twin Labs and GatorPro (not Gatorade, but "pro" for protein) by the Quaker Oats Company. It is important to reemphasize the point that these supplements should be used as an adjunct to an otherwise balanced nutritional plan, not as a substitute.

Other protein substances such as spirulina (algae), brewer's yeast, specific enzymes, and even DNA have been advocated as means to improve physical performance. However, there appears to be no research available to support their effectiveness. Spirulina and brewer's yeast are good sources of protein and a variety of vitamins and minerals but convey no magical ergogenic qualities. The enzymes and DNA would be degraded in the digestive process and thus could not be utilized for the purpose for which they were ingested.

Table 6.8 Costs of protein found in various food sources

Source	Serving size	Grams of protein/ serving	Cost per serving	Cost per 8 grams of protein
Powdered milk	23 grams	8	$0.13	$0.13
Egg	1	6	$0.10	$0.13
Turkey breast	4 ounces	28	$0.75	$0.21
Skim milk	8 fluid ounces	8	$0.20	$0.20
Protein capsules	8 capsules	8	$1.20	$1.20
MetRx Bar	1 3.5 ounce bar	27	$2.50	$0.74
Boost	8 fluid ounces	10	$1.10	$0.88
Avalanche Power Drink	16 fluid ounces	40	$3.00	$0.60

Are amino acid, amine, and related nitrogen-containing supplements effective ergogenic aids?

In recent years amino acid supplements have become increasingly available and popular in certain athletic circles. Weight lifters are consuming various amino acids in attempts to stimulate the release of growth hormone from the pituitary gland, hoping that the growth hormone will then stimulate muscle development. Amino acids have also been used to stimulate the release of insulin from the pancreas; insulin is also considered to be an anabolic hormone because it facilitates the uptake of amino acids by the muscle cells. Indeed, certain amino acid mixtures have been advertised to be more potent than anabolic steroids, one of the most popular drugs used by strength and power athletes. Anabolic steroids are discussed in Chapter 12. Other amino acids have been advertised in magazines for endurance athletes, suggesting that they may be utilized as a fuel during training or help prevent fatigue by altering the formation of neurotransmitters in the brain. Still other amino acid mixtures and related compounds such as creatine and inosine have been used in attempts to increase ATP or PC levels in the muscle or to help athletes lose body weight for competition.

Scientific research has shown that individual amino acid supplements may induce specific physiological responses in the body, particularly the formation of certain chemicals in the brain needed for nerve impulse transmission as well as secretion of hormones. However, amino acid metabolism is very complex. It depends upon a variety of factors such as the concentration in the blood, competition with other amino acids, feedback control mechanisms, and the presence in the diet of other nutrients. Consumption of specific amino acid mixtures or even high-protein diets may actually lead to nutritional imbalances, as an overload of one amino acid may inhibit the absorption of others into the body.

Because purified amino acids, known as free-form amino acids, amines such as creatine, and other nitrogen-containing substances have become commercially available for athletes, they have been the focus of increased research activity by sports medicine scientists. However, although the number of studies is increasing relative to the effect of amino acid supplementation upon physical performance, with the exception of creatine the data are still somewhat limited. Moreover, some investigators combine several amino acids or use commercial supplements that may contain not only several amino acids but other nutrients as well, which may cloud the possible ergogenic effect of any one specific amino acid. The following discussion highlights some of the current key findings regarding specific amino acids, various combinations of amino acids, amines, and nitrogen-containing compounds that have been studied for their potential ergogenic effect.

Arginine, Lysine, and Ornithine   Research has shown that infusing any of a number of amino acids into the blood potentiates the release of **human growth hormone (HGH),** a polypeptide. HGH is released from the pituitary gland into the bloodstream, affecting all tissues. One of its effects is to stimulate the production of another hormone, insulin-like growth factor-1, that spurs growth of tissue, including muscle tissue. Some amino acids may also stimulate the release of insulin from the pancreas.

Although more than a half-dozen amino acids may stimulate HGH release when infused, the effect of oral supplementation is less clear. However, Jacobson has reported that the oral administration of selected amino acids may lead to HGH release similar to that promoted by infusion. Bucci, in his book on nutritional ergogenics, also notes that oral intake of amino acids, particularly arginine and ornithine, may increase HGH release, while others have suggested lysine may elicit similar effects. Recent research by Bucci and his colleagues has supported the effect of ornithine to increase serum HGH levels. Using dosages of 40, 100, and 170 milligrams per kilogram body weight, only the highest dose of ornithine increased HGH levels, but it caused intestinal distress (osmotic diarrhea) in many of the subjects, and thus its use at this effective dose may be impractical. Moreover, in a related study, Bucci and others noted ornithine did not increase the secretion of insulin.

Arginine, lysine, and ornithine, separately or in various combinations, have received the most research attention regarding an ergogenic effect for strength/power-type athletes. They have been advertised in bodybuilding magazines as being more powerful than anabolic steroids, potent drugs used by some athletes to increase muscle mass. The advertisers apparently are capitalizing on the potential of these amino acids to enhance HGH release.

Two of the earliest published studies by Elam collectively reported that arginine and ornithine supplementation in conjunction with a weight-training program reduced body fat, increased lean body mass, and increased strength over a 5-week period. The dosage was 2 grams per day (1 gram each of arginine and ornithine), 5 days per week. Unfortunately, both studies have been criticized in the literature on the grounds of the statistical procedure by which the experimental and control groups were compared. A different analysis of the same data revealed no significant difference between the experimental and control groups in the first study. The studies have also been criticized for questionable measurement techniques and for making assumptions without adequate supporting data.

Several studies with better experimental designs have not shown any significant ergogenic effect of arginine and lysine, or other similar amino acid combinations. Lambert and others, using combinations of arginine/lysine and ornithine/tyrosine, reported no significant increases in HGH, while Fogelholm and his associates noted no significant increases in HGH or insulin secretion following supplementation with arginine, ornithine, and lysine in competitive weight lifters. Hawkins and associates, using experienced male weight lifters as subjects, reported no beneficial effects of oral arginine supplementation on various measures of muscle function, including peak torque and endurance. Suminski and others reported that although a bout of weight training would increase HGH levels in noncompetitive weight lifters, supplementation with arginine and lysine provided no additional benefit. Mitchell and others, also using experienced weight lifters, reported that 8 weeks of supplementation with arginine and lysine elicited no significant effect on HGH secretion, body composition, or various strength measures. Thus, currently there are no sound data supporting an ergogenic effect of arginine, ornithine, or lysine supplementation as a means to enhance muscular development, strength, or power via increased secretion of HGH.

Tryptophan   Although tryptophan is one of the amino acids that may increase the release of HGH, its theoretical ergogenic effect is based upon another function. Two neurotransmitters in the brain, serotonin and 5-hydroxytryptamine, are derived from tryptophan. These neurotransmitters may induce sleepiness and elicit a mellow mood, and Segura and Ventura hypothesize that they may help to decrease the perception of pain. They postulate that individuals who show the best tolerance of or resistance to pain may be able to delay the onset of fatigue, and that tryptophan supplementation therefore might improve exercise performance. In their study, twelve healthy athletes exercised to exhaustion on a treadmill at 80 percent of their VO_2 max under two conditions: A placebo was compared with a dosage of 1,200 milligrams of L-tryptophan consumed in 300-mg doses over the 24 hours prior to testing, the last dose being 1 hour prior to the test. They reported no significant improvement in peak oxygen uptake or heart rate response but did note a significant improvement in time to exhaustion (49 percent) and a decreased rating of perceived exertion (RPE) following the L-tryptophan trial. The times to exhaustion were extremely variable among the individual subjects, ranging from 2.5–18 minutes, suggesting some of the individuals may not have been well trained.

Stensrud and his associates challenged the results of this study, indicating a 49 percent increase in performance would be rather phenomenal in trained athletes. Thus, they decided to replicate this study using forty-nine well-trained male runners and better control conditions, although they had their subjects run to exhaustion at 100 percent VO_2 max, not 80 percent. In contrast to the study by Segura and Ventura, they reported no significant effect of tryptophan supplementation on performance. Other research from the University of Maastricht revealed no effect of tryptophan supplementation on endurance performance at 70–75 percent of VO_2 max.

Based on these limited data, tryptophan does not appear to be an effective ergogenic in either short-term or prolonged exercise tasks. Some adverse health effects have been associated with tryptophan supplementation and are discussed in the next section.

Branched-Chain Amino Acids (BCAA)   Eric Newsholme, a biochemist at Oxford University, proposed the central fatigue hypothesis, postulating that high levels of serum free-tryptophan (fTRP) in conjunction with low levels of branched-chain amino acids (BCAA), or a high fTRP:BCAA ratio, may be a major factor in the etiology of fatigue during prolonged endurance exercise. Research with animals has shown that a high fTRP:BCAA ratio may lead to an increased production of serotonin. Newsholme suggested that serum BCAA levels eventually decrease in endurance exercise, such as marathon running, because they may be used for energy production. Such an effect would possibly increase the fTRP:BCAA ratio, facilitating the transport of tryptophan into the brain and increasing serotonin production, which could lead to fatigue because increased serotonin levels may depress central nervous system functions. Some, but not all, research with humans supports this finding. Blomstrand and others have shown in several studies that prolonged endurance exercise, such as the 26.2 mile (42.2 kilometer) marathon, increases the fTRP:BCAA ratio, but Conlay and others noted no change in this ratio in experienced runners immediately following completion of the Boston Marathon.

The central fatigue hypothesis and BCAA supplementation have received considerable research attention since Newsholme proposed his hypothesis in the late 1980s, and these studies have served as the basis for several reviews, most notably by J. Mark Davis of the University of South Carolina. Based on these reviews, and research studies published subsequent to these reviews, the following appear to be the key points regarding the central fatigue hypothesis and the effects of nutritional interventions, particularly BCAA and carbohydrate supplementation.

Support for the hypothesis   Animal studies support the concept of central fatigue during prolonged exercise tasks. Fatigue appears to be associated with increases in brain serotonin, but fatigue is also correlated to changes in other brain neurotransmitters as well, such as dopamine. Some human data also suggest serotonin may be involved in the development of fatigue. Several drugs, approved for use with humans, may block the removal of serotonin from its active sites, thus magnifying its effects. In several studies involving running or cycling at 70 percent VO_2 max, these drugs either impaired performance or increased the psychological perception of effort, both negative findings.

However, Davis points out that although the central fatigue hypothesis has some support from experimental data, the underlying mechanism has not been determined. Investigators are studying this issue, looking not only at mechanisms associated with serotonin, but other brain neurotransmitters as well, such as dopamine.

BCAA supplementation and the fTRP:BCAA ratio   If serum BCAA fall during prolonged exercise, then BCAA supplementation might be a preventive measure. It is known that BCAA are metabolized primarily in the muscle, not the liver, and thus may provide an energy source during exercise. Some research has shown that oral supplementation with BCAA will increase the serum levels of BCAA, the BCAA may possibly be used as an energy source during exercise, the BCAA may prevent or decrease the rate of endogenous protein degradation during exercise, and the BCAA may help to maintain a normal fTRP:BCAA ratio during prolonged exercise.

BCAA supplementation and mental performance   Several sports, such as tennis and soccer, involve prolonged, high-intensity intermittent bouts of exercise in which mental alertness must be maintained. In such events, the fTRP:BCAA ratio may increase, as documented by Struder and associates in a study involving nationally-ranked tennis players involved in 4 hours of continuous tournament tennis.

As evaluated by several tests of cognitive performance, several studies by Blomstrand and her associates reported that BCAA supplementation improved mental performance in national-class soccer players after a game and in runners after a 30-kilometer race. However, other investigators reported no effect of BCAA supplementation on mental acuity following a 40-kilometer cycle performance test. These are interesting field studies, and additional similar research is merited, complemented by well-controlled laboratory studies.

Somewhat related to mental performance is the psychological perception of effort, or how mentally stressful the subject perceives a given exercise task to be. This psychological effort is usually evaluated by Borg's Rating of Perceived Exertion Scale, or RPE. In recent research, Blomstrand and others reported that BCAA supplementation, compared to a placebo trial, reduced the RPE and mental fatigue of endurance-trained cyclists during a 60-minute ride at 70 percent VO_2 max followed by another 20 minutes of maximal exercise. The fTRP:BCAA ratio increased in the placebo trial, but remained unchanged or even decreased in the BCAA trial. Conversely, other well-controlled studies have reported no significant effect of BCAA supplementation on RPE during intense exercise, such as during a 40-kilometer cycling performance test and 90 minutes of exercise at a 2-millimole lactate threshold.

BCAA supplementation and physical performance   Investigators have studied BCAA supplementation with acute dosages administered to subjects just before and during the exercise task, and chronic dosages provided to the subject for several weeks prior to and during the exercise task. Dosages have varied, ranging from 5–20 grams per day. When provided with liquids, the dosages ranged up to 7 grams per liter.

In one of the first reports of acute supplementation, Blomstrand and her colleagues studied the performance of 193 marathoners, separated into placebo and BCAA supplement groups. Overall, there was no significant difference in marathon performance between the placebo group and the BCAA group. However, using some debatable statistical tactics, they reported that BCAA supplementation significantly improved performance in the "slower" runners in the race (3:05–3:30 hours) but had no effect on the performance of the "faster" runners (<3:05 hours). They suggested that the slower runners may have depleted their muscle glycogen earlier, therefore decreasing their serum BCAA levels earlier in the race and benefiting more from the supplementation. Although this was an interesting field study, it has been criticized by Davis for several problems with experimental methodology.

Most well-controlled laboratory studies and field studies involving acute BCAA supplementation have reported no significant ergogenic effects on exercise performance. In many of these studies, the BCAA supplement was compared to a carbohydrate supplement, usually involving three trials: carbohydrate alone, BCAA alone, and BCAA with carbohydrate. An analysis of about ten studies revealed that acute BCAA supplementation, particularly when compared to carbohydrate solutions, had no effect on time to exhaustion in running or cycling tests ranging in intensities from 70–85 percent VO_2 max, performance cycling tests of 40 kilometers and 100 kilometers, intermittent, prolonged high-intensity 20-second anaerobic running performance, and prolonged shuttle-run performance tasks comparable to energy expenditure in soccer. Even the study by Blomstrand and others that reported decreased RPE and mental fatigue in endurance-trained cyclists did not find any significant improvement in performance as measured by the total work done in the 20-minute maximal test.

Research regarding the effects of chronic BCAA supplementation on exercise performance is more limited, but in one study conducted at the University of Virginia, researchers reported an improvement in 40-kilometer cycling performance following 14 days of BCAA supplementation. Several other studies used a commercial supplement containing BCAA along with glutamine and carnitine. In general, these laboratory studies reported no significant effects on total time to complete a simulated half-Ironman triathlon (2-km swim; 90-km bike; 21-km run), prolonged aerobic endurance exercise at 65 percent VO_2 max, or cycle ergometer time to exhaustion at 120 percent VO_2 peak. Although these last three studies have shown no beneficial effect, subjects in the triathlon study ran the last segment 12.8 minutes faster while on the supplement, although this time was not significant due to highly variable performances. This finding, combined with the University of Virginia study, indicates additional research relative to chronic BCAA supplementation and exercise performance is merited.

Importance of carbohydrate Although research with BCAA supplementation is merited to help understand the underlying causes of fatigue in prolonged aerobic endurance exercise, endurance athletes apparently do not need to take BCAA supplements in attempts to enhance performance. In most studies that compared carbohydrate solutions, carbohydrate/BCAA solutions, and placebo solutions, both solutions with carbohydrate improved endurance performance compared to the placebo solution, but there were no differences between the carbohydrate solution and the carbohydrate/BCAA solution. In general, the carbohydrate solution attenuates the increase in the fTRP:BCAA ratio. However, Davis points out that the mechanism whereby carbohydrate supplements prevent fatigue during prolonged exercise is not clear; it may prevent fatigue centrally by ameliorating brain functions, or it may prevent fatigue peripherally by providing energy substrate for the contracting muscle.

Carbohydrate still appears to be the preferential fuel for athletes to consume before and during prolonged intermittent and continuous endurance exercise tasks.

Glutamine Glutamine is the most abundant amino acid in the plasma. Glutamine, like alanine, is synthesized in the muscle tissue and is a major means for removing excess amino groups from the muscle, delivering the amino groups to the kidneys for excretion as ammonia. Glutamine also has other metabolic fates, and one of them is utilization as a fuel by cells of the immune system.

Overtraining, or staleness, in athletes is characterized by a number of signs and symptoms, referred to as the overtraining syndrome. Subjective symptoms such as fatigue, irritability, sleep disturbance, heaviness, and depression are associated with decreases in physical performance. Overtrained athletes are also thought to be more susceptible to various infections, particularly upper respiratory tract infections, possibly because of an impaired immune system. In a recent review, Rowbottom and others indicated that impaired glutamine status may be associated with the overtrained state.

Parry-Billings and others studied forty overtrained, international-class athletes at the British Olympic Medical Centre; most of the overtrained athletes were involved in endurance-type events. The investigators noted a decreased plasma glutamine level compared to control athletes not regarded as being overtrained. They also noted that prolonged strenuous exercise, such as a marathon, reduces plasma glutamine levels. Although they had no explanation for the decreased glutamine levels, they hypothesized that because glutamine is a prime fuel for cells in the immune system, decreased levels might impair immune function. In this study they did not note any differences between the overtrained and control groups of athletes relative to various markers of immune function. However, citing some of their previous research, they noted that BCAA supplementation prevented the decrease in plasma glutamine normally seen after a marathon.

Parry-Billings and others note that glutamine supplements have been used in attempts to enhance immune function following injury, but few data are available to evaluate their effect on the overtraining syndrome or performance.

Shewchuk and others recently reported that 21 days of glutamine supplementation had little effect on lymphocyte metabolism or function in rats that were trained to swim 2–4 hours a day. Although they provided a substantial dose of glutamine, there were no changes in plasma glutamine levels, possibly because most of the oral glutamine was used by the intestinal epithelial cells, one of the prime users of glutamine. These data do not support a beneficial effect of glutamine supplementation with animals, and the limited research data involving humans are ambivalent.

Kreider and his associates did study the effect of a commercial supplement containing BCAA, glutamine, and carnitine on markers of immune function and incidence rate of sickness in collegiate swimmers over a competitive season. Twenty swimmers were matched, ten each consuming either the supplement or the placebo; a control group of nonswimmers was also studied. Of eight markers of immune function studied (lymphocytes, immunoglobulin, mitogen stimulations), two were more favorable in the supplemented swimmers compared to the placebo group. Also, although there were no significant differences between the groups in total number or severity of sicknesses, the supplemented group reported fewer symptoms of upper respiratory tract infections such as chest congestion or frequency of coughing. Kreider and others indicated these findings provide preliminary support that glutamine and/or BCAA availability may enhance immune function during intense, prolonged training. Conversely, Castell and others reported that glutamine supplementation did not appear to have an effect on immune function, as measured by lymphocyte distribution, following completion of the Brussels Marathon.

Some investigators suggested that glutamine concentrations may fall after muscle glycogen is depleted, which could occur during prolonged periods of intense training. Again, adequate daily dietary carbohydrate could possibly prevent muscle glycogen depletion, help maintain normal glutamine status, and prevent overtraining. In a recent study, compared to a glucose-only solution, adding glutamine to a glucose drink did not provide any additional benefits on muscle glycogen resynthesis following muscle glycogen depletion.

Although Sharp and Koutedakis recommend glutamine supplements for athletes who undergo intense exercise training and some preliminary research suggests glutamine supplementation may reduce the incidence of respiratory infections in athletes, additional research is needed to provide supporting data.

Aspartates Potassium and magnesium aspartate are salts of aspartic acid, a nonessential amino acid. Although the mechanism has not been clearly documented, these substances have been postulated to improve aerobic and anaerobic exercise performance, possibly by enhancing fatty acid metabolism and thereby sparing glycogen, by reducing accumulation of ammonia (metabolic by-product of protein), or simply by improving psychological motivation. The ammonia hypothesis has been tested in several studies since increases in serum ammonia have been associated with muscular fatigue, although, as noted previously, the mechanism is not clear.

Research findings relative to the ergogenic effect of aspartates are equivocal. A number of both early and contemporary studies have reported no beneficial effects of aspartate supplementation. For example, Maughan and Sadler had eight males ride to exhaustion on a bicycle ergometer at 75–80 percent of their VO$_2$ max following either a placebo or 3,000 milligrams each of potassium and magnesium aspartate consumed in the 24 hours prior to testing. No beneficial effects upon blood concentrations of energy substrates or ammonia were found, nor were any significant effects on physiological or psychological variables important to aerobic exercise performance reported. In an anaerobic exercise task, Tuttle and others reported no significant effect of aspartate supplementation (approximately 10 grams) on plasma ammonia concentrations, ratings of perceived exertion during a resistance training workout, or performance in a bench press repetition test to failure at 65 percent of maximal bench press strength.

On the other hand, an equal number of early and contemporary studies have found some beneficial applications of aspartates. Although several of these studies possessed flaws in experimental design, increases in aerobic endurance of 21–50 percent have been reported. More recently, Wesson and others, using a double-blind, placebo protocol, revealed that the ingestion of 10 grams of aspartates over a 24-hour period increased endurance capacity by over 15 percent when subjects exercised at 75 percent of their VO$_2$ max. These researchers also reported increased blood levels of free fatty acids and decreased levels of blood ammonia.

It appears that additional quality research is needed to evaluate the ability of aspartates to exert an ergogenic effect. Dosage may be a key factor, for dosages of about 10 grams have usually been associated with improved performance.

Glycine and Gelatin Glycine is a nonessential amino acid. Because it is involved in the formation of creatine phosphate, it could theoretically be an ergogenic aid. Gelatin is derived from collagen, a protein substance in connective tissue. Although gelatin is not a complete protein because it lacks several essential amino acids, it is composed of approximately 25 percent glycine. Several studies conducted a half-century ago suggested a beneficial effect of gelatin supplements upon strength, but the experiments were poorly designed. More contemporary research with proper experimental design and relatively large doses of glycine revealed no beneficial effects upon physical performance. Because gelatin is derived from connective tissue, and because connective tissue degradation is theorized to be a cause of muscle soreness, gelatin supplements have been advocated to prevent the development of soreness following exercise. However, experiments have not supported this view.

Creatine Creatine is not an amino acid, but a nitrogen-containing compound known as an amine. Creatine is found in some foods, particularly meat products, and it may be formed in the kidney and liver from glycine and arginine. Creatine may be delivered to the muscle, where it may combine readily with phosphate to form phosphocreatine, a high-energy phosphagen in the ATP-PC energy system that is stored in the muscle. As you may recall, the ATP-PC energy system is important for rapid energy production, such as in speed and power events. Creatine supplements have recently been marketed for athletes, and they are one of the hottest sellers to strength- and power-trained athletes.

Although creatine has been known for years to play an important role in energy metabolism, it is only within this decade that considerable research has been devoted to evaluate the potential ergogenic effect of creatine supplementation. Numerous studies and several reviews have been published in recent years, and the following represent some of the key points regarding the effects of creatine supplementation.

Supplementation protocol, effects on total muscle creatine and phosphocreatine (PC), and theory The average individual needs to replace about 2 grams of creatine per day to maintain normal total creatine and creatine phosphate (PC). The normal daily intake of creatine approximates 1 gram for those who consume meat, but may be virtually zero for pure vegetarians. Endogenous formation of creatine helps complement dietary sources to achieve 2 grams, but because of inadequate dietary intake, vegetarians may have lower amounts of total creatine in the body.

Several supplementation strategies have been used in attempts to increase total body creatine stores. One very effective strategy is to consume a total of 20–30 grams of creatine, usually pure creatine monohydrate, in four equal doses (5–7 grams per dose) over the course of the day (morning, noon, afternoon, evening). Significant effects have been observed even after only 2 days of creatine loading. Paul Greenhaff, one of the leading researchers with creatine, noted that this supplementation protocol will enhance muscle creatine storage. Excessive amounts will not be stored. Longer-term supplementation with lower doses, such as 4 weeks at a dose of 3 grams per day, has been shown to be as effective. However, one study providing 2 grams per day for 6 weeks showed no beneficial effects on either muscle creatine stores or PC levels.

Research by Greenhaff and Harris has shown that individuals who increase muscle creatine levels most are those who have low levels before supplementation, such as vegetarians. Individuals who have somewhat higher levels of muscle creatine are less responsive to creatine supplementation. However, recent research by Green and others has shown that combining creatine with a simple carbohydrate, such as glucose, will increase creatine transport into the muscle even in subjects with near-normal levels of muscle creatine, possibly via an insulin-mediated effect. The solution used in Green's study consisted of 5 grams of creatine and about 90 grams of simple carbohydrate, consumed 4 times per day. Once creatine is in the muscle, it is locked there and gradually disappears over several weeks.

In general, although not all studies are in agreement, well-controlled research by Greenhaff, Harris, Casey and their associates has shown that an appropriate creatine loading protocol will increase total muscle creatine, including free creatine and phosphocreatine. Casey and others suggest that any performance benefits may be related to increased creatine within the Type II muscle fibers.

Most of the creatine in the body is found in the muscles. About 60 percent of the total muscle creatine is PC, and the remainder is free creatine. Theoretically, increasing the amount of PC will provide more substrate for generating ATP during high-intensity exercise, and higher levels of free creatine will help resynthesize PC.

Effect on exercise performance Most research has investigated the effect of creatine supplementation on short-term, maximal exercise tasks of less than 30 seconds, those highly dependent on the ATP-PC energy system. Many studies also incorporated repetitive exercise tasks with short recovery intervals, which could evaluate the possible effect of enhanced PC resynthesis during recovery. However, some research has also investigated the effect of creatine supplementation on exercise performance tasks of somewhat longer duration, including those that would be dependent on the lactic acid energy system (anaerobic glycolysis) and the oxygen, or aerobic glycolytic energy, system.

ATP-PC energy system As with most research evaluating the effectiveness of ergogenic aids, all studies are not in agreement. However, many studies with creatine, conducted at some leading universities throughout the world, have provided some strong evidence supportive of a positive ergogenic effect of creatine supplementation in certain exercise endeavors, primarily those characterized by repetitive high-intensity exercise bouts with brief recovery periods. Using appropriate research methodology, recent studies have shown significant improvement in the following exercise tasks following creatine supplementation.

- Improvement in peak torque on five bouts of thirty maximal isometric muscle contractions

- Improvement in total and maximal force in twenty 30-second isometric muscle contractions

- Increased maximal one repetition maximum (1-RM) in the biceps curl

- Increased endurance in isokinetic bench press test

- Increased upper body strength test and sprint performance in football players

- Increased total work completed over six 6-second cycle sprints and increased peak power

- Improved performance in the 7–10 repetition of ten 6-second maximal cycling tests

- Improvement in a 10-second maximal cycling test following five 6-second maximal tests

- Increased peak power in the last 5–6 repetitions of six 10-second cycle sprints

- Increased peak and mean power output in three 30-second isokinetic cycling tests

- Increased anaerobic capacity on three 30-second Wingate tests

- Increased watt production on five maximal 30-second Wingate tests

- Increased total work in two 30-second maximal isokinetic cycling tests

These are certainly impressive findings, but similar well-controlled studies have not shown any significant effects of creatine supplementation on the following exercise tasks:

- No effect on lower body muscle strength tests

- No effect on isokinetic leg press endurance

- No effect on muscle strength or muscle endurance in upper extremity tests in females

- No effect on seven 10-second bouts of maximal cycling sprints

- No effect on two 10-second maximal cycling bouts

- No effect on two 15-second maximal cycling bouts

- No effect on single 30-second Wingate test

- No effect on 25- or 50-meter swim sprints (two studies)

- No effect on three 60-meter run sprints

The majority of the studies suggest that creatine supplementation may help enhance performance, particularly in repetitive, short-term, high-intensity tasks in which the body mass is not moved from point to point, such as cycle ergometry and various forms of resistance exercise. Creatine supplementation has not been shown to improve performance in events where the body is moved, such as swim and run sprints; theoretically, creatine supplementation should, and more research along these lines is recommended.

Lactic acid energy system Fewer studies have evaluated the effect of creatine supplementation on high-intensity exercise tasks associated with the lactic acid energy system, or anaerobic glycolysis. The results of these studies are somewhat equivocal. One field study, conducted in Estonia with ten trained middle-distance runners, involved four repetitions each of 300- and 1,000-meter runs. Although no changes were observed in the placebo group, those in the creatine group who consumed 30 grams of creatine for 6 days ran faster in the final 300-meter run, the final 1,000-meter run, and the total time for the four 1,000-meter runs. Other research has shown that creatine supplementation increased cycle ergometer ride time to exhaustion at 120 percent VO_2 max. Conversely, other studies have shown no effect of creatine supplementation on treadmill run time to exhaustion at 120 percent VO_2 max, treadmill run time to exhaustion at about 7.5 miles per hour and grades up to 20 percent, performance on a fifth cycle ergometer ride to exhaustion at 120–125 percent VO_2 max following four 60-second rides at the same intensity, or time to swim 100 meters.

Whether or not creatine supplementation may improve performance in events such as 100–200 meter swims or 400–800 meter runs, or other exercise tasks dependent primarily on anaerobic glycolysis, is uncertain and additional well-controlled research is needed to help resolve this issue.

Oxygen system There are limited data regarding the effect of creatine supplementation on aerobic endurance performance. Several studies indicate that creatine supplementation does not increase cycle ergometer VO_2 peak or energy metabolism when treadmill running at 50–90 percent of VO_2 max. Swedish investigators also reported that creatine supplementation did not improve, but actually impaired, performance in a 3.6-kilometer forest terrain run. However, creatine supplementation did affect 1,000-meter rowing time in trained rowers, improving performance by 2.3 seconds. The total time of the 1,000-meter row was about 3.5 minutes, which although primarily an aerobic exercise task, may have an anaerobic component to it, particularly in a final surge.

Body mass One of the consistent findings associated with creatine supplementation is an increase in body mass, as much as several kilograms within a week. By attracting water, creatine may increase intramuscular water stores as reported by Ziegenfuss and others, which may be an explanation for the rapid increase in body mass. However, several studies, using various techniques to assess body composition, have shown that creatine supplementation combined with a resistance-training program may increase lean muscle mass over time more so than resistance training with a placebo. Theoretically, an enhanced ability to resistance train more intensely following creatine supplementation may eventually stimulate increases in lean body mass.

Caffeine and creatine Several recent studies by Vandenberghe and others have shown that when caffeine, about 2.5 milligrams per kilogram body weight, is consumed with creatine, the caffeine negates the potential ergogenic effect of creatine. In their studies, both creatine and creatine with caffeine increased muscle creatine and PC stores, but muscular performance only improved with the creatine supplement. They reported that in some way the caffeine inhibited PC resynthesis during recovery, which would decrease ATP resynthesis and impair muscle contraction.

Because some athletes may take both creatine and caffeine in attempts to enhance performance, these preliminary findings merit additional research to substantiate this possible detrimental effect of caffeine.

Safety None of the studies using creatine supplements for up to 6 weeks have reported any acute adverse side effects. The breakdown product of creatine is creatinine, which is excreted by the kidneys. Individuals with impaired kidney function may be at risk, but the healthy kidney should be able to excrete the excess creatinine provided daily hydration is adequate. However, Greenhaff indicates we have no information on possible adverse effects of chronic creatine supplementation.

Some anecdotal reports indicate creatine supplementation may lead to muscle cramps and possible muscle tears. An increase in intramuscular water content could dilute electrolytes, possibly leading to cramps, and a tightened musculature associated with intracellular swelling could predispose to muscle tears. However, these data are only anecdotal. This potential problem has not been studied scientifically.

Several reviews have appeared in recent years, and most suggest that creatine supplementation may enhance performance in events where the amount of muscle CP may be a limiting factor. The interested reader is referred to the reviews by Balsom and others, Greenhaff, Maughan, and Williams and Branch.

HMB (Beta-Hydroxy-Beta-Methylbutyrate)

Beta-hydroxy-beta-methylbutyrate (HMB) is not a nutrient per se, but a by-product of leucine metabolism in the human body. The body produces about 0.2–0.4 gram of HMB per day depending on dietary leucine intake. HMB is being marketed as a dietary supplement salt, calcium-HMB, primarily to strength-trained and power-trained athletes. HMB supplementation is theorized to increase lean muscle mass, decrease body fat, and increase muscular strength and power. Although the underlying mechanism is not known, investigators who developed HMB speculate that it may inhibit the breakdown of muscle tissue during strenuous exercise.

Initially, in attempts to increase the nutritional quality of animal meat, research with various farm animals has indicated that HMB supplementation may increase lean muscle mass and decrease body fat. However, knowledge of the effect of HMB supplementation in humans is in its infancy, and only one study has been published at this point, although about a half-dozen research papers have been presented at national meetings, most notably the Federation of American Societies of Experimental Biology.

In the published report by Nissen and others, which contained two studies, HMB supplementation significantly increased lean body mass and strength in untrained males who initiated a resistance-training program for 3 weeks. Subjects consumed either 0 (placebo), 1.5 grams (low), or 3.0 grams (high) of HMB daily, and although all subjects increased lean muscle mass and strength with the resistance-training program, the HMB groups gained more than the placebo group, and the high group gained more than the low group. As measured by urinary 3-methylhistidine levels, the HMB groups also experienced less muscle tissue catabolism. Also in this same report, HMB supplementation (3.0 grams per day) did not increase total body mass, decrease body fat, or improve performance in two of three strength tests in physically active males who continued resistance training several hours per day over a 50-day period. Although the HMB group experienced favorable changes in lean body mass at various points over the course of the study, there were no significant differences between the placebo and HMB group at the completion of the study.

These published findings are somewhat inconsistent, as are the findings from unpublished research papers presented at national scientific meetings, some of which showed possible ergogenic effects while others did not, as the following highlights from these studies indicate. HMB supplementation (3.0 grams per day) was reported to increase lean body mass, decrease body fat, and increase bench press strength in both trained and untrained subjects over a 4-week period of resistance training. However, in this same study, HMB had no significant effect on other measures of strength. Compared to a placebo, HMB supplementation had no effect on the body composition of nonexercising females, but did increase lean body mass and bench press strength in females engaged in a 4-week resistance-training program. In a study with older men and women, the HMB group lost more fat over 8 weeks of resistance training, but the changes in lean body mass were not significantly different from the placebo group. Two separate reports, using the same football players undergoing resistance training as subjects, compared a placebo, HMB, and HMB plus creatine on various measures of body composition and strength. In general, the HMB supplementation provided no beneficial effect on body mass, lean body mass, body fat, or total work output and lifting volume.

Although these findings are intriguing, they are equivocal. Moreover, several problems exist with the experimental methodology in some of the studies, including questionable techniques to measure strength, use of an inappropriate placebo, and less-valid techniques to evaluate body composition. These problems do not detract from the possible importance of these studies, but they do suggest that the data currently available regarding the effects of HMB supplementation on body composition and exercise performance are preliminary, and more well-controlled research is needed to help resolve these uncertain findings.

Choline

Choline, an amine, is a nitrogen-containing substance found in various foods, particularly as lecithin (phosphatidylcholine) in animal foods such as egg yolks and organ meats like liver, and free choline in plants such as nuts, wheat germ, cauliflower, and soybeans. Commercial choline products are available as lecithin or choline salts, but the actual choline content may vary. Check the labels for actual choline content. Choline is also marketed as a powder with carbohydrate and electrolytes to make a sports drink for athletes

Choline is involved in the formation of acetylcholine, an important neurotransmitter in the central nervous system. Because plasma choline levels have been reported to be significantly reduced following exhaustive exercise such as marathon running, a possible reduction in acetylcholine levels in the nervous system may be theorized to be a contributing factor to the development of fatigue.

Research has shown that choline supplementation, either as choline salts or lecithin preparations, will increase blood choline levels at rest and during prolonged exercise. Some preliminary field and laboratory research has suggested increased plasma choline levels are associated with a significantly decreased time to run 20 miles and improved mood states of cyclists 40 minutes after completion of a cycle ergometer ride to exhaustion. On the other hand, well-controlled laboratory research has revealed that choline supplementation, although increasing plasma choline levels, exerted no effect on either brief, high-intensity anaerobic cycling tests lasting about 2 minutes, or on more prolonged aerobic exercise tasks lasting about 70 minutes.

These findings are equivocal and several reviewers, Anderson and Kanter and Williams, recommend more research with choline supplementation, particularly controlled laboratory research involving prolonged aerobic endurance exercise tasks greater than 2 hours duration.

Inosine Inosine is not an amino acid but is classified as a nucleoside. It is included for discussion here because it is associated with the development of **purines,** nonprotein nitrogen compounds that have important roles in energy metabolism. On the basis of animal research and studies of blood storage techniques, writers in popular magazines have theorized that inosine may be an effective ergogenic aid for a variety of athletes. Advertisements have suggested that inosine may improve ATP production in the muscle and thus be of value to strength-type athletes. Additionally, inosine is thought to enhance oxygen delivery to the muscles, thus being beneficial to aerobic endurance athletes.

There are no data to support these claims. No studies investigating the effect of inosine upon strength or power have been uncovered. Research from our laboratory at Old Dominion University has revealed no ergogenic effect of inosine on aerobic endurance, but on the contrary, a possible decrement in performance. Nine highly-trained runners consumed either a placebo or 6 grams of inosine prior to several tests of performance, including a peak oxygen uptake test and a 3-mile run on the treadmill conducted to simulate an all-out race. Although there were no differences in 3-mile run performance, peak oxygen uptake, or a variety of hematological

and psychological variables, time to exhaustion during the peak oxygen uptake test was longer in the placebo condition. We speculated that inosine may impair the ability of fast-twitch muscle to function optimally in very high-intensity exercise, which occurs in the latter stages of tests of maximal or peak oxygen uptake. Recent research from Ball State University revealed similar findings. Starling and his colleagues investigated the effect of 5,000 milligrams of inosine daily for 5 days on the performance of competitive male cyclists on three tests: a Wingate bike test, a 30-minute self-paced cycling performance test, and a supramaximal cycling sprint to fatigue. Compared to the placebo trial, they reported no significant effect of inosine supplementation on any performance measures in the three tests, and actually reported an impaired performance in the supramaximal test following inosine supplementation. Thus, on the basis of the available data, inosine does not appear to be an effective ergogenic aid.

Summary A balanced diet containing 12–15 percent of the Calories as protein will provide amounts of the individual amino acids more than adequate to obtain the estimated RDA, even for those who exercise extensively. For example, some reports suggest that endurance athletes need more leucine because they may use about 850 mg, or 87 percent of the estimated leucine RDA, in a 2-hour workout. However, one glass of milk contains 950 mg of leucine, while over 5,000 mg are consumed in a normal daily diet. Similar comparisons could be made with other amino acids.

However, companies that market amino acid supplements for athletes indicate that amino acids found in food are liberated slowly in the digestive processes, somewhat like a time-release tablet, and may not elicit similar effects compared to consumption of free-form amino acids. Whether or not such individual amino acids confer any ergogenic effect is still questionable at best. Although several amino acids have received some research attention, the available reputable scientific data are still somewhat limited. Additional research is merited with several purported ergogenic amino acids, particularly aspartic acid salts and the BCAA. Creatine supplementation appears to be an effective ergogenic aid for repetitive, high-intensity, short-duration exercise tasks, but additional research is needed to evaluate the effectiveness of acute or chronic creatine supplementation as applied to specific sport events. Moreover, more research is needed to explore the effect of creatine supplementation on performance in events characterized by anaerobic and aerobic glycolysis. Research findings regarding the ergogenic effect of choline and HMB are ambiguous. Additional research is needed to study the effect of choline supplementation on prolonged aerobic endurance capacity and the effect of HMB supplementation on body composition, strength, power, and related sports events.

Dietary Protein: Health Implications

Although increases in dietary carbohydrate and decreases in dietary fat in the typical American diet may be recommended for health reasons, the general recommendation is to maintain adequate protein intake. Some health problems may be associated with extremes of protein intake, however, as well as with the consumption of individual amino acid supplements.

Does a deficiency of dietary protein pose any health risks?

A short-term protein deficiency (several days) is not likely to cause any serious health problems, but because protein is the source of the essential amino acids, a prolonged deficiency could be expected to cause serious health problems. Such is the case in certain parts of the world where protein intake is inadequate for political, economic, or other reasons. Protein–Calorie malnutrition is one of the major nutritional problems in the world today, particularly for young children. Physical and mental growth may be permanently retarded. Protein deficiency may also occur in individuals who abuse sound nutritional practices, such as drug addicts, chronic alcoholics, and extreme food faddists, but adults are more likely to recover fully with adequate nutrition. Elderly individuals, those over 65 years, may be more prone to protein undernutrition because they may eat less protein-rich food and may use protein less efficiently. Lesourd indicated protein undernutrition in the elderly may impair immune function, making them more susceptible to infections.

Individuals who are on a low-protein diet plan, or young athletes who are on modified starvation diets to lose weight for such sports as gymnastics, ballet, or wrestling, may experience periods of protein insufficiency. During this time, the individual may be in negative nitrogen balance; that is, more nitrogen is being excreted from the body than is being ingested. Body tissues such as muscles and hemoglobin may be lost with a possible reduction in strength and endurance capacity. Adequate protein intake is essential for proper physiological functioning, both in the inactive and active individual.

Several major health problems associated with excessive weight loss, both in nonathletes and athletes, are related to both energy and protein balance. These topics are discussed in Chapter 10.

Does excessive protein intake pose any health risks?

The National Research Council, in its recent book *Diet and Health: Implications for Reducing Chronic Disease Risk*, reported that the current high protein consumption in the United States appears to be safe, since the human body has a very efficient system for disposal of excess nitrogen. However, the NRC did recommend that individuals consume no more than twice the RDA. Recent surveys in the United States have revealed average protein intakes of more than 100 grams per day, with nearly 70 grams being derived from animal protein. This amount, about twice the RDA, does not appear to be harmful but is on the borderline of the NRC recommendation. On the other hand, some individuals, mainly athletes, are on high-protein diets that may contain over 200 grams of protein per day. One report cited a daily intake of 400 grams of protein in a bodybuilder. Are such diets potentially harmful? Possibly, for several reasons.

One point to consider is that the protein in many foods is often accompanied by substantial quantities of saturated fat and cholesterol. You should be selective in the types of protein foods you eat. For example, a glass of whole milk and a glass of skim milk both have 8 grams of protein, but the whole milk also has 8 grams of fat compared to less than 1 gram in the skim milk. Nutritionally, skim milk is 40 percent protein Calories while the whole milk is 22.5 percent. One general recommendation is to obtain a greater proportion of daily protein intake from plant foods. In a recent detailed meta-analysis of the available scientific data, Anderson and others concluded that when soy protein is substituted for animal protein, individuals may experience significant decreases in serum total cholesterol, LDL cholesterol, and triglycerides, all factors that may help protect against coronary heart disease.

Individuals with a personal or family history of liver or kidney problems may be susceptible to adverse reactions from excessive dietary protein. As you may recall, the liver is the major organ involved in protein metabolism. Excess dietary protein may be converted to carbohydrate or fat, with the excess nitrogen being converted to urea for excretion from the body via the kidneys. High-protein diets may also lead to excessive production of ketones, which also must be excreted by the kidneys to prevent an increase in blood acidity, known as ketosis. Thus, individuals with inadequate liver or kidney function may experience a host of health problems due to the accumulation of urea or ketones in the blood or other metabolic consequences. Because diabetics are prone to kidney disorders, the American Diabetic Association recommends they consume no more than the daily RDA for protein.

Because both urea and ketone bodies need to be eliminated by the kidneys, dehydration could occur from excessive fluid loses. Such an effect could compromise the ability to deal with warm environmental temperatures, which is discussed further in Chapter 9.

Gout, a painful inflammation of the joints, may be aggravated by high-protein diets containing substantial quantities of purines, which are metabolized to uric acid (not the same as urea). The uric acid may accumulate in the joints and cause inflammation.

Earlier research had suggested that high levels of protein intake, in the form of purified proteins, would increase the urinary excretion of calcium and possibly lead to decreased bone density. However, the National Research Council and recent reviews have revealed that when protein is consumed with adequate amounts of phosphorus, as in meat and other protein foods in the typical American diet, urinary calcium losses are not increased, even on a diet with over 100 grams of protein daily. However, Heaney recently noted that increased dietary phosphorus increases release of endogenous calcium into the intestines with small increases in calcium loss via the feces. In general, some research indicates that we may lose 1 milligram of calcium for every gram of protein, which is relatively insignificant. Nevertheless, Feskanich and others recently reported that women who consumed more than 95 grams of protein, particularly animal protein, per day experienced about a 20 percent increase in forearm fractures compared to women who consumed less than 68 grams of protein per day. However, they also reported no association between dietary protein intake and hip fractures. Although individuals on a high-animal-protein and low-calcium diet may be more susceptible to bone fractures, adequate dietary calcium may help maintain normal calcium levels in the body and prevent osteoporotic fractures. The topic of calcium balance is presented in Chapter 8.

Does the consumption of individual amino acids pose any health risks?

In a recent review, Victor Herbert stated that there are no significant amounts of free-form amino acids in the foods we eat, nor is there any specific nutritional value of eating free amino acids. Free amino acids have been manufactured to serve as a drug, to be given to patients intravenously for adequate protein nutrition. They may also be used as food additives to enhance the protein quality of foods deficient in specific amino acids. Herbert indicated that the Food and Drug Administration (FDA) actually classifies amino acids as non-GRAS, or not generally recommended as safe, meaning they should not be sold as over-the-counter supplements.

Individuals should be aware that a recent epidemic of eosinophilia-myalgia syndrome (EMS), a neuromuscular disorder characterized by weakness, fever, edema, rashes, bone pain, and other symptoms, has been attributed to consumption of purified L-tryptophan. This epidemic was apparently caused by a contaminant in a specific brand of L-tryptophan, but Herbert indicated that L-tryptophan itself has not been totally absolved as the causative agent. More than 1,500 cases of EMS have been directly related to L-tryptophan, and its sale is currently banned in the United States. Interestingly, Canada banned its sale years ago and did not experience the epidemic of EMS seen in the United States in 1989. The interested reader is referred to the articles by Herbert and by Teman and Hainline regarding L-tryptophan supplementation.

Slavin and her colleagues have noted that amino acids taken in large doses are essentially drugs with unknown effects. The long-term effects of even moderate doses are also unknown, as noted previously in regard to arginine and its effect on HGH secretion. One problem is that excessive reliance on free-form amino acids, in comparison to dietary protein, may lead to a diet deficient in key vitamins and minerals that are normally found in protein foods, such as iron and zinc in meat, fish, and poultry. Some evidence from human and animal research indicates individual amino acids may interfere with the absorption of other essential amino acids; suppress appetite and food intake; precipitate tissue damage; contribute to kidney failure; lead to osteoporosis; cause gastrointestinal distress such as nausea, vomiting, and diarrhea; or create unfavorable psychological changes.

So what's the bottom line? At the present time there are inadequate scientific data to support either an ergogenic or a health benefit of supplementation with individual amino acids in the healthy individual. Adequate amounts of each amino acid may be obtained in a diet containing protein in amounts consistent with the Healthy North American Diet, and because such a diet may confer some benefits relative to physical performance and health, it should be the source of amino acid nutrition. Additional research is needed to evaluate both the ergogenic effectiveness and the health implications of supplementation with individual amino acids.

References

Books

Bucci, L. 1993. *Nutrients as Ergogenic Aids for Sports and Exercise.* Boca Raton, FL: CRC Press.

Di Pasquale, M. 1997. *Amino acids and proteins for the athlete— The anabolic edge.* Boca Raton, FL: CRC Press.

Garrett, W., and Malone, T. 1988. *Report of the Ross Symposium on Muscle Development: Nutritional Alternatives to Anabolic Steroids.* Columbus, OH: Ross Laboratories.

Hunt, S., and Groff, J. 1990. *Advanced Nutrition and Human Metabolism.* St. Paul, MN: West.

National Research Council. 1989. *Recommended Dietary Allowances.* Washington, DC: National Academy Press.

National Research Council. 1989. *Diet and Health: Implications for Reducing Chronic Disease Risk.* Washington, DC: National Academy Press.

Williams, M. 1998. *The Ergogenics Edge: Pushing the Limits of Sports Performance.* Champaign, IL: Human Kinetics.

Wolinsky, I., and Hickson, J. 1994. *Nutrition in Exercise and Sport.* Boca Raton, FL: CRC Press.

Reviews

Anderson, J., et al. 1995. Meta-analysis of the effects of soy protein intake on serum lipids. *New England Journal of Medicine* 333:276–82.

Anderson, O. 1996. Can choline supplements knock minutes off your marathon time? *Running Research News* 12 (7): 1, 4–6.

Anderson, O. 1993. Creatine propels British athletes to olympic gold medals: Is creatine the one true ergogenic aid? *Running Research News* 9 (January/February): 1–4.

Applegate, L. 1996. Protein primer. *Runner's World* 31 (11): 24–25.

Balsom, P., et al. 1994. Creatine in humans with special reference to creatine supplementation. *Sports Medicine* 18:268–80.

Bannister, E., and Cameron, B. 1990. Exercise-induced hyperammonemia: Peripheral and central effects. *International Journal of Sports Medicine* 11: Supplement 2P, S129–S142.

Benevenga, N., et al. 1993. Role of protein synthesis in amino acid catabolism. *Journal of Nutrition* 123:332–36.

Benevenga, N., and Steele, R. 1984. Adverse effects of excessive consumption of amino acids. *Annual Review of Nutrition* 4:157–81.

Brouns, F. 1997. Functional foods for athletes. *Insider* 5 (3): 1–8.

Butterfield, G. 1991. Amino acids and high protein diets. In *Perspectives in Exercise Science and Sports Medicine. Ergogenics: Enhancement of Sports Performance,* eds. D. Lamb and M. Williams. Indianapolis, IN: Benchmark Press.

Campbell, W. 1996. Dietary protein requirements of older people: Is the RDA adequate? *Nutrition Today* 31 (5): 192–97.

Clark, N. 1996. The power of protein. *Physician and Sportsmedicine* 24 (4): 11–12.

Consumers Union. 1994. Do we eat too much protein? *Consumer Reports on Health* 6: 1–3.

Cowart, V. 1992. Dietary supplements: Alternatives to anabolic steroids? *The Physician and Sportsmedicine* 20 (March): 189–96.

Crim, M., and Munro, H. 1994. Proteins and amino acids. In *Modern Nutrition in Health and Disease,* eds. M. Shils et al. Philadelphia: Lea and Febiger.

Davis, J. M. 1996. Carbohydrates, branched-chain amino acids and endurance: The central fatigue hypothesis. *Sports Science Exchange* 9 (2): 1–5.

Davis, J. M. 1995. Carbohydrates, branched-chain amino acids and endurance: The central fatigue hypothesis. *International Journal of Sport Nutrition* 5:S29–S38.

Ekblom, B. 1996. Effects of creatine supplementation on performance. *American Journal of Sports Medicine* 24:S38–S39.

Evans, W. 1993. Exercise and protein metabolism. *World Review of Nutrition and Dietetics* 71:21–33.

Fernstrom, J. 1994. Dietary amino acids and brain function. *Journal of the American Dietetic Association* 94:71–77.

Fitts, R., and Metzger, J. 1993. Mechanisms of muscular fatigue. In *Principles of Exercise Biochemistry,* ed. J. Poortmans. Basel, Switzerland: Karger.

Graham, T., and MacLean, D. 1992. Ammonia and amino acid metabolism in human skeletal muscle during exercise. *Canadian Journal of Physiology and Pharmacology* 70:132–41.

Graham, T., et al. 1997. Effect of endurance training on ammonia and amino acid metabolism in humans. *Medicine and Science in Sports and Exercise* 29:646–53.

Grandjean, A. 1993. What are the protein requirements of athletes? *Food and Nutrition News* 65 (March/April): 11.

Greenhaff, P. 1997. Creatine supplementation and implications for exercise performance. In *Advances in Training and Nutrition for Endurance Sports,* eds. A. Jeukendrup, M. Brouns, and F. Brouns. Maastricht: Novartis Nutrition Research Unit.

Greenhaff, P. 1995. Creatine and its application as an ergogenic aid. *International Journal of Sport Nutrition* 5:S100–S110.

Heaney, R. 1993. Protein intake and the calcium economy. *Journal of the American Dietetic Association* 93:1259–60.

Henriksson, J. 1991. Effect of exercise on amino acid concentrations in skeletal muscle and plasma. *Journal of Experimental Biology* 160:149–65.

Herbert, V. 1992. L-tryptophan: A medicolegal case against over-the-counter marketing of supplements of amino acids. *Nutrition Today* 27 (March/April): 27–30.

Hickson, J., and Wolinsky, I. 1994. Research directions in protein nutrition for athletes. In *Nutrition in Exercise and Sport,* eds. I. Wolinsky and J. Hickson. Boca Raton, FL: CRC Press.

Jacobson, B. 1990. Effect of amino acids on growth hormone release. *Physician and Sportsmedicine* 18 (January): 63–70.

Kanter, M., and Williams, M. 1995. Antioxidants, carnitine, and choline as putative ergogenic aids. *International Journal of Sport Nutrition* 5:S120–S131.

Kleiner, S. 1995. The role of meat in an athlete's diet. *Sports Science Exchange* 8 (5): 1–6.

Kopple, J. 1994. Nutrition, diet, and the kidney. In *Modern Nutrition in Health and Disease,* eds. M. Shils et al. Philadelphia: Lea and Febiger.

Kreider, R., et al. 1993. Amino acid supplementation and exercise performance: Analysis of the proposed ergogenic value. *Sports Medicine* 16:190–209.

Laymon, D., et al. 1994. Amino acid metabolism during exercise. In *Nutrition in Exercise and Sport,* eds. I. Wolinsky and J. Hickson. Boca Raton, FL: CRC Press.

Lemon, P. 1996. Is increased dietary protein necessary or beneficial for individuals with a physically active lifestyle? *Nutrition Reviews* 54:S169–S175.

Lemon, P. 1995. Do athletes need more dietary protein and amino acids? *International Journal of Sport Nutrition* 5:S39–S61.

Lemon, P. 1994. Protein requirements of soccer. *Journal of Sports Sciences* 12:S17–S22.

Lesourd, B. 1995. Protein undernutrition as the major cause of decreased immune function in the elderly: Clinical and functional implications. *Nutrition Reviews* 53:S86–S94.

Maughan, R. 1995. Creatine supplementation and exercise performance. *International Journal of Sport Nutrition* 5:94–101.

McLarney, M. 1996. Pattern of amino acid requirements in humans: An interspecies comparison using published amino acid requirement recommendations. *Journal of Nutrition* 126:1871–82.

Newsholme, E., et al. 1992. Physical and mental fatigue: Metabolic mechanisms and importance of plasma amino acids. *British Medical Bulletin* 48:477–95.

Obarzanek, E., et al. 1996. Dietary protein and blood pressure. *Journal of the American Medical Association* 275:1598–1603.

Parkhouse, W. 1988. Regulation of skeletal muscle myofibrillar protein degradation: Relationships to fatigue and exercise. *International Journal of Biochemistry* 20:769–75.

Paul, G. 1989. Dietary protein requirements of physically active individuals. *Sports Medicine* 8:154–76.

Poortmans, J. 1993. Protein metabolism. In *Principles of Exercise Biochemistry,* ed. J. Poortmans. Basel, Switzerland: Karger.

Reeds, P., and Hutchens, T. 1994. Protein requirements: From nitrogen balance to functional impact. *Journal of Nutrition* 124:1754S–1764S.

Rennie M., et al. 1994. Physical activity and protein metabolism. In *Physical Activity, Fitness, and Health,* eds. C. Bouchard, et al. Champaign, IL: Human Kinetics.

Rowbottom, D., et al. 1996. The emerging role of glutamine as an indicator of exercise stress and overtraining. *Sports Medicine* 21:80–97.

Sahlin, K., and Katz, A. 1993. Adenine nucleotide metabolism. In *Principles of Exercise Biochemistry,* ed. J. Poortmans. Basel, Switzerland: Karger.

Slavin, J., et al. 1988. Amino acid supplements: Beneficial or risky? *Physician and Sportsmedicine* 16 (March): 221–24.

Tarnopolsky, M. 1993. Protein, caffeine, and sports. Guidelines for active people. *Physician and Sportsmedicine* 21 (March): 137–49.

Teman, A., and Hainline, B. 1991. Eosinophilia-myalgia syndrome. *Physician and Sportsmedicine* 19:80–86.

Williams, M. 1995. Nutritional ergogenics in athletics. *Journal of Sports Sciences* 13:S63–S74.

Williams, M. 1993. Nutritional supplements for strength trained athletes. *Sports Science Exchange* 6 (6): 1–6.

Williams, M., and Branch, J. 1997. Creatine supplementation and exercise performance. *Journal of the American College of Nutrition.* In press.

Wolfe, R., and George, S. 1993. Stable isotopic tracers as metabolic probes in exercise. *Exercise and Sport Sciences Reviews* 21:1–31.

Yoshimura, H. 1970. Anemia during physical training (sports anemia). *Nutrition Review* 28:251–53.

Young, V. 1991. Soy protein in relation to human protein and amino acid nutrition. *Journal of the American Dietetic Association* 91:828–35.

Young, V., et al. 1990. Assessment of protein nutritional status. *Journal of Nutrition* 120:1496–1502.

Specific Studies

Almada, A., et al. 1997. Effects of calcium β-HMB supplementation with or without creatine during training on strength and sprint capacity. *FASEB Journal* 11:A374.

Balsom, P., et al. 1995. Skeletal muscle metabolism during short duration high-intensity exercise: Influence of creatine supplementation. *Acta Physiologica Scandinavica* 154:303–10.

Balsom, P., et al. 1993. Creatine supplementation per se does not enhance endurance exercise performance. *Acta Physiologica Scandinavica* 149:521–23.

Balsom, P., et al. 1993. Creatine supplementation and dynamic high-intensity exercise. *Scandinavian Journal of Medicine and Science in Sports* 3:143–49.

Barnett, C., et al. 1996. Effects of oral creatine supplementation on multiple sprint cycle performance. *Australian Journal of Science and Medicine in Sport* 28:35–39.

Bazzarre, T., et al. 1992. Plasma amino acid responses of trained athletes to two successive exhaustion trials with and without interim carbohydrate feeding. *Journal of American College Nutrition* 11:501–11.

Becque, M., et al. 1997. Effect of creatine supplementation during strength training on 1RM and body composition. *Medicine and Science in Sports and Exercise* 29:S146.

Bigard, A., et al. 1996. Branched-chain amino acid supplementation during repeated prolonged skiing exercises at altitude. *International Journal of Sport Nutrition* 6:295–306.

Bigard, A., et al. 1993. Effects of protein supplementation during prolonged exercise at moderate altitude on performance and plasma amino acid pattern. *European Journal of Applied Physiology* 66: 5–10.

Biolo, G., et al. 1995. Increased rates of muscle protein turnover and amino acid transport after resistance exercise in humans. *American Journal of Physiology* 268:E514–E520.

Birch, R., et al. 1994. The influence of dietary creatine supplementation on performance during repeated bouts of maximal isokinetic cycling in man. *European Journal of Applied Physiology* 69:268–76.

Blomstrand, E., and Newsholme, E. 1992. Effect of branched-chain amino acid supplementation on the exercise-induced change in aromatic amino acid concentration in human muscles. *Acta Physiologica Scandinavica* 146:293–98.

Blomstrand, E., et al. 1997. Influence of ingesting a solution of branched-chain amino acids on perceived exertion during exercise. *Acta Physiologica Scandinavica* 159:41–49.

Blomstrand, E., et al. 1995. Effect of branched-chain amino acid and carbohydrate supplementation on the exercise-induced change in plasma and muscle concentration of amino acids in human subjects. *Acta Physiologica Scandinavica* 153:87–96.

Blomstrand, E., et al. 1991. Administration of branched-chain amino acids during sustained exercise—Effects on performance and on plasma concentration of some amino acids. *European Journal of Applied Physiology* 65:83–88.

Blomstrand, E., et al. 1991. Effect of branched-chain amino acid supplementation on mental performance. *Acta Physiologica Scandinavica* 143:225–26.

Blomstrand, E., et al. 1988. Changes in plasma concentrations of aromatic and branched-chain amino acids during sustained exercise in man and their possible role in fatigue. *Acta Physiologica Scandinavica* 133:115–21.

Brannon, T., et al. 1997. Effects of creatine loading and training on running performance and biochemical properties of rat skeletal muscle. *Medicine and Science in Sports and Exercise* 29:489–95.

Bucci, L., et al. 1992. Ornithine supplementation and insulin release in bodybuilders. *International Journal of Sport Nutrition* 2:287–91.

Bucci, L., et al. 1990. Ornithine ingestion and growth hormone release in bodybuilders. *Nutrition Research* 10:239–45.

Burke, L., et al. 1996. Effect of oral creatine supplementation on single-effort sprint performance in elite swimmers. *International Journal of Sport Nutrition* 6:222–33.

Casey, A., et al. 1996. Creatine ingestion favorably affects performance and muscle metabolism during maximal exercise in humans. *American Journal of Physiology* 271:E31–E37.

Castell, L., et al. 1997. Some aspects of the acute phase response after a marathon race, and the effects of glutamine supplementation. *European Journal of Applied Physiology* 75:47–53.

Castell, L., et al. 1996. Does glutamine have a role in reducing infections in athletes? *European Journal of Applied Physiology* 73:488–90.

Chandler, R., et al. 1994. Dietary supplements affect the anabolic hormones after weight-training. *Journal of Applied Physiology* 76:839–45.

Chesley, A., et al. 1992. Changes in human muscle protein synthesis after resistance exercise. *Journal of Applied Physiology* 73:1383–88.

Conlay, L., et al. 1989. Effects of running the Boston marathon on plasma concentrations of large neutral amino acids. *Journal of Neural Transmission* 76:65–71.

Cooke, W., et al. 1995. Effects of oral creatine supplementation on power output and fatigue during bicycle ergometry. *Journal of Applied Physiology* 78:670–73.

Davis, J., et al. 1992. Effects of carbohydrate feedings on plasma free tryptophan and branched-chain amino acids during prolonged cycling. *European Journal of Applied Physiology* 65:513–19.

Dawson, B., et al. 1995. Effects of oral creatine loading on single and repeated maximal short sprints. *Australian Journal of Science and Medicine in Sport* 27:56–61.

Devolve, K., et al. 1997. Effects of carbohydrate and branch-chain amino acid ingestion on intermittent, high intensity running. *Medicine and Science in Sports and Exercise* 29:S125.

Earnest, C., et al. 1995. The effect of creatine monohydrate ingestion on anaerobic power indices, muscular strength and body composition. *Acta Physiologica Scandinavica* 153:207–9.

Elam, R. 1988. Morphological changes in adult males from resistance exercise and amino acid supplementation. *Journal of Sports Medicine and Physical Fitness* 28:35–39.

Elam, R., et al. 1989. Effects of arginine and ornithine on strength, lean body mass and urinary hydroxyproline in adult males. *Journal of Sports Medicine and Physical Fitness* 29:52–56.

Febbraio, M., et al. 1995. Effect of creatine supplementation on intramuscular TCr, metabolism and performance during intermittent, supramaximal exercise in humans. *Acta Physiologica Scandinavica* 155:387–95.

Ferrando, A., et al. 1996. Prolonged bed rest decreases skeletal muscle and whole body synthesis. *American Journal of Physiology* 270:E627–E633.

Ferreira, M., et al. 1997. Effects of ingesting a supplement designed to enhance creatine uptake on strength & sprint capacity. *Medicine and Science in Sports and Exercise* 29:S146.

Feskanich, D., et al. 1996. Protein consumption and bone fractures in women. *American Journal of Epidemiology* 143:472–79.

Fogelholm, G. M., et al. 1993. Low-dose amino acid supplementation: No effects on serum human growth hormone and insulin in male weightlifters. *International Journal of Sport Nutrition* 3:290–97.

Fry, A., et al. 1993. Endocrine and performance responses to high volume training and amino acid supplementation in elite junior weightlifters. *International Journal of Sport Nutrition* 3:306–22.

Green, A., et al. 1996. Carbohydrate ingestion augments creatine retention during creatine feeding in humans. *Acta Physiologica Scandinavica* 158:195–202.

Greenhaff, P., et al. 1994. Effect of oral creatine supplementation on skeletal muscle phosphocreatine resynthesis. *American Journal of Physiology* 266:E725–E730.

Greenhaff, P., et al. 1993. Influence of oral creatine supplementation of muscle torque during repeated bouts of maximal voluntary exercise in man. *Clinical Science* 84:565–71.

Greenhaff, P., et al. 1992. Energy metabolism in single muscle fibers during maximal sprint exercise in man. *Journal of Physiology* 446:528P.

Hamilton-Ward, K., et al. 1997. Effect of creatine supplementation on upper extremity anaerobic response in females. *Medicine and Science in Sports and Exercise* 29:S146.

Harris, R., et al. 1993. The effect of oral creatine supplementation on running performance during maximal short term exercise in man. *Journal of Physiology* 467:74P.

Harris, R., et al. 1992. Elevation of creatine in resting and exercised muscle on normal subjects by creatine supplementation. *Clinical Science* 83:367–74.

Harris, R., et al. 1992. The effect of oral creatine supplementation on running performance during maximal short term exercise in man. Queen Mary and Westfield College Meeting, 17–18 December.

Hassmen, P., et al. 1994. Branched chain amino acid supplementation during 30-km competitive run: Mood and cognitive performance. *Nutrition* 10:405–10.

Hawkins, C., et al. 1991. Oral arginine does not affect body composition or muscle function in male weight lifters. *Medicine and Science in Sports and Exercise* 23:S15.

Hefler, S., et al. 1995. Branched-chain amino acid (BCAA) supplementation improves endurance performance in competitive cyclists. *Medicine and Science in Sports and Exercise* 27:S149.

Hernandez, M., et al. 1996. The protein efficiency ratios of 30:70 mixtures of animal: Vegetable protein are similar or higher than those of the animal foods alone. *Journal of Nutrition* 126:574–81.

Hilsendager, D., and Karpovich, P. 1964. Ergogenic effect of glycine and niacin separately and in combination. *Research Quarterly* 35:389–92.

Horswill, C., et al. 1990. Changes in the protein nutritional status of adolescent wrestlers. *Medicine and Science in Sports and Exercise* 22:599–604.

Hultman, E., et al. 1996. Muscle creatine loading in men. *Journal of Applied Physiology* 81:232–37.

Kirksey, K., et al. 1997. The effects of six weeks of creatine monohydrate supplementation in male and female track athletes. *Medicine and Science in Sports and Exercise* 29:S145.

Kreider, R., et al. 1997. Effects of calcium β-HMB supplementation with or without creatine during training on body composition alterations. *FASEB Journal* 11:A374.

Kreider, R., et al. 1997. Effects of ingesting a supplement designed to enhance creatine uptake on body composition during training. *Medicine and Science in Sports and Exercise* 29:S145.

Kreider, R., et al. 1996. Effects of ingesting supplements designed to promote lean tissue accretion on body composition during resistance training. *International Journal of Sport Nutrition* 6:234–46.

Kreider, R., et al. 1993. Effects of amino acid and carnitine supplementation on immune status and symptoms of infection during an intercollegiate swim season. *Medicine and Science in Sports and Exercise* 25:S123.

Lambert, M., et al. 1993. Failure of commercial oral amino acid supplements to increase serum growth hormone concentrations in male bodybuilders. *International Journal of Sport Nutrition* 3:298–305.

Lemon, P., et al. 1992. Protein requirements and muscle mass/strength changes during intensive training in novice bodybuilders. *Journal of Applied Physiology* 73:767–75.

Liappis, N., et al. 1979. Quantitative study of free amino acids in human eccrine sweat excreted from the forearms of healthy trained and untrained men during exercise. *European Journal of Applied Physiology* 42:227–34.

MacLean, D., and Graham, T. 1992. Branched chain amino acid supplementation augments ammonia responses during prolonged exercise in humans. *Medicine and Science in Sports and Exercise* 24:S150.

MacLean, D., et al. 1996. Stimulation of muscle ammonia production during exercise following branched-chain amino acid supplementation in humans. *Journal of Physiology* (London): 493:909–22.

Madsen, K., et al. 1996. Effects of glucose, glucose plus branched-chain amino acids, or placebo on bike performance over 100 km. *Journal of Applied Physiology* 81:2644–50.

Maughan, R., and Sadler, D. 1983. The effects of oral administration of salts of aspartic acid on the metabolic response to prolonged exhausting exercise in man. *International Journal of Sports Medicine* 4:119–23.

Mero, A., et al. 1997. Influence of leucine supplementation on serum amino acid concentration and anaerobic running performance. *Medicine and Science in Sports and Exercise* 29:S192.

Mitchell, M., et al. 1993. Effects of supplementation with arginine and lysine on body composition, strength and growth hormone levels in weightlifters. *Medicine and Science in Sports and Exercise* 25:S25.

Mitchell, M., et al. 1991. Effects of amino acid supplementation on metabolic responses to ultraendurance triathlon performance. *Medicine and Science in Sports and Exercise* 23:S15.

Mujika, I., et al. 1996. Creatine supplementation does not improve sprint performance in competitive swimmers. *Medicine and Science in Sports and Exercise* 28:1435–41.

Newsholme, E., and Blomstrand, E. 1996. The plasma level of some amino acids and physical and mental fatigue. *Experientia* 52:413–15.

Nissen, S., et al. 1997. Effect of feeding calcium β-hydroxy-β-methylbutyrate (HMB) on body composition and strength of women. *FASEB Journal* 11:A150.

Nissen, S., et al. 1996. Effect of leucine metabolite β-hydroxy-β-methylbutyrate on muscle metabolism during resistance-exercise training. *Journal of Applied Physiology* 81:2095–2104.

Odland, L., et al. 1997. Effect of oral creatine supplementation on muscle [PCr] and short-term maximum power output. *Medicine and Science in Sports and Exercise* 29:216–19.

Pannemans, D., et al. 1997. The effect of prolonged moderate intensity exercise on protein metabolism of trained men. *Medicine and Science in Sports and Exercise* 29:S224.

Parry-Billings, M., et al. 1992. Plasma amino acid concentrations in the overtraining syndrome: Possible effects on the immune system. *Medicine and Science in Sports and Exercise* 24:1353–58.

Philen, R., et al. 1992. Survey of advertising for nutritional supplements in health and bodybuilding magazines. *Journal of the American Medical Association* 268:1008–11.

Pivarnik, J., et al. 1989. Urinary 3-methylhistidine excretion increases with repeated weight training exercise. *Medicine and Science in Sports and Exercise* 21:283–87.

Poortmans, J., et al. 1996. Postexercise proteinuria in childhood and adolescence. *International Journal of Sports Medicine* 17:448–51.

Redondo, D., et al. 1996. The effect of oral creatine monohydrate supplementation on running velocity. *International Journal of Sport Nutrition* 6:213–21.

Robertshaw, M., et al. 1993. Protein excretion after prolonged exercise. *Annals of Clinical Biochemistry* 30:34–37.

Rossiter, H., et al. 1996. The effect of oral creatine supplementation on the 1000-m performance of competitive rowers. *Journal of Sports Sciences* 14:175–79.

Sakkas, C., et al. 1995. Effect of choline supplementation in trained cyclists. *Medicine and Science in Sports and Exercise* 27:668–73.

Schena, F., et al. 1992. Branched-chain amino acid supplementation during trekking at high altitude. The effects on loss of body mass, body composition, and muscle power. *European Journal of Applied Physiology* 65:394–98.

Segura, R., and Ventura, J. 1988. Effect of L-tryptophan supplementation on exercise performance. *International Journal of Sports Medicine* 9:301–5.

Sharp, N., and Koutedakis, Y. 1992. Sport and the overtraining syndrome: Immunological aspects. *British Medical Bulletin* 48:518–33.

Sharp, R., et al. 1988. Effect of a protein supplement on adaptations to combined aerobic and anaerobic training. *Medicine and Science in Sports and Exercise* 20:S3.

Shewchuk, L., et al. 1997. Dietary L-glutamine does not improve lymphocyte metabolism or function in exercise-trained rats. *Medicine and Science in Sports and Exercise* 29:474–81.

Starling, R., et al. 1996. Effect of inosine supplementation on aerobic and anaerobic cycling performance. *Medicine and Science in Sports and Exercise* 28:1193–98.

Stensrund, T., et al. 1992. L-tryptophan supplementation does not improve running performance. *International Journal of Sports Medicine* 13:481–85.

Stochero, C., and Gomes, P. 1997. Acute effects of BCAA supplementation on some biochemical indicators and the performance of long-distance runners. *Medicine and Science in Sports and Exercise* 29:S250.

Struder, H., et al. 1996. Alterations in plasma free tryptophan and large neutral amino acids do not affect perceived exertion and prolactin during 90 min of treadmill exercise. *International Journal of Sports Medicine* 17:73–79.

Struder, H., et al. 1995. Amino acid metabolism in tennis and its possible influence on the neuroendocrine system. *British Journal of Sports Medicine* 29:28–30.

Suminski, R., et al. 1997. Acute effect of amino acid ingestion and resistance exercise on plasma growth hormone concentration in young men. *International Journal of Sport Nutrition* 7:48–60.

Tarnopolsky, M., et al. 1992. Evaluation of protein requirements for trained strength athletes. *Journal of Applied Physiology* 73:1986–95.

Tarnopolsky, M., et al. 1991. Whole body leucine metabolism during and after resistance exercise in fed humans. *Medicine and Science in Sports and Exercise* 23:326–33.

Thompson, C., et al. 1996. Effect of creatine on aerobic and anaerobic metabolism in skeletal muscle in swimmers. *British Journal of Sports Medicine* 30:222–25.

Tuttle, J., et al. 1995. Effect of acute potassium-magnesium aspartate supplementation on ammonia concentrations during and after resistance training. *International Journal of Sport Nutrition* 5:102–9.

Vandenberghe, K., et al. 1997. Inhibition of muscle phosphocreatine resynthesis by caffeine after creatine loading. *Medicine and Science in Sports and Exercise* 29:S249.

Vandenberghe, K., et al. 1996. Caffeine counteracts the ergogenic action of muscle creatine loading. *Journal of Applied Physiology* 80:452–57.

van Hall, G., et al. 1995. Ingestion of branched-chain amino acids and tryptophan during sustained exercise in man: Failure to affect performance. *Journal of Physiology* 486:789–94.

Varnier, M., et al. 1994. Effect of infusing branched-chain amino acid during incremental exercise with reduced muscle glycogen content. *European Journal of Applied Physiology* 69:26–31.

Vukovich, M., et al. 1997. The effect of dietary β-hydroxy-β-methylbutyrate (HMB) on strength gains and body composition changes in older adults. *FASEB Journal* 11:A376.

Vukovich, M., et al. 1997. Effects of a low-dose amino acid supplement on adaptations to cycling training in untrained individuals. *International Journal of Sport Nutrition* 7:298–309.

Wagenmakers, A., et al. 1997. Glutamine does not stimulate glycogen resynthesis in human skeletal muscle. *Medicine and Science in Sports and Exercise* 29:S280.

Weideman, C., et al. 1990. Effects of increased protein intake on muscle hypertrophy and strength following 13 weeks of resistance training. *Medicine and Science in Sports and Exercise* 22:S37.

Welsh, R., et al. 1997. Carbohydrate and branched-chain amino acid feedings suppress brain 5-HT during prolonged exercise. *Medicine and Science in Sports and Exercise* 29:S192.

Wesson, M., et al. 1988. Effects of oral administration of aspartic acid salts on the endurance capacity of trained athletes. *Research Quarterly for Exercise and Sport* 59:234–39.

Wiles, J., et al. 1991. Effect of pre-exercise protein ingestion upon VO_2, R, and perceived exertion during treadmill running. *British Journal of Sports Medicine* 25:26–30.

Williams, M., et al. 1990. Effect of oral inosine supplementation on 3-mile treadmill run performance and VO_2 peak. *Medicine and Science in Sports and Exercise* 22:517–22.

Zawadzki, K., et al. 1992. Carbohydrate–protein complex increases the rate of muscle glycogen storage after exercise. *Journal of Applied Physiology* 72:1854–59.

Ziegenfuss, T., et al. 1997. Acute creatine ingestion: Effects on muscle volume, anaerobic power, fluid volumes, and protein turnover. *Medicine and Science in Sports and Exercise* 29:S127.

CHAPTER 7

Vitamins: The Organic Regulators

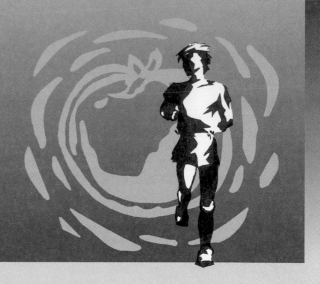

KEY TERMS

alpha-tocopherol
  equivalents
bee pollen
beta-carotene
bioavailability
biotin
coenzyme
CoQ_{10}
enzymes
folic acid (folate)
free radicals
ginseng
hypervitaminosis
megadose
niacin
niacin equivalents (NE)
osteomalacia
pantothenic acid
retinol
retinol equivalents (RE)
riboflavin (vitamin B_2)
subclinical malnutrition
thiamin (vitamin B_1)
vitamin A
vitamin B_6 (pyridoxine)
vitamin B_{12}
  (cyanocobalamin)
vitamin B_{15}
vitamin C (ascorbic acid)
vitamin D
vitamin D_3 (cholecalciferol)
vitamin E (alpha-
  tocopherol)
vitamin K (phylloquinone/
  menoquinone)
xerophthalmia

KEY CONCEPTS

• Vitamins are complex organic compounds that function in the body in a variety of ways. Some act as coenzymes to help regulate metabolic processes; others are antioxidants that protect cell membranes; and one is even classified as a hormone.

• Vitamins do not contain energy per se, such as Calories, but they do help regulate energy processes in the body.

• The water-soluble vitamins consist of those in the B complex and vitamin C, while the fat-soluble vitamins are A, D, E, and K.

• Although most vitamins must be obtained from the food we eat, several may be manufactured in the body.

• The RDA for vitamins have been established to prevent vitamin-deficiency diseases like scurvy, but the new vitamin RDA may be modified to help prevent chronic diseases, such as osteoporosis, cancer, and coronary heart disease.

• There may be four stages in a vitamin deficiency: the preliminary stage, the biochemical deficiency stage, the physiologic deficiency stage, and the clinically manifest deficiency stage.

• Although several national surveys have reported that some Americans are receiving less than the RDA for several vitamins, actual vitamin deficiencies resulting in disease are rare.

• Women of childbearing age should consume 400 micrograms of folic acid daily in order to prevent the possibility of birth defects in the newborn.

• A vitamin deficiency may impair physical performance, usually by interfering with some phase of the energy-producing process. In some cases, impairment may be seen in 2–4 weeks on a deficient diet.

• Vitamin supplements are not necessary for the individual on a balanced diet, but they may be recommended for those on a very low-Calorie diet, including athletes who are attempting weight reduction, and others with special dietary needs.

• Controlled research, in general, supports the conclusion that vitamin supplements will not improve athletic performance in individuals on a balanced diet. However, additional research is needed to help resolve some conflicting data with several vitamins and other vitamin-like substances.

• Epidemiologic data strongly suggests that diets rich in fruits and vegetables are associated with lower risks of certain chronic diseases, such as heart disease and cancer, and that some of this effect may be due to the antioxidant vitamin content of fruits and vegetables.

• Preliminary research indicates antioxidant vitamin supplementation may elicit some favorable health responses, but more research is needed before specific recommendations may be offered.

• Megadoses of some vitamins may be potentially harmful.

INTRODUCTION

Vitamins are a diverse class of thirteen known specific nutrients that are involved in almost every metabolic process in the human body. Although we need only minute amounts of vitamins in our daily diet, they are one of our most critical nutrients. Noticeable symptoms of a deficiency may appear in 2-4 weeks for several of the vitamins, and major debilitating diseases may occur with prolonged deficiencies. Vitamin deficiencies appear to be widespread in many developing countries, and according to Bouls, they affect a greater number of people in the world than does protein-energy malnutrition. Hopefully, plant breeding of commonly eaten food crops, such as wheat, rice, and corn, to fortify them with vitamins and minerals may help alleviate this major health problem. On the other hand, vitamin deficiencies are very rare in most industrialized societies. Several of the major nutrition surveys conducted in the United States have indicated that the vast majority of the population is receiving the RDA for all vitamins in the daily diet, which may be attributed to our high caloric intake and to vitamin fortification of processed foods. Moreover, about one-third of the population take vitamin supplements. However, certain segments of the population may not be receiving the RDA for several vitamins and thus may have marginal vitamin deficiencies, predisposing them to various health risks.

In general, most studies reveal that athletes, like the general population, are receiving the RDA for vitamins in their daily diet. However, certain athletic groups, particularly those who are on weight-reduction programs to qualify for competition or to enhance performance, may not receive adequate vitamin nutrition. Furthermore, individual athletes in generally well-nourished athletic groups may have a suboptimal vitamin intake.

As noted throughout this chapter, adequate vitamin nutrition is essential for both optimal health and athletic performance. But, if you do not obtain the RDA for a specific vitamin or vitamins, will your health or physical performance suffer? Will vitamin supplements above and beyond the RDA improve your health or performance? A major purpose of this chapter is to provide you with factual data, based upon the available research, to help answer these two very general questions.

A slightly different approach is used in this chapter and in Chapter 8. The first section provides some basic facts about the general role of vitamins in the human body. The next two sections cover the fat-soluble and water-soluble vitamins, respectively, with each individual vitamin discussed in terms of its RDA, food sources that provide ample amounts, metabolic functions in the body with particular reference to health and the physically active individual, and the findings of research relative to the impact of deficiencies and supplementation. The fourth section focuses on ergogenic aspects of special vitamin preparations, while the final section highlights some health implications of vitamin supplementation.

Basic Facts

What are vitamins and how do they work?

Vitamins are a class of complex organic compounds that are found in small amounts in most foods. They are essential for the optimal functioning of many different physiological processes in the human body. The activity levels of many of these physiological processes are increased greatly during exercise, and an adequate bodily supply of vitamins must be present for these processes to function best.

Coenzyme Functions For the fundamental physiological processes of the body to proceed in an orderly, controlled fashion, a number of complex chemicals known as **enzymes** are necessary to regulate the diverse reactions involved. Hundreds of enzymes have been identified in the human body. Enzymes are necessary to digest our foods, to make our muscles contract, to release the energy stores in our bodies, to help us transport body gases such as carbon dioxide, to help us grow, to help clot our blood, and so on. Enzymes serve as catalysts; that is, they are capable of inducing changes in other substances without changing themselves.

Enzymes are chemicals that generally consist of two parts. One part is a protein molecule and to it is attached the second part, a **coenzyme.** For the enzyme to function properly, both parts must be present. The coenzyme often contains a vitamin or some related compound (Figure 7.1). The enzyme is not used up in the chemical process that it initiates or in which it participates, but enzymes may deteriorate with time. Coenzymes also may be degraded through body metabolism. It is now known that the B complex vitamins are essential in human nutrition because of their role in the activation of enzymes, and thus a fresh supply of these water-soluble vitamins is constantly needed.

Antioxidant Functions Various oxidative reactions in the body produce substances called free radicals. **Free radicals** are chemical substances that contain a lone, unpaired electron in the outer orbit. The superoxide radical ($O_2^{\bullet-}$) and hydroxyl radical ($OH^{\bullet}$) are true free radicals. Two other related substances, referred to as non-radical oxygen species, are hydrogen peroxide (H_2O_2) and singlet oxygen ($^1O_2$). For the purpose of our discussion, we shall refer to them collectively as free radicals.

Free radicals are unstable compounds that possess an unbalanced magnetic field that affects molecular structure and chemical reactions in the body. Free radicals may be very reactive with body tissues. Although oxidative processes are essential to life, some oxidations may cause cellular damage by oxidation of unsaturated fats in cellular and subcellular membranes. Free radicals may cause such undesirable oxidations. Halliwell indicated that free radicals may damage DNA, lipids, proteins, and other molecules, and may be involved in the development of cancer, cardiovascular disease, and possibly neurodegenerative disease. Fortunately, although free radicals are formed naturally in the body, the body produces a number of antioxidant enzymes, such as superoxide dismutase, glutathione peroxidase, and catalase, to help neutralize them and prevent cellular damage. To function properly, these enzymes, often referred to as free radical-scavenging enzymes, must contain certain nutrients such as copper, zinc, and selenium. Comparable to these enzymes, as depicted in Figure 7.2, vitamins E, C, and beta-carotene possess antioxidant properties. These antioxidant vitamins have received recent research attention relative to effects on health and physical performance and are discussed at appropriate points later in this chapter.

Hormone Functions Although vitamin D exists in vitamin form, it undergoes several conversions in the body and in its active form functions as a hormone. After being produced in the kidney, vitamin D circulates in the blood like other hormones and exerts its functions on various tissues to promote bone metabolism. Other vitamins, such as A and K, may be produced in the liver and intestines, respectively, and exert functions in other parts of the body, but they are normally not referred to as hormones. Some vitamins may be critical in the formation of various hormones—such as the role vitamin C plays in the formation of epinephrine—but are not classified as hormones. Only vitamin D is assigned hormonal status in its active form.

Energy Although vitamins are indispensable for regulating many body functions and for the maintenance of optimal health, they are not a source of energy. They do not have any caloric value. Moreover, they make no significant contribution to the structure of the body, as do protein and some minerals.

What vitamins are essential to human nutrition?

The existence of vitamins was deduced from their physiological actions before their chemical structures had been identified. In assigning names to vitamins, the alphabet was used in order of their time of discovery. In some cases, a large time gap existed between the discovery of the vitamin and determination of its chemical structure. In others, the chemical nature was discovered rapidly, and the chemical name came into early use.

At present the human body is known to need an adequate supply of thirteen different vitamins. A well-balanced diet will satisfy all the vitamin requirements of

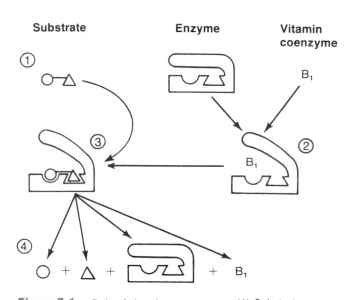

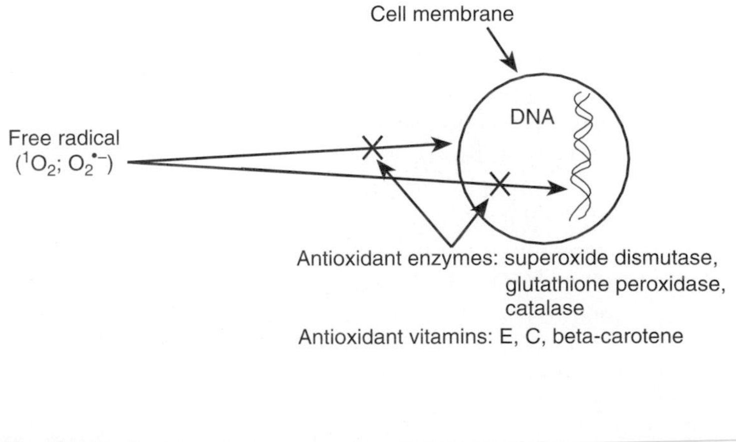

Figure 7.1 Role of vitamin as coenzyme. (1) Substrates, such as pyruvate, need enzymes to be converted into more usable compounds. However, many enzymes need to be activated before a reaction may occur. Note that the enzyme is in a closed position. (2) An enzyme and a vitamin coenzyme (B_1) combine to form an activated complex, in essence opening up the enzyme. (3) The open, activated enzyme accepts the substrate and (4) splits it into two compounds while releasing the enzyme and coenzyme.

Cell membrane

DNA

Free radical
($^1O_2$; $O_2^{\bullet -}$)

Antioxidant enzymes: superoxide dismutase,
glutathione peroxidase,
catalase
Antioxidant vitamins: E, C, beta-carotene

Figure 7.2 The antioxidant role of vitamins. To protect against the destructive nature of free radicals such as singlet oxygen and superoxides, the cells contain a number of different enzymes (superoxide dismutase, glutathione peroxidase, catalase) to help neutralize them, thus helping to prevent disintegration of cell membranes or the genetic material within the cell. Additionally, several vitamins (E, C, beta-carotene) may serve as antioxidants. Such vitamins are theorized to be protective against cancer, heart disease, and adverse effects of aging.

most individuals. Four of these vitamins are soluble in fat and are obtained primarily from the fat in our diet, while the other nine water-soluble vitamins are distributed rather widely in a variety of foods. Although most vitamins must be obtained from the food we eat, several of them may be formed in the body from other ingested nutrients, by the action of ultraviolet rays from sunlight on our skin, or by the activity of some intestinal bacteria.

A number of other substances mistakenly have been classified as vitamins. Included in this group are inositol, para-amino benzoic acid (PABA), vitamin B_{15} or pangamic acid, and vitamin B_{17} or laetrile. Although these substances have been suggested to have vitamin activity, their essentiality in the diet has not been established. Other substances have been attributed vitamin-like activity and professed to enhance health or physical performance, such as bee pollen, coenzyme Q_{10} (CoQ_{10}), ginseng, and ginkgo, but these also are not essential vitamins.

Table 7.1 presents an overview of the thirteen essential vitamins with commonly used interchangeable synonyms, the RDA, major food sources, major functions in the body, and symptoms associated with deficiencies or excessive consumption. The health and performance effects of the essential vitamins and selected vitamin-like substances are covered in the following sections.

In general, how do deficiencies or excesses of vitamins influence health or physical performance?

Whether or not a vitamin deficiency affects one's health or physical performance may depend on the magnitude of the deficiency. Hornig and his associates have described four stages of vitamin deficiency associated with the duration of undernourishment and inadequate vitamin intake.

1. A *preliminary stage* is associated with inadequate amount or availability of the vitamin in the diet. For example, a drastic change in the diet may influence vitamin **bioavailability** (the amount of a nutrient that the body absorbs), whereas pregnancy may increase the need for several vitamins.

2. *Biochemical deficiency.* In this stage, the body's pool of the vitamin is decreased. For a number of vitamins, biochemical deficiency can be identified by blood or tissue tests. For example, deficiencies of riboflavin may be detected by the activity of an enzyme in the red blood cells.

3. *Physiologic deficiency* is associated with the appearance of unspecific symptoms such as loss of appetite, weakness, or physical fatigue.

These first three stages are known as latent or marginal vitamin deficiency, or **subclinical malnutrition.** Whether or not these stages impair physical performance may depend upon the nature

of the sport, but weakness or physical fatigue would certainly be counterproductive to optimal performance.

4. *Clinically manifest vitamin deficiency.* In this final stage, specific clinical symptoms are observed. For example, anemia is a clinical symptom associated with a deficiency of several vitamins, such as folic acid and vitamin B_6. Both health and performance would be adversely affected with a clinically manifest vitamin deficiency.

In the past, RDA for vitamins have been established to prevent vitamin-deficiency diseases. However, Lachance indicated that future deliberations regarding vitamin RDA may incorporate the role of vitamins in health promotion. As noted later, the new RDA for vitamin D has been modified to help prevent osteoporosis. This raises the possibility that the RDA for other vitamins may be modified, as supported by scientific research, to help prevent chronic diseases such as cancer and cardiovascular diseases. If the RDA for some vitamins are increased as a possible means to achieve health promotion objectives, the most likely recommendation will be to obtain the increased amounts from natural foods. However, supplementation may be recommended for a few vitamins.

Except for consumption of large amounts of certain foods, such as cod liver oil, it is very difficult to obtain excessive amounts of vitamins through the diet to the point that health or performance is impaired. Even when supplements are taken, the body may rapidly excrete several vitamins, keeping body functions normal. However, **hypervitaminosis** may occur when vitamins are not excreted effectively and accumulate in the tissues, beginning to function as a drug instead of a nutrient. Toxic reactions specific to the vitamin overdose may occur.

Fat-Soluble Vitamins

The four fat-soluble vitamins are A, D, E, and K. Because they are soluble in fat but not in water, dietary sources include foods that have some fat content. The body may contain appreciable stores of each fat-soluble vitamin, and several of them may be manufactured by the body, so deficiencies are relatively rare in industrialized societies. On the other hand, excessive intake may be toxic. With the exception of vitamin E, very little research has been conducted relative to deficiency or supplementation effects upon physical performance.

Vitamin A (retinol)

Vitamin A is a fat-soluble, unsaturated alcohol. The physiologically active form of vitamin A is known as **retinol.** The human body is capable of forming retinol from provitamins known as carotenoids, primarily **beta-carotene.** Both preformed vitamin A, or retinol, and beta-carotene are found in the foods we eat.

Table 7.1 Essential vitamins

Vitamin name (Other terms)	RDA or ESADDI for adults over age 25*	Major sources
Fat-soluble vitamins		
Vitamin A (retinol: provitamin carotenoids)	1000 RE ♂ 800 RE ♀ (RE = retinol equivalents)	Retinol in animal foods: liver, whole milk, fortified milk, cheese. Carotenoids in plant foods; carrots, green leafy vegetables, sweet potatoes, fortified margarine from vegetable oils.
Vitamin D (cholecalciferol)	200–600 IU or 5–15 micrograms	Vitamin D fortified foods like dairy products and margarine, fish oils. Action of sunlight on the skin.
Vitamin E (tocopherol)	10 mg ♂ alpha-TE 8 mg ♀ alpha-TE (TE = tocopherol equivalents)	Vegetable oils, margarine, green leafy vegetables, wheat germ, whole-grain products, egg yolks.
Vitamin K (phylloquinone; menoquinone)	80 micrograms ♂ 65 micrograms ♀	Pork and beef liver, eggs, spinach, cauliflower. Formation in the human intestine by bacteria.
Water-soluble vitamins		
Thiamin (vitamin B_1)	1.5 mg ♂ 1.1 mg ♀	Ham, pork, lean meat, liver, whole-grain products, enriched breads and cereals, legumes.
Riboflavin (vitamin B_2)	1.7 mg ♂ 1.3 mg ♀	Milk and dairy products, meat, enriched grain products, green leafy vegetables, beans.
Niacin (nicotinamide, nicotinic acid)	19 mg ♂ 15 mg ♀	Lean meats, fish, poultry, whole-grain products, beans. May be formed in the body from tryptophan, an essential amino acid.
Vitamin B_6 (pyridoxal, pyridoxine, pyridoxamine)	2 mg ♂ 1.6 mg ♀	Protein foods: liver, lean meats, fish, poultry, legumes. Green leafy vegetables.
Vitamin B_{12} (cobalamin; cyanocobalamin)	2 micrograms	Animal foods only: meat, fish, poultry, milk, eggs.
Folic acid (folate)	200 micrograms ♂ 180 micrograms ♀	Liver, green leafy vegetables, legumes, nuts.
Biotin	30–100 micrograms	Meats, legumes, milk, egg yolk, whole-grain products, most vegetables.
Pantothenic acid	4–7 mg	Beef and pork liver, lean meats, milk, eggs, legumes, whole-grain products, most vegetables.
Vitamin C (ascorbic acid)	60 mg	Citrus fruits, green leafy vegetables, broccoli, peppers, strawberries, potatoes.

Major functions in the body	Deficiency symptoms	Symptoms of excessive consumption
Fat-soluble vitamins		
Maintains epithelial tissue in skin and mucous membranes; forms visual purple for night vision; promotes bone development.	Night blindness, intestinal infections, impaired growth, xerophthalmia.	Nausea, headache, fatigue, liver and spleen damage, skin peeling, pain in the joints.
Acts as a hormone to increase intestinal absorption of calcium and promote bone and tooth formation.	Rare. Rickets in children and osteomalacia in adults.	Loss of appetite, nausea, irritability, joint pain, calcium deposits in soft tissues such as the kidney.
Functions as an antioxidant to protect cell membranes from destruction by oxidation.	Extremely rare. Disruption of red blood cell membranes, anemia.	General lack of toxicity with doses up to 400 mg. Some reports of headache, fatigue, or diarrhea with megadoses.
Essential for blood coagulation processes.	Increased bleeding and hemorrhage.	Possible clot formation (thrombosis), vomiting.
Water-soluble vitamins		
Serves as a coenzyme for energy production from carbohydrate; essential for normal functioning of the central nervous system.	Poor appetite, apathy, mental depression, pain in calf muscles, beriberi.	General lack of toxicity.
Functions as a coenzyme involved in energy production from carbohydrates and fats; maintenance of healthy skin.	Dermatitis, cracks at the corners of the mouth, sores on the tongue, damage to the cornea.	General lack of toxicity.
Functions as a coenzyme for the aerobic and anaerobic production of energy from carbohydrate; helps synthesize fat and blocks release of FFA; needed for healthy skin.	Loss of appetite, weakness, skin lesions, gastrointestinal problems, pellagra.	Nicotinic acid causes headache, nausea, burning and itching skin, flushing of face, liver damage.
Functions as a coenzyme in protein metabolism; necessary for formation of hemoglobin and red blood cells; needed for glycogenolysis and gluconeogenesis.	Nervous irritability, convulsions, dermatitis, sores on tongue, anemia.	Loss of nerve sensation, impaired gait.
Functions as a coenzyme for formation of DNA, RBC development, and maintenance of nerve tissue.	Pernicious anemia, nerve damage resulting in paralysis.	General lack of toxicity.
Functions as coenzyme for DNA formation and RBC development.	Fatigue, gastrointestinal disorders, diarrhea, anemia, neural tube defects in newborns.	May prevent detection of pernicious anemia caused by B_{12} deficiency.
Functions as coenzyme in the metabolism of carbohydrates, fats, and protein.	Rare. May be caused by excessive intake of raw egg whites. Fatigue, nausea, skin rashes.	General lack of toxicity.
Functions as part of coenzyme A in energy metabolism.	Rare. Only produced clinically. Fatigue, nausea, loss of appetite, mental depression.	General lack of toxicity.
Forms collagen essential for connective tissue development; aids in absorption of iron; helps form epinephrine; serves as antioxidant.	Weakness, rough skin, slow wound healing, bleeding gums, scurvy.	Diarrhea, possible kidney stones, rebound scurvy.

*RDA values for other age groups are found in Appendix A or in the discussion of each individual vitamin.

RDA The RDA for vitamin A may be obtained by consuming retinol, beta-carotene and other carotenoids, or a combination of the two. The RDA may be expressed in several ways, usually as **retinol equivalents (RE)** or as international units (IU). The RDA is 1,000 retinol equivalents, or 5,000 IU, for adult males and 800 retinol equivalents, or 4,000 IU, for adult females. The adult male RDA value is the equivalent of 1 milligram of retinol or 6 milligrams of beta-carotene. Slightly lesser amounts are needed by children. The RDA for specific ages may be found in Appendix A. The Reference Daily Intake (RDI) is 5,000 IU, or 1,000 RE.

Food Sources Preformed vitamin A is found in substantial amounts in some animal foods such as liver, butter, cheese, egg yolks, fish liver oils, and fortified milk. Provitamin A, as beta-carotene, is found in dark-green leafy and yellow-orange vegetables as well as in some fruits such as oranges, limes, pineapples, prunes, and cantaloupes. Fortified margarine also contains beta-carotene. One glass of milk provides 10 percent of the RDA, while one medium carrot will supply nearly 200 percent and a serving of liver a whopping 900 percent of the RDA.

Major Functions Vitamin A is essential for maintenance of the epithelial cells, those cells covering the outside of the body and lining the body cavities. It is also essential for proper visual function, such as night vision and peripheral vision. Vitamin A also has a variety of other physiological roles in the body that are not well understood, although it is considered essential for maintaining optimal function of the immune system. Beta-carotene may function as an antioxidant and has been theorized to confer some health benefits.

Deficiency Vitamin A is stored in the body in relatively large amounts. However, an inadequate intake of vitamin A could have serious health implications if prolonged. The gradual loss of night vision is one of the first symptoms of vitamin A deficiency. Other symptoms of mild deficiencies include increased susceptibility to infection and skin lesions. Epidemiological research also has suggested that a deficient intake of beta-carotene could predispose the individual to the development of cancer in the epithelial tissues such as the skin, lungs, breasts, and intestinal lining. Although severe deficiencies are not common in industrialized nations, they do occur in some parts of the world and lead to blindness through destruction of the cornea of the eye, a condition known as **xerophthalmia.** Vitamin A deficiency has been associated with higher mortality rates in children of third world countries, and some, but not all, studies have shown that vitamin A supplementation may decrease the death rate, possibly by strengthening the immune system.

Theoretically, vitamin A deficiency could affect physical performance. Some investigators have suggested that a deficiency may impair the process of gluconeogenesis in the liver, which may be an important consideration for the endurance athlete in the latter stages of competition. Others have implied a reduction in the synthesis of muscle protein and impaired vision, which could negatively affect strength athletes or those involved in sports requiring eye alertness. Very little research is available to support these theoretical views.

Supplementation In general, supplements of vitamin A are not recommended. Excessive amounts of vitamin A, generally caused by self-medication with megadoses, can cause a condition known as hypervitaminosis A. Symptoms may include weakness, headache, loss of appetite, nausea, pain in the joints, peeling of skin, and liver damage. Similar symptoms were reported in a young soccer player who took about 100,000 IU daily for 2 months in an attempt to improve performance. The symptoms were relieved when he stopped taking the supplements. Extremely large doses of vitamin A may be fatal. As noted by Olson, excessive vitamin A during pregnancy may be teratogenic, causing deformities in the developing embryo or fetus. Recent research by Rothman and others has indicated that vitamin A doses as low as four times the RDA can markedly increase a pregnant woman's chances of having a baby with birth defects, such as a cleft palate, heart defects, or other problems. Although this amount would not be consumed with a normal diet, it could be obtained by someone who takes a daily supplement, drinks substantial amounts of milk, eats liver, and has several servings of fortified cereals.

Beta-carotene supplements are not believed to be toxic but may cause harmless yellowing of the skin when taken in excess because the beta-carotene may accumulate in the fat tissues. Beta-carotene has been combined with other antioxidants in an attempt to prevent muscle damage during exercise. This research is discussed later in this chapter.

Prudent Recommendations In summary, vitamin A supplementation to the diet of the active individual does not have a sound theoretical basis. Moreover, the research conducted with vitamin A and physical performance has shown no beneficial effect. Hence, there appears to be no advantage for the active individual to supplement the diet with vitamin A, particularly not with megadoses that may have undesirable effects. The advisability of beta-carotene supplementation for its antioxidant properties is discussed in the later sections of this chapter dealing with ergogenic and health issues.

Vitamin D (cholecalciferol)

Vitamin D, a term representing a number of compounds, has been classified as both a fat-soluble vitamin and as a hormone. The physiologically active form is calcitriol, which is the hormone of this vitamin. In brief, the ultraviolet rays from sunshine convert a compound found in the skin into **cholecalciferol (vitamin D₃),** a prohormone, which is released into the blood and is eventually converted by the liver and kidneys into the active hormone, calcitriol.

RDA The RDA for vitamin D is given in micrograms of cholecalciferol or as IU. One microgram of cholecalciferol is the equivalent of 40 IU. The RDA for vitamin D is higher during bone growth periods, up to age 25, being 10 micrograms, or 400 IU, daily. The recommended amount for adults is 200 IU, but given the potential role of vitamin D to optimize bone health, the National Academy of Sciences recently updated the RDA to 400 IU for those aged 51–70 and to 600 IU for those over age 70. See Appendix A for particulars. The RDI is 400 IU.

Food Sources Most foods do not contain any vitamin D. Fish liver oils are good sources, and small amounts are found in eggs, tuna, and salmon. Several foods are fortified with vitamin D, such as milk, margarine, and some breakfast cereals. One glass of fortified milk will provide 25 percent of the RDA for a child.

The RDA for vitamin D may be obtained by exposing the hands, arms, and face to 10–20 minutes of summer sunshine about 2–3 times per week. Total sunblocking agents prevent vitamin D formation, but their use by individuals concerned with skin cancer due to sun exposure is still recommended because even very small amounts of sunshine will promote vitamin D formation. Longer periods of exposure may be necessary in the winter, and it may be difficult to obtain adequate vitamin D by sunlight in northern latitudes, even in northern portions of the United States. Aging also decreases the formation of vitamin D from sunlight.

Major Functions Vitamin D plays a central role in bone metabolism through its effect on calcium and phosphorus, whose roles in bone metabolism are discussed in the next chapter. It works in conjunction with several other hormones, particularly parathormone secreted by the parathyroid gland. In particular, vitamin D helps to absorb calcium from the intestinal tract and the kidneys, helping to maintain normal serum calcium levels and proper bone metabolism. Vitamin D also helps regulate phosphorus metabolism, another mineral essential in bone formation. Besides the classical actions of vitamin D in bone metabolism, it is also involved in the development of the skin and has been used in the treatment of psoriasis, a chronic skin disorder. For a detailed review of vitamin D metabolism, the interested reader is referred to the recent reviews by Fraser and Holick.

Deficiency Deficiencies of vitamin D are unusual in most temperate climates because the body possesses adequate stores in the liver and can manufacture it through exposure to the sun. However, deficiencies may occur in individuals who have little exposure to sunshine, such as elderly people who are homebound. Deficiencies may lead to inadequate calcium metabolism and bone deformities known as rickets, especially in children. This was a major concern years ago but has nearly been eradicated through the use of vitamin D-fortified foods, primarily milk. However, in a recent interview, Holick indicated that adults do not drink much milk and many are not getting enough Vitamin D to satisfy their body requirements, predisposing them to bone loss. Loss of bone tissue may occur in adults, leading to **osteomalacia,** or a softening of the bones, accompanied by muscular weakness. The muscle weakness has been theoretically linked with an impairment of calcium metabolism in the muscle.

Supplementation In general, vitamin D supplements in amounts greater than the RDA are not recommended. Because vitamin D is fat soluble, megadoses may lead to increased storage in the body, and pathological results have been reported, even in doses five times the RDA, or 1,000 IU. Hypervitaminosis D may lead to vomiting, diarrhea, weight loss, loss of muscle tone, and possible damage to soft tissues such as the kidney, heart, and blood vessels due to deposits of calcium. Although adequate amounts of vitamin D are needed for prevention of osteomalacia and osteoporosis, Moon and others hypothesized that chronic excess intake may induce osteoporosis and also exacerbate atherosclerosis by increasing the calcium content in plaque. Exposure to the sun and a balanced diet, unless the food is improperly fortified, will not lead to hypervitaminosis D, but supplements may.

There is very little theoretical basis for athletes to take vitamin D supplements. For this reason, only a few studies have been conducted with vitamin D supplementation and physical performance, and they revealed no beneficial effect, either through single megadoses or supplementation over a 2-year period. Some recent research has revealed that weight training increases the serum concentration of vitamin D, and the investigators theorized this could be related to the increased bone mass which is developed through exercise. However, this study does not suggest that vitamin D supplementation would be ergogenic.

Prudent Recommendations As with vitamin A, there appear to be sound medical reasons for healthy individuals not to use vitamin D supplements. Some elderly women may merit supplementation, but only to complement dietary intake to obtain 400–600 IU.

Vitamin E (alpha-tocopherol)

Vitamin E is a fat-soluble vitamin. Its physiological activity is derived from a number of different tocopherols and tocotrienols found in the diet, **alpha-tocopherol** being the most active.

RDA The RDA for vitamin E is given in **alpha-tocopherol equivalents,** or alpha-TE, although you may also see it expressed in IU. One alpha-TE is the equivalent of 1 mg of alpha-tocopherol or about 1.5 IU. The current RDA is 10 alpha-TE (10 mg or 15 IU) for adult males and 8 alpha-TE (8 mg or 12 IU) for females. The amount is slightly less for children. See Appendix A for specific values. The RDI, however, is 30 IU.

Food Sources Vitamin E is found primarily in the small fat content in various vegetables. The most common dietary sources are polyunsaturated vegetable oils such as corn, soybean, and safflower oils, and margarines made from these oils; one tablespoon contains about 3–5 IU. Other good sources of vitamin E include fortified ready-to-eat cereals, whole-grain products, wheat germ oil, and eggs. One ounce of a fortified cereal may include about 10–45 IU of vitamin E, while a tablespoon of wheat germ oil contains about 40 IU. Moderate to small amounts are found in meats, dairy products, fruits, and vegetables, particularly sweet potatoes and dark-green leafy vegetables. Four spears of asparagus contain 2 IU. The fat substitute, Olestra, may retard the absorption of vitamin E found in natural foods. Nutritionists have recommended that foods containing Olestra should be fortified with vitamin E. The RDA for vitamin E actually increases as the amount of polyunsaturated oils in the diet increases. Fish oil supplements may be contraindicated in this regard since they are high in polyunsaturated fatty acids, but low in vitamin E unless fortified.

Major Functions Although the total function of vitamin E in human nutrition is unclear, its principal role is to serve as an antioxidant. Vitamin E helps prevent the oxidation of unsaturated fatty acids in cell membrane phospholipids and thereby protects the cell from damage. It may also help prevent the oxidation of vitamin A. Other claims, extrapolated from research with animals, have suggested that vitamin E may also play a key role in the synthesis of hemoglobin or serve a pro-oxidant effect by activating enzymes in the mitochondria to improve cellular oxygen utilization, but these claims are not well documented in humans. Some of the vitamin E antioxidant effects are theorized to help prevent the development of several chronic diseases. The related mechanisms are discussed later in this chapter.

Deficiency Because vitamin E is rather widely distributed in foods, and because it is also stored in the body, a true vitamin E deficiency in humans is rare. In one experiment prisoners were fed a vitamin E-deficient diet for 13 months and evidenced no symptoms of a deficiency. However, certain individuals with genetic diseases, such as the inability to absorb fat, do experience a deficiency. In such cases, anemia may occur because the membranes of the red blood cells (RBC) are oxidized and release their hemoglobin. Deficiency symptoms noted in animals include nutritional muscular dystrophy and damage to the heart and blood vessels. Because of its role in preventing cellular damage from free radical oxidation, a deficiency of vitamin E has been theorized to contribute to the development of heart disease and cancer in humans. Some studies have suggested that a deficiency will lead to premature aging and decreased fertility.

Supplementation Although vitamin E deficiency is rare in humans, several authors have used the data from research with animals and those humans with genetic defects to support the need for supplementation by athletes. They suggest that a vitamin E deficiency may lead to impaired oxygen transport due to RBC damage and to reduced oxidative capacity within the muscle cell. These effects would reduce VO_2 max and lead to a decrease in aerobic endurance capacity.

Over a dozen studies have been conducted to investigate the effect of vitamin E supplementation upon physical performance, especially VO_2 max and aerobic endurance capacity. Some of the early studies showed a beneficial effect, particularly at higher altitudes, but the experiments were poorly designed. However, one very well-planned experiment by Kobayashi, using a double-blind, placebo protocol, found that 1,200 IU of vitamin E supplements daily for 6 weeks improved VO_2 max, reduced blood lactic acid during submaximal exercise, and increased aerobic endurance at altitudes of 5,000 and 15,000 feet. The vitamin E was theorized to prevent the increased rate of oxidation of the RBC membrane that might occur while exercising at altitude. Although this was a well-designed study, the subjects were sedentary and were not in a state of training, so it may not be applicable to athletes. More recent research by Simon-Schnass and Pabst has supported these earlier findings. These researchers reported that 400 milligrams of vitamin E given to high-altitude mountain climbers over a 10-week period improved the anaerobic (lactate) threshold. Additional research would appear to be warranted with athletes at altitude.

Moreover, one investigator has noted a similar situation may exist with athletes exercising in high-smog areas, where some of the pollutants in the air could damage the RBC. With the magnitude of sports conducted in cities such as Los Angeles, this topic also might benefit from such research. Given these findings, and the possible effects of vitamin E on exercise-induced muscle damage discussed later in this chapter, Simon-Schnass noted in a recent review that athletes should consume 100–200 IU daily and that it would be bordering on malpractice not to point out the benefits of such supplementation to athletes.

On the other hand, the majority of the recent well-designed studies, using doses from 400–1,200 IU and using athletes in training as subjects, revealed no significant effect upon physiological functions such as VO_2 max or tests of aerobic endurance when performed at sea level. One possible reason for this finding is that the plasma level of vitamin E appears to rise significantly during intense exercise, as reported by Pincemail and others. But even when 5 months of vitamin E supplementation, as compared to a placebo treatment, significantly increased serum vitamin E levels in national class racing cyclists, Rokitzki and others noted no improvement in VO_2 max and other cycling performance measures.

Although the potential ergogenic effect of vitamin E supplementation at altitude needs additional research, Tiidus and Houston recently reviewed the scientific literature and concluded that while supplementation may increase tissue or serum vitamin E concentration, there is currently a lack of conclusive evidence that exercise performance or recovery in either elite or recreational athletes would benefit in any significant way.

Like beta-carotene, vitamin E has been theorized to prevent muscle damage during exercise, and this topic is covered later in this chapter.

Prudent Recommendations As a means to enhance physical performance, vitamin E supplements are not recommended. However, as noted later in this chapter, although most health professionals recommend increased attention to foods rich in vitamin E, others may recommend supplements for possible prevention of various chronic diseases.

Vitamin K (phylloquinone; menoquinone)

Vitamin K is a fat-soluble vitamin. It is often called the blood coagulation vitamin or antihemorrhagic vitamin.

RDA An RDA was established for vitamin K in 1989; for adults it is 65 and 80 micrograms per day for women and men, respectively.

Food Sources Vitamin K is found in a variety of plant and animal foods. **Phylloquinone** is the plant form of vitamin K, while **menoquinone** is the animal form. Good plant sources include green and leafy vegetables, such as peas, broccoli, and spinach, while meats and milk contain lower amounts. One-half cup of cooked broccoli contains about 110 milligrams. The typical American diet contains about 200–300 micrograms per day. Additionally, vitamin K (menoquinone) is also formed in the intestines by bacteria, so a deficiency is unlikely.

Major Functions Vitamin K is needed for the formation of four compounds that are essential in two steps of the blood-clotting process. In addition, vitamin K appears to enhance the function of osteocalcin, a protein that plays an important role in strengthening bones. Suttie has provided a recent review of the role of vitamin K in human nutrition.

Deficiency A deficiency of vitamin K impairs blood clotting and leads to hemorrhage. Although controversial, Binklely and Suttie indicated vitamin K insufficiency may affect kidney excretion of calcium and be involved in the etiology of osteoporosis. Although deficiency states are rare, they may occur in some individuals when antibiotic medications kill the intestinal bacteria that produce the vitamin.

Supplementation No supplementation studies are available to evaluate the effect of vitamin K on physical performance because it does not appear to play an important role in this regard. The National Research Council has noted that, unlike vitamins A and D, vitamin K is not very toxic when consumed in large doses. However, some synthetic forms may be toxic in large doses. Moreover, vitamin K supplements are available by prescription only.

Prudent Recommendations There is no evidence available that supports vitamin K supplementation as a means to improve the health status of the average individual or to improve performance in athletes. Therefore, vitamin K supplements are not recommended unless under the guidance of a physician.

Water-Soluble Vitamins

There are nine water-soluble vitamins, including eight in the vitamin B complex and vitamin C (ascorbic acid). The B complex vitamins include thiamin, riboflavin, niacin, B_6, B_{12}, folic acid, biotin, and pantothenic acid. Being water soluble they are not, with a few exceptions, stored to any significant extent in the body. The effects of a deficiency may be noted in 2–4 weeks for some of these vitamins, often reducing physical performance capacity. Excess supplements of these vitamins are usually excreted in the urine and are generally considered to be relatively harmless. However, there are some exceptions.

Because several of the B vitamins work closely together in energy metabolism, many studies have investigated the effect of a deficiency or supplementation of multiple vitamins from the B complex. A summary of this research follows a discussion of each individual vitamin.

Figure 7.3 provides a broad perspective on the major sites of activity of the water-soluble vitamins, highlighting sites for vitamin E and other antioxidants as well.

Thiamin (vitamin B₁)

Thiamin, also known as **vitamin B_1,** is a water-soluble vitamin and is also known as the antiberiberi or antineuritic vitamin. It was one of the first vitamins discovered.

RDA The RDA for thiamin varies according to the intake of Calories, being approximately 0.5 mg per 1,000 Calories. The average adult male needs approximately 1.5 mg/day,

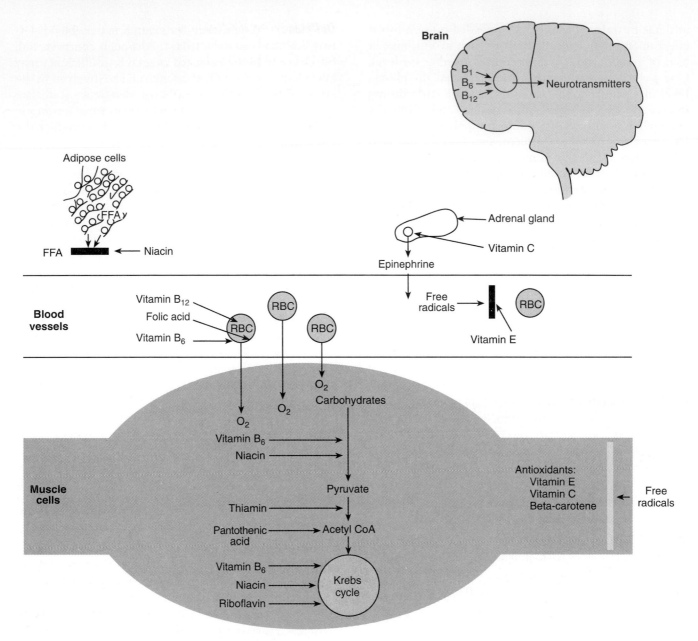

Figure 7.3 Roles of vitamins important to sports performance. A number of B vitamins, including thiamin, riboflavin, niacin, B₆, and pantothenic acid are essential for the conversion of carbohydrate into energy for muscular contraction. Vitamin B₁₂ and folic acid are essential for the development of the red blood cells (RBC), which deliver oxygen to the muscle cell. Vitamin E helps protect the RBC membrane from destruction by free radicals. Vitamin E and other antioxidant vitamins are theorized to prevent free radical damage in muscle cells during exercise. Vitamin C is needed for the formation of epinephrine (adrenaline), a key hormone during strenuous exercise. Niacin may actually block the release of free fatty acids from the adipose tissue, which could be a disadvantage for ultraendurance athletes. Finally, several of the B vitamins are also involved in the formation of neurotransmitters in the brain, which may induce a relaxation effect.

while the adult female needs about 1.1 mg/day. See Appendix A for other age groups. The RDI is 1.5 mg.

Food Sources Thiamin is widely distributed in both plant and animal tissues. Good sources include whole-grain cereals, beans, seeds, nuts, pork, and many fruits and vegetables. There also is some limited synthesis of thiamin by bacteria in the intestinal tract. One lean pork chop contains 30 percent of the RDA. Several fortified ready-to-eat cereals contain 100 percent of the RDA for thiamin, as well as most of the other B vitamins.

Major Functions Thiamin has a central role in the metabolism of glucose. It is part of a coenzyme known as thiamin pyrophosphate, which is needed to convert pyruvate to acetyl CoA for entrance into the Krebs cycle. Thiamin is essential for the normal functioning of the nervous system and energy derivation from glycogen in the muscles.

Deficiency Deficiency symptoms may occur in several weeks, including loss of appetite, mental confusion, muscular weakness, and pain in the calf muscles. Prolonged deficiencies lead to beriberi, a serious disease involving damage to the nervous system and the heart. Fortunately, thiamin deficiency is not very common, although it may be rather prevalent among the homeless, alcoholics, and other special groups.

Of importance to the athlete, two factors that increase the need for thiamin are exercise and high-carbohydrate intake. A deficiency of thiamin could prove to be detrimental to the active individual who might rely on high levels of carbohydrate metabolism for aerobic energy production during exercise, such as endurance athletes. Indeed, some well-controlled research conducted during World War II noted decreased endurance capacity after several weeks of a thiamin-deficient diet. More contemporary research has also investigated the role of thiamin deficiency upon exercise performance, but in conjunction with riboflavin and niacin deficiencies. These reports are discussed below under vitamin B complex.

Supplementation Unfortunately, no contemporary research appears to exist relative to the effect of thiamin supplementation upon physical performance, although results from a number of studies conducted more than 50 years ago are available. Following a careful review of these studies, many with problems in establishing a proper experimental design, there appears to be no conclusive evidence to support the contention that vitamin B_1 intake above and beyond the normal RDA will enhance performance.

Although not using thiamine, Doyle and others recently reported that 5 days of supplementation with allithiamine, a thiamin derivative, did not improve muscular strength and endurance.

Thiamin, as indicated, is important for normal neurological functions. In a recent study from Japan, Suzuki and Itokawa reported that 100 milligrams of thiamine for 3 days increased serum thiamin levels and reduced subjective complaints of fatigue from subjects following a strenuous exercise task. As noted later under the B-complex section, thiamin was one of the vitamins proposed to improve neurological function in pistol shooting. These are interesting observations and merit additional research.

As noted above, physical activity, particularly high-intensity, endurance-type activity, increases the need for thiamin in the diet; this exercise training also increases the need for caloric intake. With proper selection of foods, the increased thiamin need may be met by the content in the additional foods eaten. An adequate thiamin intake is one of the reasons physically active individuals need to select foods that are dense in nutrients, and in general to avoid those foods that provide Calories but few nutrients.

Prudent Recommendations Although thiamin supplements are not needed by the individual who is consuming an adequate diet, megadoses of thiamin up to 1,000 mg appear to have no detrimental effect. The excess will be excreted in the urine.

Riboflavin (vitamin B₂)

Riboflavin is also known as **vitamin B_2**. It is a water-soluble vitamin and is a component of the B complex.

RDA The RDA for riboflavin is slightly higher than that of thiamin, being about 0.6 mg per 1,000 Calories. It averages about 1.7 mg for the adult male and 1.3 mg for the adult female. Appendix A contains the RDA for other age groups. The RDI is 1.7 mg.

Food Sources Riboflavin is distributed widely in foods. A major source is milk and other dairy products; one glass of milk contains 20 percent of the RDA. Other good sources include liver, eggs, dark-green leafy vegetables, wheat germ, yeast, whole-grain products, and enriched breads and cereals.

Major Functions Riboflavin is important for the formation of several oxidative enzymes known as flavoproteins, which are involved in energy production from carbohydrate and fats in the body cells. It is also involved in protein metabolism and maintenance of healthy skin tissue.

Deficiency Deficiencies are very rare but have been seen in alcoholics and those adhering to various fad diets. Early signs of deficiency may include glossitis (an inflammation of the tongue), cracks at the corners of the mouth, and dry, scaly skin at the corners of the nose, symptoms common in individuals who experience multiple nutrient deficits.

Although the effect of a riboflavin deficiency upon physical performance has not been studied directly, research from Cornell University suggests that physically untrained women who initiate an aerobic training program may need a higher intake of riboflavin to synthesize more flavoproteins in the muscles. Using a blood test, the investigators determined that the RDA did not maintain proper riboflavin status in the early stages of training, but they suggested a value of about 1.1 mg per 1,000 Calories would be sufficient. It should be noted that no data were reported relative to the effect of this deficiency upon performance. Haralambie also reported a possible deficiency in trained athletes but did not relate it to performance.

Supplementation Reviews by Keith and van der Beek reveal only one reputable study of the effects of riboflavin supplementation on physical performance. Tremblay and others, studying elite swimmers, reported that 60 mg of riboflavin daily for 16–20 days did not improve VO_2 max, anaerobic (lactate) threshold, or swim performance.

Prudent Recommendations Considering the available research data and the absence of riboflavin deficiency in most individuals, one must conclude that riboflavin supplementation will not enhance physical performance. No adverse effects of riboflavin megadoses have been reported. Excess riboflavin is apparently excreted.

Niacin

Niacin is also known as nicotinic acid, nicotinamide, or the antipellagra vitamin. It is a water-soluble vitamin in the B complex and is sometimes erroneously referred to as vitamin B_3.

RDA Niacin is found naturally in many foods, but it also may be formed in the body from excess amounts of dietary tryptophan, an essential amino acid. Therefore, the RDA is expressed in **niacin equivalents,** or **NE.** One NE equals 1 mg of niacin or 60 mg of tryptophan, because 1 mg of niacin can be produced from that amount of tryptophan. The RDA for niacin is based upon energy intake, approximating 6.6 mg per 1,000 Calories, which totals about 19 NE for adult males and 15 NE for adult females. The requirement is different for other age groups, and specific values may be obtained from Appendix A. The RDI is 20 mg.

Food Sources Niacin is found in foods that have a high protein content. It is most abundant in lean meats, organ meats, fish, poultry, whole-grain cereal products, legumes such as beans and peanuts, and enriched foods. Milk and eggs contain almost no niacin, but they contain moderate amounts of tryptophan. One-half of a chicken breast contains over 60 percent of the RDA of niacin.

Major Functions Niacin serves as a component of two coenzymes concerned with energy processes within the cell. One of these coenzymes is important in the process of glycolysis, which is the means by which muscle glycogen produces energy both aerobically and anaerobically. The other coenzyme is involved in fat metabolism by promoting fat synthesis in the body.

Deficiency Although niacin deficiency was prevalent in the past, the enrichment of foods with niacin has nearly eliminated this problem. Deficiency symptoms include loss of appetite, skin rashes, mental confusion, lack of energy, and muscular weakness. Serious deficiencies lead to pellagra, a disease characterized by severe dermatitis, diarrhea, and symptoms of mental illness.

In theory, physical performance would be impaired by a niacin deficiency because the production of energy from carbohydrate could be impaired. Both aerobic- and anaerobic-type performances could be affected. However, no research has been uncovered that has directly studied the effects of such a deficiency on exercise performance.

Supplementation Because of the role of niacin in energy metabolism, a number of experiments have been conducted relative to niacin supplementation and physical performance capacity. However, several recent reviews concluded that niacin supplementation has not been shown to be an effective ergogenic aid for well-nourished athletes, having no effect on various exercise endeavors, including performance in a 10-mile run and in a 3.5-mile cycle time trial following 2 hours of cycling.

As a matter of fact, niacin supplementation is not recommended for most athletes, particularly those involved in endurance-type exercise such as marathon running because excessive niacin intake (3–9 grams/day) can block the release of FFA from the adipose tissue. This will decrease the supply of FFA to the muscle, which may lead to an increased dependence on carbohydrate as an energy source during exercise, as recently shown by Heath and others. This could lead to a more rapid depletion of muscle glycogen, an important energy source during exercise. As noted by Bulow, niacin supplements may reduce endurance capacity.

Niacin supplements may also increase blood flow to the skin due to a histamine-like effect. In one experiment, Kolka and Stephenson found that such an effect could lower the sweat rate and decrease body heat storage during exercise. These effects could possibly be ergogenic to athletes exercising in the heat, but further investigation is needed.

Megadoses of niacin have been used in attempts to treat several health problems, being relatively ineffective in the treatment of mental disease and somewhat successful in reducing high serum lipid levels. Niacin may not only lower total and LDL cholesterol but may also lower triglycerides and raise HDL cholesterol. Some health professionals consider niacin the drug of first choice in the treatment of high blood cholesterol, but with cautions as noted below.

Although niacin is generally considered to be non-toxic, large doses in the form of nicotinic acid may cause flushing, with burning and tingling sensations around the face, neck, and hands occurring within 15–20 minutes after ingestion (i.e., the histamine-like effect). Taken over long periods, niacin may contribute to liver problems such as hepatitis and peptic ulcers. In particular, timed-release niacin preparations have been implicated as a cause of hepatitis. The Center for Science in the Public Interest recommends that no one take niacin to lower blood cholesterol without guidance from a physician.

Prudent Recommendations Unless under the treatment of a physician, niacin supplements are not recommended for a physically active individual on a balanced diet. Excessive intake may actually impair certain types of athletic performance and elicit adverse health effects.

Vitamin B₆ (pyridoxine)

Vitamin B₆ is a collective term for three naturally occurring substances that are all metabolically and functionally related. They are pyridoxine, pyridoxal, and pyridoxamine. **Pyridoxine** is most often used as a synonym. Vitamin B₆ is water-soluble.

RDA   The adult RDA for vitamin B₆ is 2 mg/day. Slightly different amounts are needed at different age levels. Consult Appendix A for specific RDA. Actually, the RDA for vitamin B₆ is based on protein intake, so requirements may increase with high-protein diets. The RDI is 2 mg.

Food Sources   Vitamin B₆ is widely distributed in foods. The best sources are protein foods such as meats, poultry, fish, wheat germ, whole-grain products, brown rice, and eggs. One-half of a chicken breast contains over 25 percent of the RDA.

Major Functions   In its coenzyme form (primarily pyridoxal phosphate), vitamin B₆ is critically involved in the metabolism of protein, but it is also involved in carbohydrate and fat metabolism. It functions with more than sixty enzymes in such processes as the synthesis of dispensable amino acids, the conversion of tryptophan to niacin, the formation of neurotransmitters in the nervous system, and the incorporation of amino acids into body proteins such as hemoglobin, myoglobin, and oxidative enzymes. It is also involved in the breakdown of muscle glycogen as well as gluconeogenesis in the liver. Interested readers are directed to the review by Melinda Manore for more details on the metabolic functions of vitamin B₆.

Deficiency   Vitamin B₆ deficiency is not considered to be a major health problem. The average American diet appears to provide an adequate amount of the vitamin, but poor diets do not. The use of diuretics and oral contraceptives has been associated with deficiencies. Most studies report that male athletes have adequate dietary intakes of vitamin B₆, whereas some females, especially those with low energy intakes, appear to have low vitamin B₆ intakes. Deficiency symptoms include nausea, impaired immune function, skin disorders, mouth sores, weakness, mental depression, anemia, and epileptic-like convulsions.

Theoretically, a B₆ deficiency could adversely affect endurance activities dependent upon oxygen, for it is involved in the formation of protein compounds such as hemoglobin that are essential to oxidative processes. Its role in carbohydrate metabolism, particularly muscle glycogen utilization, is also important to the endurance athlete. Its role in the formation of neurotransmitters could be important to athletes engaged in fine motor control sports, such as archery and riflery. In addition, the requirement for B₆ increases with protein intake, which may have some implications for those athletes who may be on high-protein diets. However, since B₆ is found in protein products, it should be easily obtainable in such a diet.

No research has been uncovered that has directly studied the effect of a B₆ deficiency upon physical performance. One report did suggest that runners who covered 5–10 miles per day appear to use more B₆ than their sedentary counterparts, but these investigators also noted that exercise may actually promote storage of the vitamin in the athlete, thus helping to prevent a deficiency state. Serum levels of B₆ actually increase during exercise. Hoffman and others noted the source of serum B₆ remains to be identified, but it may be derived from the B₆-dependent enzyme phosphorylase, which breaks down muscle glycogen.

In general, exercise does not appear to cause excessive losses of vitamin B₆ from the body. For example, Rokitzki and others estimated a loss of only 1 milligram over the course of a marathon, an amount that could easily be replaced in the diet.

Supplementation   Several reports relative to the effect of B₆ supplementation upon physical performance are available. Although the muscle may store B₆, Coburn and others recently noted that B₆ supplementation did not markedly increase muscle stores. Moreover, in general, the studies reveal no significant effect upon metabolic functions during exercise or the capacity to do more work. One investigator suggested B₆ may actually be detrimental to endurance athletes because it may facilitate the use of muscle glycogen and lead to an earlier depletion in prolonged events. Although this theory has not been tested, in one of the more recent studies from the laboratory at Oregon State University, Manore and Leklem recommended that athletes not supplement their high-carbohydrate diets with B₆ above the RDA.

Vitamin B₆ supplementation has been used to treat the nausea of pregnancy, mental depression associated with the use of oral contraceptives, and premenstrual syndrome (PMS), but its effectiveness for these purposes has received mixed reviews. There appears to be little or no toxicity associated with moderate doses, but several recent case studies of individuals using 2–6 grams daily revealed such problems as loss of natural sensation from the limbs and an impaired gait. The National Research Council noted neurological symptoms with smaller dosages, averaging 117 mg per day for 6 months to 5 years.

Prudent Recommendations   Vitamin B₆ supplementation does not appear to be warranted for the physically active individual, and may be associated with some health risks if consumed in large doses for prolonged periods.

Vitamin B₁₂ (cyanocobalamin)

Vitamin B₁₂ (cyanocobalamin) is a water-soluble vitamin. It is part of the B complex and is the latest vitamin to be discovered.

RDA The adult RDA for B_{12} is 2 micrograms per day. The average diet contains about 5–15 micrograms. Slightly different allowances are made for other age groups; see Appendix A. The RDI is 6 micrograms.

Food Sources Vitamin B_{12} is found in good supply only in animal foods such as meat, fish, poultry, cheese, eggs, and milk. One glass of milk contains nearly 30 percent of the RDA. It is not found in plant foods such as fruits, vegetables, beans, and grains. However, it is present in microorganisms such as bacteria and yeast, which may be found in some plant foods, but the bioavailability of B_{12} from these sources is uncertain. Although B_{12} may be produced by microorganisms in the human bowel, the site of production is below the point of absorption.

Major Functions Vitamin B_{12} is a part of coenzymes present in all body cells and is essential in the synthesis of DNA. It works closely with folic acid, and both have important roles in the development of red blood cells. Vitamin B_{12} is also essential for the formation of the protective sheath around nerve fibers (the myelin sheath).

Deficiency Deficiency of vitamin B_{12} in humans due to inadequate dietary intake is rare. Even strict vegetarians appear to receive enough in their diet, either through the consumption of microorganisms or the use of fortified products. The body also stores a considerable amount in the liver, which may last for years. A deficiency normally is caused by the lack of an intrinsic factor in the gastrointestinal tract that is needed for B_{12} to be absorbed into the body. The major symptoms are a severe form of anemia, known as pernicious anemia, and nerve damage that may cause paralysis. Pregnant women, particularly vegans, need to obtain adequate B_{12} because a deficit may impair myelination in the newborn.

Because of its role in the formation of RBC, a deficiency of B_{12} resulting in pernicious anemia would be theorized to decrease aerobic endurance capacity. No research is available relative to the effect of a vitamin B_{12} deficiency upon performance, but other types of anemia have been shown to impair exercise performance.

Supplementation Relative to supplementation, vitamin B_{12} is one of the most abused vitamins in the athletic world, with some reports of athletes receiving large amounts by injection just prior to competition. The belief probably exists that if a little vitamin B_{12} can prevent anemia, then a lot of it will do something magical to increase performance capacity. However, several well-controlled studies have been conducted with B_{12} supplementation with the general conclusion that it will not help to increase metabolic functions, such as VO_2 max, or endurance performance.

A coenzyme form of B_{12}, known as Dibencobal, has been advertised for bodybuilders to increase muscle growth and strength. However, in a review for the National Strength and Conditioning Association, Williams noted the claims were based upon fallacious data and no data were available to support an ergogenic effect of Dibencobal.

Megadoses of vitamin B_{12} are considered to be relatively harmless. B_{12} megadoses may be an effective medical treatment for a particular type of anemia, but do not appear to benefit the active individual on a balanced diet.

Prudent Recommendations Vegans should consume food products fortified with vitamin B_{12}, such as fortified breakfast cereals or similar products. Individuals who consume animal products normally do not need vitamin B_{12} supplements, and there are no sound data that supplementation will enhance sport performance.

Folic acid (folate)

Folic acid, or **folate,** is a water-soluble vitamin. It is part of the B complex.

RDA The RDA for folic acid is 0.2 mg/day, or 200 micrograms, for adult males, and 180 micrograms for adult females. During pregnancy the RDA is increased to 400 micrograms per day, and it is 280 micrograms during the early stages of lactation.

However, as shall be noted below, some professional health organizations recommend the RDA be raised to about 400 micrograms for rather large segments of the population. Interestingly, the RDA for folate was 400 micrograms before 1989, the last time the RDA were revised. The RDI is 400 micrograms.

Food Sources Folic acid derives its name from foliage because it is found in green leafy vegetables like spinach. Other good sources include organ meats such as liver and kidney, dry beans, whole-grain products, and some fruits like oranges and bananas. One banana provides almost 10 percent of the RDA. Many breakfast cereals are fortified with folic acid, and some health professionals are recommending fortification of more cereal/grain products.

Major Functions Folic acid serves as part of a coenzyme that plays a critical role in the formation of DNA, the genetic material that regulates cell division. It is essential for maintaining normal production of RBC, one of the most rapidly dividing cells in the body. Folic acid is also critical during the very early stages of pregnancy when cells in the fetus divide rapidly. Researchers indicate during periods of rapid cell division large amounts of folic acid are needed to make DNA.

Deficiency   One national survey has reported folic acid intakes below the RDA for some Americans. Individuals who consume large quantities of alcohol and women who take oral contraceptives may experience deficiencies in folic acid, as these drugs may impair absorption of the vitamin. One of the major effects of folic acid deficiency is anemia, attributed to inadequate RBC regeneration. Anemia could impair delivery of oxygen and significantly impair performance in aerobic endurance events.

Women who are folic acid-deficient and become pregnant may give birth to children with neural tube defects (NTD) such as spina bifida, an incomplete closure of the tissue surrounding the spinal cord; such defects may cause paralysis and severe disabling conditions in the child. Approximately 2,500 infants are affected each year.

Folic acid deficiency is also associated with high plasma levels of homocysteine, an amino acid linked to vascular disease. In a recent meta-analysis of thirty-eight studies, Boushey reported strong evidence supporting high plasma homocysteine levels as a risk factor of vascular disease, such as coronary heart disease (CHD), stroke, and peripheral vascular disease (PVD).

Supplementation   One advocate of vitamin supplementation to athletes has reported that runners need additional folic acid to replace RBC that may be destroyed in heavy training programs. Unfortunately, no evidence is available to support this theory, nor are there any data that folic acid supplements will benefit physical performance. Only one study has been uncovered related to folate supplementation to athletes. Matter and her colleagues provided therapy (5 mg/day for 11 weeks) to female marathon runners who were diagnosed as being folate deficient. Although the folate therapy restored serum folate levels to normal, no improvements were noted in VO_2 max, maximum treadmill running time, peak lactate levels, or running speed at the lactate anaerobic threshold.

To be sure, anemia resulting from a folic acid deficiency could have serious consequences for endurance performance, but a balanced diet should prevent this condition from developing.

The United States Public Health Service has recommended that all women who have the potential to become pregnant should consume 400 micrograms of folic acid daily. Currently women consume about 200–300 micrograms per day, so they would either have to increase their intake of folate-rich foods or take a daily supplement containing about 200 micrograms. Because many women do not consume folic acid-rich foods, many health professionals recommend supplementation with either folic acid or multivitamin tablets. Oakley indicates adequate folic acid intake could prevent about 1,000 birth defects a year.

Adequate folic acid intake may also reduce homocysteine levels. Boushey indicates that 400 micrograms of folic acid appears to be sufficient to reduce plasma homocysteine levels maximally, and no additional effect is observed with larger doses. Although Oakley has estimated that adequate folic acid intake could prevent as many as 50,000 premature deaths from CHD, experts on folic acid note that research is needed to determine whether or not increased folic acid intake, including the use of folic acid supplements, could reduce the risk of CHD and other vascular diseases.

Megadoses of folic acid are considered harmless, although it is remotely possible that they could mask a vitamin B_{12} deficiency by preventing the development of anemia that would otherwise be discovered by a blood test. Unfortunately, folic acid does not prevent nerve damage, so the B_{12} deficiency may lead to paralysis if not detected.

Prudent Recommendations   All individuals should increase their intake of folic acid-rich foods, particularly vegetable sources, not only to obtain adequate folate but other healthful nutrients as well. Women in their childbearing years should obtain 400 micrograms daily, using a supplement to complement natural dietary sources if needed. Relative to the risk of vascular diseases, 400 micrograms again appears to be a reasonable amount that may be obtained through the diet, particularly with folic acid-fortified cereals, or with the use of a daily supplement. Those at risk for vascular disease might have their homocysteine level measured by a physician and undertake appropriate dietary strategies to reduce it if high.

Pantothenic acid

Pantothenic acid is a water-soluble vitamin. It is a factor in the B complex. Pantothenate is a salt of pantothenic acid.

RDA   The Food and Nutrition Board does not list the RDA of pantothenic acid in the main table, but the recommended ESADDI is 4–7 mg. The RDI is 10 mg.

Food Sources   Pantothenic acid is distributed widely in foods. It is found in all natural animal and plant products, but best sources include organ meats, eggs, legumes, yeasts, and whole grains. It should also be noted that highly refined, processed foods have lost most of the pantothenate content.

Major Functions   Pantothenic acid is an essential component of coenzyme A (CoA), which plays a central role in energy metabolism. You may recall acetyl CoA, which may be derived from carbohydrate, fat, and protein metabolism, is the principal substrate for the Krebs cycle. Pantothenic acid is also involved in gluconeogenesis, in the synthesis and breakdown of fatty acids, and in the synthesis of acetylcholine, a chemical released by the motor neuron to initiate muscle contraction.

Deficiency Except under experimentally induced conditions, deficiencies are not seen in humans. In such cases deficiencies have been reported to cause a variety of symptoms, including fatigue, muscle cramping, and impairment of motor coordination.

On a theoretical basis, pantothenic acid appears crucial to the active individual because it has an important function at the center of energy pathways. Several investigators have suggested that a deficiency would decrease the availability of acetyl CoA for the Krebs cycle and thus shift energy production to anaerobic glycolysis, which is less efficient. Because deficiencies of pantothenic acid have not been observed, such effects upon physical performance have not been studied.

Supplementation Research findings regarding the effect of pantothenic acid supplementation on physical performance are equivocal. Data from one well-designed study with supplements of pantothenic acid—2 grams per day for 14 days—suggested a beneficial effect by reducing oxygen consumption and lactate production during a submaximal exercise task at 75 percent VO_2 max for 40 minutes. This would suggest that pantothenic acid increased the efficiency of the exercise task. No data on maximal performance were provided. Unfortunately this report was available only as a brief abstract and very few details were presented. Conversely, another well-designed study revealed that 1 gram of pantothenic acid given daily for 2 weeks had no effect upon various blood measures or maximal performance in highly-trained distance runners. In his review, Keith analyzed six animal and human studies and suggested a possible relationship between exercise and pantothenic acid metabolism. However, only two studies involved humans, and the results were equivocal as noted above. Thus, more research is desirable.

Supplements of pantothenic acid appear to be relatively nontoxic. However, large doses of 10–20 grams have been known to cause diarrhea.

Prudent Recommendations Given the fact that pantothenic acid deficiency is rather nonexistent and there is little research to support a beneficial effect on health or physical performance at this time, supplementation is not recommended. A balanced diet should provide adequate pantothenic acid for the healthy, physically active individual.

Biotin

Biotin is a water-soluble vitamin in the B complex.

RDA No RDA has been established for biotin, but the recommended ESADDI is 30–100 micrograms. The RDI is 300 micrograms.

Food Sources Good dietary sources of biotin include organ meats such as liver, egg yolk, legumes such as peas and beans, and dark-green leafy vegetables. It is also synthesized in significant amounts in the intestines by bacteria.

Major Functions Biotin serves as a coenzyme for a variety of enzymes involved in amino acid metabolism and the synthesis of glucose and fatty acids. Because biotin is an important coenzyme for gluconeogenesis, it may have some implications relative to endurance performance.

Deficiency Deficiency states are rare but may occur when the diet contains large amounts of raw egg whites; a protein in the raw egg white binds biotin and prevents its absorption into the body. In such cases symptoms include loss of appetite, mental depression, dermatitis, and muscle pain. For athletes who consume eggs for their protein content it may be important to know that cooking the egg white eliminates this problem while providing the same amount of high-quality protein. It should also be mentioned in passing that raw eggs pose a risk of salmonella, a type of bacteria associated with food poisoning.

Supplementation No research into the effects of biotin supplementation and physical performance has been uncovered. Thus, there is no evidence that biotin supplementation increases physical performance capacity. Supplements of biotin appear to be harmless.

Prudent Recommendations It would appear that biotin supplements are unnecessary for the physically active individual.

Vitamin B complex

Because several of the vitamins in the B complex work together in energy metabolism, a number of studies have investigated the effect of either a deficiency or supplement of more than one vitamin upon physical performance. Several of these studies were well-controlled experiments during World War II, but contemporary evidence is also available.

Deficiency As might be expected from evidence presented on deficiencies of individual vitamins, a deficiency of several B vitamins together would negatively affect physical performance. This theory has been supported by those studies in which daily intake was reduced to less than 50 percent of the RDA. Several studies by van der Beek from the Netherlands have shown that a daily intake of less than one-third of the Dutch RDA for several of the B vitamins (B_1, B_2, B_6) and vitamin C leads to a dramatic decrease of VO_2 max and the anaerobic threshold in less than 4 weeks. The reduction in performance occurred even when other vitamins in the diet were supplemented at twice the RDA. In the most recent study VO_2 max decreased by 10 percent and the onset of blood lactate accumulation (anaerobic threshold) decreased approximately 20 percent after 8 weeks of a deficient diet. The findings support earlier research showing a significant decrease in endurance capacity with a B complex deficiency.

Supplementation   In general, research supports the idea that individuals who obtain adequate vitamins through a balanced diet will not improve performance through the use of B complex supplements. However, a number of studies, several with children, have shown that when a deficiency state is corrected by vitamin supplements, physical performance is restored to normal. Moreover, some research with large dosages of B_1, B_6, and B_{12} (about 60–200 times the RDA) has shown increases in fine motor control and performance in pistol shooting. Bonke suggested the beneficial effect was related to the role of these vitamins in promoting the development of neurotransmitters that induce relaxation. Additional research is needed to confirm this finding.

Several of the principal Dutch investigators in this area, such as van Erp-Baart and Saris, suggest that B complex supplementation may be useful in sports with a high energy expenditure if these athletes consume large amounts of foods with empty Calories—high-sugar and high-fat foods. This again stresses the importance of eating foods that are high in nutrient value.

Prudent Recommendations   Vitamin B complex supplementation does not appear to be needed for the individual consuming a balanced diet of wholesome, natural foods. However, athletes involved in intensive training for endurance type sports and consuming highly processed foods may benefit from a B complex supplement.

Vitamin C (ascorbic acid)

Vitamin C, or **ascorbic acid,** is a water-soluble vitamin. Its alleged effects upon health and physical performance have been the subject of much controversy.

RDA   The adult RDA and RDI for vitamin C is 60 mg/day. Slightly lower amounts are recommended for children. See Appendix A for specific recommendations.

Food Sources   The best food sources of vitamin C are fruits and vegetables, primarily the citrus fruits and the leafy parts of green vegetables. Excellent sources include oranges, grapefruit, broccoli, and salad greens. Other good sources are green peppers, potatoes, strawberries, and tomatoes. One orange contains the RDA. Milk, meats, and grain products are low in vitamin C.

Major Functions   Although vitamin C does not directly participate in enzyme-catalyzed conversions of substrate to product, Padh suggests it modifies mineral ions in the enzymes to make them active. Vitamin C has a number of different functions in the body, some of which have important implications for the active individual. Its principal role is in the synthesis of collagen, which is necessary for the formation and maintenance of the connective tissues of the body such as cartilage, tendon, and bone. Vitamin C is also involved in the formation of certain hormones and neurotransmitters, such as epinephrine (adrenaline), which are secreted during stressful situations like exercise. It helps absorb some forms of iron from the intestinal tract—about a two to fourfold increased absorption—and is involved in the synthesis of RBC. Vitamin C helps regulate the metabolism of folic acid, cholesterol, and amino acids. It is also important in the healing of wounds through the development of scar tissue. Finally, vitamin C is a powerful antioxidant.

Deficiency   Serious deficiencies of vitamin C are rare in industrialized societies because fresh or frozen fruits and vegetables are abundant. Also, the human body has a pool of vitamin C ranging from 1.5–3.0 grams. However, smoking, aspirin, oral contraceptives, and stress may increase the need for this vitamin. The major deficiency disease is scurvy, a disintegration of the connective tissue in the gums, skin, tendons, and cartilage that may develop in a month on a vitamin C-free diet. Typical symptoms include bleeding gums, rupture of blood vessels in the skin, impaired wound healing, muscle cramps, and weakness. Anemia also may develop.

It is obvious that many of these symptoms of a vitamin C deficiency would impair physical performance. Sensations of weakness could adversely affect all types of performance, whereas anemia would hamper aerobic endurance. Data available from several studies with vitamin C-deficient subjects do suggest such an effect, particularly the widely known Minnesota starvation experiments during World War II, directed by Ancel Keys.

Some epidemiological research has indicated that individuals with low plasma levels of vitamin C, most often associated with a vitamin deficiency, had a higher incidence of CHD. This may be related to the antioxidant effect of vitamin C, or to observations by Ness and others that adequate vitamin C intake is associated with increased serum HDL levels and reduced serum triglycerides.

Supplementation   The effect of vitamin C supplementation upon physical performance has received considerable attention, mainly because it is one of the vitamins that athletes consume in rather substantial quantities. Both early and contemporary research have shown that vitamin C supplementation improves physical performance in subjects who were vitamin C-deficient, but a thorough analysis of these studies supports the general conclusion that vitamin C supplementation does not increase physical performance capacity in subjects who are not vitamin deficient. No solid experimental evidence supports the use of megadoses of 5–10 grams that some athletes take. The interested reader may consult the reviews by Gerster and Keith.

On the other hand, because exercise is a stressor, some investigators have recommended that the active individual may need slightly more vitamin C than the RDA, for example, 200–300 milligrams per day. Some research with runners doing 5–10 miles a day does not support this viewpoint; in any case, this amount could easily be obtained by wise selection of foods high in vitamin C content. Keith also suggests vitamin C supplementation may be beneficial to heat acclimation, a topic that merits additional research with trained athletes.

Megadoses of vitamin C also have been claimed to have significant health benefits, particularly prevention of colds. Some research suggests the antihistamine effects of vitamin C may decrease the severity of some symptoms of a cold. For example, Peters and others reported 600 milligrams of vitamin C supplementation for 21 days prior to an ultramarathon reduced symptoms of respiratory tract infections, and in a recent review, Hemila reported other research with physically active individuals supporting these findings. However, recent research revealed that 200 milligrams of vitamin C daily will lead to full saturation of plasma and white blood cells, which should optimize immune functions associated with vitamin C. It may be possible that smaller amounts of vitamin C, such as 200 milligrams, may provide effects comparable to those seen with larger doses. In general, although the severity of the symptoms may be reduced, most studies find no effect of vitamin C supplementation to prevent colds.

Vitamin C supplementation has also been suggested to help prevent cardiovascular disease and cancer. Because vitamin C is an antioxidant, we will discuss it later in conjunction with the alleged effects of other vitamin antioxidants—vitamin E and beta-carotene.

There is some debate regarding the safety of megadoses of vitamin C. Several investigators have found that excessive amounts of vitamin C, such as 5–10 grams daily, may produce some undesirable side effects such as diarrhea; destruction of vitamin B_{12} in the diet; excessive excretion of vitamin B_6; decreased copper bioavailability; predisposition to gout, creating pain in the joints; and formation of kidney stones from oxalate salts, one of the breakdown products of vitamin C. Although for some individuals, increased iron absorption is a beneficial effect of vitamin C, it may be a major health problem for individuals prone to iron-storage disease, discussed in the next chapter. Excessive amounts of vitamin C also may interfere with the correct interpretation of certain blood and urine tests. Finally, several case studies revealed the development of a condition known as rebound scurvy when the individual stopped taking the supplements. The researchers suggested a mechanism whereby the increased activity of an enzyme in the body that destroys excess vitamin C during the supplement stages continued after the supplements were stopped, leading to a deficiency and symptoms of scurvy.

Conversely, others have reported megadoses to be relatively harmless because excessive amounts are excreted by the kidneys. They criticize the research upon which claims of adverse effects are based, noting that some of the conclusions rest on isolated case studies. Others support a middle viewpoint, noting that larger doses may be harmless to many, but certain individuals may be prone to problems, such as those who have a family history of kidney stones. For example, in a recent highly-controlled supplementation study, Levine and others saw evidence of oxalates appearing in the urine when subjects were supplemented with 1,000 milligrams of vitamin C per day. This was a short-term study and no observations of kidney stones were detected, but increased oxalates could lead to stone formation over time in those at risk. However, in a longer prospective study involving men between the ages of 40 and 75 with no history of kidney stones, Curhan and others found that after 6 years of follow-up there was no association between vitamin C intake—up to levels of 250–1,500 milligrams per day—and kidney stone formation. The National Research Council recommends against the routine use of large supplements. Megadose supplementation with vitamin C remains controversial, and the interested reader is referred to the opposing viewpoints presented by Herbert and Enstrom.

Prudent Recommendations   Recent reviews by the Consumers Union and by Weber and others suggest that adequate vitamin C intake may be associated with various health benefits for certain individuals. The amounts recommended approximate 200 milligrams per day, an amount easily obtained in the diet. Currently, the Consumers Union indicates it is premature to recommend vitamin C supplements, but it does recommend a diet rich in fruits and vegetables, which as previously noted, contain not only substantial amounts of vitamin C but other healthful substances as well. This is a solid recommendation for both the sedentary and physically active individual.

Vitamin Supplements: Ergogenic Aspects

Like the general population, the vast majority of athletes receive the RDA for vitamins in their daily diet. It is true that some studies report that certain groups of athletes receive less than the RDA for some vitamins or even have indicators of a biochemical deficiency, but Sarah Short of Syracuse University, in her exhaustive review of dietary surveys with athletes, and Larry Armstrong and Carl Maresh in their recent review, found that vitamin deficiency symptoms rarely are reported. Moreover, in his review, Michael Fogelholm reported that most studies have not found the vitamin status of athletes to be different from untrained controls. Nevertheless, elite endurance athletes, such as Tour de France cyclists, and the majority of both high school and college athletes believe vitamins are essential for success, and it is a matter of fact that many consume vitamin supplements either as nutritional insurance or in the hope of improving performance. For example, in a review of over fifty-one studies involving data on more than ten thousand male and female athletes in fifteen sports, Sobol and Marquart reported that the overall mean prevalence of athletes' supplement use was 46 percent. Elite athletes use supplements more than college or high school athletes, and women more often than men. Athletes appear to use supplements more than the general population, and some take high doses that may lead to nutritional problems.

In recent years some vitamin manufacturers have turned their attention to the physically active individual, suggesting through advertisements that their special product enhances athletic performance. In her review, Priscilla Clarkson of the University of Massachusetts suggested such advertisements were a major reason for the use of vitamin supplements by athletes.

Should physically active individuals take vitamin supplements?

There may be some good reasons for physically active individuals to take vitamin supplements. For example, in certain types of athletic activity such as wrestling, gymnastics, and ballet, participants may undertake prolonged semi-starvation or starvation diets. As discussed in Chapter 10, this is not a recommended procedure, but some athletes may do it to obtain or maintain an optimal body weight for competition. In such cases, when the energy intake may be well below 1,200–1,600 Calories per day, many surveys have shown that the athlete may not be receiving enough vitamins. Research suggests that vitamin depletion, mainly the water-soluble vitamins, can occur rapidly in humans on low-Calorie diets and that these vitamins should be replaced daily. Athletes may also need vitamin supplementation if they are subsisting on poor diets, as discussed in the next section.

However, as is obvious from the evidence presented in this chapter, the athlete who is on a balanced diet has no need for vitamin supplementation to improve performance. Nevertheless, some interesting hypotheses suggest antioxidant vitamin supplements may help prevent muscle tissue damage during training, and a variety of special vitamin-like compounds have been marketed specifically for athletes.

Can the antioxidant vitamins prevent muscle damage during training?

It has been known for years that certain forms of physical training for sports, particularly intense training, can induce muscle damage and soreness. Eccentric muscle contractions, such as those incurred in the quadriceps muscle when running downhill, may cause mechanical trauma to the muscle and connective tissue resulting in soreness dur-

ing the following days. Research also suggests that exhaustive maximal exercise induces free radical generation, and excessive production of free radicals may induce lipid peroxidation, possibly damaging the integrity of cellular and subcellular membranes in the muscles, leading to muscle soreness. However, ongoing physical training itself increases the activity of the free radical-scavenging enzymes, such as superoxide dismutase, to help minimize recurrent damage and thus provides a protective effect. For example, Niess and others recently reported that although exhaustive exercise could induce free radical damage to DNA, trained subjects, compared to untrained subjects, experienced less damage.

For several reasons, in recent years considerable research attention has been devoted to the effect of various antioxidant supplements to reduce exercise-induced muscle damage. Although antioxidants have not been shown to reliably improve physical performance, theoretically, prevention of muscle tissue damage may enable the athlete to train more effectively, the desired result being improvement in competition. Some endurance athletes will train at altitude in attempts to enhance their oxygen-delivery ability, and as noted earlier in this chapter, vitamin E supplements may convey some benefits when exercising at altitude. Additionally, older individuals may be more susceptible to oxidative stress during exercise, for optimal functioning of the free radical-scavenging enzymes appears to decline with the aging process. Millions of older individuals perform aerobic exercise for the related health benefits and often become involved in various forms of athletic competition. With increasing focus on competition for older athletes, for example, international competition for athletes over age 40, it may not be just coincidental that one of the most popular vitamin supplements for masters runners is vitamin E. Olympic athletes are reported to take antioxidant supplements and some companies are taking advantage of athletes' interest in antioxidants, marketing a product with "live enzyme foods" called Runners Edge and Exercise Edge. Because there may be some harm associated with excess antioxidant supplements, the United States Olympic Committee recently issued some guidelines recommending that athletes should consider limiting their intake of beta-carotene to 3–20 mg, vitamin C to 250–1,000 mg, and vitamin E to 150–400 IU.

Numerous studies have been conducted to evaluate the effect of antioxidant supplements on exercise-induced muscle damage and, in some studies, on performance. The designs of these studies have varied, including differences in subjects (animals versus humans), methods to induce muscle soreness (e.g., downhill running versus level running), the type and amount of supplement given, and the biochemical markers used to assess muscle damage. The most common supplements used were vitamins E and C, and beta-carotene, but coenzyme Q10, selenium, and other substances have also been used. Some studies used "antioxidant cocktails" consisting of approximately 800 IU of vitamin E, 1,000 milligrams of vitamin C, and 10–30 milligrams of beta-carotene. The markers of muscle tissue damage include serum enzymes that may leak from the muscle such as creatine kinase (CK) and lactic acid dehydrogenase (LDH), end products of lipid peroxidation such as malondialdehyde (MDA), myoglobin leakage from the muscle tissue, and others.

Overall, the results of these studies may be regarded as promising. A number of studies have shown some beneficial effects of antioxidant supplementation, that is, reduced markers of muscle tissue damage when compared to the placebo treatment. Benefits have been reported for both young and old physically active individuals. On the other hand, other studies have reported no significant benefits. Most studies used multiple markers of muscle tissue damage, and in some cases one marker of muscle damage would be improved by the antioxidant supplements but another would be unaffected. Some studies compared different antioxidants, for example, C versus E, reporting a beneficial effect of one but not the other.

The role of antioxidants in exercise was the subject of several recent reviews, with somewhat diverging opinions regarding the ability of antioxidant supplementation to prevent muscle tissue damage. Summarizing the research presented at an American College of Sports Medicine symposium, Alan Goldfarb noted that although the literature suggests trained individuals have a greater need for antioxidants, further investigations are needed to determine the viability of antioxidant supplements in preventing exercise-induced lipid peroxidation and muscle damage. This viewpoint has been reinforced by other experts, such as Mitchell Kanter, who noted recently that although consuming an antioxidant supplement to ward off the possible ill-effects of exercise has much theoretical merit, the facts remain to be determined. However, in their analysis of human studies, Dekkers and others concluded that dietary supplementation with antioxidant vitamins has favorable effects on lipid peroxidation, and although several points of discussion still exist, they believe antioxidant vitamins do play a role in exercise-induced muscle damage and that vitamin supplementation can be recommended to individuals performing regular, heavy exercise. Nevertheless, all reviewers indicate more research is needed to address this issue and to provide guidelines for recommendations to athletes.

Although Kanter and others recently noted that short-term vitamin E supplementation (1,000 IU for 1 week) had no effects on markers of muscle tissue damage following prolonged aerobic exercise, the investigators indicated it may generate some health-related benefits by reducing the sensitivity of LDL to oxidation. As you may recall, oxidized LDL is believed to be associated with the development of atherosclerosis. The role of vitamin E and other antioxidants in preventing chronic diseases is discussed in the section on health aspects of vitamin supplementation.

Prudent Recommendations Although Kim LeBlanc, a sports-oriented physician, noted there is no conclusive data to support antioxidant supplementation to improve athletic performance, he also indicated it is not unreasonable to support supplementation for limiting the effects of oxidative stress. Nevertheless, the recommended strategy is to obtain vitamins naturally from food. Increasing the consumption of fruits, fruit juices, and vegetables will enable athletes to obtain the recommended amounts of beta-carotene (10–30 milligrams) and vitamin C (250–1,000 milligrams) but it would be difficult to obtain 150–400 IU of vitamin E through natural dietary sources. For the athlete who wants to supplement vitamin E, inexpensive over-the-counter preparations are available in 100 and 400 IU capsules.

How effective are the special vitamin supplements marketed for athletes?

Special athletic vitamin packs have been appearing on the market—even in single packets at your local convenience store—that have been advertised as a means for the athlete to reach peak performance. Many of these have simply been multivitamin-mineral supplements, while others have been special concoctions like bee pollen and ginseng. Five such products will be highlighted.

Multivitamin-Mineral Supplements Because in human metabolism vitamins often work together, and often in conjunction with minerals, the ergogenic potential of multivitamin-mineral compounds has been studied for half a century. In a review of the older research, Williams reported that although results of a number of studies suggested ergogenic effects, the experimental designs were usually poorly controlled. In contrast, contemporary research indicates that such supplements, consumed for substantial periods, are not ergogenic for the athlete on a balanced diet. Barnett and Conlee found that 4 weeks of supplementation with a multivitamin-mineral compound (including additional amino acids) had no influence on maximal oxygen uptake. From Timothy Noakes' laboratory in South Africa, Weight conducted a thorough 9-month double-blind, placebo, crossover study. Although multivitamin-mineral supplements did raise blood levels of some vitamins, the authors reported that 3 months of supplementation did not improve maximal oxygen uptake, the anaerobic (lactate) threshold, treadmill run time to exhaustion, or running performance in a 15-kilometer time trial. Similar results have been reported by Labadarios, also from Noakes' laboratory. A recent well-designed double-blind placebo study conducted by Schrijver and others, using a supplement containing ten times the RDA for iron and all vitamins except K for 4 months, revealed no beneficial effect upon physical performance capacity as measured by heart rate, VO_2 max, or running performance in the Cooper test (1.5 miles). Anita Singh and her colleagues provided either a high-potency multivitamin-mineral supplement or a placebo to 22 healthy, physically active males for 90 days. The vitamin dosages ranged from 300 to 6,000 percent of the RDA. Although serum levels of many of the vitamins increased, there were no significant effects on physiological variables during a 90-minute run, nor were there any effects on maximal heart rate, VO_2 max, or time to exhaustion. Finally, Richard Telford, the chief exercise physiologist and nutritionist at the Australian Institute of Sport, and his colleagues matched 82 nationally ranked Australian athletes and assigned them to either a supplement or placebo treatment. The supplement contained an assortment of vitamins and minerals, ranging from about 100 to 5,000 percent of the RDA. The supplement was taken for approximately 7–8 months, and the subjects were tested on a variety of sport specific tests (e.g., swim bench) as well as common tests of strength (torque), anaerobic power (400-meter run), and aerobic endurance (12-minute run and VO_2 max). These investigators reported no significant effect of the supplement on any measure of physical performance when compared with athletes whose vitamin and mineral RDA were met by dietary intake.

Thus, all of the current reputable research refutes an ergogenic effect of multivitamin-mineral supplements in adequately nourished athletes.

Prudent recommendations Although multivitamin-mineral supplements may not enhance athletic performance in well-nourished athletes, those involved in weight-control sports with limited caloric intake might consider taking a simple one-a-day supplement with no more than 100 percent of the RDA for the essential vitamins and minerals.

Bee Pollen Bee pollen has been marketed almost specifically for athletes, primarily runners, as a means to improve performance. Chemical analysis of bee pollen reveals it is a mixture of vitamins, minerals, amino acids, and other nutrients. Although no specific physiological effects of bee pollen have been documented, theoretical ergogenic effects are based on some of the roles that vitamins have in the body. Advertising claims for bee pollen cite questionable research: a field study showing faster recovery rates in athletes who took pollen supplements. However, six well-designed studies using double-blind placebo protocols revealed that supplementation with bee pollen had no significant effect upon VO_2 max, other physiological responses to exercise, endurance capacity, or rate of recovery from exhausting exercise.

Prudent recommendations Bee pollen supplements are not recommended for physically active individuals. Moreover, caution is necessary as some individuals may experience an allergic reaction.

Vitamin B₁₅ Another product advertised to improve athletic performance is **vitamin B₁₅.** It should be noted, however, that B₁₅ is not considered to be a vitamin because no specific disease state is associated with a deficiency. Indeed, vitamin B₁₅ and products marketed with vitamin B₁₅ qualities do not appear to have any definite chemical identity but may be composed of a number of different substances. Pangamic acid is a term often used in conjunction with B₁₅; one patented form of B₁₅ is calcium pangamate, a mixture of calcium gluconate and dimethylglycine (DMG), an amino acid. These substances have been labeled as the active ingredients in vitamin B₁₅.

The increasing popularity and use of vitamin B₁₅ as an ergogenic aid in the 1980s was based upon Soviet research with rats, suggesting an improvement in aerobic oxidative processes during exercise. Claims of its effectiveness by a world-champion boxer and a professional football team helped bolster its sales to athletes. However, these claims are not supported by reputable research. Four studies revealed that B₁₅ supplementation does not improve cardiovascular or metabolic responses during exercise, VO_2 max, or endurance capacity. Thus, contemporary research supports the viewpoint that B₁₅ is not an effective ergogenic aid.

Prudent recommendations Vitamin B₁₅ supplements are not recommended for physically active individuals. Moreover, analysis of several vitamin B₁₅ products revealed the presence of several compounds that could be hazardous to one's health.

CoQ₁₀ The compound **CoQ₁₀,** also known as coenzyme Q_{10} and ubiquinone, is actually a lipid but has characteristics common to vitamins; its chemical structure is similar to vitamin K. CoQ₁₀ is found in the mitochondria of all mammalian tissues, but concentrations are relatively high in the heart and other organs in humans. It plays an important role in oxidative metabolism within the mitochondria, facilitating the aerobic generation of ATP as part of the electron transfer system. CoQ₁₀ also appears to function as an antioxidant. It has been used therapeutically for treatment of cardiovascular disease since 1965 because it may protect heart tissue from damage associated with inadequate oxygen, although Webb recently noted that not all scientists agree it has shown beneficial applications.

Because some studies have shown that CoQ₁₀ may improve heart function, maximal oxygen uptake, and exercise performance in cardiac patients, it has been theorized to be ergogenic for athletes. Moreover, Bucci has cited a number of studies indicating that CoQ₁₀ levels are lower in trained athletes compared to sedentary controls and that oral supplementation with CoQ₁₀ will increase tissue levels, two factors providing theoretical support for its role as an ergogenic. Theoretically, CoQ₁₀ should benefit endurance performance because of its role in aerobic metabolism. However, Demopoulous and others suggest CoQ₁₀ might actually be ergolytic, indicating that when taken orally it may actually auto-oxidize, producing free radicals and damaging the mitochondria.

Are CoQ_{10} supplements ergogenic? In his book on nutritional ergogenics, Bucci cites results from six studies with sedentary young men, sedentary middle-aged women, aerobically trained volleyball players, male professional basketball players, and endurance runners supporting an ergogenic effect of CoQ_{10}, noting improvements in one or more of the following: VO_2 max, exercise performance, indicators of enhanced aerobic capacity, and improved antioxidant function. Most of these studies were presented in a book entitled *Biomedical and Clinical Aspects of Coenzyme Q* and do not appear to have been published in refereed scientific journals. Moreover, a careful review of these studies indicated each suffered one or more flaws in proper experimental design, including no control group, no placebo, no randomization of order in which CoQ_{10} or placebo was given, and use of a submaximal heart rate exercise task to predict maximal oxygen uptake.

There are few published studies regarding the effect of CoQ_{10} on exercise performance, but those that are available do not support its effectiveness as an ergogenic. For example, Weston and others, using 1 milligram of CoQ_{10} per kilogram body weight daily for 28 days, reported no beneficial effects on oxygen uptake, substrate use, or cycle ergometer exercise time to exhaustion in trained male cyclists and triathletes. Although serum CoQ_{10} levels were increased, Braun and others reported no effect of 100 milligrams daily for 8 weeks on submaximal physiological indicators of enhanced aerobic capacity, VO_2 max, time to exhaustion on a bicycle ergometer, or lipid peroxidation, indicating no effect on either aerobic metabolism or antioxidant function. In a well-designed, double-blind, placebo, crossover study, Laaksonen and others supplemented both young and old physically trained males with 120 milligrams of CoQ_{10} per day for 6 weeks, and reported no significant effect on maximal oxygen uptake or on time to exhaustion in a progressive cycling task following 60 minutes of submaximal cycling. Actually, performance time in the placebo trial was significantly greater than the CoQ_{10} trial. Additionally, there were no effects of the CoQ_{10} supplement on MDA, a marker of lipid peroxidation. In yet another study from the Karolinska Institute in Sweden, Malm and others reported that CoQ_{10} supplementation (120 milligrams per day for 20 days) exerted no effect on fifteen high-intensity, anaerobic 10-second sprint tests on a cycle ergometer with 50 seconds recovery between each sprint. These investigators noted that, compared to the placebo groups, subjects taking the CoQ_{10} supplement showed evidence of muscle tissue damage. In actuality, the placebo group improved their performance in the cycle sprints, but the supplement group did not.

CoQ_{10} is also one of the ingredients in a supplement (also containing vitamin E, inosine, and cytochrome C) widely advertised for endurance athletes, particularly triathletes. In a recent double-blind, placebo, crossover study, Snider and others reported that 4 weeks of supplementation with this commercial product had no ergogenic effect on an endurance task that consisted of a 90-minute treadmill run at 70 percent VO_2 max followed by a cycling test to exhaustion at 70 percent VO_2 max.

At the present time, research findings appear to be equivocal relative to the ergogenic efficacy of CoQ_{10}, but the published well-designed studies do not support an ergogenic effect. Bucci presents some questionable data supportive of an ergogenic effect of CoQ_{10} supplementation, but some of the studies showing no ergogenic effect may not have been available at the time of his review. The effect of CoQ_{10} supplementation on physical performance merits additional research efforts, and Bucci even notes that although CoQ_{10} is poised to be an ergogenic, more research is needed to confirm its effect on sports performance. Bucci notes that the long-term safety of CoQ_{10} has been thoroughly documented.

Prudent recommendations   Given these findings, CoQ_{10} supplementation is not recommended for the physically active individual.

Ginseng   Extracts derived from the plant family Araliaceae contain numerous chemicals that may influence human physiology, the most important being the glycosides, or ginsenosides. Collectively, these extracts are referred to as **ginseng,** and their physiologic effects vary depending on the plant species, the part of the plant used, and the place of origin. The most common forms of ginseng include Chinese or Korean (Panax ginseng), American (Panax quinquefolium), Japanese (Panax japonicum), and Russian/Siberian (Eleutherococcus senticosus). Eleutherococcus senticosus is recognized by some as a legitimate form of ginseng and its ginsenosides are also referred to as eleutherosides.

Ginseng has been marketed in various forms as a means to enhance health and physical performance. Although the underlying mechanisms are unknown, ginseng is believed to influence neural and hormonal activity in the body. The most prevalent theory suggests ginseng may stimulate the hypothalamus, the part of the brain that controls the pituitary gland, an endocrine gland often referred to as the master gland. The pituitary gland releases hormones that influence other endocrine glands in the body, such as the adrenal gland. The adrenal gland releases cortisol, a hormone involved in the response to stress. The Russians conducted much of the early research with ginseng, and used the term "adaptogens" to characterize its ability to increase resistance to the catabolic effects of stress. Because excessive stress is believed to influence the development of a number of chronic diseases, particularly coronary heart disease, ginseng has been used for its alleged therapeutic properties.

The Russians believed that ginseng helped develop resistance not only to mental stress, but also to the physical stress of intense exercise training. Other theories suggest ginseng supplementation may influence physical performance in other ways as well, such as increased cardiac function, blood flow, and oxygen transport during exercise; increased oxygen utilization and decreased lactic acid levels during exercise; enhanced muscle glycogen synthesis after exercise; and a positive effect on nitrogen or protein balance. In essence, given these theorized anti-stress effects, restorative effects, and metabolic effects, ginseng supplementation is theorized to enhance sport performance by allowing athletes to train more intensely and by influencing physiological processes associated with an antifatiguing effect that increase stamina during competition. It should be noted that although numerous theories have been advanced in attempts to explain the alleged ergogenic effects of ginseng supplementation, an underlying mechanism has yet to be determined.

Although numerous studies investigated the ergogenic possibilities of ginseng supplementation, few were well-controlled. Research design flaws included no control or placebo group, no double-blind protocol, no randomization of order of treatment, and no statistical analysis. Highlighting these methodological problems in a recent extensive review of the ergogenic effect of ginseng supplementation, Michael Bahrke and William Morgan concluded that there is a lack of controlled research demonstrating the ability of ginseng to improve or prolong performance.

Subsequent to the review by Bahrke and Morgan, several well-controlled studies evaluated the ergogenic effects of both standardized ginseng extracts and commercial products and reported no significant effects. For example, Dowling and others reported no effect of Eleutherococcus senticosus on metabolic (oxygen uptake and lactic acid accumulation), physiologic (heart rate and ventilation), or psychologic (ratings of perceived exertion) responses to submaximal and maximal running. Using a similar research protocol but with cycling, Engels and Wirth reported no ergogenic effect of Panax ginseng. Other well-controlled studies have found no ergogenic effect of other forms of ginseng on cycling or running time to exhaustion.

Currently, well-controlled research does not support the effectiveness of ginseng supplementation as a sports ergogenic. Moreover, although most commercial ginseng preparations appear to have relatively low acute or chronic toxicity when taken in dosages recommended by the manufacturer, a ginseng-abuse syndrome has been reported, with such symptoms as high blood pressure, nervousness, and sleeplessness. These effects may be attributed to the postulated stimulant effect of ginseng, or possibly to additional substances in the commercial preparation, such as the stimulant ephedrine. For athletes involved in sports that may use drug testing, the use of ginseng products containing ephedrine could lead to disqualification.

Some research suggests long-term ginseng supplementation may prevent some adverse effects of stress on the immune system. Although not studied extensively in athletes, a healthier immune system could help prevent illness or some of the symptoms of the overtraining syndrome during high-intensity training.

Prudent recommendations Given the available scientific evidence, ginseng supplements cannot be recommended. The consumer should also be aware that commercial ginseng products may suffer from quality control. A recent assay of fifty commercial ginseng preparations indicated that over 10 percent of the products contained no detectable ginsenosides, and the amount in the remaining products varied from 1.9–9.0 percent.

Individuals who desire to experiment with long-term ginseng supplementation should consult with their physicians, because ginseng use may exacerbate various health problems, such as high blood pressure. Long-term use may also lead to the ginseng-abuse syndrome in some individuals.

What's the bottom line regarding vitamin supplements for athletes?

Given the available scientific data, there does not appear to be a very strong case supporting an ergogenic effect of any single vitamin, vitamin-mineral combinations, or the various vitamin-like compounds. As noted, additional research is warranted for those that have some limited support as an ergogenic, for example, the effect of vitamin E on performance at altitude. At the present time, the recommended advice is to obtain adequate vitamin nutrition through a well-planned diet. For athletes who feel they need to take a vitamin-mineral supplement, the typical one-a-day supplement containing 50–150 percent of the RDA for all vitamins (except K) and minerals may be recommended.

However, as discussed in the next section, some physicians recommend athletes involved in intensive exercise training should consume antioxidant vitamin supplements, not for their possible ergogenic effects but rather for health reasons.

Vitamin Supplements: Health Aspects

Vitamins continue to be one of the most used and abused supplements in the United States today. Certain segments of the population may have a vitamin intake below the RDA, but no disease states are usually associated with these lower intakes, probably because of the safety factor incorporated in the RDA. The vast majority of Americans receive the RDA for all vitamins in their daily diets. Nevertheless, certain vitamin pill manufacturers and advertisers have perpetuated the myth that the average American diet contains insufficient amounts of vitamins, a potential cause of many health problems. We now have vitamin supplements on the market that have been designed, or so the manufacturers imply, to combat the stress of everyday life, prevent the common cold, reduce blood cholesterol, and prevent baldness, aging, arthritis, and a host of other diseases, including cancer. These are enticing claims. It is no wonder that approximately 35–40 percent of the U.S. population spends over five billion dollars yearly on vitamin supplements. Vitamins are big business. They are marketed for all segments of the population, from infant formulas to geriatric supplements.

In the preceding sections we have already covered each individual vitamin and the possible effects of deficiencies and supplementation upon health (review Table 7.1 for a broad overview). This section summarizes prudent dietary recommendations for optimal vitamin nutrition, including the possible use of supplements, relative to health.

Can I obtain the vitamins I need through my diet?

If you read the advertisements of vitamin supplement manufacturers, you are left with the impression that it is difficult, if not impossible, to obtain adequate vitamin nutrition through the typical American diet. In contrast, the American Medical Association (AMA) and the National Research Council support the view that a balanced diet will satisfy all nutrient needs of the healthy individual. There is some truth to both positions, for the typical diet of some individuals may not be a balanced diet.

Vitamin intake may be inadequate for several reasons. First, the refining process of many foods removes vitamins. For example, the preparation of flour for white bread removes many of the vitamins found in the outer parts of the grain. Although some of these vitamins are returned by an enrichment process, not all are restored. Thus, many processed foods may be lower in total vitamin content than their natural counterparts. In some cases, however, processing actually increases the vitamin content of foods. Examples include the fortification of milk with vitamins A and D and use of vitamin C as an antioxidant preservative in some foods. Second, improper storage of foods may lead to vitamin losses. Once fruits and vegetables are harvested, the vitamin content begins to diminish. In general, such foods should be refrigerated or frozen in airtight containers as applicable and stored in dark places to minimize vitamin losses caused by exposure to air, heat, and light. Third, improper preparation may also lead to significant vitamin losses from foods. Prolonged cooking, excessive heat, and cooking vegetables in water should be avoided. Steaming, microwave cooking, and the use of boiling bags and waterless cookware will help retain the natural vitamin content of foods. Thus, the individual who consumes a diet high in processed foods with empty Calories and does not prepare foods properly may receive less than the RDA for several vitamins.

The key to adequate vitamin nutrition is to consume a balanced diet of natural foods that have a high nutrient density. Buy foods in their natural state and store them properly as soon as possible. Prepare them to eat so as to minimize vitamin losses.

The position of the ADA is that the best nutritional strategy for promoting optimal health and reducing the risk of chronic disease is to obtain essential nutrients through a wide variety of foods. In this way, other nutrients, particularly minerals, will be obtained at the same time, as they also are natural constituents of the food we eat. Vitamins often work in conjunction with minerals, such as vitamin D and calcium, vitamin B_6 and magnesium, and vitamin E and selenium. By obtaining vitamins through the selection of a balanced diet, we may be assured of receiving sufficient amounts of other nutrients necessary for optimal physiological functioning, in addition to various phytochemicals that may also confer some health benefits. Moreover, it is recommended that the active individual be selective in choosing foods. The stress of exercise can increase the utilization of some water-soluble vitamins, but these can be replaced easily if the extra Calories expended during exercise are replaced by foods with high nutrient density, that is, foods rich in vitamins and minerals. Table 7.2 presents a quick overview of foods containing substantial amounts of the major vitamins, while Table 7.3 presents a list of ten foods, totaling approximately 1,200 Calories, that will provide at least 100 percent of the RDA for every vitamin, assuming adequate sunlight for vitamin D and intestinal synthesis of biotin and vitamin K.

Why are vitamin supplements often recommended?

There are many bona fide reasons for vitamin supplementation. For example, pregnancy and lactation increase the RDA for all vitamins, so many physicians recommend a general vitamin supplement. In addition, certain diseases or disorders increase the need for a specific vitamin. An impaired ability to absorb fat decreases the availability of the fat-soluble vitamins, while a lack of the intrinsic factor necessitates injections of vitamins B_{12}. An intolerance to certain foods, such as milk, may limit the intake of several important vitamins, such as riboflavin and vitamin D. Drugs taken to treat or prevent illness may lead to problems, such as antibiotics that kill intestinal bacteria and decrease the production of vitamin K. In such cases, specific vitamins are prescribed by physicians.

Vitamin supplements also have been recommended for individuals who may be at risk for a deficiency because of their particular life-style. Individuals who are on low-Calorie diets, particularly less than 1,200 Calories, may need a vitamin supplement in order to obtain the RDA. Even if adequate in Calories, a poor diet in itself will also contain an insufficient amount of some vitamins. Other practices, such as smoking, alcohol consumption, and the use of drugs such as aspirin and oral contraceptives, increase the need for certain vitamins. In such cases, if an individual feels he or she is not receiving a balanced diet for some reason, most medical authorities agree that a simple, balanced vitamin supplement containing 50–150 percent of the RDA will not do any harm. There are a

Table 7.2 High-vitamin-content foods

Vitamin	Foods
Vitamin A	Beef liver, fish liver oils, egg yolks Milk, butter, cheese, fortified margarine Orange vegetables (carrots, sweet potatoes) Green vegetables (spinach, collards)
Thiamin (Vitamin B₁)	Pork, legumes (dried peas and beans) Milk Nuts Whole-grain and enriched cereal products (bread) All vegetables Fruits
Riboflavin (Vitamin B₂)	Meats, liver, kidneys, eggs Milk, cheese Whole-grain and enriched cereal products Wheat germ Green leafy vegetables
Niacin	Lean meats, organ meats (liver), poultry Legumes, peanuts, peanut butter Whole-grain and enriched cereal products
Vitamin B₆ (Pyridoxine)	Meat, poultry, fish Whole-grain cereals, seeds Vegetables
Pantothenic acid	Meats, poultry, fish Milk, cheese Legumes Whole-grain products
Folic Acid	Meats, liver, eggs Milk Legumes Whole wheat products Green leafy vegetables
Vitamin B₁₂ (Cyanocobalamin)	Meats, poultry, fish, eggs Milk, cheese, butter (not found in plant foods)
Biotin	Meats, liver, egg yolks Legumes, nuts Vegetables
Vitamin C	Citrus fruits, oranges, grapefruit, melons, berries, tomatoes Broccoli, brussels sprouts, cabbage, salad greens, green peppers, cauliflower
Vitamin D	Liver, tuna, salmon, cod liver oil, eggs Fortified milk and margarine
Vitamin E	Legumes, nuts, seeds Margarine, salad oils, wheat germ oil Green leafy vegetables
Vitamin K	Pork, liver, meats Green leafy vegetables, cauliflower, spinach, cabbage

Table 7.3 1,200 Calorie diet containing at least 100% of the RDA for each vitamin

Food	Amount
Milk, skim, fortified with vitamins A and D	2 cups
Carrot	1 medium
Orange	1 average
Bread, whole wheat	4 slices
Chicken breast, roasted	3 ounces
Broccoli	1 stalk
Margarine	1 tablespoon
Cereal, Grape-Nuts	2 ounces
Tuna fish, in water	3 ounces
Cauliflower	1/2 cup

number of preparations on the market that contain the daily RDA of most vitamins. However, the American Dietetic Association recommends low levels that do not exceed the RDA for those who chose to use supplements, and the American Medical Association suggests that use of larger amounts be under medical supervision. Nevertheless millions of Americans consume vitamin megadoses without such supervision.

Why do individuals take vitamin megadoses?

We have all heard of the adage "if a little bit is good, more is better." As already noted, vitamin nutrition for optimal health can be obtained from a proper diet. The RDA for all thirteen vitamins totals approximately 100 milligrams, yet some individuals are consuming prodigious amounts of vitamins—thousands of milligrams—via supplements, for a variety of health reasons, particularly to help deter the effects of aging and the development of various chronic diseases. For example, as discussed previously, niacin supplements may be useful therapy for reducing serum cholesterol levels. In general, however, Kim and others reported no increase in longevity among vitamin and mineral supplement users in the United States. Nevertheless, vitamins C and E are the two most popular supplements, and many individuals are taking beta-carotene supplements probably because all three possess antioxidant properties. Although most authorities indicate that much needs to be learned, they also note that some interesting data are emerging in relation to the health aspects of antioxidants.

Do foods rich in antioxidant vitamins help deter disease?

As discussed on pages 209–210, free radicals may be very reactive with body tissues, causing cellular damage by oxidation of unsaturated fats in cellular and subcellular membranes. Free radicals are theorized to contribute to the aging process and to the development of more than sixty diseases, including cardiovascular disease and cancer. Discussing the free radical theory of aging, Koltover estimated that our life span could be 250 years, but for the damages due to free radicals. Various antioxidant enzymes in the cells counteract undesirable effects of free radicals, but there is increasing evidence that what we eat may also help to prevent certain adverse health effects associated with free radicals.

Numerous epidemiological studies have indicated that diets rich in vegetables and fruits are associated with lower risk for subsequent development of several forms of cancer. Several recent reviews, including those by Gaziano and Hennekens and by Steinmetz and Potter indicated that the evidence for a protective effect of increased consumption of vegetables and fruits, foods rich in antioxidant vitamins, is consistent for cancers of the stomach, esophagus, lung, endometrium, pancreas, and colon, and that the most effective are raw vegetables. The precise mechanism underlying this possible protective effect is not known, although phytochemicals found in some vegetables may block tumor formation. Other investigators believe the antioxidant vitamins (vitamin C, vitamin E, beta-carotene) found naturally in vegetables and fruits may confer the protective effect, for various epidemiologic studies have shown that high serum levels of some antioxidant vitamins are associated with a decreased risk of cancer. In a review, Gladys Block presented biochemical data suggesting that optimal antioxidant intake may protect against environmental factors, such as cigarette smoke and polluted air, that may generate free radicals and subsequent cancer. Antioxidant vitamins may also strengthen the immune system, a major defense against cancer, particularly as we grow older. Meydani indicated cells of the immune system have a very high content of polyunsaturated fatty acids, which makes them susceptible to oxidative damage. When oxidized, polyunsaturated fats may produce PGE_2, an eicosanoid that may suppress immune function by interfering with several major functions, such as the activity of T cells. Meydani indicated vitamin E supplementation may enhance T cell-mediated immune functions.

Research also suggests that dietary antioxidant vitamins may help to prevent cardiovascular disease. Two recent epidemiologic studies indicated high intakes of vitamin E are associated with a reduced risk for coronary heart disease. Rimm and others reported a reduced risk in men, while Kushi and Stampfer, with their associates, reported a reduced risk in women. Prevention of oxidation of LDL cholesterol and the subsequent formation of atherosclerosis is theorized to be the primary underlying mechanism. Antioxidants may also reduce factors that may lead to blood clot formation, including platelet aggregation and coagulability.

Other health problems, such as cataracts and age-related macular degeneration in the eyes, may be prevented by optimal antioxidant nutrition, particularly vitamin E. The current recommendation associated with the Healthy North American Diet is to eat more fruits and vegetables, and the National Cancer Institute has recently sponsored a campaign called "Five a Day for Better Health," meaning to eat at least five servings of fruits and vegetables daily. The point is stressed that five is the minimum number of servings and more should be consumed, hopefully five servings *each* of fruits and vegetables.

Do antioxidant vitamin supplements help deter disease?

If the vitamin antioxidants in fruits and vegetables do provide some protection against the development of chronic diseases, such as cancer and heart disease, will supplements provide any additional benefit? Although the epidemiological and intervention data are very limited, and although the results are equivocal, some investigators indicate that the data are promising, but more research is needed.

Limited epidemiological data are available regarding the association between antioxidant vitamin supplementation and health. Kushi and others reported reduced risk of breast cancer in women who took 500 milligrams of vitamin C or 10,000 IU of vitamin A, but the reduction was not statistically significant. Other studies also have documented a weak role of dietary antioxidant intake in the prevention of breast cancer. However, in a recent review of the relationship between vitamin E and breast cancer, Kimmick and others noted that the epidemiologic study results have been inconsistent, and further study is warranted because of this inconsistency. Relative to other forms of cancer, Gridley and others indicated that individuals who took supplements of individual vitamins, such as C and E, had a significantly lower risk for oral and pharyngeal cancer. Losonczy and others reported that vitamin E supplementation was associated with about a 50 percent reduction in overall cancer mortality.

In the studies cited previously headed by Rimm, Stampfer, and Losonczy, the greatest reduction in risk of coronary heart disease was associated with those groups of subjects who took vitamin E supplements. In support of these findings, Hodis and others found that men with dietary intakes of vitamin E greater than 100 IU per day may experience reduced plasma LDL levels and angiographic evidence of coronary artery lesion progression, as compared to men with lower vitamin E intake.

These epidemiologic studies and reviews are encouraging, but the investigators stress the point that such studies only document an association, not a cause and effect relationship that needs to be supported by intervention studies.

Some intervention data are available. In a year-long study using a daily multivitamin-mineral compound containing relatively small amounts of sixteen vitamins and minerals, but four times the normal daily intake of vitamin E and beta-carotene, Chandra reported an improved immunity in elderly subjects. Meydani and others also noted improved immune responsiveness in elderly subjects who were given 800 milligrams of vitamin E daily for 1 month or 200 milligrams daily for 4 months. Improved immune functions may help prevent cancer, as reported by Shibata and others, who found that women, but not men, who supplemented with antioxidant vitamins were at lower risk for cancer of the bladder and colon. On the other hand, in a recent review Mayne concluded that supplementation with beta-carotene is of little or no value in prevention of the major cancers in healthy nonsmokers, and may actually increase the risk in smokers. One major intervention study designed to evaluate the possible protective effect of beta-carotene supplementation against lung cancer in high-risk smokers was stopped when it was discovered that the incidence of lung cancer increased in the subjects taking the supplement.

Mayne reviewed the available scientific literature and concluded that beta-carotene supplements do not prevent cardiovascular disease. However, preliminary data by Plotnick and others indicates that vitamins C and E, when consumed with a high-fat meal, may prevent one of the initial events associated with the development of atherosclerosis. Moreover, in a recent review regarding vitamin E and the incidence of cardiovascular disease, Tangney noted that several small intervention studies have shown some beneficial effects associated with supplementation. In one study with heart patients, varying doses of 400–800 IU resulted in a 35 percent reduction in major cardiovascular events and a 66 percent reduction in nonfatal myocardial infarctions. However, there was no effect on cardiovascular death or total mortality.

One intervention study suggested that vitamin E supplementation—2,000 IU daily for 2 years—may delay by 7 months the onset of the major debilitating effects associated with Alzheimer's disease. However, Sano and her colleagues cautioned that the data are preliminary and that healthy people should not consume such high doses of vitamin E.

The theory of a health-protective effect of antioxidant supplementation is enticing. Gaziano indicated that the results of current intervention trials do not prove or disprove any benefits of antioxidant supplements, nor do they incriminate them as harmful. Currently, a number of clinical intervention trials are underway to evaluate the health benefits of antioxidant vitamin supplementation, including studies with individual vitamins such as vitamin E, and combinations of antioxidants, such as beta-carotene and vitamins C and E. In essence, these studies and others are evaluating whether or not nutrients may function as drugs, or nutraceuticals. Hopefully, data from these long-term clinical trials will be available in the near future to provide us with information as to whether or not antioxidant vitamin supplementation confers any significant health benefits above and beyond those associated with the Healthy North American Diet.

Are vitamin megadoses harmful?

A **megadose** generally is defined as an amount ten times the RDA, but may be lower for vitamin A (only 5 times) and vitamin D (only 2 times). If the vitamin content of the body is adequate, excessive vitamin intake serves no useful purpose and may even be harmful in certain situations. As noted previously, vitamins function primarily as coenzymes. When a vitamin enters the body, it travels through the bloodstream to a particular body cell and then forms part of the enzyme complex within that cell. The cell has a limited capacity to produce these enzymes, and when that capacity is reached, the vitamin cannot be used for its basic purpose. It may now have other fates. It may be excreted from the body if in excess, particularly if it is a water-soluble vitamin; it may be stored in some body tissue, particularly if it is a fat-soluble vitamin; or it may begin to function in uncharacteristic ways, as a drug instead of a nutrient.

Although the positive health effects of the antioxidant vitamins look promising, some investigators note that additional research is needed before specific doses may be recommended. There may be an appropriate balance between free radicals and antioxidants in the body, and upsetting this balance may elicit negative effects. If negative effects do occur, it may take years before they become clinically evident. Nevertheless, Garewal and Diplock noted that beta-carotene and vitamins C and E are relatively safe, except in unusual circumstances. For example, vitamin E supplements may aggravate bleeding tendency in individuals taking anticoagulation drugs.

As noted throughout this chapter, megadoses of several vitamins may be pathological, particularly A, D, niacin, and B_6. There are more than 4,000 cases of vitamin/mineral overdose in the United States each year, resulting in about thirty fatalities. Although most of these cases occur in children, the literature contains some case reports of serious health problems with adults, including athletes taking vitamin megadoses in attempts to improve athletic performance. Several good reviews of possible adverse effects of excessive vitamin supplementation are presented by Hathcock, Snodgrass, and Cook and McDermott.

If I want to take a vitamin-mineral supplement, what are some prudent guidelines?

Unfortunately, scientific data are not available to provide specific guidelines relative to the amounts of each particular vitamin needed to promote optimal health. For those who desire to take vitamin supplements, the American Dietetic Association recommends low levels that do not exceed the RDA. To reiterate, excess amounts of some vitamins (A, D, niacin and B_6) can be toxic, as can excess amounts of some minerals (calcium, phosphorus, iron, chromium, selenium, and zinc) as discussed in the next chapter. However, other organizations, such as the Center for Science in the Public Interest (CSPI), used an educated guess approach to offer some prudent guidelines. The following are the highlights of the CSPI recommendations, as reported in an article written by Bonnie Liebman. The recommendation for vitamin E is also in accord with recommendations offered by the Consumers Union, publishers of *Consumer Reports on Health*.

1. Buy supplements high in beta-carotene and low in vitamin A. Avoid supplements with more than 5,000 IU of vitamin A.

2. Buy supplements rich in vitamin C, about 250–500 milligrams.

3. Buy supplements rich in vitamin E, about 100–400 IU.

4. Buy a supplement with about 200 micrograms of folic acid. This is especially important for women who are capable of bearing children. The supplement will complement the diet to provide about 400 micrograms per day.

5. Buy a supplement with 400 IU of vitamin D if you are either elderly or are a postmenopausal woman who does not drink adequate amounts of vitamin D-fortified milk or does not get enough sunshine in the winter.

6. Buy a supplement with 6 micrograms of vitamin B_{12} if you are a vegan.

7. Buy a supplement limited in the minerals iron, copper, and zinc; no more than the Reference Daily Intake for each.

8. Buy a supplement with calcium if you are female and do not consume adequate dietary calcium.

9. Buy a supplement with chromium and selenium, at least 50 micrograms but less than 200 micrograms.

10. Buy the inexpensive house brand of vitamins. Most companies that market vitamins buy their vitamins from the same manufacturers, so the contents in national brands and house brands are similar. In a recent evaluation of vitamin supplements, the Consumers Union recommended that if you decide to take vitamins, including antioxidants, go for the bargain price.

Although the CSPI published these recommendations, they, along with most investigators researching the health implications of vitamin supplementation, note there is no guarantee of improved health. Almost all health professionals note we should obtain our vitamin nutrition through consumption of a wide variety of healthful, natural foods, particularly fruits and vegetables. Remember, vitamin supplements do not supply all of the nutrients and other substances, such as phytochemicals, present in foods that are believed to be important to health.

References

Books

Bucci, L. 1993. *Nutrients as Ergogenic Aids for Sports and Exercise.* Boca Raton, FL: CRC Press.

Cooper, K. 1994. *Antioxidant Revolution.* Nashville: Thomas Nelson Publishers.

Council for Responsible Nutrition. 1997. *Vitamin and Mineral Safety.* Washington, DC: Council for Responsible Nutrition.

Fogelholm, M. 1992. *Vitamin and Mineral Status in Physically Active People.* Turku, Finland: Social Insurance Institution.

Jacobs, M. 1991. *Vitamins and Minerals in the Prevention and Treatment of Cancer.* Boca Raton, FL: CRC Press.

Keys, A. 1950. *Human Starvation.* Minneapolis, MN: West.

Lee, R., and Nieman, D. 1993. *Nutritional Assessment.* Madison, WI: Brown and Benchmark.

Machlin, L., ed. 1991. *Handbook of Vitamins.* New York and Basel: Marcel Dekker, Inc.

Moslen, M., and Smith, C., eds. 1992. *Free Radical Mechanism of Tissue Injury.* Boca Raton, FL: CRC Press.

National Research Council. 1989. *Diet and Health: Implications for Reducing Chronic Disease Risk.* Washington, DC: National Academy Press.

National Research Council. 1989. *Recommended Dietary Allowances.* Washington, DC: National Academy Press.

Sauberlich, H., and Machlin, L., eds. 1992. *Beyond Deficiency. New Views on the Function and Health Effects of Vitamins,* Volume 669. New York: The New York Academy of Sciences.

Shils, M., eds. 1994. *Modern Nutrition in Health and Disease.* Philadelphia: Lea and Febiger.

Walter, P., et al. eds. 1989. Elevated dosages of vitamins: Benefits and hazards. *International Journal for Vitamin and Nutrition Research,* Supplement 30.

Wolinsky, I., and Driskell, J. 1996. *Sports Nutrition: Vitamins and Trace Elements.* Boca Raton, FL: CRC Press.

Wolinsky, I., and Hickson, J., eds. 1994. *Nutrition in Exercise and Sport.* Boca Raton, FL: CRC Press.

Reviews

Alessio, H. and Blasi, E. 1997. Physical activity as a natural antioxidant booster and its effect on a healthy life span *Research Quarterly for Exercise and Sport* 68:292–302.

American Dietetic Association. 1996. Position of the American Dietetic Association: Vitamin and mineral supplementation. *Journal of the American Dietetic Association* 96:73–77.

American Medical Association, Council on Scientific Affairs. 1987. Vitamin preparations as dietary supplements and as therapeutic agents. *Journal of the American Medical Association* 257:1929–36.

Armstrong, L., and Maresh, C. 1996. Vitamin and mineral supplements as nutritional aids to exercise performance and health. *Nutrition Reviews* 54:S148–S158.

Bahrke, M. S., and Morgan, W. P. 1994. Evaluation of the ergogenic properties of ginseng. *Sports Medicine* 18:229–48.

Bendich, A. 1992. Safety issues regarding the use of vitamin supplements. *Annals of the New York Academy of Sciences* 669:300–312.

Beyer, R. 1992. An analysis of the role of coenzyme Q in free radical generation and as an antioxidant. *Biochemistry and Cell Biology* 70:390–403.

Binkley, N., and Suttie, J. 1995. Vitamin K nutrition and osteoporosis. *Journal of Nutrition* 125:1812–21.

Block, G. 1992. The data support a role for antioxidants in reducing cancer risk. *Nutrition Reviews* 50:207–13.

Block, G. 1992. Vitamin C status and cancer. Epidemiologic evidence of reduced risk. *Annals of the New York Academy of Sciences* 669:280–92.

Brooks, G. 1992. Proceedings of the panel discussion: Antioxidants and the elite athlete. American College of Sports Medicine Meeting, Dallas, Texas.

Bouis, H. 1996. Enrichment of food staples through plant breeding: A new strategy for fighting micronutrient malnutrition. *Nutrition Reviews* 54:131–37.

Boushey, C., et al. 1995. A quantitative assessment of plasma homocysteine as a risk factor for vascular disease: Probable benefits of increasing folic acid intakes. *Journal of the American Medical Association* 274:1049–57.

Bulow, J. 1993. Lipid mobilization and utilization. In *Principles of Exercise Biochemistry,* ed. J. Poortmans. Basel, Switzerland: Karger.

Butterworth, C., and Bendich, A. 1996. Folic acid and the prevention of birth defects. *Annual Reviews in Nutrition* 16:73–97.

Carr, C. J. (1986). Natural plant products that enhance performance and endurance. In *Enhancers of Performance and Endurance,* eds. C. J. Carr and E. Jokl. Hillsdale, NJ: Lawrence Erlbaum Associates.

Clarkson, P. 1995. Antioxidants and physical performance. *Critical Reviews in Food Science and Nutrition* 35:131–41.

Clarkson, P. 1991. Vitamins, iron and trace minerals. In *Perspectives in Exercise Science and Sports Medicine. Ergogenics: The Enhancement of Sports Performance,* eds. D. Lamb and M. Williams. Indianapolis, IN: Benchmark.

Consumers Union. 1996. Is E for you? *Consumer Reports on Health* 8:121–24.

Consumers Union. 1994. Can vitamin C save your life? *Consumer Reports on Health* 6:2527.

Consumers Union. 1994. Taking vitamins: Can they prevent disease? *Consumer Reports* 59: 561–69.

Cook, M., and McDermott, R. 1991. Vitamin supplementation: Changing the view that more is better. *Journal of Health Education* 22:217–23.

Dawson-Hughes, B. 1996. Calcium and vitamin D nutritional needs of elderly women. *Journal of Nutrition* 126:1165S–1167S.

Dekkers, J., et al. 1996. The role of antioxidant vitamins and enzymes in the prevention of exercise-induced muscle damage. *Sports Medicine* 21:213–38.

Demopoulous, H., et al. 1986. Free radical pathology: Rationale and toxicology of antioxidants and other supplements in sports medicine and exercise science. In *Sport, Health and Nutrition,* ed. F. Katch. Champaign, IL: Human Kinetics.

Enstrom, J. 1993. Counterpoint: Vitamin C and mortality. *Nutrition Today* 28 (May/June): 39–42.

Flynn, M. 1996. Vitamin E: Does evidence defy usual advice to rely on foods, not pills. *Environmental Nutrition* 19 (9): 1, 6.

Fogelholm, M. 1995. Indicators of vitamin and mineral status in athletes' blood: A review. *International Journal of Sport Nutrition* 5:267–84.

Fraser, D. 1995. Vitamin D. *The Lancet* 345:104–7.

Garewal, H., and Diplock, A. 1995. How 'safe' are antioxidant vitamins? *Drug Safety* 13:8–14.

Gaziano, J. 1996. Antioxidants in cardiovascular disease: Randomized trials. *Nutrition* 12:583–88.

Gaziano, J., and Hennekens, C. 1996. Update on dietary antioxidants and cancer. *Pathological Biology* 44:42–45.

Gershoff, S., ed. 1997. Vitamin D toxicity may be widespread. *Tufts University Health and Nutrition Letter* 15(8): 1.

Gershoff, S. 1993. Vitamin C (ascorbic acid): New roles, new requirements. *Nutrition Reviews* 51:313–26.

Gerster, H. 1989. Review: The role of vitamin C in athletic performance. *Journal of the American College of Nutrition* 8:636–43.

Goldfarb, A. 1993. Antioxidants: Role of supplementation to prevent exercise-induced oxidative stress. *Medicine and Science in Sports and Exercise* 25:232–36.

Gray, M., and Titlow, L. 1982. B_{15}: Myth or miracle? *Physician and Sportsmedicine* 10 (January): 107–12.

Halliwell, B. 1996. Antioxidants in human health and disease. *Annual Reviews in Nutrition* 16:33–50.

Halliwell, B. 1996. Oxidative stress, nutrition and health. Experimental strategies for optimization of nutritional antioxidant intake in humans. *Free Radical Research* 25:57–74.

Hathcock, J. 1997. Vitamins and minerals: Efficacy and safety. *American Journal of Clinical Nutrition* 66:427–37.

Hawley, J., et al. 1995. Nutritional practices of athletes: Are they suboptimal? *Journal of Sports Sciences* 13:S75–S87.

Haymes, E. 1991. Vitamin and mineral supplementation to athletes. *International Journal of Sport Nutrition* 1:146–69.

Hemila, H. 1996. Vitamin C and common cold incidence: A review of studies with subjects under heavy physical stress. *International Journal of Sports Medicine* 17:379–83.

Herbert, V. 1993. Viewpoint: Does mega-C do more good than harm, or more harm than good? *Nutrition Today* 28 (January/February): 28–32.

Holick, M. 1997. Vitamin D deficiency: The silent epidemic. *Nutrition Action Health Letter* 24 (8): 1–6.

Holick, M. 1996. Vitamin D and bone health. *Journal of Nutrition* 126:1159S–1164S.

Hornig, D., et al. 1988. Vitamin C. In *Modern Nutrition in Health and Disease,* eds. M. Shils and V. Young. Philadelphia: Lea and Febiger.

Jacob, R. 1994. Vitamin C. In *Modern Nutrition in Health and Disease.* eds. M. Shils, et al. Philadelphia: Lea and Febiger.

Jenkins, R. 1993. Introduction: Oxidant stress, aging, and exercise. *Medicine and Science in Sports and Exercise* 25:210–12.

Ji, L. 1992. Antioxidant enzyme response to exercise and aging. *Medicine and Science in Sports and Exercise* 25:225–31.

Kagan, V., et al. 1994. The significance of vitamin E and free radicals in physical exercise. In *Nutrition in Exercise and Sport,* eds. I. Wolinsky and J. Hickson. Boca Raton, FL: CRC Press.

Kanter, M. 1995. Free radicals and exercise: Effects of nutritional antioxidant supplementation. *Exercise and Sport Sciences Reviews* 23:375–98.

Kanter, M. 1995. Free radicals and exercise: How much do we know? *American Medical Athletic Association Quarterly* 9 (3): 9–10.

Kanter, M., and Williams, M. 1995. Antioxidants, carnitine and choline as putative ergogenic aids. *International Journal of Sport Nutrition* 5:S120–S131.

Keith, R. 1994. Vitamins and physical activity. In *Nutrition in Exercise and Sport,* eds. I. Wolinsky and J. Hickson. Boca Raton, FL: CRC Press.

Kimmick, G., et al. 1997. Vitamin E and breast cancer: A review. *Nutrition and Cancer* 27:109–17.

Koltover, V. 1992. Free radical theory of aging: View against the reliability theory. *EXS* 62:11–19.

Lachance, P. 1996. Future vitamin and antioxidant RDAs for health promotion. *Preventive Medicine* 25:46–47.

LeBlanc, K. 1996. Antioxidants as ergogenic aids. *American Medical Athletic Association Quarterly* 1 (1): 6–10.

Leklem, J. 1994. Vitamin B$_6$. In *Modern Nutrition in Health and Disease,* eds. M. Shils, et al. Philadelphia: Lea and Febiger.

Liebman, B. 1993. The ultra mega vitamin guide. *Nutrition Action Newsletter* 20 (January/February): 7–9.

Lowe, K., and Norman, A. 1992. Vitamin D and psoriasis. *Nutrition Reviews* 50:138–47.

Machlin, L., and Sauberlich, H. 1994. New views on the function and health effects of vitamins. *Nutrition Today* 29 (January/ February): 25–29.

Manore, M. 1994. Vitamin B$_6$ and exercise. *International Journal of Sport Nutrition* 4:89–103.

Mansfield, L., and Goldstein, G. 1981. Anaphylactic reaction after ingestion of local bee pollen. *Annals of Allergy* 47:154–56.

Mar, S. 1995. The "adaptogens" (Part I): Can they really help your running? *Running Research News* 11 (5): 1–5.

Mar, S. 1995. Can adaptogens help athletes reduce their risk of infections and overtraining? *Running Research News* 11 (9): 1–7.

Mayne, S. 1996. Beta-carotene, carotenoids, and disease prevention in humans. *FASEB Journal* 10:690–701.

Meydani, S. 1995. Vitamin E enhancement of T cell-mediated function in healthy elderly: Mechanisms of action. *Nutrition Reviews* 53:S52–S58.

Meydani, S. 1993. Vitamin/mineral supplementation, the aging immune response, and risk of infection. *Nutrition Reviews* 51:106–15.

Moon, J., et al. 1992. Hypothesis: Etiology of atherosclerosis and osteoporosis: Are imbalances in the calciferol endocrine system implicated? *Journal of the American College of Nutrition* 11:567–83.

National Strength and Conditioning Association. 1989. Popularized ergogenic aids. *National Strength and Conditioning Association Journal* 11:10–14.

Oakley, G., et al. 1996. More folic acid for everyone, now. *Journal of Nutrition* 126:751S–755S.

Olson, J. 1994. Vitamins: The tortuous path from needs to fantasies. *Journal of Nutrition* 124:1771S–1776S.

Olson, J. 1994. Vitamin A, retinoids, and carotenoids. In *Modern Nutrition in Health and Disease,* eds. M. Shils, et al. Philadelphia: Lea and Febiger.

Padh, H. 1991. Vitamin C: Newer insights into its biochemical functions. *Nutrition Reviews* 49:65–70.

Painter, P., et al. 1990. Megavitamin abuse: Vitamin toxicity in an athlete. *Diagnostics and Clinical Testing* 28:24–29.

Perera, F. 1996. Uncovering new clues to cancer risk. *Scientific American* 274 (5): 54–62.

Picciano, M., et al. 1994. The folate status of women and health. *Nutrition Today* 29 (6): 20–29.

Rivlin, R., and Dutta, P. 1995. Vitamin B$_2$ (riboflavin). *Nutrition Today* 30 (2): 62–67.

Rock, A. 1995. Vitamin hype: Why we're wasting $1 of every $3 we spend. *Money* September:83–91.

Rock, C., et al. 1996. Update on the biological characteristics of the antioxidant micronutrients: Vitamin C, vitamin E, and the carotenoids. *Journal of the American Dietetic Association* 96:693–702.

Schaumburg, H., et al. 1983. Sensory neuropathy from pyridoxine abuse. *New England Journal of Medicine* 309:445–48.

Short, S. 1994. Surveys of dietary intake and nutrition knowledge of athletes and their coaches. In *Nutrition in Exercise and Sport,* eds. I. Wolinsky and J. Hickson. Boca Raton, FL: CRC Press.

Sies, H., et al. 1992. Antioxidant functions of vitamins: Vitamins E and C, beta-carotene, and other carotenoids. *Annals of the New York Academy of Sciences* 669:7–20.

Simon-Schnass, I. 1993. Vitamin requirements for increased physical activity: Vitamin E. In *Nutrition and Fitness for Athletes* 71:144–53, eds. A. Simopoulos and K. Pavlou. Basel, Switzerland: Karger.

Snodgrass, S. 1992. Vitamin neurotoxicity. *Molecular Neurobiology* 6:41–73.

Sobol, J., and Marquart, L. 1994. Vitamin/mineral supplement use among athletes: A review of the literature. *International Journal of Sport Nutrition* 4:320–34.

Stein, A. 1993. Magic bullets. Do cyclists need vitamins? *Bicycling* 34:68–69.

Steinmetz, K., and Potter, J. 1996. Vegetables, fruit, and cancer prevention: A review. *Journal of the American Dietetic Association* 96:1027–39.

Suttie, J. 1992. Vitamin K and human nutrition. *Journal of the American Dietetic Association* 92:585–90.

Swain, R., and St. Clair, L. 1997. The role of folic acid in deficiency states and prevention of disease. *Journal of Family Practice* 44:128–144.

Tangney, C. 1997. Vitamin E and cardiovascular disease. *Nutrition Today* 32 (1): 13–21.

Tiidus, P., and Houston, M. 1995. Vitamin E status and response to exercise training. *Sports Medicine* 20:12–23.

Tufts University. 1996. The trials of beta-carotene: Is the verdict in? *Tufts University Diet & Nutrition Letter* March: 4–6.

Ubbink, J. 1994. Vitamin nutrition status and homocysteine: An atherogenic risk factor. *Nutrition Reviews* 52:383–93.

van der Beek, E. 1991. Vitamin supplementation and physical exercise performance. *Journal of Sports Sciences* 92:77–79.

Webb, D. 1997. Coenzyme Q$_{10}$: Miracle nutrient or merely promising? *Environmental Nutrition* 20 (11): 1, 4.

Weber, P., et al. 1996. Vitamin C and human health: A review of recent data relevant to human requirements. *International Journal of Vitamin and Nutrition Research* 66:19–30.

Williams, M. 1989. Vitamin supplementation and athletic performance. *International Journal for Vitamin and Nutrition Research,* Supplement 30:161–91.

Yetley, E., and Rader, J. 1996. The challenge of regulating health claims and food fortification. *Journal of Nutrition* 126:765S–772S.

Young, V. 1996. Evidence for a recommended dietary allowance for vitamin C from pharmacokinetics: A comment and analysis. *Proceedings of the National Academy of Sciences* 93:14344–48.

Specific Studies

Alpha-tocopherol, Beta-carotene Cancer Prevention Study Group. 1994. The effect of vitamin E and beta-carotene on the incidence of lung cancer and other cancers in male smokers. *New England Journal of Medicine* 330:1029–35.

Barnett, D., and Conlee, R. 1984. The effects of a commercial dietary supplement on human performance. *American Journal of Clinical Nutrition* 40:586–90.

Bonke, D. 1986. Influence of vitamin B$_1$, B$_6$ and B$_{12}$ on the control of fine motoric movements. *Bibliotheca Nutritio et Dieta* 38:104–9.

Braun, B., et al. 1991. The effect of coenzyme Q10 supplementation on exercise performance, VO_2 max, and lipid peroxidation in trained cyclists. *International Journal of Sport Nutrition* 1:353–65.

Chandler, J., and Hawkins, J. 1984. The effect of bee pollen on physiological performance. *International Journal of Biosocial Research* 6:107–14.

Chandra, R. 1992. Effect of vitamin and trace-element supplementation on immune responses and infection in elderly subjects. *Lancet* 340:1124–27.

Coburn, S., et al. 1990. Effect of vitamin B_6 intake on the vitamin content of human muscle. *FASEB Journal* 4:A365.

Curhan, G., et al. 1996. A prospective study of the intake of vitamin C and B_6, and the risk of kidney stones in men. *Journal of Urology* 155:1847–1851.

Dowling, E. A., et al. 1996. Effect of Eleutherococcus senticosus on submaximal and maximal exercise performance. *Medicine and Science in Sport and Exercise,* 28:482–489.

Doyle, M., et al. 1997. Allithiamine ingestion does not enhance isokinetic parameters of muscle performance. *International Journal of Sport Nutrition* 7:39–47.

Dreon, D., and Butterfield, G. 1986. Vitamin B_6 utilization in active and inactive young men. *American Journal of Clinical Nutrition* 43:816–24.

Engels, H., and Wirth, J. 1997. No ergogenic effect of ginseng (Panax genseng C.A. Meyer) during graded maximal aerobic exercise. *Journal of the American Dietetic Association* 97:1110–15.

Faber, M., and Spinnler Benade, A.J. 1991. Mineral and vitamin intake in field athletes (discus-, hammer-, javelin-throwers and shotputters). *International Journal of Sports Medicine* 12:324–27.

Ghosh, M., et al. 1996. Vitamin C prevents oxidative damage. *Free Radical Research* 25:173–179.

Gilois, C., et al. 1992. The hematological and electrophysiological effects of cobalamin. Deficiency secondary to vegetarian diets. *Annals of the New York Academy of Sciences* 669:345–48.

Godsen, R., and Bell, N. 1987. The effect of weight training on vitamin D and mineral metabolism. *Medicine and Science in Sports and Exercise* 21:S21.

Gridley, G., et al. 1992. Vitamin supplement use and reduced risk of oral and pharyngeal cancer. *American Journal of Epidemiology* 135:1083–92.

Haralambie, G. 1976. Vitamin B_2 status in athletes and the influence of riboflavin administration on neuromuscular irritability. *Nutrition and Metabolism* 20:1–8.

Heath, E., et al. 1993. Effect of nicotinic acid on respiratory exchange ratio and substrate levels during exercise. *Medicine and Science in Sports and Exercise* 25:1018–23.

Hellsten, Y., et al. 1996. Effect of sprint cycle training on activities of antioxidant enzymes in human skeletal muscle. *Journal of Applied Physiology* 81:1484–87.

Hennekens, C., et al. 1996. Lack of effect of long-term supplementation with beta carotene on the incidence of malignant neoplasms and cardiovascular disease. *New England Journal of Medicine* 334:1145–49.

Hodis, H., et al. 1995. Serial coronary angiographic evidence that antioxidant vitamin intake reduces progression of coronary artery atherosclerosis. *Journal of the American Medical Association* 273:1849–54.

Hoffman, A., et al. 1989. Plasma pyridoxal phosphate concentrations in response to ingesting water or glucose polymer during a two hour run. *Medicine and Science in Sports and Exercise* 21:S59.

Jacobus, C., et al. 1992. Hypervitaminosis D associated with drinking milk. *The New England Journal of Medicine* 326:1173–77.

Kanter, M., et al. 1997. Effects of short term vitamin E supplementation on lipid peroxidation, inflammation & tissue damage during & following exercise. *Medicine and Science in Sports and Exercise* 29:S40.

Kim, I., et al. 1993. Vitamin and mineral supplement use and mortality in a U.S. cohort. *American Journal of Public Health* 83:546–50.

Knekt, P., et al. 1992. Serum antioxidant vitamins and risk of cataract. *British Medical Journal* 305 (6866): 1392–94.

Kobayashi, Y. 1974. Effect of vitamin E on aerobic work performance in man during acute exposure to hypoxic hypoxia. Unpublished doctoral dissertation. University of New Mexico.

Kolka, M., and Stephenson, L. 1990. Skin blood flow during exercise after niacin ingestion. *FASEB Journal* 4:A279.

Kushi, L., et al. 1996. Dietary antioxidant vitamins and death from coronary heart disease in postmenopausal women. *New England Journal of Medicine* 334:1156–62.

Kushi, L., et al. 1996. Intake of vitamins A, C, and E and postmenopausal breast cancer: The Iowa Women's Health Study. *American Journal of Epidemiology* 144:165–74.

Laaksonen, R., et al. 1995. Ubiquinone supplementation and exercise capacity in trained young and older men. *European Journal of Applied Physiology* 72:95–100.

Labadarios, D., et al. 1989. The effects of vitamin and mineral supplementation on running performance in trained athletes. *American Journal of Clinical Nutrition* 49:1133.

Levine, M., et al. 1997. Vitamin C pharmacokinetics in healthy volunteers: Evidence for a recommended dietary allowance. *Proceedings of the National Academy of Sciences* 93:3704–9.

Losonczy, K., et al. 1996. Vitamin E and vitamin C supplement use and risk of all cause and coronary heart disease mortality in older persons: The Established Populations for Epidemiologic Studies of the Elderly. *American Journal of Clinical Nutrition* 64:190–96.

Lukert, B., et al. 1992. Menopausal bone loss is partially regulated by dietary intake of vitamin D. *Calcified Tissue International* 51:173–79.

Malm, C., et al. 1996. Supplementation with ubiquinone-10 causes cellular damage during intense exercise. *Acta Physiologica Scandinavica* 157:511–12.

Manore, M., and Leklem, J. 1988. Effect of carbohydrate and vitamin B_6 on fuel substrates during exercise in women. *Medicine and Science in Sports and Exercise* 20:233–41.

Matter, M., et al. 1987. The effect of iron and folate therapy on maximal exercise performance in female marathon runners with iron and folate deficiency. *Clinical Science* 72:415–22.

Meydani, M., et al. 1993. Protective effect of vitamin E on exercise-induced oxidative damage in young and older adults. *American Journal of Physiology* 264:R992–R998.

Mitra, S., et al. 1996. Neuropharmacological studies on Panax ginseng. *Indian Journal of Experimental Biology* 34:41–47.

Morris, A., et al. 1996. No ergogenic effect of ginseng ingestion. *International Journal of Sport Nutrition* 6:263–71.

Murray, R., Bartoli, W. P., Eddy, D. E., and Horn, M. K. 1995. Physiological and performance responses to nicotinic-acid ingestion during exercise. *Medicine and Science in Sports and Exercise* 27:1057–62.

Ness, A., et al. 1996. Vitamin C status and serum lipids. *European Journal of Clinical Nutrition* 50:724–29.

Ness, A., et al. 1996. Vitamin C status and blood pressure. *Journal of Hypertension* 14:503–8.

Nice, C., et al. 1984. The effects of pantothenic acid on human exercise capacity. *Journal of Sports Medicine and Physical Fitness* 24:26–29.

Niess, A., et al. 1996. DNA damage after exhaustive treadmill running in trained and untrained men. *International Journal of Sports Medicine* 17:397–403.

Nyyssonen, K., et al. 1997. Vitamin C deficiency and risk of myocardial infarction: Prospective study of men from eastern Finland. *British Medical Journal* 314:634–38.

Omenn, G. 1996. Effects of a combination of beta carotene and vitamin A on lung cancer and cardiovascular disease. *New England Journal of Medicine* 334:1150–55.

Peters, E., et al. 1993. Vitamin C supplementation reduces the incidence of postrace symptoms of upper-respiratory-tract infection in ultramarathon runners. *American Journal of Clinical Nutrition* 57:170–74.

Pincemail, J., et al. 1988. Tocopherol mobilization during intensive exercise. *European Journal of Applied Physiology* 57:188–91.

Plotnick, G., et al. 1997. Effect of antioxidant vitamins on the transient impairment of endothelium-dependent brachial artery vasoactivity following a single high-fat meal. *Journal of the American Medical Association* 278:1682–6.

Powers, H., et al. 1985. Effects of a multivitamin and iron supplement on running performance in Gambian children. *Human Nutrition: Clinical Nutrition* 39:427–37.

Rauma, A., et al. 1995. Vitamin B-12 status of long-term adherent of a strict uncooked vegan diet ("living food diet") is compromised. *Journal of Nutrition* 125:2511–15.

Retsky, K., et al. 1993. Ascorbic acid oxidation product(s) protect human low density lipoprotein against atherogenic modification. Anti- rather than pro-oxidant activity of vitamin C in the presence of transition metal ions. *Journal of Biological Chemistry* 268:1304–9.

Rimm, E., et al. 1993. Vitamin E consumption and the risk of coronary heart disease in man. *New England Journal of Medicine* 328:1450–56.

Rokitzki, L., et al. 1994. Acute changes in vitamin B_6 status in endurance athletes before and after a marathon. *International Journal of Sport Nutrition* 4:154–65.

Rokitzki, L., et al. 1994. α-tocopherol supplementation in racing cyclists during extreme endurance training. *International Journal of Sport Nutrition* 4:253–64.

Rothman, K., et al. 1995. Teratogenicity of high vitamin A intake. *New England Journal of Medicine* 333:1369–73.

Sano, M., et al. 1997. A controlled trial of selegiline, alpha-tocopherol, or both as treatment for Alzheimer's disease. The Alzheimer's Disease Cooperative Study. *New England Journal of Medicine* 336:1245–47.

Sastre, J., et al. 1992. Exhaustive physical exercise causes oxidation of glutathione status in blood: Prevention by antioxidant administration. *American Journal of Physiology* 263:R992–95.

Schmid, A., et al. 1996. Effect of physical exercise and vitamin C on absorption of ferric sodium citrate. *Medicine and Science in Sports and Exercise* 28:1470–73.

Schrijver, J., et al. 1987. Effect of vitamin and iron supplementation on physical performance. Presented at International Symposium on Elevated Dosages of Vitamins: Benefits and Hazards, September, Interlaken, Switzerland.

Seddon, J., et al. 1994. Dietary carotenoids, vitamins A, C, and E, and advanced age-related macular degeneration. *Journal of the American Medical Association* 272:1413–20.

Shibata, A., et al. 1992. Intake of vegetables, fruits, beta-carotene, vitamin C and vitamin supplements and cancer incidence among the elderly: A prospective study. *British Journal of Cancer* 66:673–79.

Simon-Schnass, I., and Pabst, H. 1988. Influence of vitamin E on physical performance. *International Journal for Vitamin and Nutrition Research* 58:49–54.

Singh, A., et al. 1992. Chronic multivitamin-mineral supplementation does not enhance physical performance. *Medicine and Science in Sports and Exercise* 24:726–32.

Singh, A., et al. 1992. Vitamin and mineral status in physically active men: Effects of a high-potency supplement. *Journal of Clinical Nutrition* 55:1–7.

Slesinski, M., et al. 1996. Dietary intake of fat, fiber and other nutrients is related to the use of vitamin and mineral supplements in the United States: The 1992 National Health Interview Survey. *Journal of Nutrition* 126:3001–8.

Snider, I., et al. 1992. Effects of coenzyme athletic performance system as an ergogenic aid on endurance performance to exhaustion. *International Journal of Sports Nutrition* 2:272–86.

Squires, R., et al. 1992. Low-dose, time-release nicotinic acid: effects in selected patients with low concentrations of high-density lipoprotein cholesterol. *Mayo Clinic Proceedings* 69:855–60.

Stampfer, M., et al. 1993. Vitamin E consumption and the risk of coronary heart disease in women. *New England Journal of Medicine* 328:1444–49.

Stephens, N., et al. 1996. Randomized controlled trial of vitamin E in patients with coronary disease: Cambridge Heart Antioxidant Study (CHAOS). *The Lancet* 347:781–86.

Suboticanec, K., et al. 1990. Effects of pyridoxine and riboflavin supplementation on physical fitness in young adolescents. *International Journal of Vitamin and Nutrition Research* 60:81–88.

Suzuki, M., and Itokawa, Y. 1996. Effects of thiamine supplementation on exercise-induced fatigue. *Metabolism in Brain Diseases* 11:95–106.

Telford, R., et al. 1992. The effect of 7 to 8 months of vitamin/mineral supplementation on athletic performance. *International Journal of Sport Nutrition* 2:135–53.

Telford, R., et al. 1992. The effect of 7 to 8 months of vitamin/mineral supplementation on the vitamin and mineral status of athletes. *International Journal of Sport Nutrition* 2:123–34.

Tiidus, P., et al. 1996. Lack of antioxidant adaptation to short-term aerobic training in human muscle. *American Journal of Physiology* 271:R832–R836.

Tremblay, A., et al. 1984. The effects of a riboflavin supplementation on the nutritional status and performance of elite swimmers. *Nutrition Research* 4:201.

Tsui, J., and Nordstrom, J. 1990. Folate status of adolescents: effects of folic acid supplementation. *Journal of the American Dietetic Association* 90:1551–56.

van der Beek, E., et al. 1984. Effect of marginal vitamin intake on physical performance of man. *International Journal of Sports Medicine* 5 (Suppl): 28–31.

van der Beek, E., et al. 1988. Thiamin, riboflavin, and vitamins B-6 and C: impact of combined restricted intake on functional performance in man. *American Journal of Clinical Nutrition* 48:1451–62.

van Erp-Baart, A., et al. 1989. Nationwide survey on nutritional habits in elite athletes. *International Journal of Sports Medicine* 10 (Suppl 1): S11–S16.

Weight, L., et al. 1988. Vitamin and mineral status of trained athletes including the effects of supplements. *American Journal of Clinical Nutrition* 47:186–91.

Weight, L., et al. 1988. Vitamin and mineral supplementation: effect on the running performance of trained athletes. *American Journal of Clinical Nutrition* 47:192–95.

West, K., et al. 1991. Efficacy of vitamin A in reducing preschool child mortality in Nepal. *Lancet* 338:67–71.

Weston, S., et al. 1997. Does exogenous coenzyme Q_{10} affect aerobic capacity in endurance athletes? *International Journal of Sport Nutrition* 7:197–206.

Woodhouse, M., et al. 1987. The effects of varying doses of orally ingested bee pollen extract upon selected performance variables. *Athletic Training* 22:26–28.

CHAPTER 8

Minerals: The Inorganic Regulators

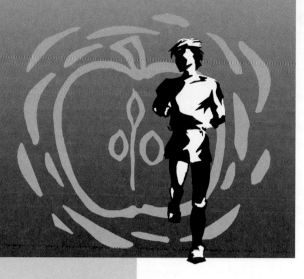

- Minerals perform two of the three major functions of food, including the formation of several body tissues and the regulation of numerous physiological processes.
- Calcium is most prevalent in the milk food group.
- In particular, children, adolescents, and all women should obtain adequate dietary calcium.
- Although calcium supplements are not necessary for the average individual, they may be recommended for some females, including athletes.
- Two keys to the prevention of osteoporosis are weight-bearing exercise and adequate calcium in the diet; hormone-replacement or appropriate drug therapy may be recommended for some women.
- Phosphate salts have been used for more than 60 years in attempts to improve athletic performance, but the research is equivocal. Recent studies supporting ergogenic effects need confirmation by additional research.
- A deficiency of magnesium may be associated with muscle cramps. At the present time, the data are too limited to support an ergogenic effect from magnesium supplementation.
- Iron deficiency, particularly among women and young children, is a major nutritional health concern, so iron-rich foods such as lean meats and beans should be stressed in the diet.

- Iron supplementation may be recommended for certain individuals, particularly female endurance athletes and those on low-Calorie diets.
- Iron supplementation may improve performance in individuals with iron-deficiency anemia, but not in individuals with normal iron status; studies also suggest those with iron deficiency without anemia will also realize no improvement in performance.
- Zinc deficiency has been shown to impair the growth process in children, so it may be a problem for young athletes who incur heavy sweat losses and are on low-Calorie diets, such as wrestlers, dancers, or gymnasts.
- Chromium supplements have been marketed to increase muscle mass and decrease body fat, but research does not support these claims.
- There does not appear to be much valid scientific evidence to support an ergogenic effect of trace mineral supplementation including zinc, copper, boron, selenium, and vanadium.
- Megadoses of minerals are not recommended.
- A diet that provides the RDA for iron, calcium, and Calories from a balanced selection of foods throughout the different food groups will provide adequate amounts of both the major and trace minerals.

athletic amenorrhea
electrolytes
female athlete triad
ferritins
hematuria
heme iron
hemochromatosis
hemolysis
ions
iron-deficiency anemia
iron deficiency without anemia
macrominerals
metalloenzymes
mineral
osteoporosis
peak bone mass
secondary amenorrhea
trabecular bone
trace minerals

INTRODUCTION

You may recall the periodic table of the elements hanging on the wall in your high school or college chemistry class. At latest count there were 112 known elements, seventy-eight of them occurring naturally and the remainder being synthetic. Many of the natural elements, including a wide variety of minerals, are essential to human bodily structure and function.

Much research attention is currently being devoted to the role of mineral nutrition in health and disease, including both epidemiological and laboratory research. For example, using the RDA as a basis for comparison, national surveys among the general population have revealed that either an inadequate dietary intake of some minerals or an excessive dietary intake of others in certain segments of the population may be contributing to several health problems. Laboratory studies using either animals or humans as subjects have explored the roles of both deficiencies and supplementation of minerals on human health and disease processes.

An increasing number of research studies have been conducted with athletes to evaluate the effect of mineral nutrition on physical performance and the converse—the effect of exercise on mineral metabolism. Because some minerals function similarly to vitamins, a deficiency state could adversely affect performance. Moreover, exercise in itself may be a contributing factor to mineral deficiencies or impaired mineral metabolism in some types of athletes. Additionally, several mineral supplements are being marketed specifically for physically active individuals.

This chapter is especially important to all females because it addresses two of their major dietary concerns, obtaining sufficient calcium and iron. These key minerals are of particular interest to females who participate in sports or are otherwise physically active. The female athlete triad—disordered eating, amenorrhea, and osteoporosis—is introduced in this chapter with the major focus on osteoporosis because of its relationship to calcium metabolism. An expanded discussion of eating disorders is presented in Chapter 10. Female endurance athletes also need to obtain adequate dietary iron intake because of its important role in the oxygen energy system.

The major purpose of this chapter is to analyze the available data relative to the effect of mineral nutrition on physical performance and health. The first section discusses some basic facts about the general role of those minerals that are essential to human nutrition. The second and third sections cover, respectively, the major minerals and the trace minerals. In these two sections, each of the minerals is discussed in terms of its RDA, good dietary sources, metabolic functions in the body with particular reference to the physically active individual, an evaluation of the research pertaining to the effects of deficiencies or supplementation, and prudent recommendations. The last section summarizes dietary mineral nutrition guidelines for those who exercise for health or sport.

Basic Facts

What are minerals, and what is their importance to humans?

A **mineral** is an inorganic element found in nature, and the term is usually reserved for those elements that are solid. Hence, a mineral is an element, but an element is not necessarily a mineral. For example, oxygen is an element, but it is not classified as a mineral. In nutrition, the term mineral is usually used to classify those dietary elements essential to life processes.

Minerals serve two of the three basic functions of nutrients in foods. First, many are used as the building blocks for body tissues such as bones, teeth, muscles, and other organic structures. Second, a number of minerals are components of enzymes known as **metalloenzymes,** which are involved in the regulation of metabolism. Several other minerals exist as **ions,** or **electrolytes,** which are small particles carrying electrical charges. They are important components or activators of several enzymes and hormones. Some of the physiological processes regulated or maintained by minerals include muscle contraction, oxygen transport, nerve impulse conduction, acid-base balance of the blood, maintenance of body water supplies, blood clotting, and normal heart rhythm. Minerals do not provide a source of caloric energy, which is the third function of nutrients.

Minerals are found in the soil and are eventually incorporated in growing plants. Animals get their mineral nutrition from the plants they eat, whereas humans obtain their supply from both plant and animal food. Drinking water also may be a good source of several minerals. As minerals are excreted daily from the body in sweat, urine, or feces, they must be replaced. Inadequate mineral nutrition has been associated with a variety of human diseases, including anemia, high blood pressure, diabetes, cancer, tooth decay, and osteoporosis. Thus, proper dietary intake of essential minerals is necessary for optimal health and physical performance.

What minerals are essential to human nutrition?

Of all the elements in the periodic table, only twenty-five are currently known to be, or presumed to be, essential in humans. Five of these elements which make up the carbohydrate, fat, and protein that we eat and the water we drink, constitute over 96 percent of the body weight. In

Table 8.1 Minerals essential to humans, with RDA or estimated safe and adequate daily dietary intakes (ESADDI) for adults*

Mineral	Symbol	RDA or ESADDI (mg)		Amount in adult body (g)
Calcium	Ca	800♂	800♀	1,500
Phosphorus	P	800♂	800♀	850
Potassium	K	2,000♂	2,000♀	180
Chloride	Cl	750♂	750♀	75
Sodium	Na	500♂	500♀	65
Magnesium	Mg	350♂	280♀	25
Iron	Fe	10♂	15♀	5
Fluoride	F	1.5–4.0♂	1.5–4.0♀	2.5
Zinc	Zn	15♂	12♀	2
Copper	Cu	1.5–3.0♂	1.5–3.0♀	0.1
Selenium	Se	0.070♂	0.055♀	0.013
Manganese	Mn	2.0–5.0♂	2.0–5.0♀	0.012
Iodine	I	0.15♂	0.15♀	0.011
Molybdenum	Mo	0.075–0.25♂	0.075–0.25♀	0.009
Chromium	Cr	0.05–0.2♂	0.05–0.2♀	0.006

The values for sodium, chloride, and potassium are estimated minimum requirements.

*See Appendix A for extended table values.

varying combinations, hydrogen, oxygen, carbon, sulfur, and nitrogen are the components of the body water, protein, fat, and carbohydrate stores. The remaining twenty minerals compose less than 4 percent of the body weight but are equally important.

Table 8.1 lists those minerals considered to be essential to humans. RDA have been established for seven minerals, and the estimated safe and adequate daily dietary intakes (ESADDI) are available for five others, while an estimated minimal requirement has been established for sodium, chloride, and potassium.

Other minerals such as boron, nickel, silicon, and vanadium, among others, are found in animal tissues and also may be important to human nutrition, but their roles have not yet been completely elucidated.

In general, how do deficiencies or excesses of minerals influence health or physical performance?

Similar to vitamin deficiencies, mineral deficiencies may occur in several stages. The first three stages (preliminary, biochemical deficiency, and physiological deficiency) may be termed subclinical malnutrition and may or may not have significant effects on health or physical performance. In the clinically manifest deficiency state, however, health and performance most likely will suffer.

The interaction of exercise and mineral nutrition may pose some special health problems, as we shall see in later sections of this chapter. In regard to the preliminary stage, some athletes may reduce their mineral intake as they shift toward a low-Calorie diet. Changes in food selection may also be important, for the bioavailability of many minerals is markedly influenced by the form in which they are consumed. In general, most minerals are poorly absorbed from the intestine. For example, the RDA for iron is ten times the amount actually needed by the body, because only about 10 percent of dietary iron from the average American diet is absorbed. Moreover, mineral absorption may be inhibited by certain compounds in foods, and supplementation with one mineral may impair the absorption of another. In athletes, factors that lower intake and absorption may be compounded because athletic activity may raise some mineral requirements. Additional minerals may be needed for the synthesis of new tissues associated with physical training, or to replace losses in the sweat, urine, and feces often observed during and following intense exercise training.

Sports nutritionists are becoming concerned that the presence of these factors during the preliminary stage of a mineral deficiency could lead to the subsequent stages of subclinical malnutrition or even to a clinical deficiency. Based on dietary surveys and clinical studies with biochemical measures of mineral status, Pennington reported there is some concern for adequate calcium, iron, and zinc nutrition in some segments of United States population, and conflicting opinions about the need for concern regarding copper and magnesium nutrition. Most dietary surveys indicate athletes, particularly males, are obtaining the RDA for all minerals. However, a number of studies have reported athletes with inadequate dietary intake and biochemical deficiencies of several minerals, predominately athletes involved in weight-control sports such as gymnastics and wrestling. Switching to a vegetarian diet for 1 year also decreased plasma levels of several minerals. Experts disagree about the potential adverse effects of such dietary or biochemical deficiencies, but certain physiologic and clinically manifest mineral deficiencies are known to have impaired physical performance.

The human body possesses a very effective control system for some minerals. When a deficiency occurs, the body absorbs more of the mineral from the food in the intestine and excretes less via routes such as the urine. When an excess is consumed the opposite is true; less is absorbed and more is excreted. On the other hand, the body has a limited ability to excrete certain minerals, so excessive consumption may cause a number of health problems, even in relatively small dosages. Additionally, a few minerals not important to human nutrition, such as lead, mercury, cadmium, arsenic, and some industrial forms of chromium, may be extremely toxic to the human body.

Macrominerals

The seven **macrominerals** (major minerals) are calcium, phosphorus, magnesium, potassium, sodium, chloride, and sulfur. Minerals are classified as macrominerals if the RDA or ESADDI is greater than 100 mg per day or the body contains more than 5 grams. In general, the human body maintains a proper balance of these minerals through precise hormonal control mechanisms, but deficiencies or excesses may occur and disturb normal physiological functions, thus impairing health or physical performance. Because potassium, sodium, and chloride are the major electrolytes in sweat, and in some sports drinks, they are covered in the following chapter dealing with water and temperature regulation.

Calcium (Ca)

Calcium, a silver-white metallic element, is the most abundant mineral in the body, representing almost 2 percent of the body weight.

RDA The RDA for calcium has recently been updated by the National Academy of Sciences. The RDA for calcium is now intended to provide optimal amounts for health, particularly for bone health and the prevention of osteoporosis. The new daily recommendations, in parentheses, are given for several selected age groups: children 1–3 years (500 mg); youths 4–8 years (800 mg); youth and adolescents 9–18 years (1,300 mg); adults 19–50 (1,000 mg); adults 50 and older (1,200 mg). Pregnant and breastfeeding women should get the amount recommended for their age group, not more as was recommended in the 1989 RDA. The RDI is 1,000 mg.

Food Sources Calcium content is highest in dairy products. One 8-ounce glass of skim milk, which contains about 300 mg of calcium, supplies about one-third of the RDA for an adult and one-fourth for adolescents and adults 50 and over. It is used as the basis of comparison for other foods. Other equivalent dairy foods are 1½ ounces of cheese, 1 cup of yogurt, and 1¾ cups of ice cream. Other good sources are fish with small bones such as sardines and canned salmon, dark-green leafy vegetables (particularly broccoli, kale, and turnip greens), tofu, legumes, and nuts. Incorporation of milk or cheese into foods such as soups, pasta dishes, and pizza is an excellent way to obtain dietary calcium. For individuals with lactose intolerance, the use of yogurt, lactase enzymes, or smaller portions of milk may be helpful. Calcium is also used as a preservative in some foods, such as breads, which may provide small amounts. Additionally, some food products such as orange juice and sodas are now being fortified with calcium. Foods high in calcium are listed in Table 8.2.

Calcium is one of the key nutrients listed on food labels, and although the food label does not indicate the milligrams of calcium per serving, you can calculate the amount fairly easily. The Daily Value (DV) for calcium is 1,000 milligrams, and the label will provide you with the percentage of the calcium DV contained in one serving. All you need to do is multiply the percentage, as a decimal, times 1,000 milligrams. For example, if a glass of calcium-fortified orange juice provides you with 30 percent of the DV, then it contains 300 milligrams of calcium (0.30 × 1,000 milligrams = 300 milligrams).

Some nutrients in food may influence calcium absorption or excretion. The calcium in milk appears to be absorbed more readily than calcium in plant foods. The vitamin D and lactose in milk facilitate absorption, whereas phytates (phytic acid compounds) found in legumes and oxalates in green leafy vegetables like spinach may diminish somewhat the absorption of calcium from those foods. Dietary fiber may reduce calcium absorption, although the effect is rather variable and presumably small. Dietary phosphorus may also decrease calcium absorption, but decreases its excretion by the kidney as well, so its effect on calcium balance is somewhat neutral. Excess sodium intake increases calcium excretion. As mentioned

Table 8.2 Major minerals: calcium, phosphorus, and magnesium

Major mineral	Major food sources	Major body functions	Deficiency symptoms	Symptoms of excessive consumption
Calcium (Ca)	All dairy products: milk, cheese, ice cream, yogurt; egg yolk; dried beans and peas; dark-green leafy vegetables; cauliflower	Bone formation; enzyme activation; nerve impulse transmission; muscle contraction; cell membrane potential	Osteoporosis; rickets; impaired muscle contraction; muscle cramps	Constipation; inhibition of trace mineral absorption. In susceptible individuals: heart arrhythmias; kidney stones; calcification of soft tissues
Phosphorus (P)	All protein products: meat, poultry, fish, eggs, milk, cheese, dried beans and peas; whole-grain products; soft drinks	Bone formation; acid–base balance; cell membrane structure; B vitamin activation; organic compound component, e.g., ATP–PC, 2, 3–DPG	Rare. Deficiency symptoms parallel calcium deficiency. Muscular weakness	Rare. Impaired calcium metabolism; gastrointestinal distress from phosphate salts
Magnesium (Mg)	Milk and yogurt; dried beans; nuts; whole-grain products; fruits and vegetables, especially green leafy vegetables	Protein synthesis; metalloenzyme; 2, 3–DPG formation; glucose metabolism; smooth muscle contraction; bone component	Rare. Muscle weakness; apathy; muscle twitching; muscle cramps; cardiac arrhythmias	Nausea; vomiting; diarrhea

in Chapter 6, excessive protein intake may lead to calcium excretion, an estimate cited by the National Dairy Council being 1 milligram of calcium lost for every gram of protein consumed.

Overall, however, calcium balance in the body is attributed mostly to adequate calcium intake. Although certain food constituents may impair the absorption of calcium, the effect is not as great as once believed. In general, the amounts of protein, phosphorus, fiber, phytates, and oxalates found in the average North American diet do not appear to pose a problem for calcium absorption. For example, research has revealed that vegetarian diets provide adequate calcium nutrition as measured by body stores. High intakes of coffee and alcohol may increase calcium loss from the body, although one to two cups of coffee and moderate alcohol consumption appear to have little effect on calcium balance.

As we shall see below, the major factor underlying calcium deficiency is inadequate calcium intake, but some of these other dietary factors may also influence calcium balance if taken to excess.

Major Functions The vast majority of body calcium, 98 percent, is found in the skeleton, where it gives strength by the formation of salts such as calcium phosphate. One percent is used for tooth formation. The remainder, which exists in an ionic state or in combination with certain pro-

teins, exerts considerable influence over human metabolism. Calcium ions (Ca^{2+}) are involved in all types of muscle contraction, including that of the heart, skeletal muscle, and smooth muscle found in blood vessels such as the arteries. Calcium activates a number of enzymes; in this capacity it plays a central role in both the synthesis and breakdown of muscle glycogen and liver glycogen. Calcium also helps regulate nerve impulse transmission, blood clotting, and secretion of hormones. It should be noted that the skeletal content of calcium is not inert. The physiological functions of calcium, such as nerve cell transmission, take precedence over formation of bone tissue. If the diet is low in calcium for a short time, the body can mobilize some from the skeleton through the action of hormones, such as parathormone and the hormonal form of vitamin D, to maintain an adequate amount in ionic form.

Deficiency Calcium balance in the human body is rather complex. Figure 8.1 depicts the fate of an intake of 800 mg. Only 300 mg (about 40 percent) is absorbed while the remaining 500 mg is excreted in the feces. The calcium that is absorbed into the blood interacts with the current body stores, the net result being the excretion of 300 mg through the intestines, kidneys, and sweat to balance the amount originally absorbed. Calcium deficiency may develop from inadequate dietary intake or increased excretion.

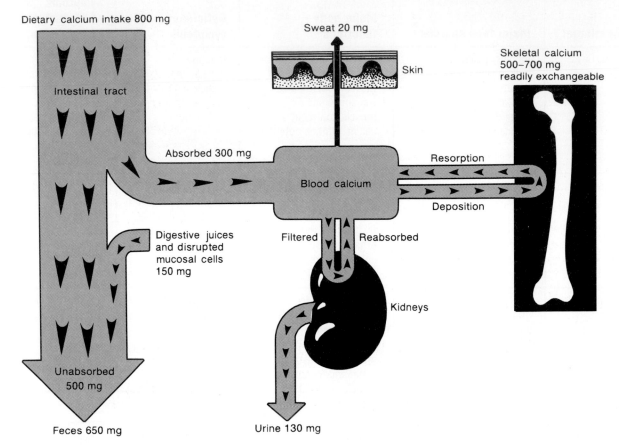

The body's maintenance of calcium
balance on a daily dietary calcium
intake of 800 milligrams

Figure 8.1   Calcium balance in an adult. On an intake of 800 mg, only about 300 mg are absorbed into the body, the remaining 500 mg being excreted in the feces. To maintain calcium balance, 300 mg are excreted including an additional 150 mg in the feces, 130 mg through the kidneys to the urine, and 20 mg in sweat. See text for further discussion.

As noted previously, nationwide surveys have revealed that many Americans, particularly females, are not obtaining the RDA for calcium. In one report, over 50 percent of women consumed less than 70 percent of the RDA. However, surveys with athletic groups reveal some athletes are getting well above the RDA, particularly males. Nevertheless, Clarkson and Haymes indicated many female athletes are also consuming less than the RDA, and in a Canadian study, Webster and Barr noted that although the mean value of calcium intake for a group of gymnasts met the Canadian RDI, many individual gymnasts within the group consumed considerably less. Many athletes trying to obtain a low body weight for competition, such as female gymnasts, long-distance runners, and ballerinas, have substandard intakes.

Strenuous exercise may also increase sweat losses of calcium. In a recent study, Klesges and others, studying primarily African American basketball players, reported losses of greater than 400 milligrams of calcium per daily training session. Such a loss would match or exceed the amount normally absorbed from the daily diet.

The effect of a calcium deficiency depends on whether calcium levels are low in the blood or in the bones. Serum calcium levels are usually regulated by several hormones in the average individual. The body can adapt to low dietary intake by increasing the rate of absorption from the intestines and decreasing the rate of excretion by the kidneys. Because the skeleton is a large reservoir of body calcium, low serum levels are rare. When they do occur, it usually is because of hormonal imbalances rather than dietary deficiencies.

Nevertheless, owing to the diverse physiological roles of calcium, a low serum level could be expected to cause a number of problems. For the athlete, impaired muscular contraction would certainly affect sport performance. One symptom may be muscle cramping due to an imbalance of calcium in the muscle and in the surrounding body fluids. Fortunately, serious deficiencies of serum calcium are rare in athletes because hormones may extract calcium from the bone as needed.

An inadequate dietary intake of calcium has been associated with several health problems, most notably colon cancer, high blood pressure, and osteoporosis.

Some evidence indicates that low levels of dietary calcium may contribute to the development of cancer of the colon. Calcium is believed to combine with bile salts or fatty acids, forming an insoluble complex and helping to excrete them in the feces, thereby reducing their potential carcinogenic effect on the walls of the colon, something akin to the role of dietary fiber. In a recent study, Lupton and others noted that calcium supplements could lead to a "healthier" bile profile, providing support for this viewpoint. Although some animal and human studies have indicated dietary calcium, including supplements, may decrease the proliferation of colonic epithelial cells, Zimmerman recently noted that the available research data are inconsistent and more research is needed. Subsequent to this review, Kearney and others reported that the intake of calcium from foods and supplements was inversely associated with colon cancer risk, but this trend was no longer statistically significant after adjusting for confounding variables. Nevertheless, the relative risk for those consuming the most calcium was reduced by 25 percent, and the authors concluded that although calcium intake may not be strongly protective against colon cancer risk, a modest association cannot be excluded.

One theory also suggests that calcium deficiency is involved in the development of high blood pressure through the mechanism of contraction of the smooth muscles in the arterioles. However, the National Research Council reports that the relationship of dietary calcium to high blood pressure is weak and the data are inconclusive. Nevertheless, in a recent review, McCarron noted that individuals who meet or exceed the RDA for dietary calcium, along with potassium and magnesium, may experience a reduced risk of sodium chloride-induced hypertension. The role of sodium in the development of hypertension is discussed in more detail in the next chapter.

The major health problems associated with impaired calcium metabolism involve diseases of the bones. A number of factors are involved in the formation, or mineralization, of bone tissue including mechanical stresses such as exercise; hormones such as parathormone, calcitonin, vitamin D (calcitriol), and estrogen; and dietary calcium. An imbalance in any one of these factors could lead to bone demineralization, resulting in the development of rickets in children and osteoporosis in adults.

Osteoporosis (thinning and weakening of the bones related to loss of calcium stores) is a debilitating disease that is primarily age- and gender-related, afflicting more than 60 percent of postmenopausal women between the ages of 55 and 64 and even higher percentages with older age groups. The National Osteoporosis Foundation indicates 28 million Americans, 80 percent of them women, are at risk for or have osteoporosis, and one reviewer estimated there would be 500,000 fractures of the hip in the United States by the year 2000. Although the percentage of men who develop osteoporosis is much lower than

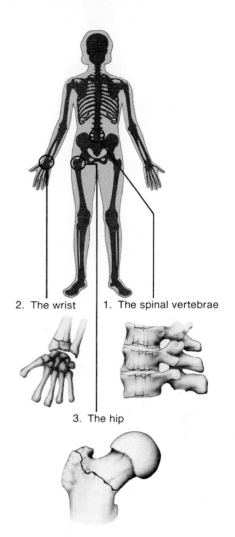

Figure 8.2   Three principal sites of osteoporosis fractures.

that for women, millions of men do have osteoporosis and suffer the same debilitating effects as women. A positive family history, or heredity, and low levels of estrogen are the two primary risk factors in women. Caucasian and Asian women are at higher risk for osteoporosis than women of African ancestry. Following menopause, estrogen production is diminished. Estrogen is a hormone essential for optimal calcium balance in women. Bone receptors for estrogen have been identified, indicating an active role in bone metabolism. In general, reduced levels of estrogen lead to negative calcium balance and a rapid onset of bone demineralization. This softening of the bones predisposes to fractures, particularly in the spine, the end of the radius in the forearm, and the neck of the femur at the hip joint, as illustrated in Figure 8.2. These latter two fractures may be completely debilitating to the older individual. The spinal fracture is more common since the vertebrae are composed of **trabecular bone,** a spongy type of bone more susceptible to calcium loss than the more dense compact bone. However, both types of bone may be lost during osteoporosis as depicted in Figure 8.3.

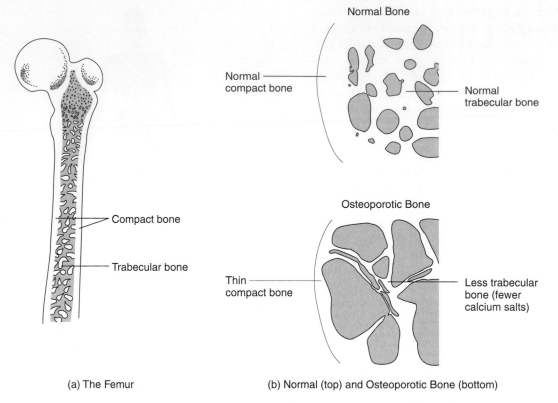

Normal Bone

Normal compact bone

Normal trabecular bone

Osteoporotic Bone

Thin compact bone

Less trabecular bone (fewer calcium salts)

Compact bone

Trabecular bone

(a) The Femur

(b) Normal (top) and Osteoporotic Bone (bottom)

Figure 8.3   In osteoporosis, impaired calcium metabolism may decrease the external compact bone thickness and the strength of the internal trabecular bone lattice network.

Although heredity and estrogen status are strong risk factors for osteoporosis, some life-style factors may impair optimal bone metabolism. Both physical inactivity and inadequate dietary intake of calcium are risk factors for osteoporosis, but so too are cigarette smoking, excess consumption of coffee and alcohol, stress, and various medications. Table 8.3 highlights the risk factors for osteoporosis.

Because the prevention and treatment of osteoporosis may include calcium supplementation, this topic is covered below.

Supplementation   Contemporary treatment for osteoporosis usually involves three components—calcium supplements, exercise, and hormone replacement or nonhormonal drug therapy.

Calcium Supplements   Calcium supplements come in a variety of forms, such as calcium carbonate, calcium lactate, and calcium gluconate, and are found in certain antacids, such as Tums. The bioavailability may vary considerably according to the brand, and there is speculation that antacids may actually interfere with calcium absorption. Be sure to check the label for the calcium content per tablet, which may range from 50–600 mg depending on the brand. For those who desire to take a calcium supplement, it may be wise to take a tablet with about 200 mg at meals three times a day, rather than one tablet with 600 mg, for it appears more calcium is

Table 8.3 Risk factors for osteoporosis	
Heredity	Positive family history
Race	White or Asian
Gender	Female
Menstrual status	Postmenopausal; amenorrheic
Age	Advanced age
Exercise	Physical inactivity; bed rest
Diet	Inadequate calcium; inadequate vitamin D; excessive coffee; excessive alcohol
Tobacco	Cigarette smoking
Alcohol	Excessive use
Stress	Excessive stress; anxiety
Medications	Certain medications increase calcium losses
Hormonal status	Low estrogen; low testosterone

absorbed when the intake is spread throughout the day. Moreover, when the supplement is combined with meals, gastric acidity and slower transit time in the gut promote calcium absorption. A daily total supplement of 600 mg calcium, combined with a dietary intake of 500–600 mg, should provide adequate calcium nutrition for most individuals. However, the point should be stressed that careful selection of foods will provide all of the calcium you need from the daily diet, thus eliminating the need for supplements.

Although supplements up to 600 mg per day do not appear to pose much danger, excessive amounts may contribute to abnormal heart contractions, constipation, and the development of kidney stones in susceptible individuals, particularly those with a family history of kidney problems. For those susceptible to kidney stones, Curhan and others evaluated data from the Nurses' Health Study and found that dietary calcium does not contribute to kidney stone formation because it reduces the absorption of oxalate in foods, preventing the formation of calcium oxalates, or kidney stones. Calcium supplements taken without food do not exert this effect, and thus may contribute to kidney stone formation. Moreover, excessive dietary calcium or calcium supplements may interfere with the absorption of other key minerals, notably iron and zinc. The National Research Council recommends against supplementation to a total much above the RDA, but the updated RDA for some age groups (1,000–1,300 milligrams) may require supplementation for some individuals.

Although the use of calcium supplements alone in the treatment of osteoporosis has been the subject of debate, several recent studies and reviews provide some positive data. Recker and Devine, and their associates, indicated that calcium supplementation greater than 1,200 milligrams per day prevented the loss of bone density at the ankle and hip and reduced the incidence of spine fractures. In a recent review, Teegarden and Weaver cited a meta-analysis of studies examining the relationship between calcium intake and bone density in adults, indicating a significant positive correlation with a stronger relationship in premenopausal than in postmenopausal women. In their review, they also cited research that calcium supplementation may increase bone mineral density and content in adolescent girls as well. Although some indicate more research is needed, Avioli, an authority on calcium metabolism, has noted that until more data are available, we must acknowledge that calcium supplements may retard the rate of bone loss in women just prior to or after menopause.

Exercise   Exercise places a mechanical stress on the bone, facilitating its development and the deposition of calcium salts. Recent data support the role of various physical activities as a means to stimulate bone development. Studies by Dook and others and by Cassell and others have indicated high impact sport activities, such as gymnastics, volleyball, and basketball, and medium impact sport activities, such as running and field hockey, increased bone mineral density in female athletes more so than females in non-impact sports, such as swimming, or sedentary females.

According to Kelley, a recent meta-analysis of eleven studies suggested that exercise can be used to help maintain and increase regional bone mineral density in postmenopausal women.

The American College of Sports Medicine recently developed a position stand on osteoporosis and exercise with the following key points.

1. Weight-bearing exercise is essential for the normal development and maintenance of a healthy skeleton.

2. Sedentary women may increase bone mass slightly by becoming more active, but the primary benefit of the increased activity may be the avoidance of further loss of bone that occurs with inactivity.

3. Exercise cannot be recommended as a substitute for hormone replacement therapy at the time of menopause.

4. The optimal program for older women would include activities that improve strength, flexibility, and coordination that may decrease the incidence of osteoporotic fractures by lessening the likelihood of falling.

Similar recommendations have been presented by the Osteoporosis Society of Canada.

Hormone replacement or drug therapy   In postmenopausal women, estrogen therapy may be necessary, possibly combined with progesterone. However, according to the editors of *HealthNews*, a reputable newsletter, estrogen therapy may pose increased risks for breast cancer in women. Calcitonin, a hormone secreted by the thyroid gland, helps deposit calcium in the bone and may be useful as a means to deter bone loss.

Additionally, recently developed drugs can help prevent bone loss and yet do not have the potential risks of estrogen. Bisphosphonates are nonhormonal agents with a high affinity for bone mineral. One common brand is Fosamax. Bisphosphonates inhibit bone resorption, but do not inhibit bone mineralization, thus preventing bone loss and possibly increasing bone mineral density. They are to be used only by postmenopausal women, and in a recent review Isenbarger and Chapin indicated they may be very useful in the treatment of established osteoporosis or for women in the early postmenopausal period. The FDA recently approved use of raloxifene (brand name Evista), a selective estrogen receptor modulator that appears to act like estrogen on the skeleton but blocks estrogen's effect on the breast and uterus. There may be some esophageal or gastrointestinal problems associated with use of these drugs, but following proper directions may prevent them.

Osteoporosis in Sports   Although osteoporosis occurs primarily in older individuals, investigators are expressing serious concern regarding disturbed calcium metabolism in young female athletes, particularly endurance athletes and those involved in weight-control sports. The **female athlete triad**—disordered eating, amenorrhea, osteoporosis—has been reported in numerous studies. As noted previously, a properly planned exercise program may actually help to prevent osteoporosis and is one of the three major components of a treatment program. However, when research first began to show that amenorrhea and osteoporosis were associated with excessive exercise, such as in female distance runners, exercise was thought to be one of the causative factors.

However, other theories prevail today. Although the exact cause has not been identified, the underlying behavior appears to be disordered eating, as will be discussed in Chapter 10. Females who attempt to lose body weight in order to improve their appearance or competitive ability in sports may modify their diets, decreasing energy and protein intake. They may also exercise excessively to burn Calories. Restrictive diets and excessive exercise regimens may affect hormone status in various ways, including disturbed functioning of the hypothalamus and pituitary gland, two glands that significantly influence overall hormone status in the body including female reproductive hormones, and decreased levels of body fat, which may lead to a reduced production of estrone, a form of estrogen. **Secondary amenorrhea** (cessation of menses for prolonged periods) is a classic sign of disturbed hormonal status associated with disordered eating in postpubertal females, as seen in patients with anorexia nervosa. When observed in athletic females, secondary amenorrhea is often referred to as **athletic amenorrhea.** In young female athletes, athletic amenorrhea is often associated with osteoporosis.

Sophisticated techniques have been used to assess bone density, or bone mineral content. In a number of these studies, amenorrheic athletes were found to have significantly less bone mineral content in the spine and other bones, including the femur, than sedentary women and athletes who were menstruating normally. Moreover, these young, amenorrheic athletes had a higher incidence of stress fractures. As with postmenopausal women, the decreased estrogen is believed to be the causative factor in loss of bone density. Some evidence suggests that when amenorrheic athletes resume normal menstruation, bone mineral content increases. On the other hand, Barbara Drinkwater, an acknowledged authority in this area, has cited several reports that some bone loss in amenorrheic athletes is irreversible.

Although these premenopausal athletes do not need any more exercise, one investigator recommended a daily intake of 1,200–1,500 milligrams of calcium as a possible means to help prevent osteoporosis. For premenopausal athletes who become amenorrheic and estrogen depleted, oral contraceptive pills have been suggested as a practical means of getting additional estrogen. However, the medical treatment suggested for this condition depends on the point of view of the individual endocrinologist, and may include estrogen or other hormone/drug therapy. An appropriate physician, such as a sports-oriented gynecologist, should be consulted.

Although males are at less risk for developing osteoporosis than females, recent reviews by Seeman and by Bennell and others noted that low calcium intake, weight loss, low body fat, and excess alcohol intake, along with other risk factors, may adversely affect bone density in males. Low levels of testosterone, the male sex hormone, are also associated with decreased bone density in males. Interestingly, Bilanin and Ormerod, along with their colleagues, reported decreased spinal bone mass in male long-distance runners, suggesting the decreased levels of testosterone or increased levels of cortisol often seen in endurance runners could be the cause. Klesges and others also recently reported a decrease in total body bone mineral content in male basketball players involved in intense training from preseason to midseason. However, these investigators also reported that calcium supplementation was associated with significant increases in bone mineral content.

Although calcium supplementation may be useful to help maintain bone mass in some female and male athletes, research regarding the effect of calcium supplementation on physical performance is almost nonexistent. Low serum levels may impair neuromuscular functions, but such conditions are rare because the body will draw from calcium reserves in the skeleton to restore serum levels.

Prudent Recommendations To help prevent osteoporosis, postmenopausal women should obtain 1,000 milligrams of calcium daily if on estrogen therapy, or 1,200–1,500 milligrams if not. Both weight-bearing aerobic and resistance strength-training exercises are recommended. Postmenopausal women should consult with their physicians relative to hormone replacement or drug therapy. Older men should also obtain adequate calcium, exercise, and consult their physicians for appropriate drug therapy if warranted.

For younger, premenopausal women, the nonpharmacological approach is recommended. The key with younger women is prevention. They need to develop **peak bone mass,** the optimal amount within genetic limitations, prior to age 25, and attempt to keep the bone mass high in the advancing years. Anderson and others note that because evidence suggests osteoporosis is easier to prevent than to treat, initiating sound health behaviors early in life and continuing them throughout life is the best approach. Thus, it would appear prudent for young women to develop a lifetime exercise program and obtain the RDA of 1,000–1,300 milligrams for calcium in the diet. The earlier the better, for research has suggested a greater increase in bone mass when calcium supplements are given to prepubertal children, but adequate calcium intake is critical for adolescents as well. Weight-bearing exercises, such as walking or jogging, promote bone mineralization by stressing the hips and spine, while resistance strength training and modified push-ups are also excellent for the spine and for the radial bone at the wrist joint. Four glasses of skim milk provide 1,200 mg of calcium. In addition, the milk (or its equivalent) would provide 32 grams of protein, which is about 80 percent of the protein RDA for the average woman, and a variety of other vitamins and minerals in less than 400 Calories. Because coffee, alcohol, and tobacco use are secondary risk factors associated with the development of osteoporosis, moderation or abstinence is advocated. Similar strategies are recommended for males as well.

Phosphorus (P)

Phosphorus is a nonmetallic element and is the second most abundant mineral in the body after calcium.

RDA The adult RDA is 800 mg for both men and women. Higher amounts are needed between ages 11 and 25. Specific values for different age groups may be found in Appendix A. The RDI is 1,000 mg.

Food Sources As noted earlier in Table 8.2, phosphorus is distributed widely in foods, mainly as phosphate salts in conjunction with animal protein. Excellent sources include seafood, meat, eggs, milk, cheese, nuts, dried beans and peas, grain products, and a wide variety of vegetables. Phosphate is a common food additive, and soft drinks have a relatively high phosphate content. In some foods, phosphorus is also a part of phytate, which may diminish the absorption of minerals like calcium, iron, zinc, and copper by forming insoluble phosphate salts in the intestine. However, as noted previously, this is not a major problem with the typical North American diet.

Most Americans consume more than the RDA for phosphorus, and as noted previously, too little calcium. The recommended calcium:phosphorus ratio is about 1:1, that is equal amounts of each. In a recent review, Anderson and Barrett indicated too much dietary phosphorus, which may occur because of phosphate additives in food, may impair calcium metabolism and predispose to osteoporosis. Too much phosphorus may also stimulate the release of parathyroid hormone. Anderson and Barrett noted that a ratio of up to 1:1.6 may be compatible with bone health, but ratios of 1:4 may be associated with osteoporosis.

Major Functions In the human body, phosphorus occurs only as the salt phosphate, which exists as inorganic phosphate or is coupled with other minerals or organic compounds. Phosphates are extremely important in human metabolism. About 80–90 percent of the phosphorus in the body combines to form calcium phosphate, which is used for the development of bones and teeth. As with calcium, the bones represent a sizable store of phosphate salts. Other phosphate salts, such as sodium phosphate, are involved in acid-base balance. The remainder of the body phosphates are found in a variety of organic forms, including the phospholipids, which help form cell membranes, and DNA. Several other organic phosphates are of prime importance to the active individual. For example, organic phosphates are essential to the normal function of most of the B vitamins involved in the energy processes within the cell. They are also part of the high-energy compounds found in the muscle cell, such as ATP and PC, which are needed for muscle contraction. Glucose also needs to be phosphorylated in order to proceed through glycolysis. Organic phosphates also are a part of a compound in the RBC known as 2,3–DPG (2,3–diphosphoglycerate), which facilitates the release of oxygen to the muscle tissues.

Deficiency Because phosphorus is distributed so widely in foods and because hormonal control is very effective, deficiency states are rare. They have been known to occur in individuals with certain diseases and in those who use antacid compounds for long periods, as the antacid decreases the absorption of phosphorus. Symptoms parallel those of calcium deficiency, such as loss of bone material resulting in rickets or osteomalacia. Other symptoms include muscular weakness. Extreme muscular exercise may increase phosphorus excretion in the urine but has not been reported to cause a deficiency state. Phosphorus deficiency could theoretically impair physical performance, but it has not been the subject of study because such deficiencies are rare.

Supplementation Phosphate salt supplements, such as sodium phosphate and potassium phosphate, were reported to relieve fatigue in German soldiers during World War I. Other research in Germany during the 1930s suggested phosphate salts could improve physical performance. Over 50 years ago one reviewer discredited much of this early research, but he did note that phosphates probably could increase human work output when consumed in quantities exceeding the amounts found in the normal diet. Indeed, they still are advertised today in some European sports-medicine journals and continue to be a favorite among European athletes. They have also been marketed as an ergogenic aid in the United States, most recently as the main ingredient in PhosFuel, advertised to be the ultimate lactic acid buffer. Leibovitz, in a popular muscle magazine, has called phosphate the power mineral.

The results of more contemporary research relative to the ergogenic effect of phosphate supplementation are somewhat equivocal. A number of studies, using appropriate experimental methods and the recommended phosphate dosages, have shown no effects of phosphate supplementation on a variety of performance variables. Researchers at Brigham Young University reported that Stim-O-Stam, a commercial phosphate salt supplement containing other nutrients, exerted no effect upon measures of strength or anaerobic endurance tests, such as a

2- to 3-minute run to exhaustion on a treadmill. Weatherwax and others, from Robert Otto's research group at Adelphi University, also noted no effect of phosphate salt supplementation on maximal oxygen uptake, lactic acid production, or performance in an 8-kilometer (5-mile) bike race. Mannix and others recently reported that although phosphate supplementation did increase 2,3–DPG levels, it did not improve cardiovascular function or oxygen efficiency in subjects exercising at 60 percent of VO_2 max. Thompson and her associates from the University of Southern Mississippi reported no effect of phosphate salt supplementation on 2,3–DPG, hemoglobin, or VO_2 max. However, there was a nonsignificant 6 percent increase of VO_2 max in the phosphate trial compared to the placebo. These investigators generally concluded that phosphate salts were not ergogenic in nature, at least in relation to the type of performance tested in their studies.

In contrast, the results of other contemporary, well-designed studies suggest that phosphate salts may enhance exercise performance. One of the first studies reported was conducted by Robert Cade and his associates at the University of Florida. In a double-blind, placebo, crossover study, highly-trained runners took 1 gram of sodium phosphate four times a day during the experimental phase. The phosphate salts increased the 2,3–DPG in the RBC, which related very closely to an increase in VO_2 max. The amount of lactate produced at a standard exercise workload decreased, suggesting more efficient oxygen delivery to the muscles. Although no performance data were presented, the authors did report that the subjects ran longer on the treadmill during the phosphate trials. This University of Florida research group also noted a reduced sensation of psychological stress while exercising at a standard workload.

Other investigators, using a protocol similar to that of Cade and his associates, have also revealed ergogenic effects. Richard Kreider and his colleagues, using highly-trained cross-country runners as subjects, found that 4 grams of trisodium phosphate for 6 days produced a significant increase in VO_2 max, approximately 10 percent—very similar to the improvement noted in Cade's study. Changes in 2,3–DPG were not the mechanism for this increase, however, since these values did not increase. Moreover, performance in a 5-mile competitive run on a treadmill did not improve, although there was a mean speed increase of approximately 12 seconds during the phosphate trial in these highly-trained runners. Ian Stewart and his associates from Australia, using trained cyclists, reported that 3.6 grams of sodium phosphate for 3 days did significantly increase 2,3–DPG levels and also increased VO_2 max by 11 percent and time to exhaustion on a progressive workload test on a bicycle ergometer by nearly 16 percent. In a follow-up to his previous study, Kreider looked at the effect of 4 grams of trisodium phosphate, 1 gram four times daily for 3–4 days, on physiological and performance factors during a maximal cycling test and a 40-kilometer bike race on a Velodyne. The study followed a double-blind, placebo, crossover protocol. Kreider and his colleagues noted a significant 9 percent increase in VO_2 max, a significantly faster 40-km time (improving from 45.75 to 42.25 minutes), and enhanced myocardial efficiency as monitored by echocardiographic techniques. These investigators suggested that phosphate salt supplementation could possess ergogenic qualities, but in a recent review, Kreider indicated that additional research is needed to confirm these findings and the underlying mechanisms. Tremblay and others addressed methodological differences between studies (e.g., calcium versus sodium phosphate supplements) that could contribute to the equivocal results and also recommended additional research employing rigorous methodological control. These viewpoints have been reiterated in subsequent reviews by Horswill and Clarkson, although Clarkson did indicate several studies have documented ergogenic effects and the degree to which performance improved was similar among the studies.

Studies with phosphate supplementation conducted following these reviews revealed no significant benefits. Galloway and others provided an acute dose (22.2 grams) of calcium phosphate to trained cyclists and untrained subjects 90 minutes prior to a submaximal cycle test followed by a maximal exercise test, and reported no significant effects on heart rate, ventilation, oxygen uptake, or time to exhaustion. In another study, Kraemer and others had recreationally-trained cyclists and untrained subjects consume a commercial product (PhosFuel) for 3.5 days and evaluated its effect on anaerobic performance in four 30-second cycle Wingate tests with 2 minutes rest between. The supplement provided no advantage over the placebo relative to peak power or mean power. However, these studies employed procedures (acute dose and calcium phosphate; commercial supplement and anaerobic performance) unlike those studies reporting beneficial effects, which used sodium phosphate, a more prolonged supplementation protocol, and more aerobic exercise performance tests.

The effect of 5–6 days of sodium phosphate supplementation on aerobic performance merits additional research.

Adenosine triphosphate (ATP), as you may recall, is the immediate source of energy for muscle contraction. Although some entrepreneurs have marketed ATP supplements for athletes, there is no available evidence that they enhance physical performance. Most likely, enzymes in the digestive tract would catabolize the ATP before it could get into the muscle. Creatine phosphate is used to replenish ATP rapidly as a component of the ATP-PC energy system. As noted in Chapter 6, recent research with oral creatine supplementation has suggested some ergogenic effects on muscular strength and running speed. In a recent study with patients over 60 years of age who experienced muscular atrophy following fracture of the femur, creatine phosphate supplements, as compared to a placebo, significantly increased muscle mass during a rehabilitation program. As with creatine, additional research is needed to determine possible ergogenic applications of creatine phosphate to athletes.

Excesses of phosphorus in the body are excreted by the kidneys. Phosphorus excess per se does not appear to pose any problems, with the exception of individuals with limited kidney function. Subjects consuming phosphate supplements may experience gastrointestinal distress, which may be alleviated by mixing the salts in a liquid and consuming with a meal. Excessive amounts of phosphate over time may impair calcium metabolism and balance.

Prudent Recommendations Phosphate supplements are not recommended on a long-term basis as they may create calcium imbalances, possibly leading to osteoporosis. Some evidence suggests sodium phosphate salt supplementation may enhance aerobic endurance performance. An accepted protocol appears to be a total of 4 grams of trisodium phosphate per day, consumed in 1-gram portions with food and drink, for 5–6 days. If you decide to experiment with phosphate supplementation, do so in training before using it in conjunction with competition. Given the association with possible calcium imbalances, this procedure should be used sparingly. Currently, the International Olympic Committee does not prohibit the use of phosphate salts.

Magnesium (Mg)

Magnesium is the fourth most abundant element found in the body; it is a positive ion and is related to calcium and phosphorus.

RDA The adult RDA for magnesium is 350 mg for men and 280 mg for women. Slightly different amounts, found in Appendix A, are required by children and adolescents. The RDI is 400 mg.

Food Sources Magnesium is widely distributed in foods, particularly nuts, seafood, green leafy vegetables, other fruits and vegetables, and whole-grain products. One-half cup of shrimp contains about 20 percent of the RDA, and a glass of skim milk has 10 percent. Many other foods contain about 2–10 percent of the RDA per serving. About 25–60 percent of dietary magnesium is absorbed. See Table 8.2.

Major Functions The body stores about 50–60 percent of its magnesium in the skeletal system, which may serve as a reserve during short periods of dietary deficiency. Sojka and Weaver indicate magnesium influences bone metabolism and helps prevent bone fragility. A small percentage is in the serum, but the remainder is found in soft tissues such as muscle, where it is a component of over 300 enzymes. As such, magnesium plays a key role in a variety of physiological processes, many of which are important to the physically active individual, including neuromuscular, cardiovascular, and hormonal functions. For example, as a part of ATPase it is involved in muscle contraction and all body functions involving ATP as an energy source. Magnesium helps regulate the synthesis of protein and other compounds, such as 2,3–DPG, which may be essential for optimal oxygen metabolism. It is a part of an enzyme that facilitates the metabolism of glucose in the muscle. Magnesium also helps block some of the actions of calcium in the body, such as contraction in both the skeletal and smooth muscles.

Deficiency Although Elin has reported that a large segment of the United States population may have an inadequate magnesium intake, the National Research Council has reported that magnesium deficiency is rare. No purely dietary magnesium deficiency has been reported in people consuming normal diets, probably because of its wide availability in a variety of foods, an effective system of conservation by the kidneys and intestines, and a substantial storage in the bone tissue. However, certain health conditions such as kidney malfunction and prolonged diarrhea, as well as the use of diuretics and excessive alcohol, may contribute to a deficiency state. Additionally, in a recent review, Henry Lukaski reported that dietary survey findings were somewhat mixed; some studies indicated that although most male athletes equaled or exceeded the RDA for magnesium, many female athletes were obtaining only about 60–65 percent of the RDA while athletes in weight-control sports were getting only 30–35 percent. Over time, such low dietary intakes may lead to a magnesium deficiency.

Deficiency symptoms include apathy, muscle weakness, muscle twitching and tremor, muscle cramps (particularly in the feet), and cardiac arrhythmias. The muscular symptoms may occur because the low levels of magnesium are not able to block the stimulating effect of calcium on muscle contraction. In this sense, magnesium deficiency may be related to high blood pressure because excessive calcium may cause the muscles in the arterioles to constrict. Given the possible relationship of magnesium deficiency to cardiac arrhythmias and high blood pressure, Douban and Brodsky indicated magnesium deficiency may be associated with cardiovascular disease, suggesting other related factors as well, including prevention of coronary artery vasospasm. Indeed, some epidemiological research from Europe and the United States has indicated that males who consume hard drinking water, which is high in magnesium, experience fewer deaths from myocardial infarction. In a recent study, Rubenowitz and others reported a 35 percent reduction in death for those who consumed the most magnesium from municipal water supplies.

Exercise appears to influence magnesium metabolism, but in an unknown way. Deuster has noted that one of the most common research observations is a decrease in plasma levels of magnesium following exercise. It is thought that magnesium enters the tissues in response to exercise-related requirements, for example, of the muscle tissue for energy metabolism and the adipose tissue for lipolysis. Some investigators also suggested that prolonged exercise increases magnesium losses from the body via urine and sweat. However, the reported sweat losses of 4–15 mg per liter are relatively small in comparison to body stores and daily intake. Casoni and others reported significantly lower serum magnesium levels in Italian endurance athletes as compared with sedentary individuals, but the serum values were well within the normal range. One study reported a correlation between plasma levels of magnesium and VO_2 max in trained individuals, but this finding has not been replicated. Other research suggests magnesium deficiency may be associated with the chronic fatigue syndrome, characterized by unexplained fatigue or easy fatigability lasting longer than 6 months. On the basis of some of these findings, several reports have recommended that individuals undergoing prolonged, intensive physical training should increase their daily intake of magnesium, but these recommendations are within range of the United States RDA. The extra Calories consumed when energy expenditure increases during exercise should provide the additional magnesium.

There is little evidence showing a magnesium deficiency in humans severe enough to impair physical performance.

Supplementation   In their extensive review, McDonald and Keen indicated they are not aware of any data showing a positive effect of magnesium supplementation on exercise performance in individuals who are in adequate magnesium status. However, several studies published subsequent to their review have provided some preliminary data, although the results are equivocal. Gullestad and others provided oral magnesium supplements or a placebo to chronic alcoholics (among whom magnesium deficiency is common) for 6 weeks and reported magnesium led to significant improvements in muscle strength whereas the placebo group experienced no change. However, there was no exercise training involved in this study. Brilla and Haley, using untrained male and female subjects involved in 7 weeks of weight training, provided a supplement to the experimental group to complement the normal daily intake to a level approximating 8 milligrams per kilogram body weight; the placebo group consumed their normal diet plus the placebo. Strength was measured before and after the experiment on an isokinetic device, recording quadriceps torque. Both groups increased muscle strength due to the weight training, but the supplemented group had a significantly greater increase than the placebo group. The authors hypothesized the magnesium stimulated protein synthesis. However, in a more recent study, Brilla and Burkett reported that 6 weeks of supplementation with a magnesium-fortified sports drink, about 200 milligrams of magnesium, did not improve strength in American football players during spring training.

Relative to aerobic endurance, Brilla and Gunter, using a similar supplementation protocol, reported magnesium enhanced running economy at 90 percent VO_2 max because the oxygen cost of running was lower compared to a placebo condition. However, magnesium did not significantly increase run time to exhaustion in this study. Additionally, Terblanche and others, matching twenty marathon runners into two groups based on performance time, provided either a placebo or 365 milligrams of magnesium per day to the subjects 4 weeks prior to and 6 weeks after running a marathon. Their dependent variables were marathon performance and several tests of quadriceps muscular strength and fatigue during the recovery phase after the marathon. They reported no significant effects of magnesium supplementation on muscle or serum levels of magnesium, marathon performance, muscle function, or muscle recovery. They suggested excess magnesium in the diet may not be absorbed in those with normal levels in the body.

These latter two studies appear to be well designed, yet the results are equivocal. It may be possible that if a magnesium deficiency is corrected, muscle strength may be improved, as suggested in the study with alcoholics. In a case study, magnesium supplementation also helped resolve muscle cramps in a tennis player. However, at the present time the data are too limited to support an ergogenic effect of magnesium supplementation, and additional well-controlled research is justified.

In general, excessive intake of magnesium does not appear to cause major health problems, except for those with kidney disorders who cannot excrete the excess. Excessive intake may cause nausea, vomiting, and diarrhea, however. The usual cause is the ingestion of magnesium salts, such as found in milk of magnesia.

Prudent Recommendations   Physically active individuals should obtain adequate magnesium from a balanced diet containing foods rich in magnesium. For those trying to lose body weight for competition, a magnesium supplement containing the RDA may be recommended. There is no need for larger doses as they may be associated with some adverse effects.

Trace Minerals

The **trace minerals** (trace elements) are those needed in quantities less than 100 mg per day. These minerals are often known as microminerals. For several the body needs only extremely minute amounts, such as a few micrograms (millionth of a gram) per day; the term ultratrace is applied to these minerals.

Iron (Fe)

Iron is a metallic element that exists in two general forms, ferrous (Fe^{2+}) and ferric (Fe^{3+}).

RDA Depending upon age and sex, the average individual needs to replace about 1.0–1.5 mg of iron that is lost from the body daily. However, because the bioavailability of iron is very low, with only about 10 percent of food iron being absorbed, the RDA is ten times the need. Currently the RDA is 10 mg for men, 12 mg for males age 11–18, and 15 mg for female teenagers and adults. Slightly different amounts are needed by other age groups and may be found in Appendix A. Pregnant women need 30 mg, while postmenopausal women need only 10 mg. The current RDI is 18 mg. It should be noted that the 1989 RDA for women and adolescents was lowered by 3 mg, from 18 to 15 mg, compared to the 1980 RDA.

Food Sources Dietary iron comes in two forms. **Heme iron** is associated with hemoglobin and myoglobin and thus is found only in animal foods, such as meat, chicken, and fish. Nonheme iron is found in both animal and plant foods. About 20–70 percent of the iron in animal foods and 100 percent in plant foods is in the nonheme form. Heme iron has greater bioavailability, for about 10–35 percent of it is absorbed from the intestines compared to only 2–10 percent for nonheme iron. The percent absorbed depends on the iron needs of the individual. Those with higher needs will absorb more and those with lower needs will absorb less.

Excellent animal sources of dietary iron include liver, heart, lean meats, oysters, clams, and dark poultry meat. One ounce of lean meat provides about 1 mg of heme iron. Good sources of nonheme iron include dried fruits such as apricots, prunes, and raisins; beans; and whole-grain products. Six dried apricot halves or one-half cup of beans provides about 3 mg of nonheme iron, and some breakfast cereals are fortified to provide 100 percent of the RDA. Cooking in iron pots or skillets also contributes iron to the diet. On a balanced diet, about 6 mg of iron is provided in every 1,000 Calories ingested. See Table 8.4 for foods high in iron.

Certain factors in food may affect the amount of iron absorbed into the body. The muscle protein factor MPF factor found in meat, fish, poultry, is an unknown agent that facilitates the absorption of both heme and nonheme iron. The existence of such a factor is suggested by the fact that small amounts of meat added to vegetable or grain products enhance nonheme absorption. Certain peptides in meat may cause this increased absorption. Vitamin C prevents the oxidation of ferrous iron to the ferric form (ferrous iron is more readily absorbed) and thus facilitates nonheme iron absorption, but it has no effect on absorption of heme iron. Thus, for breakfast, drinking orange juice improves the bioavailability of iron in toast.

On the other hand, substances found naturally in some foods, such as tannins, phosphates, phytates, oxalates, and excessive fiber may decrease the bioavailability of nonheme iron by forming insoluble salts or by promoting rapid transport through the intestines. Tea, for example, which is high in tannins, decreases iron absorption by 60 percent. However, if the diet is balanced these factors should not pose a major problem for adequate iron nutrition. Certain mineral supplements, particularly calcium, and even the calcium in milk, when taken with a meal, may impair absorption of nonheme iron. This effect may be lessened by ingestion of vitamin C with the meal. Conversely, iron supplements may decrease the bioavailability of other minerals, such as zinc.

Major Functions The major function of iron in the body is the formation of compounds essential to the transportation and utilization of oxygen. The vast majority is used to form hemoglobin, a protein-iron compound in the RBC that transports oxygen from the lungs to the body tissues. Other iron compounds include myoglobin, the cytochromes, and several Krebs-cycle metalloenzymes, which help use oxygen at the cellular level. The remainder of the body iron is stored in the tissues, principally as protein compounds called **ferritins.** The iron in the blood, serum ferritin, is used as an index of the body iron stores, as are a number of other markers such as transferrin, protoporphyrin, and hemoglobin. Other major storage sites include the liver, spleen, and bone marrow. When ferritin levels become excessive in the liver, the iron is stored as hemosiderin, an insoluble form. Approximately 30 percent of the body iron is in storage form, while the remaining 70 percent is involved in oxygen metabolism. Because iron is so critical to oxygen use in humans, it is essential that those individuals engaged in aerobic endurance-type exercises have an adequate dietary intake. Figure 8.4 represents a brief outline of iron metabolism in humans. For a comprehensive review of iron metabolism and regulation, the interested reader is referred to the reviews by Bothwell and by Beard and others.

Deficiency According to Scrimshaw, iron deficiency is the most common nutrient deficiency in the world. Iron is one of the few nutrients commonly found to be slightly deficient in the diet of many Americans, particularly women and teenagers. The body normally loses very little iron through such routes as the skin, gastrointestinal tract, hair, and sweat. About 10 mg of dietary iron daily will replace these losses. Females also lose some additional iron in the blood flow during menstruation. They need about 15 mg of dietary iron per day to replace their total losses. Adolescent boys need about 12 mg as they are increasing muscle tissue and blood volume during this rapid period of growth. With 6 mg of iron per 1,000 Calories, the adult male has no problem meeting his requirement of 10 mg per day. With a normal intake of 2,900 Calories, he will receive 17.4 mg. With 2,200 Calories, the average intake for females, only 13.2 mg iron would be provided. This is somewhat short of the 15 mg needed.

National surveys before 1989 revealed that over 90 percent of women were receiving less than the 1980 RDA

Table 8.4 Trace minerals: iron, copper, zinc, chromium, selenium

Trace mineral	Major food sources	Major body functions	Deficiency symptoms	Symptoms of excessive consumption
Iron (Fe)	Organ meats such as liver; meat, fish, and poultry; shellfish, especially oysters; dried beans and peas; whole-grain products; green leafy vegetables; spinach; broccoli; dried apricots, dates, figs, raisins; iron cookware	Hemoglobin and myoglobin formation; electron transfer; essential in oxidative processes	Fatigue; anemia; impaired temperature regulation; decreased resistance to infection	Hemochromatosis; liver damage
Copper (Cu)	Organ meats such as liver; meat, fish, and poultry; shellfish; nuts; eggs; bran cereals; avocado; broccoli; banana	Proper use of iron and hemoglobin in the body; metalloenzyme involved in connective tissue formation and oxidations	Rare; anemia	Rare; nausea; vomiting
Zinc (Zn)	Organ meats; meat, fish, poultry; shellfish, especially oysters; dairy products; nuts; whole-grain products; vegetables, asparagus, spinach	Cofactor of many enzymes involved in energy metabolism, protein synthesis, immune function, sexual maturation, and sensations of taste and smell	Depressed immune function; impaired wound healing; depressed appetite; failure to grow; skin inflammation	Increased LDL and decreased HDL cholesterol; impaired immune system; nausea; vomiting; impaired copper absorption
Chromium (Cr)	Organ meats such as liver; meats; oysters; cheese; whole-grain products; asparagus; beer	Enhances insulin function as glucose tolerance factor	Glucose intolerance; impaired lipid metabolism	Rare from dietary sources
Selenium (Se)	Meat, fish, poultry; organ meats such as kidney, liver; seafood; whole grains and nuts from selenium-rich soil	Cofactor of glutathione peroxidase, and antioxidant enzyme	Rare; cardiac muscle damage	Nausea; vomiting; abdominal pain; hair loss

of iron (18 mg), and many of these women would still have intakes lower than the 1989 RDA (15 mg). Most have normal hemoglobin and serum ferritin status. Because the normal loss of iron from the body is relatively low, and because excessive amounts in the body may be harmful, the intestine limits the amount absorbed from the diet. On the other hand, when an individual becomes iron deficient, the intestines may increase the amount of dietary iron absorbed to above 30 percent. Nevertheless, in a recent study, Looker and others reported that iron deficiency and iron deficiency anemia are still relatively common in adolescent girls and women of childbearing age. The National Research Council has reported that the frequency of iron deficiency without anemia is much greater than that of iron-deficiency anemia. Nevertheless, about 3–5 percent of the female population has iron-deficiency anemia, the most common nutrient-deficiency disorder in the United States.

Iron deficiency occurs in stages. The first stage involves depletion of the bone marrow stores and a decrease in serum ferritin. It is referred to as the stage of iron depletion. The second stage involves a further decrease in serum ferritin and less iron in the hemoglobin, or less circulating iron. Other markers are used to evaluate iron stores in this stage, including free erythrocyte protoporphyrin (FEP), which is used to form hemoglobin.

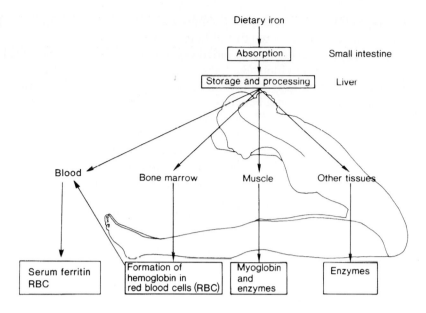

Figure 8.4 Simplified diagram of iron metabolism in humans. After digestion, iron is used in the formation of hemoglobin, myoglobin, and certain cellular enzymes, all of which are essential for transportation of oxygen in the body.

FEP in the blood increases when adequate iron is not available. Serum transferrin, a protein that carries iron in the blood, also increases. This is the stage referred to as iron-deficiency erythropoiesis. In these first two stages the hemoglobin concentration in the blood is still normal. Collectively, these stages are often alluded to as **iron deficiency without anemia.** The third stage consists of a very low level of serum ferritin and decreased hemoglobin concentration, or **iron-deficiency anemia.** Symptoms of iron-deficiency anemia include paleness, tiredness, and low vitality, and impaired ability to regulate body temperature in a cold environment.

Because iron is so critical to the oxygen energy system, it is essential for endurance athletes to have adequate iron in the diet to maintain optimal body supplies. There are some differences of opinion about the magnitude of iron deficiency in athletes. A substantial number of studies, using serum ferritin levels as a basis of iron status, revealed that 50–80 percent of female athletes, particularly endurance runners, were at risk of iron deficiency. However, the National Research Council has stated that there is currently no single biochemical indicator available to reliably assess iron adequacy, so several markers should be used. But then, Newhouse and Clement reported wide variations in these markers. In a study using serum ferritin and transferrin saturation, Risser and his associates reported no significant differences in iron status between female athletes and nonathletes—possibly owing to a wide variation in individual values—but 31 percent of the athletes and 45 percent of the nonathletes were iron deficient. In a recent review, Emily Haymes estimated the prevalence of iron depletion in runners to be about 30 percent. Although iron deficiency appears not to be a problem in most male athletes, several studies have reported poor iron status in about 15–30 percent of male distance runners. One of these studies used a bone biopsy to determine marrow stores.

After reviewing the literature, Priscilla Clarkson reported that iron deficiency to the point of decreased RBC and hemoglobin production does not appear to be prevalent in the athletic population. Some studies have reported iron-deficiency anemia occurs in female athletes at the same rate as in the general U.S. female population (about 3–5 percent) or at a higher rate. The normal hemoglobin level is 14–16 grams per deciliter (100 ml) of blood for males and 12–14 grams for females. Males have been classified as anemic with less than 13 grams, whereas values less than 11 grams, and in some cases 12 grams, have been used as the criterion for anemia in females. Randy Eichner, a hematologist involved in sports medicine, poses the interesting question of whether an athlete whose usual hemoglobin is 16 grams per deciliter is anemic if his level decreases to 14 grams.

Although there may be some debate about the magnitude of the problem of iron deficiency in athletes, most investigators concede that it may be important to monitor the diet and iron status of certain athletes, particularly if performance begins to suffer without any obvious explanation. One report noted that Greg Lemond was struggling in the first stages of the Tour of Italy until his trainer suggested iron therapy. Following several injections, Lemond finished strong in the Tour, winning the last trial race. A month later he won the Tour de France in a remarkable finish. The International Center for Sports Nutrition and the Sports Medicine and Science Division of the United States Olympic Committee recommend screening for hemoglobin and hematocrit twice yearly. Other tests of iron stores might be recommended for menstruating female athletes.

There may be a number of causes for the low iron or hemoglobin levels found in some athletes. Although adult male athletes appear to obtain sufficient dietary iron, numerous studies have revealed that dietary intake of iron may be inadequate in female and adolescent male athletes.

The type of dietary iron may also be important. Ann Snyder and her colleagues noted that although female athletes on a normal mixed diet or a modified vegetarian diet had the same iron intake (14 mg/day), the modified vegetarian diet was associated with significantly lower iron stores in the body, suggestive of a beneficial effect of heme iron. Other studies, such as by Weight and Lyle, and their colleagues, have confirmed the value of meat to help prevent decreases in iron stores during training, while Telford also stresses the value of dietary protein. Three ounces of beef per day were effective. Vegetarian athletes should be aware of the need to incorporate plant foods with high iron content in their diets. Athletes who begin to train at altitude will need to ensure adequate dietary iron intake, for the increased production of red blood cells at altitude will draw upon the body reserves.

Exercise, particularly running, may contribute to iron loss in both sexes for a variety of reasons. A condition often seen in distance runners is **hematuria,** the presence of hemoglobin or myoglobin in the urine. This may be caused by repeated foot contact with the ground, rupturing some RBC and releasing hemoglobin (a process called **hemolysis**), some of which may be excreted by the kidneys. Hemolysis has also been observed in weight lifters, attributed to the mechanical stress generated in the muscles. Prolonged running may also lead to ruptured muscle cells, releasing myoglobin, which may have the same fate. An irritation of the inner lining of the urinary bladder may also be a source of RBC loss. Even nonimpact athletes like rowers have experienced hemolysis. Several studies also have revealed increased loss of blood in the feces of endurance runners and endurance cyclists, which may be due to loss of cells in the intestinal wall or bleeding caused by the use of aspirin or other anti-inflammatory drugs to control pain. Athletes who detect blood loss in the urine or feces should see a physician, for there may be other causes that may need medical treatment.

An additional source of iron loss is the sweat. Although one study has shown that sweat losses of iron are relatively low when induced by sauna (0.02 mg per liter), according to a recent study by Waller and Haymes, the total amount of iron lost in sweat increases during exercise, more so in males than in females. This may be related to the fact that serum iron may actually increase during an exercise session and may be partially excreted in the sweat. The results of several studies, for example Aruoma and others, suggest that approximately 0.3–0.4 mg of iron is lost per liter of sweat during exercise. At a 10 percent rate of absorption, it would take 3–4 mg of dietary iron to replace the iron lost in 1 liter of sweat.

In summary, athletes in training may lose more iron than nonathletes. In a recent review, Weaver and Rajaram noted that when compared to the reference value of sedentary individuals, iron losses in the feces, urine, and sweat may be 75 percent greater in male athletes (1.75 versus 1.0 milligrams) and about 65 percent greater in female athletes (2.3 versus 1.4 milligrams). In less-athletic women engaging in a moderate exercise training program for 6 months, Rajaram and others found that training at 60–75 percent of the heart rate reserve had little effect on serum ferritin levels, although they remained below normal from the beginning to the end of the study.

As would be expected, the problem of concern to the endurance athlete is the development of iron-deficiency anemia. A number of studies have shown that anemia causes a significant reduction in the ability to perform prolonged high-level exercise. The donation of blood causes a drop in hemoglobin, which may also decrease performance capacity. This is, of course, related to the decreased ability to transport and use oxygen in the body.

One form of anemia associated with endurance training is sports anemia, mentioned previously in Chapter 6. Sports anemia is not a true anemia. Although the hemoglobin concentration is toward the lower end of the normal range, the other indices of iron status are normal. Whether sports anemia is a beneficial physiological response to endurance exercise or a condition that will hinder performance is not known. Short-term sports anemia appears to develop in some individuals during the early phases of training or when the magnitude of training increases drastically. One of the effects of endurance training is to increase both the plasma volume and the number of RBC. However, the plasma expansion appears to be greater, so there is a dilution of the RBC and a lowering of the hemoglobin concentration. This effect is believed to be beneficial to the athlete, however, because it reduces the viscosity, or thickness, of the blood and allows it to flow more easily. In many athletes the hemoglobin concentration returns to normal after the first month or so of training. Long-term sports anemia is often seen in highly-trained endurance athletes. One theory proposes that the production of RBC by the bone marrow is decreased in endurance athletes because the RBC become so efficient in releasing oxygen to the tissues. The authors of this theory suggest that sports anemia is not due to poor iron status.

In recent reviews, Eichner noted that the term sports anemia is a misnomer, while Weight also indicated the term is misleading and its use should be discouraged because athletes who develop anemia do so not because of exercise, but for the same reasons that nonathletes do, primarily inadequate dietary iron.

The effect of iron deficiency without anemia on physical performance is controversial and still under study. Lukaski and others had eleven females live in a metabolic ward for 80–100 days to induce iron deficiency without anemia. They observed a decreased rate of oxygen uptake and reduced energy production during exercise. Other research with iron-deficient, nonanemic human subjects revealed an increased lactate production during maximal exercise, indicative of reduced oxygen utilization in the muscle cells. On the other hand, research has shown that it is possible to maintain VO2 max, endurance capacity, and maximal functioning of the muscle oxidative enzymes even when the body iron stores are severely diminished or depleted. Swedish investigators, as cited by Celsing, withdrew blood over a 4-week period to create an iron deficiency. They then infused the blood back into the subjects so that they were in a condition of iron deficiency without anemia. Even though the iron status was poor, physiological functioning and endurance performance were not impaired. These investigators noted that low serum ferritin levels may not reflect low iron levels in the muscles. One might speculate that differences between these studies, that is, poor iron status due to diet versus blood withdrawal, could influence the results. However, one of the studies reporting impaired lactate metabolism with diet-induced iron deficiency also reported no effect upon VO2 max or endurance performance.

Supplementation The importance of iron to oxygen transport and endurance capacity and the possibility that many athletes, particularly females, may be iron deficient have led a number of investigators in the area of sport nutrition to recommend that more athletes take dietary iron or supplements. Others discourage the indiscriminate use of iron supplements by athletes.

Does iron supplementation improve physical performance? Many studies have been conducted in attempts to answer this question, and the answer appears to be dependent upon the iron status of the individual.

First, if the individual suffers from iron-deficiency anemia, iron therapy could help correct this condition and concomitantly increase performance capacity.

Second, most research with iron-deficient, nonanemic subjects has shown that iron supplementation may improve iron status, for example, by increasing serum ferritin, but appears to have little effect upon maximal physiological functioning as measured by VO2 max. However, in some cases small increases in hemoglobin levels have been associated with an increased VO2 max. For example, Magazanik and others reported that 160 mg of a daily oral iron supplement to young women in training had a more favorable effect on hemoglobin status and VO2 max during the first 21 days of training, but there were no differences between the supplemented and placebo group after 42 days of training. The effect of supplementation on actual physical performance is controversial, however. A recent well-controlled, double-blind, placebo study did note an improvement in running performance when iron-deficient, yet nonanemic, female high school distance runners were treated with iron supplements for 1 month. Additional beneficial effects have also been observed in several well-designed studies with iron deficient, nonanemic subjects. Hudgins and others found that 65 milligrams of iron per day improved the 5-kilometer performance of twelve female cross-country runners. Rowland and associates reported significant improvements in treadmill

endurance time in competitive runners following 4 weeks of ferrous sulfate supplementation.

Conversely, other researchers have observed no beneficial effect of iron supplementation on physical performance in subjects who had iron deficiency without anemia. Lamanca and Haymes revealed a 38 percent improvement in an endurance task following iron supplementation as compared with a 1 percent decrease in the control group; although this difference is impressive, it was not statistically significant. Matter and her associates found no improvement in the treadmill endurance performance of female marathon runners following either 1 or 10 weeks of iron supplementation, which was combined with a folate supplement. Also, Newhouse and others reported no improvement in performance on a variety of exercise tests, both aerobic and anaerobic, in physically active females following 8 weeks of oral iron supplementation. In a single-blind, placebo, crossover study, Powell and Tucker provided a placebo or 130 mg of elemental iron per day for 2 weeks to ten highly-trained female cross-country runners. The supplementation had no significant effect on metabolic variables related to running performance, but the authors noted that serum iron indices were also unaffected by the supplements. Fogelholm and others studied the effect of 100 mg iron daily for 8 weeks, versus a placebo, on a bicycle ergometer ride to exhaustion in two groups of female athletes. The supplement did increase serum ferritin levels but had no effect on performance. Klingshirn and others matched eighteen distance runners on endurance time, giving half of them 100 mg elemental iron per day and the other half a placebo for 8 weeks. The supplement improved serum iron status but did not enhance endurance capacity in a treadmill run to exhaustion, nor did it improve VO2 max. Similar findings were reported in a recent study by Karamizrak and others, who supplemented both male and female athletes with iron for 3 weeks.

Thus, the research relative to the beneficial effects of iron supplementation to those athletes who are iron deficient, yet nonanemic, is contradictory, but the majority of the studies indicate that although iron supplementation will improve iron status, performance does not appear to be enhanced. Indeed, in a recent critical review of the scientific evidence relating low iron stores to endurance performance, Garza and others concluded that although iron supplementation can raise serum ferritin levels, increases in ferritin concentration unaccompanied by increases in hemoglobin concentration have not been shown to improve endurance performance.

Third, if the individual has normal hemoglobin levels, iron supplementation offers no additional benefits. Some well-controlled research has shown that iron supplementation to highly active females in training did not raise their hemoglobin levels or the percentage of hemoglobin saturated with iron. No evidence of performance enhancement has been reported.

If you plan to take iron supplements, you should have your serum ferritin checked, for some danger may be associated with iron supplements if they lead to excessive iron in the body. Prolonged consumption of large amounts can cause a disturbance in iron metabolism in susceptible individuals. Iron then tends to accumulate in the liver as hemosiderin, which in excess can cause **hemochromatosis** in those genetically predisposed. This condition causes cirrhosis and may lead to the ultimate destruction of the liver. Of every 1,000 Americans, approximately two to three have a genetic predisposition to hemochromatosis. Other health problems associated with excessive iron intake have been detailed by Emery, and some preliminary epidemiological data reported by Wurzelmann and others suggest that high levels of iron intake may confer an increased risk for colon cancer. Excessive iron may be fatal to young children; more than thirty deaths occur each year from overdoses of iron obtained by eating large amounts of candy-flavored vitamin tablets with iron.

Some recent epidemiological research from Finland has noted an association between high levels of serum ferritin (greater than 200 micrograms per liter) and risk of heart attack. One hypothesis suggests that inflammatory processes in the coronary arteries provoke increased numbers of white blood cells, which may release iron. Iron is a prooxidant, and may possibly oxidize LDL cholesterol, a reaction believed to be one of the causes of atherosclerosis. Other observations have suggested a link between serum iron and coronary heart disease; for example, females have lower serum iron levels due to menstruation and also have lower incidence rates of heart attack compared to men, and aspirin reduces the risk of heart attack, possibly because it causes gastrointestinal bleeding and increased loss of iron. However, two recent reviews of epidemiologic data by Meyers and by Sempos and others have noted that although the Finnish hypothesis is appealing, the vast majority of data published since their original report does not support the hypothesis that high body-iron stores increase the risk of coronary heart disease. Individuals who may be concerned about high serum levels of iron should consult a physician for advice.

Prudent Recommendations   In summary, it would be wise for developing adolescent males and females of all ages to be aware of the iron content in their diets. This concern is especially important to endurance athletes, although it would appear that the extra Calories they eat to meet the additional energy requirements of training would provide the necessary iron. All active males and females should be aware of heme iron-rich foods, such as lean red meat, and be sure to include them in the daily diet, or at least two to three times a week. Mixing small amounts of meat with iron-rich plant foods, such as lean beef and chili beans, will enhance iron nutrition. Eating foods rich in vitamin C with nonheme iron-containing foods and using

iron cookware also will increase iron bioavailability. Moreover, iron supplementation by commercial preparations may be recommended for certain individuals, including female distance runners, those who experience heavy menstrual blood flow, athletes who initiate altitude training, and athletes who are on restricted caloric intake. The usual vitamin pill with iron should contain about 15 mg iron, which is 100 percent of the RDA for females and 125 percent for adolescent boys. One tablet a day may be advisable for these individuals, and it should be consumed on an empty stomach to minimize adverse effects of some foods on absorption. According to Schmid and others, ingestion of iron together with physical exercise increased serum iron concentrations more so than supplementation and rest. The individual with iron-deficiency anemia should consult a physician for iron therapy, which may consist of 100–200 mg of elemental iron per day until the condition is corrected. It is important to reemphasize that iron supplementation should not be done indiscriminately, but preferably only after determination of one's iron status.

Copper (Cu)

Copper is an essential mineral closely associated with the function of iron.

RDA   There is no RDA for copper, but the ESADDI is 1.5–3.0 mg for adults. The RDI is 2 mg.

Food Sources   Copper is widely distributed in foods and is high in seafoods, meats, nuts, beans, and grain products. One slice of whole wheat bread contains about 6 percent of the ESADDI. Copper also may be found in drinking water, particularly soft water, which leaches it from copper pipes. Some good food sources are listed in Table 8.4.

Major Functions   Copper functions in the body as a metalloenzyme and works closely with iron in oxygen metabolism. It is needed for the absorption of iron from the intestinal tract, helps in the formation of hemoglobin, and is involved in the activity of a specific cytochrome, an oxidative enzyme in the mitochondria. Copper is also a component of ceruloplasmin, a glycoprotein in the plasma, and is in superoxide dismutase (SOD), an enzyme that functions as an antioxidant to quench free radicals.

Deficiency   Copper deficiency due to inadequate dietary intake is not known to exist in humans, although a deficiency has occurred in some patients receiving prolonged intravenous feeding of a copper-free solution. The major deficiency symptom is anemia.

The effects of exercise or exercise training on serum copper levels are variable, with studies showing increases, decreases, or no changes. Several studies have reported decreases in serum copper in athletes involved in prolonged training or after an endurance exercise task. The authors theorized that the decreased levels were due to sweat or fecal losses. However, no deficiency symptoms were noted. In a recent review, Lukaski indicated that physical training does increase the copper-containing SOD, and normal body stores of copper are apparently adequate to support the increase of this antioxidant enzyme.

Supplementation   No research is available relative to copper supplementation and physical performance. Supplements are not recommended because excessive copper intake, even 5–10 milligrams, may cause nausea and vomiting. However, the National Research Council reports that toxicity from dietary sources is rare.

Prudent Recommendations   Copper supplements are not recommended for the physically active individual.

Zinc (Zn)

Zinc is a blue-white metal that is an essential nutrient for humans.

RDA   The RDA for zinc is 15 mg per day for males and 12 mg per day for adult females. The RDI is 15 mg per day.

Food Sources   Good sources of zinc are found in animal protein, such as meat, milk, and seafood, particularly oysters. Three ounces of meat contain approximately 33 percent of the RDA, whereas only one oyster will provide over 70 percent. Whole-grain products also contain significant amounts of zinc, but the phytate and fiber content will slightly decrease its bioavailability. In general, if you receive enough protein in the diet you will obtain the RDA for zinc. The MPF factor enhances zinc absorption. About 20–50 percent of dietary zinc is absorbed. Table 8.4 presents foods high in zinc.

Major Functions   Zinc is found in virtually all tissues in the body as a component of over 100 metalloenzymes. Several of these enzymes are involved in the major pathways of energy metabolism, including lactic acid dehydrogenase (LDH), which is important for the lactic acid energy system. Zinc also is involved in a wide variety of other body functions such as protein synthesis, the growth process, and wound healing. Zinc is also associated with immune functions, including optimal functioning of white blood cells and the lymphatic system.

Deficiency   Helen Lane has noted that zinc nutritional status appears to be well maintained in the average U.S. population, even with marginal intakes. However, several zinc researchers have indicated that a mild dietary zinc deficiency is not uncommon in the United States, particularly in areas where animal protein intake is relatively low and consumption of grain products is high. Zinc deficiency states have been observed in young children with

symptoms of impaired wound healing, depressed appetite, and failure to grow properly, although Prentice indicates more research is needed to determine the specific role of zinc in poor growth performance.

Most research indicates that athletes who obtain sufficient dietary Calories generally meet the RDA for zinc. Female athletes are more likely to have inadequate zinc intake as compared to males. Zinc deficiency could be a problem for certain athletes, particularly young athletes in sports that stress weight loss for optimal performance or competition. Very low-Calorie or starvation-type diets may induce significant zinc losses. In addition, sweat also may contain substantial amounts of zinc, estimated to be approximately 1 mg per liter. Although few experimental data are available, young wrestlers and gymnasts who use both dieting and sweating techniques to induce weight loss may be at risk for zinc deficiency and possible impairment of optimal growth, as suggested by Brun and others. Several studies also have reported a low serum zinc level in endurance runners and triathletes, and the cause was attributed to high sweat losses, increased urinary excretion, or low-Calorie diets. Low dietary zinc intake has been shown to depress testosterone levels, which may be related to the decreased serum testosterone often observed in endurance athletes and wrestlers. Zinc deficiency may also depress immune functions. However, no zinc deficiency symptoms were noted in these athletes or wrestlers; the authors suggested that low serum levels do not necessarily reflect low levels of zinc in the muscles. Following her review of the available literature, which is limited, Lane noted that, in general, there is no evidence that exercise causes a poor zinc status or that a marginal deficiency impairs performance. A more recent review by Lukaski supports this viewpoint.

Supplementation   Given the potential ergogenic importance of zinc, it is unusual that only limited research has been uncovered that has investigated the effect of zinc supplementation upon physical performance. In the most cited study by Krotkiewski and others, subjects were untrained women with an average age of 35 years. In a series of tests for both isometric and isokinetic strength and endurance, zinc supplements improved performance in isometric endurance and in isokinetic strength at one speed. However, performance was not affected in isokinetic endurance or in isokinetic strength at two other speeds of muscle contraction. Although the authors reported a beneficial effect of zinc supplementation and theorized it helped optimize the function of LDH in the muscle during fast contractions, it would appear additional research is needed to confirm this finding. The use of trained subjects would also be an important consideration.

Small amounts of zinc supplements do not appear to pose any major problems to the healthy individual, but larger doses may. Research has shown that zinc supplements, even 25–50 mg per day, may impair the absorption of other essential minerals, such as copper and iron. Supplements over 100 mg/day may increase the amount of LDL cholesterol and decrease the HDL cholesterol level, increasing the risk of coronary artery disease. Anemia may also result from such doses. Higher doses may impair the immune system and cause nausea and vomiting; they may even be fatal.

Prudent Recommendations   On the basis of available evidence, zinc supplementation is not warranted for most athletes. Foods rich in zinc, similar to the animal protein rich in iron, should be selected to replace the increased Calories expended through exercise. However, athletes such as wrestlers and others incurring weight losses should be exceptionally aware of high-zinc foods. If a supplement for these athletes is recommended, it should not exceed the RDA. If taken as part of a multivitamin–mineral supplement, Singh and others noted that exercise will not impair zinc absorption if the supplement is taken just before exercise.

Chromium (Cr)

Chromium is a very hard metal essential in human nutrition.

RDA   There is no RDA for chromium. The ESADDI is 50–200 micrograms per day.

Food Sources   Good sources of chromium include brewers yeast, whole grains, nuts, molasses, cheese, mushrooms, and asparagus. Beer also contains some chromium. One slice of whole wheat bread provides approximately 15 percent of the daily requirement of chromium. Cooking foods in stainless steel cookware provides negligible additional chromium. Chromium is poorly absorbed from the intestinal tract, less than 1 percent being absorbed with intakes in the ESADDI range. At lower dietary intakes, absorption is somewhat increased.

Major Functions   Chromium is considered to be an essential component of the glucose-tolerance factor associated with insulin in the proper metabolism of blood glucose. In essence, chromium potentiates the activity of insulin and thus may also influence lipid and protein metabolism. In addition to maintenance of blood glucose levels, it may be involved in the formation of glycogen in muscle tissue and may facilitate the transport of amino acids into the muscles. Chromium may also affect cholesterol metabolism.

Deficiency   Clinically manifest deficiencies of chromium are rare, but abnormally high blood glucose levels have been reported in hospital patients receiving prolonged intravenous nutrition containing no chromium. Richard Anderson, one of the principal investigators in chromium metabolism, observed that the average American intake of chromium is at the lower range of the ESADDI and suggested this may not be optimal. For example, in one study nearly one-half of subjects with impaired glucose toler-

ance improved with chromium supplementation. The role of chromium in the development of diabetes is currently being studied, and some preliminary data suggest chromium supplementation may benefit some Type II (noninsulin dependent) diabetics by reducing blood sugar and improving glucose tolerance.

Chromium deficiency could be a problem with both endurance- and strength-type athletes. Impairment in carbohydrate metabolism would not be conducive to optimal performance in endurance events, whereas decreased amino acid transport into the muscle could limit the benefits from a weight-training program. On the basis of animal experiments, Anderson has linked chromium to carbohydrate and protein metabolism during exercise, noting, for example, that chromium-deficient rats use muscle glycogen at a faster rate. Anderson believes that strenuous exercise may increase the need for chromium in humans. He noted that chromium losses are associated with stress, such as exercise, and reported increased excretion of chromium in the urine following a strenuous run. In a recent review, Lefavi speculated that athletes may incur a negative chromium balance under various conditions. One, increased intensity and duration of exercise may increase chromium excretion. Two, athletes who consume substantial amounts of carbohydrates may need more chromium to process glucose. And three, athletes who lose weight for competition may decrease dietary intake of chromium.

Supplementation   Theoretically, chromium supplementation might benefit the endurance athlete by improving insulin sensitivity and carbohydrate metabolism during exercise. Also, because chromium may enhance the anabolic effect of insulin, it may increase amino acid uptake into the muscle and modify the body composition, hopefully increasing muscle mass and decreasing body fat. Given the potential commercial application of this latter theoretical possibility to both athletes and the general population, most of the research to date has focused on the effect of chromium supplementation on body composition. Most studies have used chromium picolinate.

In the first published report of the effects of chromium supplementation on body composition, Gary Evans, a chemistry professor at Bemidji State University in Minnesota, used chromium picolinate as an adjunct to a weight-training program to investigate its effect upon body composition. Picolinate is a natural derivative of tryptophan, an amino acid, and apparently facilitates the absorption of chromium into the body. In a recent review article, Evans described two of his studies. In the first study, ten male volunteers from a weight-training class were assigned to either a placebo or a chromium supplement group. The chromium dosage was the upper level of the ESADDI, 200 micrograms. Body fat and lean body mass were determined by skinfold and girth measurements. The subjects trained with weights for 40 days, and at the conclusion

Evans found that the chromium group had increased their body weight by 2.2 kilograms, 73 percent of which was lean body mass. The placebo group had also increased their body weight by 1.25 kilograms, but Evans noted this increase was due almost totally to body fat. The second study was similar to the first, but thirty-two football players at Bemidji State University served as subjects. After a 42-day training period, the chromium group actually lost 1.2 kilograms of body weight, but most of it was fat so their proportion of lean body mass increased from 84.2 to 87.8 percent. The placebo group also lost body weight, but their lean body mass only increased from 84.6 to 85.8 percent. In both studies, Evans noted that the results were statistically significant, suggesting that chromium picolinate supplementation enhanced body composition by decreasing body fat and increasing lean body mass.

The findings of this report are certainly interesting, but several points should be noted. First, the studies were reported in a review article on the health benefits of chromium and do not appear to have been published previously in a refereed scientific journal. Second, skinfolds and girth measurements were used to assess body composition, but although these types of measurements may be helpful in weight-control programs, they are not considered to be sufficiently accurate for research purposes. Third, the dietary intake of chromium apparently was not controlled, nor were other physical activities that could affect body weight. Finally, no physical performance measures were reported.

Following the publicity associated with this report, chromium picolinate was billed in certain muscle magazines as the alternative to anabolic steroids, the advertisers suggesting that chromium's insulin-like effects may elicit significant anabolic hormone effects in the body. Advertisements also appeared in magazines targeted for the general population, suggesting chromium picolinate would facilitate the loss of body fat.

However, subsequent well-controlled research has not supported these preliminary findings. Hasten and others studied the effect of daily chromium supplementation (200 micrograms) on the body composition and strength of college-age males and females engaged in 12 weeks of weight training. Using a double-blind, placebo experimental design, no significant differences were found with the exception that females taking chromium supplements gained more body weight compared to those on the placebo. In their discussion the authors suggested the increase in body weight was lean body mass, not body fat. Although the design of this study was appropriate, one possible limitation was the use of skinfolds to predict body composition, a technique not as accurate as underwater weighing.

Hallmark and others conducted a similar study with sixteen untrained males, matching the subjects based on initial levels of strength and giving half of them a placebo and the other half 200 micrograms chromium picolinate daily for 12 weeks of progressive resistance training. Dependent variables included measures of body composition as determined by underwater weighing, and strength. The authors reported no significant effects of chromium picolinate supplementation on lean body mass, body fat, or strength. Clancy and others randomly placed twenty-one football players into either a placebo group or an experimental group receiving 200 micrograms chromium picolinate daily while involved in intensive resistance training over a 9-week period. A number of dependent variables were studied, including body composition determined by underwater weighing, anthropometrical measurements such as muscle girth, and strength. Chromium picolinate supplementation had no effect on lean body mass, body fat percentage, or strength. The studies by Hallmark and Clancy and their associates paralleled those conducted by Evans, yet the results were diametrically opposite.

Other studies have not found any significant effect of chromium supplementation on body composition. Lukaski and others compared the effects of two different types of chromium supplements, chromium chloride and chromium picolinate (about 200 micrograms each), with a placebo on body composition changes during 8 weeks of supplementation and controlled resistance strength training. Using several measures of body composition, they found no significant effects of the chromium supplements on body fat or lean muscle mass. Trent and Thieding-Cancel also reported no significant effects of chromium picolinate (400 micrograms for 16 weeks) on body weight, body fat, or lean muscle mass in either men or women engaging in aerobic exercise for 30 minutes three times a week. Moreover, seven studies presented at the most recent meeting of the American College of Sports Medicine in Denver, all involving the effect of chromium supplementation to healthy, physically active individuals or athletes, found no beneficial effect on glucose tolerance, metabolism, body composition, or various measures of physical performance.

The studies using more appropriate methods to determine body composition have not shown any beneficial effects of chromium picolinate supplementation on lean body mass, body fat, or strength. Although the scientific data are limited, these findings argue against an ergogenic effect of chromium supplementation. However, the effects of chromium supplementation on prolonged aerobic endurance remains to be investigated.

Chromium supplements may possess some health benefits. As already noted, they may help improve glucose metabolism in those with glucose intolerance. Other research has suggested that chromium may help lower total cholesterol and LDL cholesterol while raising HDL cholesterol in individuals with unhealthy serum cholesterol levels. However, Anderson has noted that chromium supplements can correct only that part of a health problem which is associated with a deficiency. In other words, individuals who have a health problem in which chromium deficiency plays a part will benefit if the deficiency is corrected, just like any nutrient-deficiency-related health problem. Anderson noted that chromium acts as a nutrient, not a therapeutic agent.

The National Research Council indicates that dietary chromium does not appear to be toxic. Amounts of 200 micrograms per day have been used safely. However, a recent review by Stearns and others indicated that prolonged or excessive chromium supplementation, such as chromium picolinate, may lead to chromium accumulation in the body to levels at which chromosomal damage (possible carcinogenic effect) has been observed in animals and in vitro. They indicated the possible long-term biological effects of chromium accumulation in humans are poorly understood. Moreover, Reading recently advised caution with chromium picolinate supplements, particularly by those with behavioral disorders, because picolinate itself may possibly adversely affect neurotransmitter functions in the central nervous system.

Prudent Recommendations In a recent review of chromium supplementation by Schardt and Schmidt, the Center for Science in the Public Interest provided a bottom line recommendation, which appears to be in accord with this presentation of the scientific data. If you are glucose intolerant or a Type II diabetic, consult your physician about chromium supplementation. In general, chromium supplementation will not help you lose weight or gain muscle. If you insist on taking a chromium supplement, it should not exceed 200 micrograms, and might best be taken as part of an inexpensive multivitamin-mineral tablet containing the other essential vitamins and minerals. The best sources of chromium, however, are whole grains, fruits, and vegetables.

Selenium (Se)

Selenium is a chemical element resembling sulfur.

RDA RDA were established for selenium in 1989, being 70 and 55 micrograms per day for males and females, respectively.

Food Sources Foods rich in selenium include seafoods, organ meats like kidney and liver, other meats, and grains grown in soil abundant in selenium. About 3 ounces of meat contains over 30 micrograms of selenium, as does 3 ounces of wheat bread.

Major Functions Selenium is a component of several enzymes, particularly glutathione peroxidase, an enzyme that helps catabolize free radicals and prevent damage to cellular structures, such as the membranes of RBC. As mentioned in the last chapter, selenium works with vitamin E as an antioxidant and has been theorized to be important in the prevention of cancer.

Deficiency The selenium content of plants depends on the selenium content of the soil. Selenium deficiency is rare in industrialized countries because foods in the diet are obtained from diverse geographical areas. However, deficiency diseases may be noted in geographical areas where the selenium content in the soil is low. Keshan disease, a cardiomyopathy, is evident in parts of China because the primary sources of food are plants grown locally in selenium-depleted soil. Other possible health effects of selenium deficiency include heart disease, possibly because of a diminished ability to prevent oxidation of LDL cholesterol. Selenium deficiency has also been linked to an impaired immune system and cancer. The interested reader is referred to the review by Oldfield.

For the athlete, selenium deficiency may impair antioxidant functions during intense exercise, possibly leading to muscle tissue or mitochondrial damage, thus impairing physical performance.

Supplementation In theory, selenium supplementation may help protect cell membranes from peroxidation. Preventing LDL oxidation may help prevent cardiovascular disease, but in a recent review Neve indicated that the therapeutic benefit of selenium administration in the prevention and treatment of cardiovascular diseases still remains insufficiently documented. Patterson and Levander cite epidemiological studies and one intervention trial that suggested selenium supplementation may prevent prostate cancer, but they indicated that the data are very preliminary and more well-controlled study evaluating the possible role of selenium supplementation in the prevention of cancer is warranted.

Although antioxidant supplements have not universally been shown to prevent peroxidation of lipids in cell membranes and other cell structures, some studies by Tessier and his associates have shown that selenium supplementation will enhance glutathione peroxidase status and reduce lipid peroxidation during prolonged aerobic exercise. Although these findings are intriguing, selenium supplementation did not improve actual physical performance, as evaluated by VO_2 max or running performance of an aerobic/anaerobic nature.

Selenium supplements within RDA levels under 100 micrograms appear to be safe, and investigators in the United States using supplements up to 200 micrograms saw no problems. However, some studies observed adverse effects at 750 micrograms per day, and accidental intakes of large amounts (over 25 milligrams per day) have been associated with nausea, vomiting, abdominal pain, hair loss, and unusual fatigue.

Prudent Recommendations Adequate selenium may be obtained on a healthful, balanced diet containing substantial amounts of grain products. In the United States and Canada, most grains are produced in the upper Great Plains, where the soil is rich in selenium. Selenium in foods is present in an organic form, which may be more effectively used by the body than inorganic selenium salt supplements. If you decide to take a selenium supplement, according to Liebman most experts agree that a selenium or multivitamin-mineral supplement with no more than 200 micrograms is safe. Larger doses are not recommended at the present time.

Boron (B)

Boron is a nonmetallic element.

RDA Although boron is an essential nutrient for plants, no RDA or ESADDI has been established. However, some scientists suggest it is of nutritional and clinical importance and most likely is an essential nutrient for humans. Nielsen indicates we probably need about 0.5–1.0 milligram per day.

Food Sources Boron is found naturally in many plant foods, particularly dried fruits, nuts, legumes, fresh vegetables, apple sauce, grape juice, and wine. One ounce of almonds contains about 0.75 milligram of boron. In the early part of this century, borate salts were used extensively as food preservatives, but their use was discontinued when their safety was questioned.

Major Functions Boron is believed to influence cell membrane structure and function in some unknown way, to influence mineral metabolism, and to be involved in the metabolism of steroid hormones, such as estrogen and testosterone.

Deficiency Barr and others recently noted that evidence on boron deficiency is scanty. In a survey by Naghii and others, Australians were estimated to consume about 2.2 milligrams per day, more than enough to prevent a deficiency if 0.5–1.0 milligram is sufficient. Although boron deficiency has been studied in relation to bone metabolism—possibly because of its potential role in estrogen metabolism—its role is poorly understood.

Supplementation Boron supplementation may not increase body stores. Hunt and others reported that a boron supplement of 3 milligrams did not accumulate in the body, but was either unabsorbed or excreted by the kidneys, suggesting that the human body maintains a stable boron level.

However, in his review, Nielsen presents an excellent example of how the results of a single study may be distorted by nutritional supplement entrepreneurs to market new products. In their study, Nielsen and his colleagues designed a diet for twelve postmenopausal women to deprive them of adequate dietary boron for nearly 4 months, and then fed them the same diet for 48 days but supplemented with 3 milligrams of boron daily, an amount

found in a diet high in fruits and vegetables. The authors reported that the boron supplements reduced the plasma concentration of calcium and the urinary excretion of calcium and magnesium, at the same time elevating the serum concentration of one form of estrogen and testosterone. The authors concluded that correcting a boron deficiency with boron supplements elicits physiological effects associated with the prevention of calcium loss and bone demineralization, suggesting dietary boron may play an important nutritional role in the prevention of osteoporosis. The major focus of this study was on the effects of boron deprivation and deficiency, not boron supplementation. The authors simply created a boron deficiency to see its physiological effects, and then restored normal dietary boron to evaluate its effects.

Nielsen notes that these findings were completely misinterpreted, the media reporting erroneously that boron could end bone disease. Commercial enterprises immediately began marketing boron supplements for prevention of osteoporosis. In his review, Nielsen negates the sensational claims the media propagated, but did indicate that boron may be one of a number of nutrients that may play a role in the prevention of osteoporosis.

One of the other findings of this study, the elevated serum testosterone levels in these postmenopausal women, was also sensationalized. Advertisements began to appear in muscle magazines indicating that boron supplements could act pharmacologically like anabolic steroids. However, Nielsen indicated that this was an erroneous extrapolation of the research data, noting that boron supplementation increased serum testosterone only after these postmenopausal women had been deprived of boron for nearly 4 months; continuation of boron supplementation did not further elevate serum testosterone levels. Moreover, Nielsen conducted other studies with males and reported no significant changes in serum testosterone levels when dietary boron intake was modified.

Limited research data are available relative to the ergogenic efficacy of boron supplementation. Ferrando and Green randomly assigned nineteen nonsteroid-using, male bodybuilders to receive either a placebo or 2.5 milligrams of a commercial boron supplement daily for 7 weeks. The bodybuilders maintained their normal diets and consumed no other supplements. The authors found that although boron supplements increased serum boron levels, there were no significant effects on total and free testosterone, lean body mass, or strength. These findings indicate that boron supplements are not ergogenic, but additional research is desirable.

Nielsen notes that 10 milligrams per day may possibly be obtained in the diet, and that this amount is probably not too high. However, he cautions that an intake of 50 milligrams per day may be toxic.

Prudent Recommendations Based on the available scientific evidence, boron supplementation does not enhance

Table 8.5 Trace minerals: cobalt, fluoride, iodine, manganese, molybdenum

Trace mineral	RDA or ESADDI*	Major food sources	Major body functions
Cobalt (Co)	**	Meat, liver, milk	Component of vitamin B_{12}; promotes development of red blood cells
Fluoride (F)	1.5–4.0 mg	Milk, egg yolks, drinking water, seafood	Helps form bones and teeth
Iodine (I)	150 micrograms	Iodized salt, seafood, vegetables	Helps in formation of thyroid hormones
Manganese (Mn)	2.0–5.0 mg	Whole-grain products, dried peas and beans, leafy vegetables, bananas	Many enzymes involved in energy metabolism; bone formation; fat synthesis
Molybdenum (Mo)	75–250 micrograms	Liver, organ meats, whole-grain products, dried beans and peas	Works with riboflavin in enzymes involved in carbohydrate and fat metabolism

*For adults. RDA or ESADDI for other age groups may be found in Appendix A.

**Essential as part of vitamin B_{12}.

athletic performance and is not recommended. However, a leading expert on boron indicated that boron deprivation for 3 weeks or more may have a negative impact on the ability to exercise. A balanced diet containing adequate amounts of plant foods will provide sufficient dietary boron, so physically active individuals who consume a typical diet should have no problem with boron deprivation.

Vanadium (V)

Vanadium is light gray metallic element.

RDA No RDA or ESADDI has been established for vanadium because it has not been deemed essential for human metabolism. Nevertheless, based on some animal research, some nutrition scientists estimate we need about 10–100 micrograms per day.

Food Sources Good sources of vanadium include shellfish, grain products, parsley, mushrooms, and black pepper. The average daily intake of vanadium in North America is about 6–20 milligrams.

Major Functions Research with animals suggests vanadium may be involved in several enzymatic reactions in the body, including the metabolism of carbohydrate and lipids. Some scientists suggest vanadium exerts an insulin-like effect on glucose and protein metabolism, inducing an anabolic effect on muscle by inhibiting protein catabolism.

Deficiency Apparently vanadium deficiency has not been detected in humans. However, if vanadium does induce an insulin-like effect, a deficiency could impair glucose metabolism.

Supplementation Vanadium supplements are available as vanadyl salts, primarily vanadyl sulfate. Boden and others found that vanadyl sulfate supplementation (100 milligrams daily for 4 weeks) improved glucose status in humans with noninsulin-dependent diabetes mellitus. These results duplicate studies with animals, and merit replication. However, the investigators noted that the safety of larger doses or the use of vanadium salts for longer periods remains uncertain.

Vanadyl salts have been marketed to athletes as a means to favorably modify body composition, comparable to the proposed effects of chromium supplementation. However, there are very limited research data with vanadium supplementation. In a well-controlled study, Fawcett and others found that supplementation with 0.5 milligrams per kilogram body weight (about 40 milligrams daily) of vanadyl sulfate to subjects undertaking strength training for 12 weeks had no effect on body fat or lean muscle mass. The investigators also studied strength gains in four tasks, a 1-repetition and 10-repetition maximal test for both the bench press and leg extension. There were no significant effects of vanadyl sulfate on three of the tests. Although subjects taking vanadyl sulfate did gain more strength on the 1-repetition maximal leg extension test during the first 4 weeks of the study, the investigators suggested this may be attributed to low scores on the pretest. The investigators concluded that vanadyl sulfate supplementation was ineffective in changing body composition, and any modest performance-enhancing effect requires further investigation.

Adverse side effects of vanadyl salt supplementation may include gastrointestinal distress, primarily diarrhea. Increased sleepiness was also an observation in one study. Excess supplementation may also cause damage to both the liver and kidney.

Deficiency symptoms	Symptoms of excessive consumption	Recommended as dietary supplement
Not found in humans	Nausea, vomiting, death	No
Higher incidence of dental cavities	Discolored teeth	No
Goiter, an enlarged thyroid gland	Depressed thyroid gland activity	No
Poor growth	Weakness; nervous system problems; mental confusion	No
Not found in humans	Rare	No

Prudent Recommendations Type II diabetics should consult with their physicians regarding the use of vanadyl salt supplementation to control blood glucose. Vanadyl salt supplementation is not recommended for the physically active individual, as it has not been found to enhance either body composition or physical performance. Moreover, excess amounts may be toxic.

Other Trace Minerals

A number of other trace minerals have physiological roles that may have important implications for health or physical performance. Food sources, RDA or ESADDI, major physiological functions, and the effects of deficiencies or excesses are summarized in Table 8.5. Only trace minerals for which an RDA or ESADDI have been developed are included. Other elements, such as nickel, tin, silicon, and arsenic may prove to be essential. It should be noted that deficiencies and excesses due to dietary sources for most of these nutrients are extremely rare. However, to help prevent a deficiency it is important to consume unprocessed foods because many of the trace elements that are removed during processing are not returned. For example, as already noted, one slice of whole wheat bread provides about 15 percent of the daily requirement of chromium, whereas a slice of white bread contains only 1 percent. Excesses may occur with use of supplements or through industrial exposure.

Two of these trace elements deserve mention for they have been shown to prevent health problems in humans. Fluoride has been shown to prevent dental caries, but excesses in children may cause mottling, or varying shades of whiteness in the outer tooth enamel. Iodine is used in the formation of thyroxine and triiodothyronine, two hormones produced in the thyroid gland. Decreased production of these hormones would lower the body's metabolism, a possible contributing factor to the development of obesity. The use of iodized salt has nearly eliminated iodine deficiency in the United States and has thereby greatly reduced the incidence of goiter, a serious iodine-deficiency disease.

Research literature relative to the effect of exercise on the metabolic fates of these trace nutrients is almost nonexistent, nor are there any studies available regarding the effects of supplements on performance. This may be understandable, as deficiencies are rare.

Mineral Supplements: Exercise and Health

Following her extensive review of dietary surveys, Sarah Short noted that both athletes and health professionals are becoming more concerned with mineral deficiencies. Perusal of athletic and health magazines marketed for the general public reveals a variety of articles and advertisements suggesting that supplementation of certain minerals will enhance athletic performance or health. As the foregoing discussion indicates, individuals who have a mineral deficiency may experience improved health or physical performance if that deficiency is corrected. In general, however, supplementation has little effect on the individual whose mineral status is adequate. This last section summarizes some key points relative to mineral nutrition, focusing on the need for supplementation.

Does exercise increase my need for minerals?

Exercise may induce mineral losses from the body by several mechanisms. Many minerals appear to be mobilized into the circulation during exercise, probably being released from body stores in the muscles or elsewhere. As they circulate, some may be removed by the kidneys and excreted in the urine, whereas others may appear in the sweat, particularly in a warm environment. Losses from the gastrointestinal tract may also occur during exercise, although the mechanism is not totally understood.

The female athlete who develops secondary amenorrhea may need additional calcium, as might the male endurance athlete in whom trabecular bone mass is decreased. The need for iron in the female athlete may decrease somewhat with the cessation of menses in secondary amenorrhea.

Because of these potential mineral losses, at least one investigator in sport nutrition has suggested that mineral supplementation should be considered for athletes. Although supplementation may be helpful for some, the first concern should be to educate the athlete about obtaining adequate mineral nutrition through dietary means.

Can I obtain the minerals I need through my diet?

As many dietary surveys have shown, many Americans are not obtaining the RDA or ESADDI for a variety of minerals, including iron, zinc, calcium, and chromium. Similar dietary deficiencies have been noted in surveys with athletes, but mainly with athletes who participate in activities such as wrestling, distance running, ballet, and gymnastics, where weight control is a concern. Let us briefly highlight the dietary recommendations that will help ensure adequate amounts of nutrients in the diet.

In general, as with all other nutrients, a balanced diet is essential. Select a wide variety of foods from all the food groups and within each group. Table 8.6 presents the percentage of the RDI provided by servings of different foods from several food groups. Note that the

percentage values for the minerals differ not only between food groups but also for some minerals in foods within the same group. For example, note that calcium is high in dairy foods but low in meats. On the other hand, iron is high in meats but low in dairy products. Also, in the meat group, pork is high in copper but beef is low. It is also important to eat foods in their natural state as much as possible. The milling of flour removes many minerals, but only iron is replaced in the enrichment process. Note the differences between whole wheat and enriched white bread in Table 8.6.

A basic principle of mineral nutrition is to eat natural foods that are rich in calcium and iron. If you select a diet to provide your RDA for these two minerals, you will receive adequate amounts of the other major and trace minerals at the same time. Dairy products and meats are excellent sources of these minerals, but other foods such as legumes and dark-green leafy vegetables also may provide significant amounts if selected wisely. Note the foods rich in calcium and iron in Tables 8.2 and 8.4, and compare the similarity to the foods listed for the other minerals in these two tables and Table 8.5.

Should physically active individuals take mineral supplements?

In general, the answer to this question for most athletes is *no* for several reasons. First, contrary to advertising claims of mineral-supplement manufacturers, you can obtain adequate mineral nutrition from the diet if you adhere to some of the guidelines presented throughout this chapter. Second, although some athletes may not be obtaining the RDA of several minerals, such as zinc and calcium, mineral deficiencies to the point of impairing physical performance are rare. Very few data are available on this

Table 8.6 Percentages of the RDI in various foods for selected minerals

Food	Serving	Calories	Ca	P	Mg	Fe	Cu	Zn
Milk, skim	1 glass	90	35	28	10	1	2	7
Cheese, cheddar	1 ounce	114	21	15	2	1	0	6
Oyster	1 average	10	1	2	1	6	28	75
Liver, beef	3 ounces	150	1	41	4	50	157	29
Beef, lean sirloin	3 ounces	176	1	22	6	21	3	33
Lamb chop, lean	1 medium	95	1	11	3	6	22	14
Beans, lima	1/2 cup	131	3	15	8	19	8	6
Broccoli	1 stalk	25	8	6	3	4	63	1
Bread, whole wheat	1 slice	80	2	5	4	3	6	3
Bread, enriched white	1 slice	80	2	2	4	2	1	1

topic, but the evidence that is available with most minerals suggests that though serum levels may be low, physical performance is not affected. An exception may be low levels of serum iron for, as noted previously, supplementation, although controversial, has been helpful to some athletes. Third, many minerals may be harmful when taken in excess. As noted throughout this chapter, the absorption rate for most minerals is relatively low. Only 40 percent of calcium is absorbed from the intestinal tract, while the percentages for iron and chromium are, respectively, 10 and 1–2 percent. This low absorption rate prevents the accumulation of excess amounts of minerals in the body, which may interfere with normal metabolism. Large supplemental doses may overload the body and cause numerous health problems, and as noted for several minerals, may be fatal.

However, it is recognized that certain athletes may not be obtaining adequate mineral nutrition from their diets and may possibly benefit from supplementation. As noted previously, athletes who are attempting to lose weight for performance are at most risk for developing a mineral deficiency. Because many of the dietary surveys of these athletes have reported intakes lower than the RDA for iron and calcium, it may be assumed that their diets are also low in other trace minerals.

If there is concern for the nutritional status of the athlete, the ideal situation would be to consult a sport nutritionist or nutritionally oriented physician for advice. Unfortunately, this approach does not appear to be common among athletes who may be in need of nutritional counseling, although the situation is improving. Some elite athletes take medically prescribed iron supplements, and dieticians with specialties in exercise physiology and sport nutrition are becoming increasingly available.

For athletes who cannot or will not seek professional advice, it may be prudent to recommend a one-a-day vitamin–mineral supplement to those who are known to have poor nutritional habits. The tablet should contain no more than 50–100 percent of the RDA for any mineral. Additionally, the point should be made to the athlete that the supplement is being recommended to help prevent a deficiency, not for any ergogenic purposes. As noted in Chapter 7, large doses of multivitamin–mineral supplements taken over prolonged periods of time have not been shown to enhance physical performance. In the meantime, efforts should be undertaken to educate the athlete concerning sound nutritional practices.

Are mineral megadoses harmful?

One of the generally accepted facts relative to mineral nutrition in the healthy individual is that the levels associated with toxicity can normally be obtained only through the use of supplements, not through dietary sources. Because they hope to improve health or physical performance, many individuals purchase supplements containing minerals. However, surveys indicate the most common preparations purchased contain the RDA or less, which should pose no health problems to the healthy individual. Unfortunately, as indicated in the last chapter, many individuals self-prescribe and may consume more than the recommended daily dosage. Although the toxicity and possible health problems associated with excessive intake of several minerals, such as calcium, iron, zinc, and copper, are fairly well documented, the level of safety for intake of a variety of other minerals, particularly some of the trace minerals suggested to be therapeutic in nature, has been more difficult to document. Nevertheless, the National Research Council has noted that all trace minerals are toxic if consumed at high doses for a long enough time.

According to Yetiv, who reviewed the literature on the relationship of minerals to health, individuals who consume mineral supplements should take only amounts similar to the RDA, or less. There are no indications for megasupplements of minerals, except for treatment of specific disease states.

Nevertheless, in a recent article, Nielsen raised the issue of an emerging new paradigm in which the determination of nutrient requirements would include consideration of the total health effects of nutrients, not just their roles in preventing deficiency pathology. The recently updated RDA for calcium and vitamin D as a possible means to prevent osteoporosis reflect this new paradigm. Although much research is needed before concrete recommendations may be made relative to mineral supplementation and purported health benefits, the recommendations presented on page 236 may be useful guidelines for healthy sedentary and physically active individuals to use in the meantime.

References

Books

Aito, A., et al., eds. 1991. *Trace Elements in Health and Disease*. Boca Raton, FL: CRC Press.

Bucci, L. 1993. *Nutrients as Ergogenic Aids for Sports and Exercise*. Boca Raton, FL: CRC Press.

Celsing, F. 1987. *Influence of Iron Deficiency and Changes in Hemoglobin Concentration on Exercise Capacity in Man*. Stockholm: Repro Print.

Council for Responsible Nutrition. 1997. *Vitamin and Mineral Safety*. Washington, DC: Council for Responsible Nutrition.

Emery, T. 1991. *Iron and your Health*. Boca Raton, FL: CRC Press.

Fogelholm, M. 1992. *Vitamin and Mineral Status in Physically Active People*. Turku, Finland: The Social Insurance Institution.

Hunt, S., and Groff, J. 1990. *Advanced Nutrition and Human Metabolism*. St. Paul, MN: West.

Kies, C., and Driskell, J. 1995. *Sports Nutrition: Minerals and Electrolytes*. Boca Raton, FL: CRC Press.

National Research Council. 1989. *Diet and Health: Implications for Reducing Chronic Disease Risk*. Washington, DC: National Academy Press.

National Research Council. 1989. *Recommended Dietary Allowances.* Washington, DC: National Academy Press.

Shils, M., et al. 1994. *Modern Nutrition in Health and Disease.* Philadelphia: Lea and Febiger.

Wolinsky, I., and Hickson, J. 1994. *Nutrition in Exercise and Sport.* Boca Raton, FL: CRC Press.

Yetiv, J. 1986. *Popular Nutritional Practices: A Scientific Appraisal.* Toledo, OH: Popular Medicine Press.

Reviews

American College of Sports Medicine. 1997. Position stand: The female athlete triad. *Medicine and Science in Sport and Exercise* 29 (5): i–ix.

American College of Sports Medicine. 1995. ACSM position stand on osteoporosis and exercise. *Medicine and Science in Sports and Exercise* 27 (4): i–vii.

Anderson, J., and Barrett, C. 1994. Dietary phosphorus: The benefits and the problems. *Nutrition Today* 29 (2): 29–34.

Anderson, J., et al. 1996. Roles of diet and physical activity in the prevention of osteoporosis. *Scandinavian Journal of Rheumatology Supplement* 103:65–74.

Anderson, R. 1988. Selenium, chromium, and manganese. (B) Chromium. In *Modern Nutrition in Health and Disease,* eds. M. Shils and V. Young. Philadelphia: Lea and Febiger.

Armstrong, L., and Maresh, C. 1996. Vitamin and mineral supplements as nutritional aids to exercise performance and health. *Nutrition Reviews* 54:S149–S158.

Atkinson, H. (Ed.) 1997. Hormone therapy: When and for how long? *HealthNews* 3 (4): 1–2.

Avioli, L. 1988. Calcium and phosphorus. In *Modern Nutrition in Health and Disease,* eds. M. Shils and V. Young. Philadelphia: Lea and Febiger.

Barr, R., et al. 1996. Boron levels in man: Preliminary evidence of genetic regulation and some implications for human biology. *Medical Hypotheses* 46:286–89.

Beard, J., et al. 1996. Iron metabolism: A comprehensive review. *Nutrition Reviews* 54:295–317.

Bennell, K., et al. 1996. Effect of altered reproductive function and lowered testosterone levels on bone density in male endurance athletes. *British Journal of Sports Medicine* 30:205–8.

Benson, J., et al. 1996. Nutritional aspects of amenorrhea in the female athlete triad. *International Journal of Sport Nutrition* 6:134–45.

Bothwell, T. 1995. Overview and mechanisms of iron regulation. *Nutrition Reviews* 53:237–45.

Burke, L. 1995. Practical issues in nutrition for athletes. *Journal of Sports Sciences* 13:S83–S90.

Clarkson, P. 1996. Nutrition for improved sports performance. *Sports Medicine* 21:393–401.

Clarkson, P. 1991. Vitamins, iron, and trace minerals. In *Perspectives in Exercise Science and Sports Medicine. Ergogenics: The Enhancement of Sport Performance,* eds. D. Lamb and M. Williams. Indianapolis, IN: Benchmark.

Clarkson, P., and Haymes, E. 1995. Exercise and mineral status of athletes: Calcium, magnesium, phosphorus, and iron. *Medicine and Science in Sports and Exercise* 27:831–45.

Clarkson, P., and Haymes, E. 1994. Trace mineral requirements for athletes. *International Journal of Sport Nutrition* 4:104–19.

Dawson-Hughes, B. 1996. Calcium and vitamin D nutritional needs of elderly women. *Journal of Nutrition* 126:1165S–1167S.

Deuster, P. 1989. Magnesium in sports medicine. *Journal of the American College of Nutrition* 8:462.

Douban, S., and Brodsky, M. 1995. Magnesium: An important nutritional element in cardiovascular health. *Journal of Optimal Nutrition* 4:9–12.

Drinkwater, B. 1989. Amenorrheic athletes: At risk for premature osteoporosis. *Proceedings of the First IOC World Congress on Sport Sciences.* Colorado Springs, CO: United States Olympic Committee.

Eichner, E. R. 1992. Sports anemia, iron supplements, and blood doping. *Medicine and Science in Sports and Exercise* 24:S315–S318.

Elin, R. 1988. Magnesium metabolism in health and disease. *Disease-A-Month* 34:161–218.

Evans, G. 1989. The effect of chromium picolinate on insulin controlled parameters in humans. *International Journal of Biosocial and Medical Research* 11:163–80.

Fairbanks, V. 1994. Iron in medicine and nutrition. In *Modern Nutrition in Health and Disease,* eds. M. Shils, et al. Philadelphia: Lea and Febiger.

Fosmire, G. 1990. Zinc toxicity. *American Journal of Clinical Nutrition* 51:225–27.

Garza, D., et al. 1997. The clinical value of serum ferritin tests in endurance athletes. *Clinics in Sport Medicine* 7:46–53.

Hathcock, J. 1997. Vitamins and Minerals: Efficacy and safety. *American Journal of Clinical Nutrition* 66:427–37.

Haymes, E. 1993. Dietary iron needs in exercising women: A rational plan to follow in evaluating iron status. *Medicine, Exercise, Nutrition, and Health* 2:203–12.

Hood, D., et al. 1992. Mitochondrial adaptations to chronic muscle use: Effect of iron deficiency. *Comparative Biochemistry and Physiology* 101A:597–605.

Horswill, C. 1995. Effects of bicarbonate, citrate, and phosphate loading on performance. *International Journal of Sport Nutrition* 5:S111–S119.

Isenbarger, D., and Chapin, B. 1997. Osteoporosis: Current pharmacological options for prevention and treatment. *Postgraduate Medicine* 101:129–42.

Keen, C., and Hackman, R. 1986. Trace elements in athletic performance. In *Sport, Health and Nutrition,* ed. F. Katch. Champaign, IL: Human Kinetics.

Kelley, G., et al. 1997. Exercise and regional bone mineral density in postmenopausal women: A meta-analysis. *Medicine and Science in Sports and Exercise* 29:S189.

King, J., and Keen, C. 1994. Zinc. In *Modern Nutrition in Health and Disease,* eds. M. Shils, et al. Philadelphia: Lea and Febiger.

Kreider, R. 1992. Phosphate loading and exercise performance. *Journal of Applied Nutrition* 44:29–49.

Lane, H. 1989. Some trace elements related to physical activity: Zinc, copper, selenium, chromium, and iodine. In *Nutrition in Exercise and Sport,* eds. J. Hickson and I. Wolinsky. Boca Raton, FL: CRC Press.

Lefavi, R. 1992. Efficacy of chromium supplementation in athletes: Emphasis on anabolism. *International Journal of Sport Nutrition* 2:111–22.

Leibovitz, B. 1990. Nutrition and performance. *Muscular Development,* 27 (July): 27.

Levander, O. 1988. Selenium, chromium, and manganese. (A) Selenium. In *Modern Nutrition in Health and Disease,* eds. M. Shils and V. Young. Philadelphia: Lea and Febiger.

Loosli, A. 1993. Reversing sports-related iron and zinc deficiencies. *Physician and Sportsmedicine* 6 (June): 70–77.

Lukaski, H. 1995. Micronutrients (magnesium, zinc, and copper): Are mineral supplements needed for athletes? *International Journal of Sport Nutrition* 5:S74–S83.

McCarron, D. 1997. Role of adequate dietary calcium intake in the prevention and management of salt-sensitive hypertension. *American Journal of Clinical Nutrition* 65:712S–716S.

McDonald, R., and Keen, C. 1988. Iron, zinc and magnesium nutrition and athletic performance. *Sports Medicine* 5:171–84.

Mertz, W. 1993. Chromium in human nutrition: A review. *Journal of Nutrition* 123:626–33.

Meyers, D. 1996. The iron hypothesis: Does iron cause atherosclerosis? *Clinics in Cardiology* 12:925–29.

National Dairy Council. 1998. Making the most of calcium: Factors affecting calcium metabolism. *Dairy Council Digest* 69:1–6.

National Dairy Council. 1997. Dietary reference intakes: Calcium and related nutrients. *Dairy Council Digest* 68:31–36.

National Dairy Council. 1996. Osteoporosis: Boning up on the latest facts. *Dairy Council Digest* 67:1–6.

Nattiv, A., and Mandelbaum, B. 1993. Injuries and special concerns in female gymnasts. Detecting, treating, and preventing common problems. *Physician and Sportsmedicine* 21 (July): 66–81.

Neve, J. 1996. Selenium as a risk factor for cardiovascular diseases. *Journal of Cardiovascular Risk* 3:42–47.

Newhouse, I., and Clement, D. 1988. Iron status in athletes: An update. *Sports Medicine* 5:337–52.

Nielsen, F. 1996. How should dietary guidance be given for mineral elements with beneficial actions or suspected of being essential? *Journal of Nutrition* 126:2377S–2385S.

Nielsen, F. 1994. Ultratrace minerals. In *Modern Nutrition in Health and Disease,* eds. M. Shils et al. Philadelphia: Lea and Febiger.

Nielsen, F. 1992. Facts and fallacies about boron. *Nutrition Today* 27:6–12.

Oldfield, J. 1991. Some implications of selenium for human health. *Nutrition Today* 26 (July/August): 6–11.

Patterson, B., and Levander, O. 1996. Naturally occurring selenium compounds in cancer chemoprevention trials: A workshop summary. *Cancer Epidemiology and Biomarkers of Prevention* 6:63–69.

Pennington, J. 1996. Intakes of minerals from diets and foods: Is there a need for concern? *Journal of Nutrition* 126:2304S–2308S.

Porter, D. 1994. Washington update: NIH Consensus Development Conference statement optimal calcium intake. *Nutrition Today* 29:37–40.

Prasad, A. 1991. Role of zinc in human health. *Contemporary Nutrition* 16:1–2.

Prentice, A. 1993. Does mild zinc deficiency contribute to poor growth performance? *Nutrition Reviews* 51:268–77.

Prior, J., et al. 1996. Prevention and management of osteoporosis: Consensus statements from the Scientific Advisory Board of the Osteoporosis Society of Canada. 5. Physical activity as therapy for osteoporosis. *Canadian Medical Association Journal* 155:940–44.

Rayssiguier, Y., et al. 1990. New experimental and clinical data on the relationship between magnesium and sport. *Magnesium Research* 3:93–102.

Reading, S. 1996. Chromium picolinate. *Journal of the Florida Medical Association* 83:29–31.

Roberts, D., and Smith, D. 1992. Training at moderate altitude: Iron status of elite male swimmers. *Journal of Laboratory and Clinical Medicine* 120:387–91.

Rowland, T. 1990. Iron deficiency in the young athlete. *Pediatric Clinics of North America* 37:1153–62.

Schardt, D., and Schmidt, S. 1996. Chromium. *Nutrition Action Healthletter* 23 (4): 10–11.

Scrimshaw, N. 1991. Iron deficiency. *Scientific American* 265 (October): 46–52.

Seeman, E. 1997. Do men suffer from osteoporosis? *Australian Family Physician* 26:135–43.

Sempos, C., et al. 1996. Iron and heart disease: The epidemiologic data. *Nutrition Reviews* 54:73–84.

Sharman, I. 1984. Need for micro-nutrient supplementation with regard to physical performance. *International Journal of Sports Medicine* 5 (Suppl): 22–24.

Short, S. 1994. Dietary surveys and nutrition knowledge. In *Nutrition in Exercise and Sport,* eds. I. Wolinsky and J. Hickson. Boca Raton, FL: CRC Press.

Shils, M. 1994. Magnesium. In *Modern Nutrition in Health and Disease,* eds. M. Shils et al. Philadelphia: Lea and Febiger.

Smith, E., and Gilligan, C. 1989. Osteoporosis, bone mineral and exercise. *American Academy of Physical Education Papers* 22:107–19.

Snow-Harter, C. 1994. Bone health and prevention of osteoporosis in active and athletic women. *Clinics in Sports Medicine* 13:389–404.

Snow-Harter, C., and Marcus, R. 1991. Exercise, bone mineral density, and osteoporosis. *Exercise and Sport Sciences Reviews* 19:351–88.

Sojka, J., and Weaver, C. 1995. Magnesium supplementation and osteoporosis. *Nutrition Reviews* 53:71–80.

Stearns, D., et al. 1995. A prediction of chromium (III) accumulation in humans from chromium dietary supplements. *FASEB Journal* 9:1650–57.

Teegarden, D., and Weaver, C. 1994. Calcium supplementation increases bone density in adolescent girls. *Nutrition Reviews* 52:171–73.

Tremblay, M., et al. 1994. Ergogenic effects of phosphate loading: Physiological fact or methodological fiction? *Canadian Journal of Applied Physiology* 19:1–11.

Turnland, J. 1994. Copper. In *Modern Nutrition in Health and Disease,* eds. M. Shils et al. Philadelphia: Lea and Febiger.

Weaver, C., and Rajaram, S. 1992. Exercise and iron status. *Journal of Nutrition* 122:782–87.

Weight, L. 1993. 'Sports anemia' Does it exist? *Sports Medicine* 16:1–4.

Whiting, S. 1995. The inhibitory effect of dietary calcium on iron bioavailability: A cause for concern? *Nutrition Reviews* 53:77.

Wurzelmann, J., et al. 1996. Iron intake and the risk of colorectal cancer. *Cancer Epidemiology and Biomarkers of Prevention* 5:503–7.

Zimmerman, J. 1993. Does calcium supplementation reduce the risk of colon cancer? *Nutrition Reviews* 51:109–11.

Specific Studies

Albertson, A., et al. 1997. Estimated dietary calcium intake and food sources for adolescent females: 1980–1992. *Journal of Adolescent Health* 20:20–26.

Anderson, R., et al. 1995. Acute exercise effects on urinary losses and serum concentrations of copper and zinc of moderately trained and untrained men consuming a controlled diet. *Analyst* 120:867–70.

Anderson, R., et al. 1986. Strenuous exercise may increase dietary needs for chromium and zinc. In *Sport, Health and Nutrition,* ed. F. Katch. Champaign, IL: Human Kinetics.

Aruoma, O., et al. 1988. Iron, copper and zinc concentrations in human sweat and plasma: The effect of exercise. *Clinica Chimica Acta* 177:81–87.

Balaban, E., et al. 1989. The frequency of anemia and iron deficiency in the runner. *Medicine and Science in Sports and Exercise* 21:643–48.

Bilanin, J., et al. 1989. Lower vertebral bone density in male long distance runners. *Medicine and Science in Sports and Exercise* 21:66–70.

Boden, G., et al. 1996. Effects of vanadyl sulfate on carbohydrate and lipid metabolism in patients with non-insulin-dependent diabetes mellitus. *Metabolism* 45:1130–35.

Brilla, L., and Burkett, R. 1997. Effect of magnesium-fortified sports drink on strength in collegiate football players. *Medicine and Science in Sports and Exercise* 29:S250.

Brilla, L., and Gunter, K., 1994. Magnesium ameliorates aerobic contribution at high intensity. *Medicine and Science in Sports and Exercise* 26:S53.

Brilla, L., and Haley, T. 1992. Effect of magnesium supplementation on strength training in humans. *Journal of the American College of Nutrition* 112:326–29.

Cade, R., et al. 1984. Effects of phosphate loading on 2, 3–diphosphoglycerate and maximal oxygen uptake. *Medicine and Science in Sports and Exercise* 16:263–68.

Casoni, I., et al. 1990. Changes in magnesium concentrations in endurance athletes. *International Journal of Sports Medicine* 11:234–37.

Cassell, C., et al. 1996. Bone mineral density in elite 7- to 9-yr-old female gymnasts and swimmers. *Medicine and Science in Sports and Exercise* 28:1243–46.

Clancy, S., et al. 1994. Effects of chromium picolinate supplementation on body composition, strength, and urinary chromium loss in football players. *International Journal of Sport Nutrition* 4:142–53.

Cook, J., et al. 1991. Calcium supplementation: Effect on iron absorption. *American Journal of Clinical Nutrition* 53:106–11.

Couzy, F., et al. 1990. Zinc metabolism in the athlete: Influence of training, nutrition, and other factors. *International Journal of Sports Medicine* 11:263–66.

Davies, K., et al. 1982. Muscle mitochondrial bioenergetics, oxygen supply, and work capacity during dietary iron deficiency and repletion. *American Journal of Physiology* 242:E418–27.

Devine, A., et al. 1997. A 4-year follow-up study of the effects of calcium supplementation on bone density in elderly postmenopausal women. *Osteoporosis International* 7:23–28.

Dook, J., et al. 1997. Exercise and bone mineral density in mature female athletes. *Medicine and Science in Sports and Exercise* 29:291–96.

Drinkwater, B., et al. 1986. Bone mineral density after resumption of menses in amenorrheic athletes. *Journal of the American Medical Association* 256:380–82.

Duffy, D., and Conlee, R. 1986. Effects of phosphate loading on leg power and high intensity treadmill exercise. *Medicine and Science in Sports and Exercise* 18:674–77.

Faber, M., and Spinnler Benade, A. 1991. Mineral and vitamin intake in field athletes (discus, hammer, javelin-throwers and shotputters). *International Journal of Sports Medicine* 12:324–27.

Fawcett, J., et al. 1996. The effect of oral vanadyl sulfate on body composition and performance in weight-training athletes. *International Journal of Sport Nutrition* 6:382–90.

Ferrando, A., and Green, N. 1993. The effect of boron supplementation on lean body mass, plasma testosterone levels, and strength in male bodybuilders. *International Journal of Sport Nutrition* 3:140–49.

Fogelholm, M., et al. 1992. Effect of iron supplementation in female athletes with low serum ferritin concentration. *International Journal of Sports Medicine* 13:158–62.

Galloway, S., et al. 1996. The effects of acute phosphate supplementation in subjects of different aerobic fitness levels. *European Journal of Applied Physiology* 72:224–30.

Gullestad, L., et al. 1992. Oral magnesium supplementation improves metabolic variables and muscle strength in alcoholics. *Alcoholism, Clinical and Experimental Research* 16:986–90.

Hallmark, M., et al. 1996. Effects of chromium and resistive training on muscle strength and body composition. *Medicine and Science in Sports and Exercise* 28:139–44.

Hasten, D., et al. 1992. Effects of chromium picolinate on beginning weight training students. *International Journal of Sport Nutrition* 2:343–50.

Hudgins, P., et al. 1990. Effects of iron supplementation on hematologic profile and performance in female endurance athletes. *FASEB Journal* 4:A1197.

Hunt, C., et al. 1997. Metabolic responses of postmenopausal women to supplemental dietary boron and aluminum during usual and low magnesium intake: Boron, calcium, and magnesium absorption and retention and blood mineral concentrations. *American Journal of Clinical Nutrition* 65:803–13.

Johnson, J., and Walker, P. 1992. Zinc and iron utilization in young women consuming a beef-based diet. *Journal of the American Dietetic Association* 92:1474–78.

Karamizrak, S., et al. 1996. Evaluation of iron metabolism indices and their relation with physical work capacity in athletes. *British Journal of Sports Medicine* 30:15–19.

Kearney, J., et al. 1996. Calcium, vitamin D, and dairy foods and the occurrence of colon cancer in men. *American Journal of Epidemiology* 143:907–17.

Kiriike, N., et al. 1992. Reduced bone density and major hormones regulating calcium metabolism in anorexia nervosa. *Acta Psychiatrica Scandinavica* 86:358–63.

Klesges, R., et al. 1996. Changes in bone mineral content in male athletes. *Journal of the American Medical Association* 276:226–30.

Klingshirn, L., et al. 1992. Effect of iron supplementation on endurance capacity in iron-depleted female runners. *Medicine and Science in Sports and Exercise* 24:819–24.

Konig, D., et al. 1997. Zinc concentrations in serum, red blood cells and urine following strenuous exercise in endurance trained athletes. *Medicine and Science in Sports and Exercise* 29:S295.

Krall, E., et al. 1993. Heritable and life-style determinants of bone mineral density. *Journal of Bone and Mineral Research* 8:1–9.

Kraemer, W., et al. 1995. Effects of multibuffer supplementation on acid-base balance and 2,3-diphosphoglycerate following repetitive anaerobic exercise. *International Journal of Sport Nutrition* 5:300–314.

Kreider, R., et al. 1992. Effects of phosphate loading on metabolic and myocardial responses to maximal and endurance exercise. *International Journal of Sport Nutrition* 2:20–47.

Kreider, R., et al. 1990. Effects of phosphate loading on oxygen uptake, ventilatory anaerobic threshold, and run performance. *Medicine and Science in Sports and Exercise* 22:250–56.

Krotkiewski, M., et al. 1982. Zinc and muscle strength and endurance. *Acta Physiologica Scandinavica* 116:309–11.

Lamanca, J., and Haymes, E. 1993. Effects of iron repletion on VO$_2$ max, endurance, and blood lactate in women. *Medicine and Science in Sports and Exercise* 25:1386–92.

Liu, I., et al. 1983. Hypomagnesemia in a tennis player. *Physician and Sportsmedicine* 11 (May): 79–80.

Looker, A., et al. 1997. Prevalence of iron deficiency in the United States. *Journal of the American Medical Association* 277:973–76.

Lukaski, H., et al. 1996. Chromium supplementation and resistance training: Effects on body composition, strength, and trace element status of men. *American Journal of Clinical Nutrition* 63:954–65.

Lukaski, H., et al. 1996. Iron, copper, magnesium and zinc status as predictors of swimming performance. *International Journal of Sports Medicine* 17:535–40.

Lukaski, H., et al. 1991. Altered metabolic response of iron deficient women during graded, maximal exercises. *European Journal of Applied Physiology* 63:140–45.

Lukaski, H., et al. 1990. Thermogenesis and thermoregulatory function of iron-deficient women without anemia. *Aviation, Space and Environmental Medicine* 61:913–20.

Lupton, J., et al. 1996. Calcium supplementation modifies the relative amounts of bile acids in bile and affects key aspects of human colon physiology. *Journal of Nutrition* 126:1421–28.

Lyle, R., et al. 1992. Iron status in exercising women: The effect of oral iron therapy vs increased consumption of muscle foods. *American Journal of Clinical Nutrition* 56:1049–55.

Magazanik, A., et al. 1991. Effect of an iron supplement on body iron status and aerobic capacity of young training women. *European Journal of Applied Physiology* 62:317–23.

Mannix, E., et al. 1990. Oxygen delivery and cardiac output during exercise following oral phosphate-glucose. *Medicine and Science in Sports and Exercise* 22:341–47.

Matter, M., et al. 1987. The effect of iron and folate therapy on maximal exercise performance in female marathon runners with iron and folate deficiency. *Clinical Science* 72:415–22.

Myburgh, K., et al. 1993. Low bone mineral density at axial and appendicular sites in amenorrheic females. *Medicine and Science in Sports and Exercise* 25:1197–1202.

Naghii, M., et al. 1996. The boron content of selected foods and the estimation of its daily intake among free-living subjects. *Journal of the American College of Nutrition* 15:614–19.

Newhouse, I., et al. 1993. Effects of iron supplementation and discontinuation on serum copper, zinc, calcium, and magnesium levels in women. *Medicine and Science in Sports and Exercise* 25:562–71.

Newhouse, I., et al. 1989. The effects of prelatent/latent iron deficiency on physical work capacity. *Medicine and Science in Sports and Exercise* 21:263–68.

Nielsen, F., and Shuler, T. 1992. Studies of the interaction between boron and calcium, and its modification by magnesium and potassium, in rats. Effects on growth, blood variables, and bone mineral composition. *Biological Trace Elements Research* 35:225–37.

Ohno, H., et al. 1990. Training effects on blood zinc levels of humans. *Journal of Sports Medicine and Physical Fitness* 30:247–52.

Ormerod, S., et al. 1990. The relationship between weekly mileage and bone density in male runners. *Medicine and Science in Sports and Exercise* 22:S62.

Pirola, V., et al. 1991. Evaluation of the recovery of muscular trophicity in aged patients with femoral fractures treated with creatine phosphate and physiokinesitherapy. *Clinica Terapeutica* 139:115–19.

Powell, P., and Tucker, A. 1991. Iron supplementation and running performance in female cross-country runners. *International Journal of Sports Medicine* 12:462–67.

Rajaram, S., et al. 1995. Effects of long-term moderate exercise on iron status in young women. *Medicine and Science in Sports and Exercise* 27:1105–10.

Recker, R., et al. 1996. Correcting calcium nutritional deficiency prevents spine fractures in elderly women. *Journal of Bone Mineral Research* 11:1961–66.

Rowland, T., et al. 1988. The effect of iron therapy on the exercise capacity of nonanemic iron-deficient adolescent runners. *American Journal of Diseases in Children* 142:165–69.

Rubenowitz, E., et al. 1996. Magnesium in drinking water and death from acute myocardial infarction. *American Journal of Epidemiology* 143:456–62.

Salonen, J., et al. 1992. High stored iron levels are associated with excess risk of myocardial infarction in Eastern Finnish men. *Circulation* 86:1036–37.

Schmid, A., et al. 1996. Effect of physical exercise and vitamin C on absorption of ferric sodium citrate. *Medicine and Science in Sports and Exercise* 28:1470–73.

Schoene, R., et al. 1983. Iron repletion decreases maximal exercise lactate concentrations in female athletes with minimal iron deficiency anemia. *Journal of Laboratory and Clinical Medicine* 102:306–12.

Singh, A., et al. 1992. Plasma zinc uptake from a supplement during submaximal running. *Medicine and Science in Sports and Exercise* 24:442–46.

Singh, A., et al. 1991. Chronic multivitamin-mineral supplementation does not enhance physical performance. *Medicine and Science in Sports and Exercise* 24:726–31.

Smith, E., et al. 1989. Deterring bone loss by exercise intervention in premenopausal and postmenopausal women. *Calcified Tissue International* 44:312–21.

Snyder, A., et al. 1989. Influence of dietary iron source on measures of iron status among female runners. *Medicine and Science in Sports and Exercise* 21:7–10.

Stewart, I., et al. 1990. Phosphate loading and the effects on VO_2 max in trained cyclists. *Research Quarterly for Exercise and Sport* 61:80–84.

Suetta, C., et al. 1996. Haematological status in elite long-distance runners: Influence of body composition. *Clinical Physiology* 16:563–74.

Telford, R., et al. 1993. Iron status and diet in athletes. *Medicine and Science in Sports and Exercise* 25:796–800.

Terblanche, S., et al. 1992. Failure of magnesium supplementation to influence marathon running performance or recovery in magnesium-replete subjects. *International Journal of Sport Nutrition* 2:154–64.

Tessler, F., et al. 1995. Selenium and training effects on the glutathione system and aerobic performance. *Medicine and Science in Sports and Exercise* 27:390–96.

Thompson, D., et al. 1990. Effects of phosphate loading on erythrocyte 2, 3–diphosphoglycerate (2, 3–DPG), adenosine 5'–triphosphate (ATP), hemoglobin (Hb), and maximal oxygen consumption (VO_2 max). *Medicine and Science in Sports and Exercise* 22:S36.

Tilyard, M., et al. 1992. Treatment of postmenopausal osteoporosis with calcitriol or calcium. *New England Journal of Medicine* 326:357–62.

Tipton, K., et al. 1993. Zinc loss in sweat of athletes exercising in hot and neutral temperatures. *International Journal of Sport Nutrition* 3:261–71.

Trent, L., and Thieding-Cancel, D. 1995. Effects of chromium picolinate on body composition. *Journal of Sports Medicine and Physical Fitness* 35:273–80.

Verde, T., et al. 1982. Sweat composition in exercise and in heat. *Journal of Applied Physiology* 53:1540–45.

Waller, M., and Haymes, E. 1996. The effects of heat and exercise on sweat iron loss. *Medicine and Science in Sports and Exercise* 28:197–203.

Weatherwax, R., et al. 1986. Effects of phosphate loading on bicycle time trial performance. *Medicine and Science in Sports and Exercise* 18:S11–12.

Webster, B., and Barr, S. 1995. Calcium intake of adolescent female gymnasts and speed skaters: Lack of association with dieting behavior. *International Journal of Sport Nutrition* 5:2–12.

Weight, L., et al. 1992. Dietary iron deficiency and sports anaemia. *British Journal of Nutrition* 68:253–60.

Wilhite, J., and Mellion, M. 1990. Occult gastrointestinal bleeding in endurance cyclists. *Physician and Sportsmedicine* 18:75–78.

Wood, R., and Zheng, J. 1997. High dietary calcium intakes reduce zinc absorption and balance in humans. *American Journal of Clinical Nutrition* 65:1803–9.

CHAPTER 9

Water, Electrolytes, and Temperature Regulation

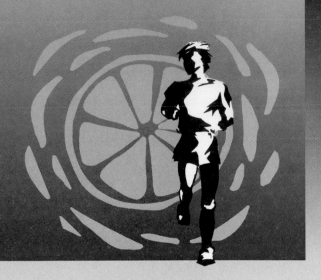

acclimatization
aldosterone
anhidrotic heat exhaustion
antidiuretic hormone (ADH)
conduction
convection
core temperature
electrolyte
evaporation
exertional heat stroke
extracellular water
glucose-electrolyte solutions (GES)
glucose-polymer solutions (GPS)
heat-balance equation
heat cramps
heat index
heat stroke
heat syncope
high blood pressure
homeostasis
hyperhydration
hyperkalemia
hypertension
hyperthermia
hypohydration
hypokalemia
hyponatremia
hypothermia
insensible perspiration
intercellular water
intracellular water
intravascular water
metabolic water

KEY CONCEPTS

• The average adult, who needs 2–3 quarts of water per day, maintains fluid balance primarily by drinking liquids, but substantial amounts of water also are obtained from solid foods in the diet.

• Normal water levels in the various body fluid compartments are maintained by a feedback mechanism involving specific receptors for osmotic pressure, the antidiuretic hormone (ADH), and the kidneys.

• Water has a number of functions in the body, but one of its most important benefits for people who exercise is the control of body temperature.

• Sodium, chloride, and potassium perform vital functions such as generating electrical impulses for contraction of muscles, including the heart. Their concentrations in the body are precisely regulated, and deficiencies or excesses are rare even in cases of heavy sweating.

• Humans are heat producers, and their body temperature, regulated by the brain's hypothalamus, is dependent upon the amount of heat they produce and how much they gain from or lose to the environment.

• High environmental temperatures, high relative humidity, or radiant heat from the sun can impose a severe heat stress to those who exercise under such conditions.

• Exercise can produce significant amounts of heat, but the body temperature usually can be regulated quite effectively by activation of heat-loss mechanisms, particularly sweating. However, both

hyperthermia and dehydration may impair endurance capacity.

• Sweat consists mainly of water and some minerals, primarily sodium and chloride. It is hypotonic compared to the body fluids.

• An effective rehydration solution is one that optimizes gastric emptying and intestinal absorption of fluid.

• Rehydration with cold water is effective in moderating body temperature during exercise in the heat, but carbohydrate solutions may be equally effective.

• Electrolyte replacement generally is not needed during exercise but may be helpful in very prolonged exercise tasks. Water alone, in combination with a balanced diet, will adequately restore normal electrolyte levels in the body on a day-to-day basis.

• Current research suggests that a 5–10 percent solution of glucose, fructose, glucose polymers, or combinations of these different carbohydrates may be effective for athletes who need carbohydrate replacement during exercise.

• Sodium bicarbonate appears to be an effective ergogenic aid in exercise tasks that depend primarily upon the lactic acid energy system.

• Heat injuries, of which heat stroke is the most potentially dangerous, may be due to increased body core temperature, loss of body fluids, or loss of electrolytes. Some individuals, such as the obese, are more susceptible to heat injury.

- The general treatment for heat-stress illnesses is to rest, drink cool liquids, and cool the body. Rapid body cooling is essential in suspected cases of heat stroke.
- If you exercise in the heat, you should be aware of signs of impending heat injury. You should also be aware of methods to reduce heat gain to the body and methods to facilitate heat loss.
- Acclimatization to exercise in the heat takes about 1–2 weeks, but endurance capacity in the heat is still limited somewhat even when one is fully acclimatized.
- Dietary practices to help prevent or treat high blood pressure include moderation in salt and sodium intake, moderation in alcohol consumption, and increased intake of fruits, vegetables, whole grains, low-fat dairy products, and foods rich in magnesium, potassium, and calcium.

normohydration
osmolality
radiation
salt-depletion heat
   exhaustion
shell temperature
sodium bicarbonate
specific heat
tonicity
water-depletion heat
   exhaustion
WBGT Index

INTRODUCTION

Water is a clear, tasteless, odorless fluid. It is a rather simple compound composed of two parts hydrogen and one part oxygen (H_2O). Of all the nutrients essential in the chemistry and functioning of living forms, it is the most important. Although humans may survive about 7 days without water under optimal conditions, rapid losses of body water through dehydration may prove fatal in a relatively short time, even within hours when young children with diarrhea lose large amounts of water and electrolytes.

Water provides no food energy, but most of the other nutrients essential to life can be used by the human body only because of their reaction with water. Water constitutes the majority of the body weight and provides the medium within which the other nutrients may function. Although water has a number of diverse functions in human metabolism, one of the most important, particularly for the athletic individual, is the regulation of body temperature. In a review of food and drink in sport, Macdonald noted that fluid is still the priority constituent that needs to be monitored.

When the body loses fluids by any route, it not only loses water but electrolytes as well. Electrolytes, particularly those discussed in this chapter (sodium, chloride, and potassium) are involved in numerous physiological functions, such as muscle contraction and fluid balance. An abnormal electrolyte status may adversely affect both health and physical performance.

Proper fluid replacement is important for both health and sport. To help decrease mortality from diarrhea, a major health problem associated with cholera in undeveloped countries, medical scientists developed oral rehydration therapy (ORT) solutions to help replace lost fluids rapidly. Today, the standard ORT solution contains sodium chloride, potassium chloride, trisodium citrate, glucose, and water,

and its application has effectively decreased mortality during epidemics of cholera. In the 1950s and 1960s, heat illnesses were widespread among military personnel and athletes, primarily because of regulations that restricted fluid intake. Research by sports medicine scientists during this time helped to identify risk factors associated with exercise under warm or hot environmental conditions, and with application of appropriate guidelines, the incidence of heat injuries declined. During these studies, scientists also noted that endurance-exercise performance declined with excessive exercise-induced sweating and fluid loss, and research into sport ORT as a means to help delay fatigue due to fluid losses increased dramatically, leading to our sports drinks of today.

Of the factors that may influence physical performance on any given day, one of the major concerns is the environmental temperature. Anyone who is physically active for prolonged periods is probably aware of the effect that temperature changes have on performance ability. In particular, as the temperature increases, the combination of the environmental heat and the increased body heat from exercise metabolism may disturb body-water supplies, electrolyte status, and temperature regulation, which at the least may prove detrimental to endurance capacity and at the extreme may have fatal consequences.

Given the seriousness of this topic, the primary focus of this chapter will be upon those problems that may confront you when exercising in the heat and how you may prevent or correct them. Topics covered include the role of water and selected electrolytes in human metabolism, the regulation of body temperature, the effect of fluid and electrolyte losses upon performance, methods of fluid and electrolyte replacement, ergogenic aids, and health-related problems such as heat illnesses and high blood pressure (hypertension).

Water

How much water do you need per day?

The requirement for body water depends on the body weight of the individual. The requirement varies in different stages of the life cycle. Under normal environmental temperatures and activity levels, the average adult needs about 1 milliliter of water per Calorie of energy intake. For the average adult female and male, this approximates 2,000 and 2,800 ml, respectively, or about 2 and 3 quarts. This amount will help maintain adequate water balance in the body.

Body-water balance is maintained when the output of body fluids is matched by the input of water. A small amount of water is lost in the feces and through the exhaled air in breathing. **Insensible perspiration** on the skin, which is not visible, is almost pure water and accounts for about 30 percent of body-water losses. Perspiration, or sweat, losses may be increased considerably during exercise and/or hot environmental conditions. Urinary output is the main avenue for water loss. It may increase through the use of diuretics, including alcohol and caffeine, or the use of a high-protein diet that produces urea, which needs to be excreted by the kidneys.

Fluid intake of beverages, such as water, soda, milk, coffee, and tea, is the main source of water to replenish losses. However, solid foods also contribute as a water source, and in two different ways. First, food contains water in varying amounts; certain foods such as lettuce, celery, melons, and most fruits contain about 90 percent water, and many others contain more than 60 percent; even bread, an apparently dry food, contains 36 percent water. Second, the metabolism of foods for energy also produces water. Fat, carbohydrate, and protein all produce water when broken down for energy. You may recall the reaction when glucose is metabolized to produce energy, with one of the by-products being **metabolic water:**

$$C_6H_{12}O_6 + 6O_2 \rightarrow Energy + 6CO_2 + 6H_2O$$

Table 9.1 summarizes the daily water loss and intake for the maintenance of water balance for an adult female. As shall be seen later, however, these amounts may change drastically under certain conditions.

It should be noted that most of the water we drink contains more than just water. In some areas, water may contain substantial amounts of various minerals, including calcium, sodium, magnesium, iron, zinc, and lead. Some minerals, like excess sodium and lead, may lead to various health problems, whereas others, such as calcium and magnesium, may be beneficial. Other substances find their way into our water supply as well. Lefferts reported that more than 700 contaminants have been found in public drinking water, including organic chemicals like pesticides. Under the Safe Drinking Water Act, the Environmental Protection Agency (EPA) has set maximum

Table 9.1	Daily water loss and intake for water balance in a sedentary adult female (60 kg)
Water loss	
Urine output	1,100 ml
Water in feces	100 ml
Lungs (exhaled air)	200 ml
Skin (insensible perspiration)	600 ml
Total	2,000 ml
Water intake	
Fluids	1,000 ml
Water in food	700 ml
Metabolic water	300 ml
Total	2,000 ml

contaminant levels for the most harmful substances, and most, but not all, municipal water treatment facilities conform to these standards. In general, municipal water supplies in the United States and Canada are safe. Water filters added to your tap may help remove unwanted substances, such as chlorine or chlorinated by-products. Many types of water filters are on the market, so if interested, have your water analyzed and then seek an appropriate filter to help purify your tap water. To get information on the quality of your water supply, you may contact the EPA or your local water utility.

In 1996, the Food and Drug Administration (FDA) effected guidelines for defining bottled waters. Artesian water is drawn from a well that taps a confined aquifer; mineral water comes from a protected underground source and must contain minerals distinguishing it from other waters; spring water flows naturally from an underground source; purified water is produced by distillation or some comparable process. Bottled waters must conform to the same safety standards as municipal water supplies. About 85 percent of bottled-water manufacturers belong to the International Bottled Water Association (IBWA), which sets even tougher standards for its members than the FDA. Individuals who drink bottled water should be aware that approximately 25 percent is simply tap water that has undergone a purification process. Also, bottled waters may not contain fluoride, a mineral added to most municipal water sources.

Where is water stored in the body?

Water is stored in several body compartments but moves constantly between compartments. About 65 percent of body water is stored inside body cells as **intracellular**

water. The remaining 35 percent is outside the cells and is termed **extracellular water.** The extracellular water is further subdivided into the **intercellular** (interstitial) **water** between or surrounding the cells, the **intravascular water** within the blood vessels, and miscellaneous water compartments such as the cerebrospinal fluid. Figure 9.1 represents the distribution of water in the body.

Water is held in the body in conjunction with protein, carbohydrate, and electrolytes. The protein content in the muscles, blood, and other tissues helps bind water to those tissues. Muscle glycogen has considerable amounts of water bound to it (about 3 grams of water per gram of glycogen), which may prove to be an advantage as discussed in Chapter 4. In essence, the metabolism of 350 grams of carbohydrate during exercise will provide nearly 1 liter of water for body functions, as recently documented by Rogers and others. The sodium in the extracellular fluid, including sodium in the circulatory system, attracts water.

Proper water and electrolyte balance within these compartments is of extreme importance to the athletic

individual. Fluid shifts such as decreases in blood volume and cellular dehydration, both of which may develop during exercise in the heat, could contribute to the onset of fatigue or heat illness.

Water comprises about 60 percent of the body weight in the average adult male and 50 percent in the adult female, but this percentage may be as low as 40 percent in obese individuals and as high as 70 percent or more in muscular individuals. The reason is that fat tissue is low in water content and muscle tissue is high in water content.

How is body water regulated?

Body water is maintained at a normal level through kidney function. Normal body-water level is called **normohydration,** or euhydration. Loss of body water results in a state of **hypohydration,** and **hyperhydration** represents a condition in which the body retains excess body fluids. Normal kidneys function very effectively to eliminate excess water during hyperhydration and conserve water during hypohydration.

Because water is so essential to life, it is indeed fortunate that the body possesses an efficient mechanism to maintain proper water balance. **Homeostasis** is the term used to describe the maintenance of a normal internal environment so that the body has the proper distribution and use of water, electrolytes, hormones, and other substances essential for life processes. Homeostatic mechanisms are extremely complex, and a full discussion is beyond the scope of this book. However, in essence, all homeostatic mechanisms work by a series of feedback devices. If these feedback devices are functioning properly, the body usually has no problem in maintaining the normal physical and chemical composition of its fluid compartments.

The main feedback device for the control of body water is the osmolality of the various body fluids. **Osmolality** refers to the amount, or concentration, of dissolved substances, known as solute, in a solution. In the body a number of different substances affect osmolality, including glucose, protein, and several electrolytes, most notably sodium. These substances are dissolved in the body water. One mole of a nonionic substance such as glucose, dissolved in a liter of water is one osmole. One millimole (1/1,000 mole) is one milliosmole. However, a mole of a substance that can dissociate into two ions, such as sodium chloride, is equivalent to two osmoles. One millimole of sodium chloride would be two milliosmoles (mOsm).

A term often used in conjunction with osmolality is **tonicity,** which means tension or pressure. When two solutions have the same osmotic pressure they are said to be isosmotic or, more commonly, isotonic. Iso means "same." When two solutions with different solute concentrations are compared, the one with the higher osmotic pressure is called hypertonic and the other is hypotonic.

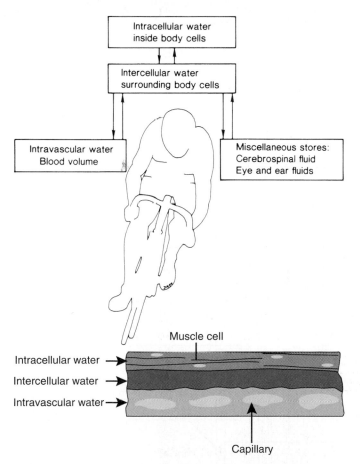

Figure 9.1 Body-water compartments. There is a constant interchange among the different body-water compartments. The water inside the body cells, the intracellular water, is important for cell functions. The other three compartments (intercellular, intravascular, and miscellaneous) are known collectively as the extracellular water. Decreases in blood volume may adversely affect endurance capacity.

When two solutions with different solute concentrations are separated by a permeable membrane, as in the human body between the fluid compartments, a potential pressure difference may develop between the solutions that will allow for water movement. This pressure is known as osmotic pressure. Water moves across the membrane from the hypotonic solution (low solute concentration and high water content) to the hypertonic solution (high solute concentration and low water content). In essence, high solute concentrations create high osmotic pressures and tend to draw water into their compartments. Figure 9.2 depicts this mechanism between the blood and the body cells.

To briefly illustrate the feedback mechanism for control of body water, let us look at what happens when you become dehydrated owing to excessive body-water losses or lowered water intake. The blood then becomes more concentrated, or hypertonic. Because maintenance of a normal blood volume is of prime importance, the blood tends to draw water from the body cells. Certain cells in the hypothalamus, called osmoreceptors, are sensitive to changes in osmotic pressure. These cells react to the more concentrated body fluids by stimulating the release of a hormone from the pituitary gland, the so-called master gland of the body. This hormone is called the **antidiuretic hormone (ADH).** The ADH travels by the blood to the kidneys and directs them to reabsorb more water. Hence, urinary output of water is diminished considerably. Figure 9.3 illustrates this feedback process that helps conserve body water and blood volume. During hyperhydration, which would produce a hypotonic condition in the body fluids, a reverse process would occur leading to increased water excretion. As we shall see below, other hormones that influence sodium balance in the body also help regulate water balance.

Osmoreceptors and other mechanisms also may stimulate the sensation of thirst, which is usually a good guide to body-water needs and is effective in restoring body water to normal on a day-to-day basis. However, thirst may not be an accurate indicator of the need for water replacement during exercise in a hot environment.

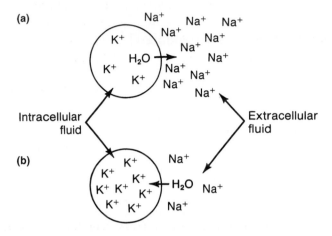

Figure 9.2 Osmosis and tonicity. (a) When the extracellular fluid contains more electrolytes or other osmotic substances, it is hypertonic to the intracellular fluid. In this case water will flow from the interior of the cell to the outside, or to an area of greater osmotic pressure. (b) When the intracellular fluid contains more electrolytes or greater osmotic pressure, water will flow into the cell from the extracellular fluid.

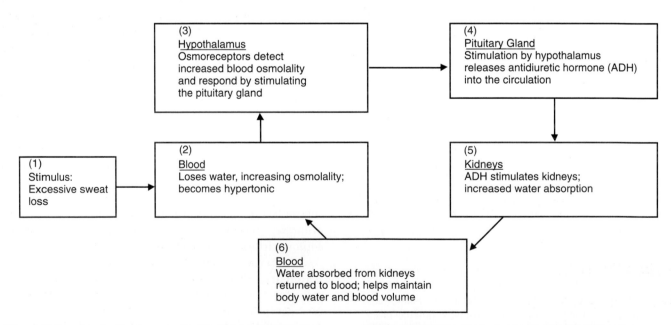

Figure 9.3 One feedback mechanism for homeostatic control of body water and blood volume. Other feedback mechanisms operate concurrently. For example, the hypothalamus also stimulates the thirst response to increase fluid intake.

What are the major functions of water in the body?

Water is essential if the other nutrients are to function properly within the human body; it is the solvent for life. It has a number of diverse functions that may be summarized as follows:

1. Water provides the essential building material for cell protoplasm, the fundamental component of all living matter.

2. Because water cannot be compressed, it serves to protect key body tissues such as the spinal cord and brain.

3. Water is essential in the control of the osmotic pressure in the body, or the maintenance of a proper balance between water and the electrolytes. Any major changes in the electrolyte concentration may adversely affect cellular function. A serious departure from normal osmotic pressure cannot be tolerated by the body for long.

4. Water is the main constituent of blood, the major transportation mechanism in the body for conveying oxygen, nutrients, hormones, and other compounds to the cells for their use, and for carrying waste products of metabolism away from the cells to organs such as the lungs and kidneys for excretion from the body.

5. Water is essential for the proper functioning of our senses. Hearing waves are transmitted by fluid in the inner ear. Fluid in the eye is involved in the reflection of light for proper vision. For the taste and smelling senses to function, the foods and odors need to be dissolved in water.

6. Of primary importance to the active individual is the role that water plays in the regulation of body temperature. Water is the major constituent of sweat, and through its evaporation from the surface of the skin, it can help dissipate excess body heat. Of all the nutrients, water is the most important to the physically active person and is one of the few that may have beneficial effects on performance when used in supplemental amounts before or during exercise. Hence, the athletic individual should know what is necessary to help maintain proper fluid balance, a topic covered in detail later in this chapter.

Electrolytes

What is an electrolyte?

An **electrolyte** is defined as a substance which, in solution, conducts an electric current. The solution itself may be referred to as an electrolyte solution. Acids, bases, and salts are common electrolytes, and they usually dissociate into ions, particles carrying either a positive (cation) or a negative (anion) electric charge. The major electrolytes in the body fluids are sodium, potassium, chloride, bicarbonate, sulfate, magnesium, and calcium. Electrolytes can act at the cell membrane and generate electrical current, such as in a nerve impulse. Electrolytes can also function in other ways, activating enzymes to control a variety of metabolic activities in the cell. In the last chapter we covered some of the important metabolic functions of calcium, phosphorus, and magnesium; in this chapter the focus is on sodium, chloride, and potassium because of their presence in sports drinks, popular beverages used to replace fluid losses in physically active people.

In later sections we shall look at the interaction of these electrolytes with exercise in warm environmental conditions, a possible ergogenic effect of certain sodium salts (comparable to sodium phosphate discussed in the last chapter), and their role in the etiology of high blood pressure. But first, let us briefly cover the function of each of these electrolytes in the human body.

Sodium (Na)

Sodium is a mineral element also known as natrium, from which the symbol *Na* is derived. It is one of the principal positive ions, or electrolytes, in the body fluids.

RDA There is no RDA for sodium. The estimated minimum requirement for sodium in adults is 500 milligrams. Common table salt (sodium chloride) is about 40 percent sodium, so only about 1,250 milligrams (1.25 grams) is needed to supply the minimum requirement. In the National Research Council book *Diet and Health*, the upper recommended intake is 2.4 grams of sodium per day, which amounts to 6 grams of table salt. There is no RDI for sodium, although 2.4 grams (2,400 milligrams) is the amount used as the Daily Value for food labels.

Food Sources Sodium is distributed widely in nature but is found in rather small amounts in most natural foods. However, significant amounts of salt, and hence sodium, are usually added from the salt shaker for flavor. One teaspoon of salt contains about 2,000 milligrams of sodium. Moreover, processing techniques add significant amounts of salt to the foods we buy. For example, a serving of fresh or frozen green peas contains only 2 milligrams of sodium, but increases to 240 milligrams in the canning process. In general, natural foods are low in sodium whereas processed foods are relatively high. Because of health concerns for some individuals with high-sodium diets, food manufacturers have been reducing the salt content in some of their products. Nevertheless, researchers have reported that the average American consumes about 10–12 grams of salt (4–4.8 grams of sodium) per day, approximately 3 grams from

Table 9.2 Sodium content of common foods

Food exchange item	Amount	Sodium (mg)
Milk		
Low-fat milk	1 c	120
Cottage cheese		
Creamed	1/2 c	320
Unsalted	1/2 c	30
Cheese, American	1 oz	445
Vegetables		
Beans, cooked fresh	1 oz	5
Beans, canned	1 oz	150
Pickles, dill	1 medium	900
Potato, baked	1 medium	6
Fruits		
Banana	1 medium	1
Orange	1 medium	1
Starch		
Bread, whole wheat	1 slice	130
Bran flakes	3/4 c	340
Oatmeal, cooked	1 c	175
Pretzels	1 oz	890
Meat		
Luncheon meats	1 oz	450
Frankfurter	1 medium	495
Chicken	3 oz	40
Beef, steak	3 oz	70
Tuna, low sodium	3 oz	35
Tuna, in oil	3 oz	800
Fish (cod, flounder)	3 oz	100
Deviled crab, frozen	1 c	2,085
Fats		
Butter, salted	1 tsp	50
Margarine, salted	1 tsp	50
Canned foods and prepared entrees		
Chop suey, canned	1 c	1,050
Spaghetti, canned	1 c	1,220
Turkey dinner, frozen	1	1,735
Chicken noodle soup	5 oz	655
Chicken noodle soup, low sodium	5 oz	120
Condiments		
Mustard	1 tbsp	195
Tomato catsup	1 tbsp	155
Soy sauce	1 tbsp	1,320

As you can see in this table, the sodium content of foods can vary greatly. In general, canned and processed foods have a much higher sodium content than do fresh foods. Eat fresh meats, fruits, vegetables, and bread products whenever possible, and prepare them with little or no salt. Avoid highly salted foods like pickles, pretzels, soy sauce, and others. Look for "sodium free" or "low sodium" labels when shopping for canned foods.

Source: U.S. Department of Agriculture.

natural foods, 3–5 grams from processed foods, and 4 grams from the salt shaker. Table 9.2 highlights the sodium content in several foods within the major food groups. Note the difference in salt content between fresh and processed foods. In one recent study, subjects obtained nearly 80 percent of their daily sodium intake from processed foods. To help reduce sodium intake from this source, read nutrition labels. Food labels must list the sodium content, both in milligrams and in percent of the Daily Value. Check the label for salt content; remember "sodium free" means less than 5 milligrams per serving, "very low sodium" means less than 40 milligrams, and "low sodium" means less than 140 milligrams. With some canned vegetables, draining and rinsing the product with fresh water removes some of the sodium. Some processed foods high in sodium are shown in Figure 9.4.

Major Functions Sodium is an important element in a number of body functions. As the principal electrolyte in the extracellular fluids, it serves primarily to help maintain normal body-fluid balance and osmotic pressure. In this regard it is essential in the control of normal blood pressure through its effect on the blood volume. The role of sodium in the etiology of high blood pressure is discussed in a later section.

In conjunction with several other electrolytes, sodium is critical for nerve impulse transmission and muscle contraction. It is also a component of several compounds, such as sodium bicarbonate, that help maintain normal acid-base balance and, as noted in a later section, may be an effective ergogenic aid. An overview of sodium is presented in Table 9.3.

Deficiency and Excess Because the maintenance of normal blood pressure is critical to life, the body has an effective regulatory feedback mechanism allowing for a wide range of dietary sodium intake. The hypothalamus helps regulate sodium as well as water balance in the body. If the sodium concentration decreases in the blood, a series of complex reactions leads to the secretion of **aldosterone,** a hormone produced in the adrenal gland, which stimulates the kidneys to retain more sodium. On the other hand, excesses of serum sodium will lead to decreased aldosterone production and increased excretion of sodium by the kidneys in the urine. Other hormones, notably ADH via its effect on water absorption in the kidneys, help maintain normal sodium equilibrium in the body fluids. During exercise, particularly intense exercise, sodium concentration increases in the blood, which helps to maintain blood volume. Exercise also leads to increased secretion of ADH and aldosterone, which helps conserve body water and sodium supplies.

Because this regulatory mechanism is so effective, deficiency states due to inadequate dietary intake are not common. Indeed, humans even have a natural appetite for salt, assuring adequate sodium intake and sodium balance over time. On the other hand, excessive losses of sodium from the body, usually induced by prolonged sweating while exercising in the heat, may lead to short-term deficiencies that may be debilitating to the athletic individual. These problems are discussed later in this chapter in the sections on fluid and electrolyte replacement and health aspects.

Chloride (Cl)

Chloride is the major negative ion in the extracellular fluids.

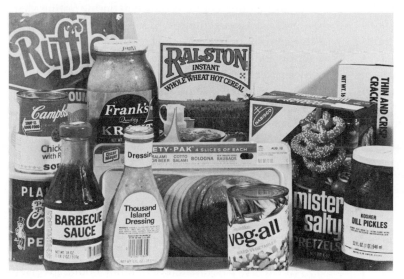

Figure 9.4 Foods with high salt (sodium) content should be reduced in the diet. Be aware of foods that have large amounts of hidden sodium.

RDA The estimated daily adult minimum requirement for chloride is 750 milligrams. There is no RDA or RDI for chloride.

Food Sources Chloride is distributed in a variety of foods. Its dietary intake is closely associated with that of sodium, notably in the form of common table salt, which is 60 percent chloride.

Major Functions Chloride ions have a variety of functions in the human body. They work with sodium in the regulation of body-water balance and electrical potentials across cell membranes. They also are involved in the formation of hydrochloric acid in the stomach, which is necessary for certain digestive processes.

Deficiency Under normal circumstances chloride deficiency is rather rare. However, because the losses of sodium and chloride in sweat are directly proportional, the symptoms of chloride loss during excessive dehydration through sweating parallel those of sodium loss. The effects of electrolyte losses and replacement, including chloride, on physical performance and health are covered in later sections of this chapter. An overview of chloride is presented in Table 9.3.

Potassium (K)

Potassium is a mineral element also known as kalium, from which the symbol K is derived. It is a positive ion.

Table 9.3 Major electrolytes: sodium, chloride, and potassium*

Major electrolyte	Estimated minimum requirement	Major functions in the body	Deficiency symptoms	Symptoms of excess consumption
Sodium	500 milligrams	Primary positive ion in extracellular fluid; nerve impulse conduction; muscle contraction; acid-base balance; blood volume homeostasis	Hyponatremia; muscle cramps; nausea; vomiting; loss of appetite; dizziness; seizures; shock; coma	Hypertension (high blood pressure) in susceptible individuals
Chloride	750 milligrams	Primary negative ion in extracellular fluid; nerve impulse conduction; hydrochloric acid formation in stomach	Rare; may be caused by excess vomiting and loss of hydrochloric acid; convulsions	Hypertension, in conjunction with excess sodium
Potassium	2,000 milligrams	Primary positive ion in intracellular fluid; same functions as sodium, but intracellular; glucose transport into cell	Hypokalemia; loss of appetite; muscle cramps; apathy; irregular heartbeat	Hyperkalemia; inhibited heart function

*Food sources for sodium and potassium may be found in Tables 9.2 and 9.4, respectively; food sources for chloride are similar to those for sodium.

RDA There is no RDA for potassium. The estimated daily adult minimum requirement for potassium is 2,000 milligrams. In *Diet and Health,* an increase in potassium intake to about 3,500 mg per day is recommended. There is no RDI for potassium.

Food Sources Potassium is found in most foods and is especially abundant in bananas, citrus fruits, fresh vegetables, milk, meat, and fish. Table 9.4 provides some data on the potassium content of several common foods in the major food groups.

Major Functions As the major electrolyte inside the body cells, potassium works in close association with sodium and chloride in the maintenance of body fluids and in the generation of electrical impulses in the nerves and the muscles, including the heart muscle. Potassium also plays an important role in the energy processes in the muscle, for it helps in the transport of glucose into the muscle cells, the storage of glycogen, and the production of high-energy compounds.

Deficiency and Excess Potassium balance, like sodium balance, is also regulated by aldosterone. A high serum potassium level stimulates the release of aldosterone from the adrenal cortex, leading to an increased excretion of potassium by the kidneys into the urine. A decrease in serum potassium levels elicits a drop in aldosterone secretion and hence a greater conservation of potassium by the kidneys. Because a potassium imbalance in the body may have serious health consequences, potassium regulation is quite precise. Deficiencies or excessive accumulation are extremely rare under normal circumstances.

Although potassium deficiencies are rare, they may occur under certain conditions such as during fasting, diarrhea, and the use of diuretics. In such cases **hypokalemia,** or low serum potassium levels, could lead to muscular weakness and even cardiac arrest due to a decreased ability to generate nerve impulses. Several deaths of individuals on unbalanced liquid-protein fasting diets several years ago were associated with potassium deficiencies.

Excessive body potassium stores also are not very common, occurring mainly in conjunction with several disease states or in individuals who overdose on potassium supplements. **Hyperkalemia,** or excessive potassium in the blood, may disturb electrical impulses, causing cardiac arrhythmias and possible death. For this reason, individuals should never take potassium supplements in large doses without the consent of a physician. An overview of potassium is presented in Table 9.3.

In theory, a potassium deficiency could adversely affect physical performance capacity. The effect of exercise on potassium losses and the need for potassium supplementation in athletic individuals have therefore been studied by several investigators. The role of potassium in the etiology of high blood pressure has also been studied. The results of this research are presented in later sections of this chapter.

Regulation of Body Temperature

What is the normal body temperature?

The temperature of different body parts may vary considerably. The skin may be very cold, but the body internally is much warmer. When we speak of body temperature, we mean the internal, or **core temperature,** and not the external shell temperature. **Shell temperature,** which represents the temperature of the skin and the tissues directly under it, varies considerably depending upon the surrounding environmental temperature.

In humans, normal body temperature is approximately 98.6° F (37° C). This core temperature may be measured in a variety of ways, but the two most common methods are orally and rectally. For research purposes, a thermocouple is inserted through the nose down into the esophagus to provide a more precise measure of core temperature. Normal body temperature at rest varies, and may

Table 9.4	Potassium content in some common foods in the major food exchanges	
Food	**Amount**	**Milligrams of potassium**
Milk		
Skim milk	8 oz glass	410
Yogurt, low-fat	1 c	530
Cheese, cheddar	1 oz	28
Meat		
Chicken breast	1 oz	70
Beef, lean	1 oz	100
Fish, flounder	1 oz	160
Starch		
Bread, whole wheat	1 slice	65
Cereal, Cheerios	1 oz	110
Fruit		
Banana	1 medium	460
Orange	1 avg	260
Apple	1 avg	35
Vegetables		
Potato, baked	1 avg	780
Broccoli	1 stalk	270
Carrot	1 medium	275

range from 97–99° F (36.1–37.2° C). At rest the rectal temperature is normally about 0.5–1.0° F higher than the oral temperature; however, following a road race one study reported that the rectal temperature was 5.5° F higher than the oral temperature, suggesting that an oral reading may not be an accurate reflection of the true body temperature in an assessment of heat injury.

Humans can survive a range of core temperatures for a short time, but optimal physiological functioning usually occurs within a range of 97–104° F (36.1–40.0° C). A variety of factors may affect body temperature, but here we are concerned with the effect exercise has on the core temperature and how our body adjusts to help maintain heat balance.

What are the major factors that influence body temperature?

Humans are warm-blooded animals and are able to maintain a constant body temperature under varying environmental temperatures. To do this, the body must constantly make adjustments to either gain or lose heat.

Humans are heat-producing machines. The basal metabolic heat production is provided through normal burning (oxidation) of the three basic foodstuffs in the body—carbohydrate, fat, and protein. A higher basal metabolic rate, infectious diseases, shivering, and exercise are several factors that might increase heat production.

The human body also has a variety of means to lose heat. Heat loss is governed by four physical means—conduction, convection, radiation, and evaporation.

Conduction—Heat is transferred from the body by direct physical contact, as when you sit on a cold seat.

Convection—Heat is transferred by movement of air or water over the body.

Radiation—Heat energy radiates from the body into the surrounding air.

Evaporation—Heat is lost from the body when it is used to convert sweat to a vapor, known as the heat of vaporization. The lungs also help to dissipate heat through evaporation.

During rest and under normal environmental temperatures, body heat is transported from the core to the shell by way of conduction and convection, the blood being the main carrier of the heat. The vast majority of the heat escapes from the body by radiation and convection, with a smaller amount being carried away by the evaporation of insensible perspiration. A cooler environment,

increased air movement such as a cool wind, increased blood circulation to the skin, or an increased radiation surface would facilitate heat loss.

On the other hand, under certain environmental conditions, such as exercising in the sunlight on a hot day, some of these processes may be reversed with the body gaining heat instead of losing it. For example, radiant energy from the sun could add heat to the body.

The well-known **heat-balance equation** may be used to illustrate these interrelationships:

$$H = M \pm W \pm C \pm R - E$$

where H = heat balance, M = resting metabolic rate, W = work done (exercise), C = conduction and convection, R = radiation, E = evaporation.

If any of these factors governing heat production or heat loss are not balanced by an opposite reaction, heat balance will be lost and the body will deviate from its normal value. During exercise, W increases heat production. Hence, compensating adjustments in C, R, and E must be made to dissipate the extra heat. Figure 9.5 illustrates heat stress factors and mechanisms of heat loss during exercise.

How does the body regulate its own temperature?

Body temperature is controlled by the autonomic division of the central nervous system. The hypothalamus is an important structure in the brain that is involved in the control of a wide variety of physiological functions,

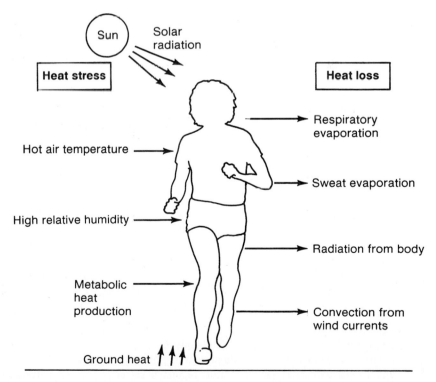

Figure 9.5 Sources of heat gain and heat loss to the body during exercise. See text for details.

including body temperature. The hypothalamus is thought to function pretty much like the thermostat in your house. If your house gets too cold, the heat comes on; if it gets too warm, the air conditioning system starts. The human body makes similar adjustments.

The temperature-regulating center in the hypothalamus receives input from several sources. First, receptors in the skin can detect temperature changes and send impulses to the hypothalamus. Second, the temperature of the blood can directly affect the hypothalamus as it flows through that structure.

In general, if the skin receptors detect a warmer temperature or the blood temperature rises, the body will make adjustments in an attempt to lose heat. Two major adjustments may occur. First, the blood will be channeled closer to the skin so that the heat from within may get closer to the outside and radiate away more easily. Second, sweating will begin and evaporation of the sweat will carry heat away from the body.

If the skin receptors detect a colder temperature or the blood temperature is lowered, then the body will react to conserve heat or increase heat production. First, the blood will be shunted away from the skin to the central core of the body. This decreases heat loss by radiation and helps keep the vital organs at the proper temperature. Second, shivering may begin. Shivering is nothing more than the contraction of muscles, which produces extra heat by increasing the metabolic rate. Figure 9.6 is a simplified schematic of body temperature control.

The hypothalamus is usually very effective in controlling body temperature. However, certain conditions may threaten temperature control. For example, an individual who falls into cold water will lose body heat rapidly, for water is an excellent conductor of heat. Such a situation may lead to **hypothermia** (low body temperature) and a rapid loss of temperature control. Hypothermia may also develop in slower runners during the latter part of a road race under cold, wet, and windy environmental conditions when heat is lost more rapidly than it is produced through exercise. Muscular incoordination and mental confusion are early signs of hypothermia.

On the other hand, the most prevalent threat to the athletic individual is **hyperthermia,** or the increased body temperature that occurs with exercise in a warm or hot environment. Hyperthermia is one of the major factors limiting physical performance and one of the most dangerous.

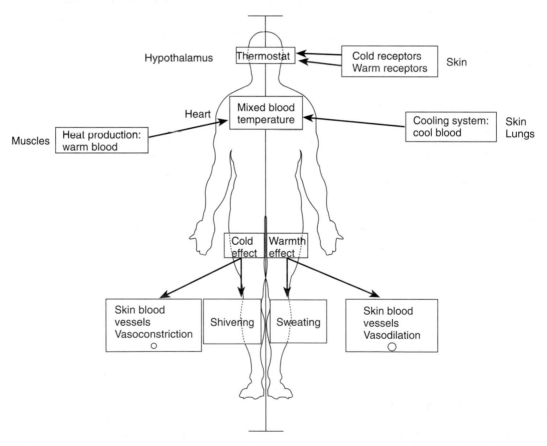

Figure 9.6 Simplified schematic of body temperature control. The temperature of the blood returning from the muscles and the skin stimulates the temperature regulation center (thermostat) in the hypothalamus, as do nerve impulses from the warmth and cold receptors in the skin. An overall cold effect will elicit a constriction of the blood vessels near the body surface and muscular shivering, thus helping to conserve body heat. An overall warmth effect will elicit a dilation of blood vessels near the skin and sweating, thus increasing the loss of body heat.

What environmental conditions may predispose an athletic individual to hyperthermia?

The interaction of four environmental factors are important determinants of the heat stress imposed on an active individual:

1. Air temperature. Caution should be advised when the air temperature is 80° F (27° C) or above. However, if the relative humidity and solar radiation are high, lower air temperatures, even 70° F, may pose a risk of heat stress during exercise.

2. Relative humidity. As the water content in the air increases, the relative humidity rises. The increased humidity impairs the ability of sweat to evaporate and thus may restrict the effectiveness of the body's main cooling system when exercising. With humidity levels from 90–100 percent, heat loss via evaporation nears zero. Caution should be used when the relative humidity exceeds 50–60 percent, especially when accompanied by warmer temperatures.

3. Air movement. Still air limits heat carried away by convection. Even a small breeze may help keep body temperature near normal by moving heat away from the skin surface.

4. Radiation. Radiant heat from the sun may create an additional heat load.

Some useful guidelines have been developed taking these four factors into consideration. The wet-bulb globe temperature (WBGT) thermometer, illustrated in Figure 9.7, measures all four. Small hand-held WBGT thermometers are available. The dry-bulb thermometer (DB) measures air temperature, the globe thermometer (G) measures radiant heat, and the wet-bulb thermometer (WB) evaluates relative humidity and air movement as they influence air temperature. The **WBGT Index** is computed as follows:

WBGT Index = 0.7 WB + 0.2 G + 0.1 DB

For example, if the WB reads 70, the G is 100, and the DB is 80, then the WBGT = $(0.7 \times 70) + (0.2 \times 100) + (0.1 \times 80) = 77°$ F.

Another indicator of heat stress is the **heat index** (Table 9.5), which combines the air temperature and relative humidity to determine the apparent temperature, or how hot it feels. Table 9.5 also contains some guidelines to prevent heat disorders based on the heat index.

The American College of Sports Medicine (ACSM) has published a position statement with guidelines for the prevention of heat, and cold, illnesses during distance running. These guidelines, which also are applicable to other athletes exercising in the heat, are incorporated in

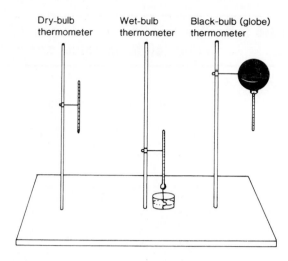

Figure 9.7 A typical setup for measurement of the wet-bulb globe temperature index (WBGT). The dry bulb measures air temperature, the wet bulb indirectly measures humidity, and the black bulb measures the radiant heat from the sun. Computerized commercial devices that measure the WBGT rapidly are also available.

the last section of this chapter. A modified version of the ACSM warnings based on the WBGT is presented in Table 9.6.

How does exercise affect body temperature?

As noted in Chapter 3, exercise increases the metabolic rate and the production of energy. Under a normal mechanical efficiency ratio of 20–25 percent, the remaining 75–80 percent of energy is released as heat. The total amount of heat produced in the body depends on the intensity and duration of the exercise. A more intense exercise will produce heat faster, while the longer the exercise lasts the more total heat is produced.

For illustrative purposes only, let us look at a hypothetical example of the body temperature changes that might occur in an exercising individual who was unable to dissipate heat. A physically conditioned person may be able to perform in a steady state for prolonged periods. If a normal-sized male, 154 lbs or 70 kg, were to jog for about an hour he could expend approximately 900 Calories. Assuming a mechanical efficiency rate of 20 percent, 80 percent, or 720 Calories (0.80×900), would be released in the body as heat.

Specific heat is defined as the heat in Calories required to raise the temperature of 1 kilogram of a substance by 1 degree Celsius. Because the specific heat of the body is 0.83, that is, 0.83 Calorie will raise 1 kg of the body 1° C, then 58 Calories (70 kg × 0.83) would raise the body temperature 1° C in this person. Thus, if this excess heat were not dissipated, his body temperature

Table 9.5 Possible heat disorders in runners and other high-risk groups based on the heat index (air temperature and relative humidity versus apparent temperature)

Relative humidity (%)

Air temperature (°F)	0	5	10	15	20	25	30	35	40	45	50	55	60	65	70	75	80	85	90	95	100
140	125																				
135	120	128																			
130	117	122	131																		
125	111	116	123	131	141																
120	107	111	116	123	130	139	148														
115	103	107	111	115	120	127	135	143	151												
110	99	102	105	108	112	117	123	130	137	143	150										
105	95	97	100	102	105	109	113	118	123	129	135	142	149								
100	91	93	95	97	99	101	104	107	110	115	120	126	132	138	144						
95	87	88	90	91	93	94	96	98	101	104	107	110	114	119	124	130	136				
90	83	84	85	86	87	88	90	91	93	95	96	98	100	102	106	109	113	117	122		
85	78	79	80	81	82	83	84	85	86	87	88	89	90	91	93	95	97	99	102	105	108
80	73	74	75	76	77	77	78	79	79	80	81	81	82	83	85	86	86	87	88	89	91
75	69	69	70	71	72	72	73	73	74	74	75	75	76	76	77	77	78	78	79	79	80
70	64	64	65	65	66	66	67	67	68	68	69	69	70	70	70	70	71	71	71	71	72

Heat index (or apparent temperature)

Heat index	Possible heat disorders for people in higher risk groups
130° or higher	Heatstroke/sunstroke highly likely with continued exposure.
105° – 130°	Sunstroke, heat cramps, or heat exhaustion likely, and heatstroke possible with prolonged exposure and/or physical activity.
90° – 105°	Sunstroke, heat cramps and heat exhaustion possible with prolonged exposure and/or physical activity.
80° – 90°	Fatigue possible with prolonged exposure and/or physical activity.

Source: Data from U.S. Department of Commerce. National Oceanic and Atmospheric Administration.

would increase over 12.4° C (720/58), or over 22° F, resulting in a body temperature of 120° F, a fatal condition. Although the core temperature does rise during exercise, it rarely hits these extreme levels. The average core temperature during exercise, even during moderately warm temperatures, may reach about 102.2–104.9° F (39–40° C). This is because of the body's cooling system.

How is body heat dissipated during exercise?

During exercise in a cold or cool environment, body heat is lost mainly through radiation and convection via the air movement around the body. Some evaporation of sweat and evaporative heat loss from the lungs may also contribute to maintenance of heat balance.

However, when the environmental temperature rises, the evaporation of sweat becomes the main means of

controlling an excessive rise in the core temperature. For example, evaporation of sweat may account for about 20 percent of total heat loss when exercising in an ambient temperature of 50° F (10° C), but increases to about 45 percent at 68° F (20° C) and 70 percent at 86° F (30° C). Although variable, the maximal evaporation rate is about 30 milliliters of sweat per minute, or 1.8 liters per hour. However, greater sweat rates may occur when sweat drops off the skin without vaporizing. Only sweat that evaporates has a cooling effect. One liter of sweat, if perfectly evaporated, will dissipate about 580 C. In our example above, the evaporation of 1.24 liters of sweat (720/580) would prevent a rise in the core temperature. However, the evaporation of sweat from the body is not perfect, as sweat can drip off the body and not carry away body heat, so more than 1.24 liters may be lost. If we assume that 2.0 liters were lost, then this individual would have lost 4.4 lbs

Table 9.6 Guidelines for preventing heat illness in runners and other athletes

Flag color/WBGT	Risk	Warnings*
Green/below 64° F (18° C)	Low	Although the risk is low, heat injury still can occur; caution still needed.
Yellow/64–72° F (18–22° C)	Moderate	Runners should closely monitor for signs of impending heat injury and slow pace if necessary; in long races, heat stress may increase during the course of the race if run in morning to early afternoon.
Red/73–82° F (23–28° C)	High	Runner must slow running pace and be very aware of warning signs of heat injury. Do not run if unfit, ill, unacclimatized, or sensitive to heat and humidity.
Black/above 82° F (28° C)	Very high	Even with considerable slowing of pace, great discomfort will be experienced. Races should be postponed or cancelled under these conditions.

WBGT = Wet-bulb globe temperature
These precautions should be noted not only by the active individual for safety, but also by those who conduct physical training sessions or athletic competition. Flag colors may be used to inform athletes of prevailing heat stress conditions. Commercial devices are available to quickly and accurately measure the WBGT and should be used to help assess environmental heat stress and modify training or competition as recommended. For those who wish to construct an inexpensive WBGT device, consult the reference cited for Spickard at the end of this chapter.

*Although these warnings are expressed in regard to running, they are also relevant to other sports involving prolonged exercise in the heat, such as soccer, field hockey, and football. Wearing additional clothing or equipment may increase the heat stress.

of body fluids during the 1-hour run; 1 liter of sweat weighs 1 kg or 2.2 lbs. It should be noted that sweat rates may vary considerably between individuals. Ron Maughan, an environmental physiologist from Scotland, studied two marathoners who completed a race in the same time and had the same fluid intake; one lost only 1 percent of his body weight while the other lost 6 percent.

Under most warm environmental circumstances, the evaporative mechanisms and the body's natural warning signals are able to keep the core temperature during exercise below 105° F (40.5° C) and prevent heat injuries. However, an excessive rise in the core temperature, above 105° F, or excessive fluid and electrolyte losses, may lead to diminished performance or serious thermal injury.

Fluid and Electrolyte Losses

How does environmental heat affect physical performance?

Although performance in strength, power, or speed events that last less than a minute does not appear to be affected adversely by warm environmental conditions, performance in more prolonged aerobic endurance activities is normally worse when compared to performance in cooler temperatures. A sprinter may not see any change in speed; a runner in a 5-kilometer race (3.1 miles) will have to slow his or her normal pace somewhat, while a marathoner will suffer a considerable impairment in performance.

In the 5-kilometer race the runner will be performing at a rather high metabolic rate and thus will be producing heat rapidly. To control an excessive rise in body temperature, blood flow to the skin will increase so as to dissipate heat to the environment. This shifting of blood to the skin will result in a lesser proportion of blood, and hence oxygen, being delivered to the active musculature. Both Nadel and Young found that under these conditions cellular metabolism changes somewhat, with greater accumulation of lactic acid if the athlete attempts to maintain the pace normally done in a cooler environment. Yaspelkis and others reported similar lactate findings, but found no increase in muscle glycogen utilization. They speculated the increased lactic acid could be associated with decreased clearance by the liver. Nevertheless, increased lactic acid could be associated with a greater sensation of stress. In some individuals, the circulatory adjustments may not be adequate and the body temperature will rise rapidly, leading to hyperthermia and symptoms of weakness. Because of these changes, and possibly others not yet identified, the runner normally must slow the pace.

Although the 5-kilometer runner will sweat heavily, the duration of the event is usually short, so an excessive loss of body fluids does not occur. However, in more prolonged events, athletes may suffer the problems noted above plus the adverse effects of dehydration. Marathoners may lose 5 percent or more of their body weight (mostly water) during a race, which may not only deteriorate performance but have serious health consequences as well.

How do dehydration and hypohydration affect physical performance?

The effect of dehydration on physical performance has been studied from two different viewpoints. Voluntary dehydration is often used by athletes such as wrestlers and boxers to qualify for lower weight classes prior to competition. In other athletes, dehydration occurs involuntarily during training or competition as the body attempts to maintain temperature homeostasis. Dehydration leads to hypohydration.

Voluntary Dehydration   Voluntary dehydration techniques used by wrestlers have included exercise-induced sweating, thermal-induced sweating such as the use of saunas, diuretics to increase urine losses, and decreased intake of fluids and food. Involuntary dehydration usually occurs via heavy sweat losses during prolonged exercise in the heat.

Much of the research with voluntary dehydration has been conducted with wrestlers. Evaluation criteria have emphasized factors such as strength, power, local muscular endurance, and performance of anaerobic exercise tasks designed to mimic wrestling. Not all studies are in agreement. Many studies conducted in this area suggest that hypohydration, even up to levels of 8 percent of the body weight, will not affect these physical performance factors in events involving brief, intense muscular effort. On the other hand, many other studies have reported significant impairments in such tasks with body weight losses of 4 percent or higher. The adverse effects on strength are not consistent, but anaerobic muscular endurance tasks lasting longer than 20–30 seconds have been impaired when subjects were hypohydrated. Suggested mechanisms of impairment include loss of potassium from the muscle and higher muscle temperatures during exercise. It should also be noted that there is no evidence that hypohydration improves performance in these exercise tasks.

Involuntary Dehydration   Involuntary dehydration is most common during prolonged physical activity, particularly under warm, humid environmental conditions. The adverse effects of involuntary dehydration are most severe on aerobic endurance performance. Hypohydration of more than 2 percent of the body weight usually will lead to decrements in performance, and Gisolfi recently indicated that deleterious effects may be observed with as little as a 1 percent weight loss. The decrease in performance also appears to be proportional to the degree of hypohydration, with greater fluid losses leading to greater impairment. In several major reviews, Michael Sawka, Kent Pandolf, and John Greenleaf have suggested that the deterioration in aerobic endurance performance appears to be related to adverse effects on cardiovascular functions and temperature regulation. They noted that hypohydration would significantly decrease maximal aerobic power by 4–8 percent with a 3 percent weight loss during exercise in a neutral environment, but the impairment would be even greater in a hot environment. Also, a reduction in the plasma volume may reduce cardiac output and blood flow to the skin and the muscles. Reductions in skin blood flow have been shown to lower the sweat rate and raise the core temperature. In a recent review, Coyle reported some of the effects of dehydration in endurance-trained cyclists. In general, he reported that skin blood flow decreased with dehydration and that the greater the level of dehydration, the greater the rise in the core temperature and heart rate and the greater the decrease in the stroke volume (amount of blood pumped by the heart per beat). The effects of dehydration on cardiovascular dynamics are depicted in Figure 9.8.

Dehydration may also be a major factor in the onset of gastrointestinal (GI) distress, according to Nancy Rehrer. GI symptoms include nausea, vomiting, bloating, GI cramps, flatulence, diarrhea, and GI bleeding, many of which could impair performance if severe enough. However, Peters and others contend that the causes of GI distress during exercise are currently unknown, and may vary depending on the individual.

Other factors associated with hypohydration may also contribute to suboptimal performance. Disturbed fluid and electrolyte balance in the muscle cells may affect energy processes, while adverse effects of hyperthermia upon mental processes may contribute to central fatigue.

How fast may an individual dehydrate while exercising?

Because the maximal sweat rate for a trained athlete is about 2–3 liters per hour, it will not take long to incur a 2–3 percent decrease in body weight. Two liters of sweat is the equivalent of 4.4 pounds (1 liter = 1 kg = 2.2 pounds), so a 150-pound runner could experience a loss of 3 percent body weight in 1 hour (4.4/150 = .03; .03 × 100 = 3%), which could cause premature fatigue as illustrated in Figure 9.9. Some athletes, like football players, may lose 5–6 kg (11–13 pounds) over a day with multiple daily workouts.

Meyer and Bar-Or indicate that while children may sweat somewhat less than adults, they still may reach hypohydration levels comparable to adults. Excessive dehydration may not only impair one's physical performance, but possibly also one's health, as discussed later in this chapter.

How can I determine my sweat rate?

The rate of sweating varies among different individuals, so some may be more prone to dehydration than others. The Gatorade Sports Science Institute has presented a method to calculate the sweat rate during exercise. To do so, one must accurately measure body weight before and after exercise, measure the amount of fluid consumed during exercise, and the amount of urine excreted, if any, during exercise.

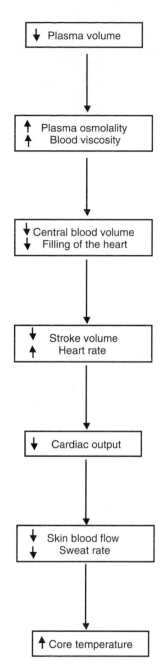

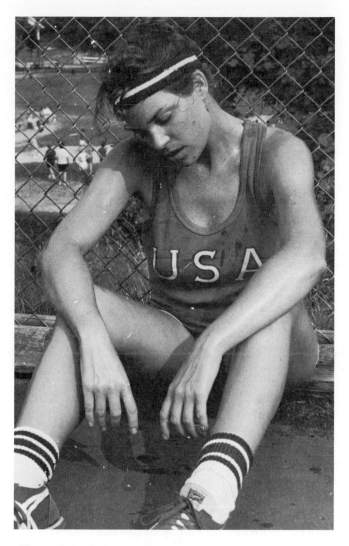

Figure 9.9 Body-water loss can be very rapid during exercise in warm or hot weather, leading to dehydration and premature fatigue and heat illness.

Figure 9.8 Some physiological effects of dehydration. The decreased blood volume and increased core temperature may contribute to premature fatigue and heat illness.

You may use the following examples as a guide to calculate your own sweat rate during exercise. The sweat rate for athlete A is calculated in the metric measurement system and for athlete B in the English system. Remember, 1 gram equals about 1 milliliter, and 1 pound equals 16 ounces.

		Athlete A	Athlete B
A.	Body weight before exercise	70.5 kg	180 lbs
B.	Body weight after exercise	68.9 kg	174 lbs
C.	Change in body weight	−1.6 kg	−6 lbs
		1600 g	96 oz
D.	Drink volume	+300 ml	16 oz
E.	Urine volume	−100 ml	0 oz
F.	Sweat loss (C + D − E)	1800 ml	112 oz
G.	Exercise time	60 min	90 min
H.	Sweat rate (F ÷ G)	30 ml/min	1.25 oz/min

What is the composition of sweat?

The human body contains two different types of sweat glands. The apocrine sweat glands are located in hairy areas of the body, such as the armpits, and secrete an oily mixture to decrease friction. We are all aware of the odor that may be generated from these sweat glands under certain conditions. Our concern here is with the eccrine sweat glands, about 2–3 million over the surface of the body, which are primarily involved in temperature regulation.

Sweat is mostly water (about 99 percent), but a number of major electrolytes and other nutrients may be found in varying amounts. Sweat is hypotonic in comparison to the fluids in the body. This means that the concentration of electrolytes is lower in sweat than in the body fluids.

The composition of sweat may vary somewhat from individual to individual and will even be different in the same individual when acclimatized to the heat, as contrasted to the unacclimatized state. The major differences are the concentrations of the solid matter in the sweat, the electrolytes or salts.

The major electrolytes found in sweat are sodium and chloride because sweat is derived from the extracellular fluids, such as the plasma and intercellular fluids, which are high in these electrolytes. You may actually note the formation of dried salt on your skin or clothing after prolonged sweating. Carl Gisolfi has reported that the concentration of salt in sweat is variable but averages 2.6 grams (45 mEq) per liter of sweat during exercise with sweat losses of about 1–1.5 liters per hour.

Other minerals lost in small amounts include potassium, magnesium, calcium, iron, copper, and zinc. As noted in Chapter 8, certain athletes, especially those who lose large amounts of sweat, may need to increase their dietary intake of certain trace minerals, such as iron and zinc, to replace losses during exercise.

Small quantities of nitrogen (N), amino acids, and some of the water-soluble vitamins also are present in sweat, but these amounts are easily restored by consuming a balanced diet.

Is excessive sweating likely to create an electrolyte deficiency?

There are two ways to look at this question. What happens to electrolyte balance during exercise? And, what happens during the recovery period on a day-to-day basis?

The concentration of electrolytes in the blood during exercise with excessive sweating has been studied under laboratory conditions as well as immediately after endurance events such as the Ironman Triathlon and a marathon run. In general, exercise raises the concentration of several electrolytes in the blood. Sodium and potassium concentrations are elevated; the sodium increase may be due to greater body-water loss than sodium loss, so a concentration effect occurs. The potassium may leak from the muscle tissue to the blood, thereby increasing the blood concentration of this ion. Chloride and calcium ion concentrations remain relatively unchanged during exercise. Magnesium levels usually fall, possibly because the active muscle cells and other tissues need this ion during exercise and it passes from the blood into the tissues. During acute, prolonged bouts of exercise then, even in marathon running, it appears that an electrolyte deficiency will not occur.

This is not to say that electrolyte replacement is not important. As we shall see in the next section, an electrolyte imbalance may occur in the body during extremely prolonged endurance events, such as ultramarathoning and Ironman-type triathlons, if proper fluid replacement techniques are not used. Moreover, what happens during the recovery period after excessive sweating may contribute to an electrolyte deficiency. Prolonged sweating has been shown to decrease the body content of sodium and chloride by 5–7 percent and potassium by about 1 percent. If these electrolytes are not replaced daily, an electrolyte deficiency may occur over time. The next section deals with the need for water and electrolyte replacement.

Fluid, Carbohydrate, and Electrolyte Replacement

Which is most important to replace during exercise in the heat—water, carbohydrate, or electrolytes?

In the 1960s Robert Cade, a scientist-physician working at the University of Florida, developed an oral fluid replacement for athletes that was designed to restore some of the nutrients lost in sweat. This product was eventually marketed as Gatorade (Gator is the nickname for University of Florida athletes) and was the first of many **glucose-electrolyte solutions (GES)** and, later, **glucose-polymer solutions (GPS)** to appear in the athletic marketplace. The three main ingredients in GES and GPS are water, carbohydrates, and electrolytes.

GES were the first commercial fluid-replacement preparations designed to replace both fluid and carbohydrate. Common brands today include All-Sport, Gatorade, Mountain Dew Sport, and Power Ade. Other than water, the major ingredients in these solutions are carbohydrates in the form of fructose, glucose, or sucrose and some of the major electrolytes. The sugar content ranges from about 5–10 percent depending on the brand. The caloric values range from about 6–12 Calories per ounce. The major electrolytes include sodium, chloride, potassium, and phosphorus. These ions are found in varying amounts in different brands. Some brands may also include some of the following: magnesium, calcium, citric acid, vitamin C, or artificial coloring and flavoring.

GPS are designed to provide carbohydrate while decreasing the osmotic concentration of the solution, thus helping to minimize the effect upon gastric emptying. Commercially available brands include GatorLode and Ultra Fuel. The concentration of the glucose polymers in commercial brands ranges from 5–20 percent although weaker or stronger concentrations may be made from the powder form. Guidelines are presented in Chapter 4 on page 114. Fructose and electrolytes are found in some brands. The contents of selected ingredients for several GES and GPS are presented in Table 9.7.

Each of the components of GES and GPS may be important to the athlete, depending on the circumstances. When dehydration or hyperthermia is the major threat to performance, water replacement is the primary consideration. In prolonged endurance events, where muscle glycogen and blood glucose are the primary energy sources, carbohydrate replacement, as noted in Chapter 4, may help improve performance. In very prolonged exercise in the heat with heavy sweat losses, such as ultramarathons, electrolyte replacement may be essential to prevent heat injury. Although the beneficial effects of carbohydrate intake during exercise were covered in Chapter 4, the role of carbohydrate as a component of the GES and GPS is stressed in this chapter.

The following questions focus on the importance and mechanisms of water, carbohydrate, and electrolyte replacement for the individual incurring sweat losses while exercising under heat stress conditions.

What are some sound guidelines for maintaining water (fluid) balance during exercise?

Athletes have used several strategies to help prevent excessive increases in body temperature, hypohydration, carbohydrate depletion, and electrolyte imbalances associated with certain types of sport competition. Depending on the sport, three commonly used practices are skin wetting, hyperhydration, and rehydration.

Skin Wetting Skin wetting techniques, such as sponging the head and torso with cold water or using a water spray have been shown to decrease sweat loss. This could be an important consideration in a long run, as body-water supplies may be depleted less rapidly. These techniques also cool the skin and offer an immediate sense of psychological relief from the heat stress, which may help to improve performance. On the other hand, skin wetting techniques as they may be used in athletic competition have not been shown to cause any major reductions in core temperature or cardiovascular responses. Moreover, some researchers have theorized that skin wetting techniques may be potentially harmful: the psychological sense of relief may encourage athletes to accelerate their pace, increasing heat production without providing for control of the body temperature. If the core temperature increases, heat illness may occur. Although some scientists suggest that skin wetting is not beneficial, many endurance athletes claim that it helps. Additional research appears to be warranted.

Hyperhydration Hyperhydration, also known as superhydration, is simply an increase in body fluids by the voluntary ingestion of water or other beverages. It is an attempt to assure that the body-water level is high before exercising in a hot environment. Rico-Sanz and others reported that soccer players training in the heat of Puerto Rico maintained higher body-water levels with mandated hyperhydration methods compared to their normal fluid replacement strategies. This extra water supply can delay the effects of dehydration and help prolong endurance capacity. Although there are few data indicating hyperhydration actually improves sport performance, research conducted with hyperhydration before exercise has revealed that it may effectively reduce the effects of heat stress on the core temperature and the cardiovascular system during exercise, but not as effectively as rehydration techniques. The American College of Sports Medicine recommends that hyperhydration be used prior to exercise in heat stress environments. If you plan to compete or do any prolonged exercise in the heat, it may be wise for you to hyperhydrate. All you need to do is consume about a pint (16 ounces) of cold water about 15–30 minutes before exercising. With experience, you may be able to tolerate larger amounts, although the diuretic effects should be kept in mind if you are to be involved in competition.

Rehydration Of the various techniques used, research has shown that rehydration is the most effective to enhance performance. Rehydration techniques have been used to replenish fluid loss associated with both voluntary and involuntary dehydration in sports such as wrestling and distance running, respectively.

One laboratory research approach to evaluate the effects of rehydration is related to the sport of wrestling, in which athletes dehydrate to qualify for a weight class and then attempt to rehydrate rapidly prior to competition. In this approach, subjects performed some exercise task, such as a measure of strength, power, or anaerobic endurance, were then dehydrated and tested again, and finally were rehydrated and tested one more time to see if rehydration could improve performance back to the pre-dehydration level. The results of such research are mixed. In some studies, no effect of rehydration was found, probably because as some studies have shown, dehydration may not impair strength, power, or local muscular endurance. Thus, rehydration would not improve performance as measured by these criteria beyond that usually seen in normohydration. However, some studies reported a partial improvement in endurance performance after rehydration, but usually not all the way back to normal. Because rehydration may possibly bring about performance improvements beyond the dehydrated level, it is therefore recommended for wrestlers.

A second approach in studying rehydration is to have subjects ingest fluids during prolonged endurance exercise, particularly in warm environments. Rehydration has been shown to minimize the rise in core temperature, to reduce stress on the cardiovascular system by minimizing the decrease in blood volume, and to help maintain an optimal race pace for a longer period. This beneficial effect

Table 9.7 Fluid replacement and high-carbohydrate* beverage comparison chart

Beverage	Flavors	Carbohydrate ingredient	Carbohydrate % (concentration)
Gatorade Thirst Quencher (The Gatorade Company)	Lemon-Lime Lemonade Fruit Punch Orange Citrus Cooler Tropical Fruit Grape Iced Tea Cooler	Powder: sucrose & glucose Liquid: sucrose & glucose/syrup solids	6
PowerAde (Coca-Cola)	Lemon-Lime Fruit Punch Orange	High-fructose corn syrup Maltodextrin	7.9
All Sport (Pepsico)	Lemon-Lime Fruit Punch Orange	High-fructose corn syrup Maltodextrin	8–9
XLR8 (Advanced Nutritional)	Lemon-Lime Orange	Glucose Fructose Glucose polymers Maltose Glycerol	5.2
Quickick (Cramer Products, Inc.)	Lemon-Lime Orange Fruit Punch	Fructose Sucrose	4.7
Hydra Fuel (Twin Labs)	Orange Fruit Punch Lemon-Lime	Glucose polymers Glucose Fructose	7
Cytomax (Champion Nutrition)	Fresh Apple Tropical Fruit Cool Citrus	Fructose corn syrup Sucrose	7–11
Coca-Cola	Regular Cherry	High-fructose corn syrup Sucrose	11
Diet Soft Drinks	All	None	0
Orange Juice	—	Fructose Sucrose	11–15
Water	—	—	0
GatorLode High Energy Carbohydrate Drink* (The Gatorade Company)	Lemon Citrus Banana	Maltodextrin Glucose	20 (47 grams per 8 oz. serving)
Carboplex* (Unipro, Inc.)	Plain	Maltodextrin	24 (55 grams per 8 oz. serving)
Ultra Fuel* (Twin Labs)	Lemon-Lime Grape Fruit Punch Orange	Maltodextrin Glucose Fructose	21 (50 grams per 8 oz. serving)

Compiled from product labels and sources provided by the Gatorade Company.

Sodium (mg) per 8 oz.	Potassium (mg) per 8 oz.	Other minerals & vitamins
110	25	Chloride Phosphorus
73 or less	33	Chloride
55	55	Chloride Phosphorus Calcium
40	30	Calcium Magnesium
116	23	Calcium Chloride Phosphorus
25	50	Chloride Magnesium Chromium Phosphorus Vitamin C
10	150	Chromium Magnesium
9.2	Trace	Phosphorus
0–25	Low	Phosphorus
2.7	510	Vitamins A & C Niacin Thiamin Riboflavin
Low	Low	Low
64	—	—
0	—	—
0	—	—

is usually attributed to decreased dehydration and the maintenance of a better water balance in the blood and other fluid compartments. Rehydration techniques, both with water alone or with carbohydrate solutions, have been shown to improve performance in exercise tasks of 1 hour or more in the heat. Hargreaves and others also reported that water intake may help reduce muscle glycogen use in prolonged exercise, another benefit.

If fluid replacement is to be effective, water has to be absorbed into the circulating blood so that the reduction in blood volume and sweat production that occurs during prolonged endurance exercise will be minimized. Research in which water was labeled with radionuclides showed that water ingested during exercise may appear in plasma and sweat within 10–20 minutes. However, the amount of the ingested fluid that enters the circulation to benefit the athlete depends on two factors: gastric emptying and intestinal absorption.

What factors influence gastric emptying and intestinal absorption?

In a later section we will discuss factors, such as palatability, that may influence how much fluid you drink during exercise. For any fluid to be of benefit during exercise it must first empty from the stomach and then be absorbed into the bloodstream from the intestines.

Gastric Emptying   A number of factors may influence the gastric emptying rate, including volume, solute or caloric density, osmolality, drink temperature, exercise intensity, mode of exercise, and dehydration.

Volume is one of the most important factors affecting gastric emptying. In a recent review, Gisolfi noted that the larger the volume of fluid ingested, up to approximately 700 milliliters, the greater the rate of gastric emptying. However, large volumes consumed during exercise may cause discomfort to the athlete because of abdominal distension.

A number of studies have shown that fluids with a 6–8 percent concentration of carbohydrate may not adversely affect gastric emptying of fluids. Thus, such solutions may provide the athlete with the best of both worlds, water and carbohydrate. However, solutions with higher concentrations, particularly above 10 percent, may impair gastric emptying. In one review, Gisolfi and Duchman noted the mechanism is not known, but may be related to the effects of carbohydrate on osmolality.

Fluids with a higher osmolality generally inhibit gastric emptying. Adding electrolytes and carbohydrates to fluids increases their osmolality, and Gisolfi indicated this effect may be attributed mostly to the carbohydrate content. Although glucose polymers have a lesser effect on osmolality than glucose, some investigators have observed little difference in gastric emptying of fluids that had marked differences in osmotic pressure created by adding electrolytes, glucose, or glucose polymers. However, Bennett and Dotson, in a review employing meta-analysis, demonstrated that a glucose polymer-fructose solution inhibited gastric emptying least. In general, cold fluids empty rapidly and may also help cool the body core.

Moderate exercise intensity facilitates emptying, whereas intense exercise greater than 70–75 percent VO$_2$ max has been reported to exert an inhibitory effect. Little difference is noted in gastric emptying between cycling and running during the first hour even at an exercise intensity of 75 percent VO$_2$ max, but some research suggests that more fluids appear to be emptied during the later stages of prolonged cycling.

Excessive dehydration also may inhibit gastric emptying, and may be associated with gastrointestinal distress experienced by some athletes who consume fluids during prolonged exercise in warm environmental conditions.

Intestinal Absorption   Factors affecting intestinal absorption of ingested fluids during exercise have not been studied as extensively as gastric emptying, but several important findings have been presented by key investigators in this area, particularly Carl Gisolfi and Ron Maughan.

Gisolfi recently indicated that the absorptive capacity of the intestines is not likely to limit the effectiveness of an oral rehydration solution. Water is absorbed fairly readily by passive diffusion, and theoretically water absorption may actually be helped by concurrent absorption of glucose and sodium. As highlighted in Figure 9.10(a), glucose and sodium interact in the intestinal wall; glucose stimulates sodium absorption, and sodium is necessary for glucose absorption. When glucose and sodium are absorbed, these solutes tend to pull fluid with them via an osmotic effect, thus facilitating the absorption of water from the intestine into the circulation. However, research by Hargreaves and others noted that beverage sodium content of either 0, 25, or 50 mmol per liter had no effect on plasma glucose levels during exercise. Gisolfi indicated that the intestines themselves contain enough sodium from body fluids, so that adding sodium to the rehydration solution provides no additional benefits. Research by Shi and others, from Gisolfi's laboratory, has shown that when compared to a single form of carbohydrate, using multiple, different forms such as glucose, fructose, and polymers, enhanced intestinal absorption of water. Each form of carbohydrate may have its own receptor for absorption and pull water with it.

However, as discussed in Chapter 4, excess carbohydrate in the intestine may cause a reverse osmotic effect, as depicted in Figure 9.10(b), leading to gastrointestinal distress with symptoms such as abdominal cramping and diarrhea.

Whether exercise impairs intestinal absorption is controversial. High-intensity exercise may compromise blood flow to the intestine, which might impair absorption. Gisolfi, in his recent review, noted some of the

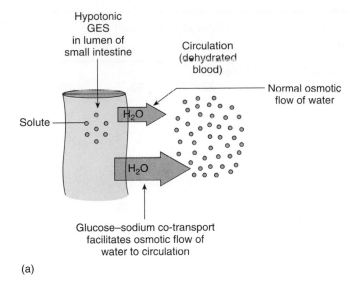

Hypotonic
GES
in lumen of
small intestine

Circulation
(dehydrated
blood)

Normal osmotic
flow of water

Solute

H₂O

H₂O

Glucose–sodium co-transport
facilitates osmotic flow of
water to circulation

(a)

Hypertonic
concentrated sugar
solution in lumen of
small intestine

Circulation

Reverse osmotic flow

H₂O

H₂O

Glucose–sodium transport

(b)

Figure 9.10   (a) Water normally diffuses from the intestine to the circulation via osmosis. Glucose and sodium in a GES enhance osmosis as shown by the larger arrow. (b) A hypertonic solution may actually reverse osmosis, moving fluid from the circulatory system to the intestines, possibly leading to gastrointestinal distress symptoms such as diarrhea.

methodological difficulties in studying this problem, citing studies showing that exercise either reduced or had no effect on intestinal absorption.

It should be noted that individual differences in both gastric emptying and intestinal absorption may be significant. In reviewing studies of gastric emptying, Costill noted some subjects could empty 80–90 percent of the ingested solution in 15–20 minutes, whereas others emptied only 10 percent. As noted above, some subjects may also develop diarrhea caused by ineffective intestinal absorption of fluids.

How should carbohydrate be replaced during exercise in the heat?

The value of carbohydrate intake during exercise as a means to improve performance was detailed in Chapter 4, primarily in relationship to performance in a cool environment. Keep in mind that carbohydrate intake may be useful primarily in prolonged exercise, under conditions where one is exercising at a high level of intensity for an hour or more. Carbohydrate is the primary fuel during such exercise tasks, and some, but not all, research suggests that warm environmental conditions may accelerate the use of muscle glycogen. Thus, carbohydrate intake may also improve performance during exercise in the heat, but if temperature regulation is of prime importance, water replacement should receive top priority. Hence, one of the goals of researchers has been to develop a fluid that will help replace carbohydrate during exercise in the heat without affecting water absorption. As discussed previously, glucose-electrolyte solutions (GES) and glucose-polymer solutions (GPS) have been developed for this purpose.

Research indicates that an appropriate amount of carbohydrate in solution may maintain body temperature as effectively as water, and may enhance performance during prolonged exercise. Water and carbohydrate complement each other to improve physical performance. In a recent unique study, Below and others found that water alone and carbohydrate alone improved 1-hour cycling performance in the heat, but the beneficial effects were additive when both were consumed together. Mindy Millard-Stafford also reported that a carbohydrate solution, in comparison to water alone, improved performance in highly-trained runners in a 15-kilometer run.

Scores of studies have compared the effectiveness of different carbohydrate combinations and concentrations in enhancing physical performance during prolonged endurance tasks. Most of this research is discussed in Chapter 4. The following are the pertinent general findings relative to GES and GPS intake during prolonged exercise under warm environmental conditions.

In general, GES and GPS solutions between 5 to 10 percent seem to empty from the stomach as effectively as water during prolonged exercise in a hot environment. They may possibly also be absorbed more readily from the intestinal tract. No significant adverse effects of these solutions upon plasma volume, sweat rate, or temperature regulation, when compared to water ingestion, have been observed. Actually, they may help maintain plasma volume, liver glycogen, and blood glucose levels during prolonged exercise, and, as noted above, most investigators report that carbohydrate intake during exercise enhances endurance capacity in a variety of prolonged tasks in the heat. Coggan and Coyle recommend about 1 gram of

Table 9.8 Fluid consumption (milliliters) at a given percent carbohydrate concentration to obtain desired grams of carbohydrate

Percent concentration	Grams of carbohydrate delivered							
	30	40	50	60	70	80	90	100
2%	1,500	2,000	2,500	3,000	3,500	4,000	4,500	5,000
4%	750	1,000	1,250	1,500	1,750	2,000	2,250	2,500
6%	500	666	833	1,000	1,166	1,333	1,500	1,666
8%	375	500	625	750	875	1,000	1,125	1,250
10%	300	400	500	600	700	800	900	1,000
12%	250	333	417	500	583	667	750	833
15%	225	300	375	450	525	600	675	750
20%	150	200	250	300	350	400	450	500

carbohydrate per minute. Additionally, there appears to be no difference between the forms of carbohydrate relative to these effects. GES and GPS seem to be equally effective.

Although higher concentrations of carbohydrates deliver more glucose to the intestine, solutions higher than 10–12 percent may significantly delay gastric emptying and possibly cause gastrointestinal distress. Peters and others indicated that excess carbohydrate may pass on to the colon, where bacterial fermentation may lead to excess gas production, flatulence, the urge to defecate, and gastrointestinal cramps, more so in runners than in cyclists. High concentrations of fructose may be particularly debilitating. However, ultraendurance athletes may experiment with higher concentrations of carbohydrate in training and may adapt to such concentrated solutions for use during competition. In a recent case study, Alice Lindeman noted that one cyclist involved in the Race Across America (RAAM) consumed a 23 percent carbohydrate solution with no gastrointestinal problems.

In summary, a recent consensus statement by leading researchers, chaired by Ronald Maughan, indicated that sports drinks containing carbohydrate as an energy source are more effective than plain water in improving performance. Water is the essential nutrient that needs to be replenished during prolonged exercise in the heat, for it will help deter some of the adverse responses to dehydration. When carbohydrate replenishment is desired, the current evidence suggests that a 5–10 percent solution of a GES, glucose polymer, or glucose polymer/fructose would be recommended. Cola-type drinks or fruit juices may be diluted by adding equal parts of water to achieve a concentration of about 5–10 percent.

Table 9.8 calculates the amount of fluid you must consume, for a given concentration, in order to obtain 30–100 grams of carbohydrate. For example, if you wanted to get 60 grams of carbohydrate per hour, you would need to drink 1 liter (1,000 ml) of a 6 percent solution, but only one-half liter (500 ml) of a 12 percent solution.

How should electrolytes be replaced during or following exercise?

Because the major solid component of sweat consists of electrolytes, considerable research has been conducted relative to the need for replacement of these lost nutrients, primarily sodium and potassium. We shall look at this question from two points of view, one dealing with the need for replacement during exercise and the other involving daily replacement.

Because sweat is hypotonic to the body fluids, the concentration of electrolytes in the blood and other body fluids actually increases during exercise and makes the body fluids hypertonic. Thus, electrolyte replacement during exercise is not necessary. Several studies have reported that even during strenuous prolonged exercise with high levels of sweat losses, like marathon running, water alone is the recommended fluid replacement to help maintain electrolyte balance, although added carbohydrate may provide some needed energy. Excessive intake of salts may actually aggravate electrolyte imbalance and impair performance capacity. On the other hand, small amounts of electrolytes have not been shown to be detrimental. The typical sports drink contains 10–25 mmol sodium per liter.

In very prolonged bouts of physical activity, such as marathons, ultramarathons, Ironman-type triathlons, or tennis tournaments where one might play off and on all day, electrolyte replacement during performance may be necessary. A number of medical case studies have reported complications resulting from a condition known as **hyponatremia,** or subnormal levels of sodium in the blood. In one Ironman triathlon, 27 percent of the competitors were diagnosed as hyponatremic after the event, but not all exhibited medical problems. Hyponatremia may be symptomatic or asymptomatic. Symptoms include epileptic-like seizures attributed to disturbed water balance in the brain; death may also occur. Although there may be several possible causes of hyponatremia, the most common observation is overhydration leading to water intoxication. Exercise-induced hyponatremia has been observed following prolonged periods of mild to moderate activity, but most cases have occurred in athletes. During competition lasting 4–5 hours or longer, athletes may lose sodium through sweating, and if they consume excessive amounts of fluids, primarily plain water, they may actually retain several liters in the body. In essence, the body fluids become diluted and the sodium level in the blood reaches very low levels. In a recent case study, Armstrong and others noted that low normal-levels of serum sodium before prolonged exercise in the heat may increase the risk of hyponatremia. To prevent the development of hyponatremia in such prolonged events, a solution with small amounts of salt may be recommended. Twenty milliequivalents of sodium and chloride may be found in some commercial sports drinks, but research by Barr and others suggests this amount may be inadequate to prevent a decrease in plasma sodium during prolonged exercise in the heat. Gisolfi recommends 20–30 mEq per liter, but even higher amounts approaching the salt content of sweat (about 40–50 mEq per liter) have been suggested. This would be approximately 2.5 grams of salt per liter. However, this may taste too salty and may not be palatable. In a major review of the hyponatremia of exercise, Timothy Noakes recommended limiting fluid intake to 500 milliliters per hour, which might be appropriate for some individuals, but not others. Again, individual differences may dictate who may be prone to developing hyponatremia during prolonged exercise, but it appears that athletes involved in ultraendurance events should consume adequate salt in their diet the days before competition to help assure normal serum sodium levels and consume fluids with added sodium during the event. Although this is a difficult area to research in the laboratory, possibly more precise recommendations will be provided in the future.

In general, heavy daily sweat losses do not lead to an electrolyte deficiency. If body levels of sodium and potassium begin to decrease, the kidneys begin to reabsorb more of these minerals and less are excreted in the urine. Research has shown that water alone, in combination with a balanced diet, will adequately maintain proper body electrolyte levels from day to day, even when an individual is exercising and is losing large amounts of sweat.

However, if electrolytes are not adequately replaced, a deficit may occur over 4–7 days of very hard training, especially in hot environmental conditions where fluid losses will tend to be high. Thus, in a recent review, Maughan noted that exercising individuals who experience heavy daily sweat losses need both adequate fluids and sodium to ensure adequate rehydration. For such individuals, adding salt to meals and drinks may help. The sodium is needed in the body to help retain water and maintain normal osmotic pressures.

A good method to check on the adequacy of fluid replenishment on a day-to-day basis is to check your body weight in the morning; it should be nearly the same every day. If you weigh several pounds less from one day to the next, it is likely you are hypohydrated.

Are salt tablets or potassium supplements necessary?

In general, the use of salt tablets to replace lost electrolytes, primarily sodium, is not necessary. As noted above, an adequate diet will replace electrolytes lost in sweat on a daily basis.

The concentrations of salt in sweat may vary; we have noted previously that the average may be about 2.6 grams of salt per liter, although there are reports as high as 4.5 grams per liter in unacclimatized individuals and as low as 1.75 grams per liter in the heat-acclimatized individual. Because salt is 40 percent sodium and 60 percent chloride, the sodium content in 2.6 grams of salt is 1 gram, in 4.5 grams of salt is 1.8 grams, and in 1.75 grams of salt is 0.7 grams. If an athlete would lose about 8–9 pounds of body fluids during an exercise period, a total of 4 liters of fluid (about 4 quarts) would be lost because a liter weighs 2.2 pounds. Four liters of sweat would contain, at the most, 7.2 grams of sodium in the unacclimatized individual, but less than 3 grams in one who was acclimatized. Because the average meal contains about 2–3 grams of sodium if well salted, three meals a day would offer 6–9 grams, about enough to just cover the losses in the sweat. However, sodium is lost through other means, primarily in the urine; thus, a slight increase in sodium intake may be reasonable for the unacclimatized athlete. Doug Hiller, a physician who has worked extensively with endurance athletes, suggests that during the week or two of acclimatization to exercising in the heat, athletes should consume about 10–25 grams of salt daily, or 4–10 grams of sodium. A more liberal salting of the food should provide an adequate amount; 1 teaspoon of salt contains about 5 grams of salt, or 2 grams of sodium. Although this recommendation is much greater than the maximal amount of 2.4 grams recommended by the National Research Council, that recommendation is based on the sedentary individual, not an athlete losing copious amounts of sodium during a period of acclimatization.

Common salt tablets contain only sodium and chloride. They are not necessary to replace lost sodium but may be recommended for unacclimatized athletes who do not replace sodium through normal dietary means in the early stages of an acclimatization program. Salt tablets should be taken only if the athlete loses substantial amounts of weight via sweat losses during a workout. Checking the body weight before and after a workout provides a good estimate of sweat loss. If we switch to the English system, 1 quart of sweat equals 2 pounds; one-half quart, or a pint, is 1 pound. One recommendation is that salt tablets should be taken only if the athlete needs to drink more than 4 quarts of fluid per day to replace that lost during sweating; that is, an 8-pound weight loss. The general rule is to take two salt tablets with each additional quart of fluid beyond the 4 quarts; this would be equal to 1 gram of sodium (the average tablet has one-half gram of sodium) per quart. Another way to look at it is to take one pint of water with every salt tablet. The use of salt tablets should be discontinued after the athlete is acclimatized, usually about 6–9 days.

Potassium supplements are not recommended for several reasons. First, research by David Costill and his associates has revealed that a deficiency of potassium is rare, even with large sweat losses and a diet low in potassium. Second, excessive potassium may be lethal as it can disturb the electrical rhythm of the heart. The moderate use of substitutes, such as potassium chloride for common table salt, may be helpful in assuring potassium replacement, but investigators recommended particular attention to the diet, citing citrus fruits and bananas as two of the many foods high in potassium. For example, a large glass of orange juice will replace the potassium lost in 2 liters of sweat.

What are some prudent guidelines relative to fluid replacement while exercising under warm or hot environmental conditions?

In sport nutrition, no other area has received as much research attention as the objective of determining the optimal formulation of an oral rehydration solution (sports drink) for individuals doing prolonged exercise under warm or hot environmental conditions. This may be so because water and carbohydrates are two nutrients that may enhance performance in such events, and water and electrolytes may also help to prevent heat-related illnesses. As discussed above in relation to the need for fluid, carbohydrate, or electrolytes, a number of factors—in particular, the intensity and duration of the exercise task, the prevailing environmental conditions, and individual differences in sweat rate, gastric emptying, and intestinal absorption—may influence the desired composition of the sports drink. Given these considerations, most of the leading investigators in this area, including Edward Coyle, Carl Gisolfi, Ron Maughan, and Timothy Noakes have all indicated there currently is no general agreement on the optimal formulation of an oral rehydration solution for all individuals who engage in prolonged exercise tasks.

However, through their concerted research efforts, these and other investigators have provided us with enough information to offer some guidelines that may be regarded as prudent—that is, they are likely to do some good and do no harm. The following guidelines for maintaining body fluid balance, improving performance in the heat, and preventing heat-related illnesses appear to be prudent as based on the current scientific knowledge. These guidelines are related to exercising under warm or hot environmental conditions and are in accord with the American College of Sports Medicine (ACSM) position stand on exercise and fluid replacement (Appendix L).

1. Cold water, about 40–50° F (4.4–10° C) is effective when carbohydrate intake is of little or no concern, for example, in endurance events less than 50–60 minutes. As noted in Chapter 4, if muscle glycogen levels are low, the intake of carbohydrate prior to the event may be helpful.

2. For longer duration events, carbohydrate may provide an important source of energy. If carbohydrate is desired in the drink, the concentration should not be excessive. As discussed above, a 6–8 percent solution appears to be effective in maintaining fluid balance while supplying carbohydrates. Studies have also shown that concentrations up to 10 percent may also be helpful, but concentrations greater than 10–12 percent may retard gastric emptying. It might be helpful to consume a carbohydrate drink that has multiple forms of carbohydrate, such as glucose, sucrose, fructose, and glucose polymers. Check the food label for ingredients.

3. The fluid should contain small amounts of electrolytes. Gisolfi recommends 460–690 milligrams of sodium per liter (20–30 mmol) and 200–400 milligrams of potassium per liter (about 5–10 mmol) of solution. According to the research group at the University of Limburg in the Netherlands, a range of about 400–1,100 milligrams of sodium per liter (approximately 20–50 mmol per liter) and 120–225 milligrams of potassium per liter (approximately 3–6 mmol per liter) would be adequate for those endurance events that could lead to excessive electrolyte losses, that is, greater than 4–5 hours in duration. Many commercial sports drinks contain electrolytes within this range; check the food label.

4. The fluid should be palatable, for research has shown that the voluntary intake of fluids increases when they are tasty. Being cold and sweet enhances palatability. Carbonated beverages do not appear to inhibit gastric emptying, nor does the use of aspartame (an artificial sweetener), but Zachwieja and others noted that certain flavorings, such as citric acid, may impair gastric emptying by as much

as 25 percent. Other research from Costill's laboratory has shown no difference between carbonated and noncarbonated beverages on temperature regulation while exercising submaximally in the heat. However, Lambert and others reported similar findings, but noted that subjects consumed less fluid when it was carbonated, suggesting a lower palatability compared to noncarbonated beverages.

5. The athlete should hyperhydrate with 10–17 ounces (300–500 milliliters) of cold fluid about 15–30 minutes before exercising. If the exercise task is prolonged, carbohydrate may be added. A concentration of 6–8 percent is advisable, but concentrations of 20 percent and higher have been used by some individuals without adverse effects.

6. Rehydrate with 6–8 ounces (180–240 milliliters) of cold fluid during exercise at 10- to 15-minute intervals. (A good rule of thumb to remember is that one normal mouthful or swallow equals about 1 ounce.) Such amounts can total to about 1 liter per hour, which could be enough to maintain fluid balance with mild to moderate sweating. It is important to realize that during periods of heavy sweating, it is very difficult to consume enough fluids to replace all of those lost. Costill has noted that, per minute, 50 milliliters of fluid may be lost through sweating (3 liters per hour), but only 20–30 milliliters per minute may be absorbed from the intestines. The sweating rate in this case is simply greater than the ability of the stomach to empty the fluid into the small intestine for absorption to occur. Although some dehydration will occur, rehydration will help maintain circulatory stability and heat balance thereby delaying deterioration in endurance capacity.

7. It is important to start rehydrating early in endurance events because thirst does not develop until about 1–2 percent of body weight has been dehydrated, by which time performance may have begun to deteriorate. Moreover, research by Nancy Rehrer, Fred Brouns, and Wim Saris and their colleagues at the University of Limburg has shown that dehydration may impair gastric emptying and may be related to a higher rate of gastrointestinal distress.

8. Drinking beverages containing caffeine should be avoided several hours before exercising because they may cause a diuretic effect, possibly leading to dehydration.

9. During recovery, consume enough fluids to regain your body-weight losses. If you have depleted much of your endogenous carbohydrate stores, consume fluids with a high carbohydrate content. Fruit juices and sports drinks are helpful when you need to replenish both fluids and carbohydrates. As noted in Chapter 4,

however, possibly combining protein and carbohydrate in the recovery drink may maximize the rate of muscle glycogen resynthesis. Be sure to consume enough sodium as well, using sports drinks or putting additional salt on your food. Weigh yourself each morning to see that your weight remains stable, a good indication of proper fluid balance.

10. Practice consuming fluids while you train. Use a trial and error approach. By consuming various formulations while you train, particularly during training comparable to the intensity and duration experienced in competition, you will be able to determine what fluids work specifically for you.

A summary of guidelines for fluid, carbohydrate, and electrolyte replacement during exercise under warm environmental conditions is presented in Table 9.9. For additional information, consult the ACSM position stand on exercise and fluid replacement or the review by Bob Murray. You may also receive a free copy of the pamphlet, *Stay Cool to Perform Best* by sending a self-addressed stamped envelope to the ACSM, P.O. Box 1440, Indianapolis, IN, 46206–1440.

Ergogenic Aspects

If preventing or correcting a nutrient deficiency is seen as an ergogenic technique, then certainly water could be construed to be an ergogenic aid. Compared to taking in no fluid before or during exercise, both hyperhydration and rehydration have been shown to enhance temperature regulation or exercise performance. On the other hand, some athletes have attempted to lose body water for ergogenic purposes. Although we have seen that hypohydration generally does not improve performance, and indeed may actually impair performance in endurance-type events, certain athletes such as high jumpers may use drugs like diuretics to lose weight rapidly without losses in power. Research has shown that diuretic-induced weight losses may improve vertical jumping ability because the athlete can develop the same power to move a lower body weight. Detailed coverage of these drugs is beyond the scope of this text. Moreover, the use of diuretics is banned by most athletic governing bodies, such as the United States Olympic Committee and the National Collegiate Athletic Association.

An electrolyte deficiency could impair physical performance, but supplements above and beyond normal electrolyte nutrition have not been shown to enhance performance.

Two possible ergogenic aids will be discussed in this section, one which has been studied only recently and another that was proposed as an ergogenic nearly 60 years ago. Glycerol supplementation has been studied in attempts to enhance endurance performance in warm environments, whereas the effect of sodium bicarbonate ingestion on anaerobic exercise performance has been investigated since the 1930s.

Table 9.9 Summary of guidelines for fluid, carbohydrate, and electrolyte replacement during exercise in warm environmental conditions

Type of event	Timing of consumption	Amount and type of beverage
Sports or exercise less than 60 minutes: 10-kilometer (6.2 miles) run 25-kilometer (15.5 miles) bike race	**Before:** 1–2 hours 15–30 minutes **During:** Every 10–15 minutes **Recovery:** Over next 24 hours	16 ounces (500 ml) cold water 10–16 ounces (300–500 ml) cold water Beverage may contain carbohydrate (6–8% solution) if there is a possibility of low muscle glycogen levels 6–8 ounces (180–240 ml) cold water Adequate fluid to replace body losses
Sports or exercise from 1 to 4 hours duration: Marathon (42.2 kilometers; 26.21 miles) Triathlon (1-mile swim, 25-mile bike, 6.2-mile run) Soccer game Field hockey game Tennis match	**Before:** 1–2 hours 15–30 minutes **During:** Every 10–15 minutes **Recovery:** Immediately after and every 2 hours for 6–8 hours	16 ounces (500 ml) GES (5–10% carbohydrate) 10–16 ounces (300–500 ml) GES (5–10% carbohydrate) 6–8 ounces (180–240 ml) GES (5–10% carbohydrate) GES or GPS to provide 1 gram carbohydrate per kilogram body weight, i.e., 50–70 grams carbohydrate. Carbohydrate/protein fluids may speed glycogen resynthesis. Solid carbohydrates and protein also may be used
Sports or exercise greater than 4 hours: Ultraendurance runs (50 miles or more) Century bike race (100 miles) Ironman-type triathlons (2.4-mile swim, 112-mile bike, 26.2-mile run)	**Before:** 1–2 hours 15–30 minutes **During:** Every 10–15 minutes **Recovery:** Immediately after and every 2 hours for 6–8 hours	16 ounces (500 ml) GES (5–10% carbohydrate) 10–16 ounces (300–500 ml) GES (5–10% carbohydrate) Higher concentrations (20–50% carbohydrate) may be used with experience 6–8 ounces (180–240 ml) GES (5–10% carbohydrate) and 20–30 milliequivalents of sodium and chloride GES or GPS to provide 1 gram carbohydrate per kilogram body weight, i.e., 50–70 grams carbohydrate. Carbohydrate/protein fluids may speed glycogen resynthesis. Solid carbohydrates and protein also may be used

These guidelines are approximations and may be modified based on individual preferences derived through personal experience in both training and competition. Body weight should be back to normal the day after training or competition.

Does glycerol supplementation enhance endurance performance during exercise under warm environmental conditions?

As discussed in Chapter 5, glycerol is an alcohol that combines with fatty acids to form a triglyceride. Glycerol has been studied as an ergogenic aid because it may serve as substrate for gluconeogenesis (new formation of glucose), but results of these studies have not supported an ergogenic effect. More recently, however, glycerol has been combined with water during hyperhydration prior to exercise to study its potential ergogenic effects on performance in prolonged endurance events, often under warm environmental conditions. Theoretically, glycerol-induced hyperhydration will increase osmotic pressure in the body fluids, helping to retain more total body water and also possibly increase the plasma volume, factors that could enhance temperature regulation and exercise performance.

Various techniques have been used to hyperhydrate subjects with glycerol. The amount used was based on either the subject's body weight, lean body mass, or body-water content. On average, for each kilogram body weight, subjects consumed 1 gram of glycerol combined with about 20–25 milliliters of water. Thus, a 70-kilogram male would consume 70 grams of glycerol in about 1.4–1.75 liters of water or similar fluid. In some studies, glycerol was also provided with carbohydrate solutions. Glycerol-induced hyperhydration protocols were normally compared to water-induced hyperhydration techniques.

Research data regarding the effects of glycerol-induced hyperhydration, compared to water-induced hyperhydration, on body-water levels are equivocal. In a series of early reports from the U.S. Army Research Institute of Environmental Medicine, Sawka, Freund, and DeLuca and their associates found that glycerol-induced hyperhydration resulted in a greater retention of fluids in the body than water hyperhydration. The investigators noted that the glycerol helped to maintain the osmolality of the blood, leading to better preservation of serum ADH levels and, hence, a lower urinary output of water. Although the plasma volume increased with glycerol-induced hyperhydration, the increase was not significantly different from that observed with water hyperhydration alone. Wendtland and others also reported that glycerol-induced hyperhydration increased fluid retention. Conversely, two more recent reports from the U.S. Army Research Institute of Environmental Medicine, by Sawka and Latzka and their associates, have not shown any advantage of glycerol-induced hyperhydration over water-induced hyperhydration on total body water. Lamb and others also recently noted no improvement in plasma volumes with glycerol-induced hyperhydration.

Research data regarding the effects of glycerol-induced hyperhydration on performance are also equivocal. Lyons and others found that glycerol-induced

hyperhydration was more effective than water-induced hyperhydration in reducing the thermal stress of moderate exercise in the heat. Montner and others reported that glycerol-induced hyperhydration significantly improved performance in a cycling endurance test to exhaustion at 65 percent VO_2 max in a neutral laboratory environment. The authors also noted a lower heart rate and rectal temperature response during the glycerol trial and speculated the benefits were due to an increased plasma volume. Montner and others also recently reported that glycerol-induced hyperhydration coupled with carbohydrate supplementation also improved cycling endurance test performance. On the other hand, Sawka and others reported that although glycerol-induced hyperhydration did improve exercise performance in the heat at 55 percent VO_2 max compared to control conditions, the improvement was not significantly greater than that noted in the water-induced hyperhydration trial. Wendtland and others reported no effects of glycerol-induced hyperhydration on cardiovascular responses or temperature regulation when exercising at 65–80 percent VO_2 max in a moderate environment (24° C; 75° F). Lamb and his colleagues compared the effect of a glycerol solution against a placebo solution and a carbohydrate solution on performance of well-trained cyclists in a cycling test at 75 percent VO_2 max to exhaustion. Although the cyclists rode significantly longer in the glycerol trial versus the placebo trial, the glycerol-trial performance was not significantly better than the carbohydrate trial, suggesting carbohydrate supplementation was as effective as glycerol supplementation as a means to enhance performance.

Although some of these studies suggest that glycerol may be an effective ergogenic aid, the research data are clearly ambivalent. However, several magazines targeted to cyclists and runners have already suggested that glycerol may be an effective ergogenic. Although it might be for cyclists, who need not be too concerned with the additional body weight associated with water retention, runners may be at a slight disadvantage because they need to expend energy to move the extra water weight. Additional research is needed to confirm these preliminary positive findings, and to determine the possible ergogenic effect on various types of sports performance.

Although the dosages used in these studies appear to be safe and Sawka indicated the total body-water increase was distributed proportionately between the intracellular and extracellular spaces, if larger doses are used there may be some concern with the possibility of excess fluid being retained in the intracellular spaces, leading to abnormal pressures and possible tissue damage. Sawka reported in one study that glycerol supplementation induced nausea and headaches.

For those who want to experiment with glycerol, a commercial product, Glycerate, is available with appropriate instructions. A sports drink, Pro Hydrator, also contains glycerol. Glycerine, sold in drug stores, is glycerol. It is not to be taken internally as sold, but should be diluted. One recommendation presented in *FitNews*, a publication of the American Running and Fitness Association, is to mix 36 milliliters of glycerol with 955 milliliters of water for each 100 pounds of body weight. This recommendation is in accord with amounts used in research. Roughly, this would be about 1.25 ounces of glycerol per quart of water. Thus, a 150-pound runner would need to consume 1.5 quarts of this concoction to hyperhydrate prior to performance.

Does sodium bicarbonate, or soda loading, enhance physical performance?

Sodium bicarbonate is an alkaline salt found naturally in the human body. Its major function is to help control excess acidity by buffering acids. Thus, it is also known as a buffer salt. Its action is comparable to that of medications you may take to control an upset stomach caused by gastric acidity. The baking soda you can purchase in a supermarket is actually sodium bicarbonate.

During high-intensity anaerobic exercise, sodium bicarbonate helps buffer the lactic acid that is produced when the lactic acid energy system is utilized. You may recall from Chapter 3 that the accumulation of excess lactic acid in the muscle cell may interfere with the optimal functioning of various enzymes and thus lead to fatigue. The natural supply of sodium bicarbonate that you have in your blood can help delay the onset of fatigue during anaerobic exercise. It may facilitate the removal of the hydrogen ions associated with lactic acid from the muscle cell, thereby mitigating the adverse effects of the increased acidity. However, fatigue is inevitable if the rate of lactic acid production exceeds the capacity of your sodium bicarbonate supply to buffer it. Theoretically, an increase in the sodium bicarbonate level in the body could delay the onset of fatigue.

Over a half-century ago, German scientists reported that the ingestion of sodium bicarbonate and other alkaline salts could help improve anaerobic work capacity. Since then, many studies have failed to support this finding, but now a substantial number of well-controlled experiments by highly respected investigators in sport nutrition research have provided supportive data.

The usual experimental protocol has been to have subjects, about 1–3 hours before the exercise task, ingest a dosage of 0.15–0.30 grams of sodium bicarbonate per kilogram body weight. Recent research by McNaughton has indicated 0.30 grams per kilogram body weight appears to be the optimum dose, with higher dosages providing no additional benefits. This amount totals less than 1 ounce for the average adult. Most studies have used a double-blind placebo design in which all subjects took all treatments. The exercise task selected was normally one that stressed the lactic acid energy system, or about 1–3 minutes of maximal exercise. Often these exercise tasks were

classified as supramaximal, because they used workloads greater than 100 percent VO_2 max. Repeated bouts of intense exercise interspersed with short rest periods have also been used, such as five 100-yard swims with a 2-minute rest between each.

Based on the available scientific data, sodium bicarbonate does not appear to be an effective ergogenic aid for exercise tasks dependent primarily upon the ATP-PC energy system, for most studies have reported no beneficial effects on performance in exercise bouts lasting less than 30 seconds or in resistive exercise tasks stressing strength, power, or short-term local muscle endurance.

The effect of sodium bicarbonate on performance in events that use primarily the oxygen energy system, such as events greater than 10 minutes in duration, needs further study. The ingestion of sodium bicarbonate has actually been suggested to depress aerobic metabolism, but few data are available to support this viewpoint. For example, several studies used exercise tests to exhaustion that lasted 9–10 minutes; such tests would stress both the lactic acid and oxygen energy systems. These results were inconclusive as to any beneficial effect of bicarbonate supplementation, but no adverse effects were noted.

Based on the available scientific evidence, sodium bicarbonate supplementation does appear to enhance performance in exercise tasks dependent upon the lactic acid energy system. A consistent finding is an increased serum pH following sodium bicarbonate supplementation, the desired effect to induce buffering of lactic acid. Regarding other factors that have been investigated, approximately half of the well-controlled laboratory studies suggest that ingestion of sodium bicarbonate will reduce acidosis in the muscle cell, decrease the psychological sensation of fatigue at a standardized level of exercise, and increase performance in high-intensity anaerobic exercise tasks to exhaustion. Various field studies have reported significant improvements in events that primarily use the lactic acid energy system, such as 400 or 800 meters in highly trained track athletes, 100-meter swims in experienced swimmers, and 5-kilometer bicycle races in trained cyclists. It should also be noted that although performance was not improved in the other half of the studies, neither was it impaired.

However, as with most research with nutritional ergogenic aids, not all studies find positive effects. For example, Kozak-Collins and her associates recently reported that sodium bicarbonate supplementation taken at moderate altitude did not improve the performance of competitive female cyclists on repeated 1-minute interval cycle tasks at 95 percent VO_2 max, nor did Potteiger and others find any beneficial effect of sodium bicarbonate supplementation to male runners on performance in a run to exhaustion at 110 percent of the lactate threshold following 30 minutes of running at the lactate threshold.

Nevertheless, several recent reviews by Linderman and Fahey, Matson and Tran, and Williams have all concluded that sodium bicarbonate is an effective ergogenic aid in events that may depend primarily on the lactic acid energy system. Matson and Tran provided the most convincing analysis, using the meta-analytic technique to statistically compare the effects reported in twenty-nine of the best studies. In general, they noted that the ingestion of sodium bicarbonate enhanced performance, and in studies that measured exercise time to exhaustion, there was a mean improvement of 27 percent. About half of the studies conducted subsequent to these reviews have indicated sodium bicarbonate or sodium citrate supplementation was an effective ergogenic aid.

The exact mechanism by which sodium bicarbonate may elicit an ergogenic effect has not been determined. As noted previously, other substances containing sodium, such as sodium citrate, have been shown to improve performance. McNaughton and Cedaro reported that sodium citrate improved performance in anaerobic tasks of 2–4 minutes. In Chapter 8 some studies were cited showing an improvement in aerobic endurance capacity with trisodium phosphate supplementation and Potteiger and others reported that sodium citrate supplementation improved 30 km cycling performance. Thus, some investigators have suggested that the buffering of lactic acid may not be the only mechanism underlying the ergogenic effect of sodium bicarbonate and that sodium itself may play a role. For example, in a recent study with horses, Hinchcliff and others compared sodium bicarbonate with sodium chloride supplementation on exercise performance and found that both improved performance compared to the control treatment. In the study cited above, Kozak-Collins and others reported no significant difference in cycling exercise performance between sodium bicarbonate and sodium chloride supplementation, possibly because they controlled the amount of sodium ingested. However, they had no control trial to see if both supplements improved performance compared to the control. In contrast to the Hinchcliff findings, Bird and others found that sodium bicarbonate supplementation did improve 1,500-meter run performance in male runners compared to both a sodium chloride-calcium carbonate placebo and a control trial. Multiple mechanisms may underlie the possible ergogenic effects of sodium bicarbonate supplementation.

The dosage of sodium bicarbonate used in most of these studies, about 300 milligrams per kilogram body weight, appears to be effective yet medically safe. Relative to possible disadvantages, several investigators have noted that some subjects developed gastrointestinal distress, including nausea and diarrhea. Excessive doses could lead to alkalosis, with symptoms of apathy, irritability, and possible muscle spasms.

The use of sodium bicarbonate (baking soda) by athletes has been dubbed "soda loading," possibly to liken it to carbohydrate loading. As you may recall, the purpose of carbohydrate loading is to increase the storage of muscle and liver glycogen as a means to prevent fatigue in prolonged endurance events. Soda loading is viewed by some in a similar context, an attempt to increase the supply of a natural body ingredient helpful as a means to delay fatigue. However, because sodium bicarbonate may be regarded as a drug, it remains to be seen whether this technique will be deemed illegal and banned by athletic governing bodies such as the International Olympic Committee. Currently there is no test to detect its use, except for urinary pH, which can also be affected by some antacids, and at present sodium bicarbonate is considered to be legal for use in sports.

Health Aspects: Heat Injuries and High Blood Pressure

For athletes or people who exercise primarily to improve their health, there are two major health considerations related to water and electrolyte balance. We have already noted some of the potential adverse effects of hypohydration and electrolyte losses on physical performance and certain health conditions, such as hyponatremia. This section concentrates on heat injuries, or heat illnesses, that may confront the physically active individual in a warm or hot environment. We shall also discuss high blood pressure, a health problem that may be aggravated by salt ingestion but ameliorated by proper exercise training.

What are the potential health hazards of excessive heat stress imposed on the body?

One of the most serious threats to the performance and health of the physically active individual is heat injury, or heat illness. Any athlete who exercises in a warm environment is susceptible to heat injury, but the increasing popularity of road racing has generated concern for runners who are not prepared for strenuous exercise in the heat, or who participate in races that are poorly organized in regard to preventing and treating heat injuries.

The individual who exercises unwisely under conditions of environmental heat stress may experience one or several of a variety of heat injuries. Three factors may contribute to these injuries: increased core temperature, loss of body fluids, and loss of electrolytes.

Figure 9.11 represents a simple flow chart of heat disorders. When a combination of exercise and environmental heat stress is imposed on the body, vasodilation and sweating increase as the body tries to cool itself. When these two adjustments begin to falter, problems develop. In essence, the circulation is attempting to regulate both body temperature and blood pressure at the same time, and when stressed excessively, control of blood pressure wins and body temperature regulation is impaired. In addition, if the exercise metabolic load is very great, heat injuries may develop independent of circulatory and sweating inadequacies.

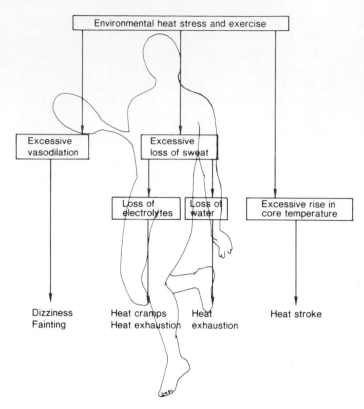

Figure 9.11 Basic flow chart for heat illnesses. The combination of environmental heat and exercise may cause an excessive vasodilation or pooling of blood. These conditions may decrease blood return to the heart and brain, causing dizziness and fainting. Excessive loss of sweat may cause significant losses of body water and electrolytes, leading to various heat illnesses. See text for details.

Excessive vasodilation may contribute to circulatory instability. The blood vessels expand and have a much greater capacity. Owing to a decreased relative blood volume, dizziness and fainting may occur. This condition is called **heat syncope.**

Although no conclusive evidence is available, **heat cramps** may be caused by excessive loss of sodium, potassium, or magnesium through profuse sweating. Cramps usually appear late in the day following ingestion of large amounts of plain water, which can dilute electrolyte concentrations, and usually involve the muscles in the calf or the abdomen. Several case studies with tennis players who consistently experienced heat cramps have shown that increased intake of either sodium or magnesium, along with adequate fluids, was effective in preventing muscle cramping during exercise.

Water-depletion heat exhaustion is a common heat injury. It resembles fainting and is caused by inadequate circulation to the brain. Fatigue and nausea are common symptoms, and the individual is usually lying down but conscious. The skin is usually pale, cool, and covered with sweat. The rectal temperature is usually below 104° F (40° C). Heat exhaustion may incapacitate the individual for a few hours but is usually responsive to body-cooling treatments.

Anhidrotic heat exhaustion resembles water-depletion heat exhaustion, except that sweating has ceased. The skin is dry. Otherwise, the symptoms and treatment are comparable to those for water-depletion heat exhaustion. If the individual continues to exercise when sweating stops, the core temperature may rise rapidly, leading to heat stroke.

Salt-depletion heat exhaustion occurs most frequently in individuals who are not acclimatized to work in the heat and do not replace the salt they have lost over a period of several days. Symptoms are similar to water-depletion heat exhaustion, although there may be a decrease in the sweat rate. Fatigue is common, and cramps may develop.

Heat stroke is the most dangerous heat injury, as it may be fatal. Heat stroke occurs primarily in the elderly and very young but may also occur in healthy, physically fit athletes. In such cases, it is classified as **exertional heat stroke,** which may be caused by too great an exercise work load under heat-stress conditions without dehydration. It can also occur after excessive loss of body water. It usually is preceded by mental changes ranging from disorientation to unconsciousness, as characterized in Figure 9.12. The skin is usually warm and red, and sweating may or may not be present. A rectal temperature over 105.8° F (41° C) is a characteristic sign. Exertional heat stroke may lead to rhabdomyolysis, damaged muscle tissue that leaks its contents into the blood eventually leading to kidney damage and possible death.

What are the symptoms and treatment of heat injuries?

The symptoms of impending heat injury are variable. Among those reported are weakness, feeling of chills, piloerection (goose pimples) on the chest and upper arms, nausea, headache, faintness, disorientation, muscle cramping, and cessation of sweating. Continuing to exercise in a warm environment when experiencing any of these symptoms may lead to heat injury. Table 9.10 presents the major heat injuries along with principal causes, clinical findings, and treatment.

Do some individuals have problems tolerating exercise in the heat?

A number of predisposing factors have been associated with heat injury, including gender, level of physical fitness, age, body composition, previous history of heat injury, and degree of acclimatization.

One of the major factors contributing to exertional heat illness is poor physical fitness. For example, in a recent study of Marine Corps recruits in training, Gardner and others found that one of the major predictors of exertional heat illness was poor aerobic fitness as measured by

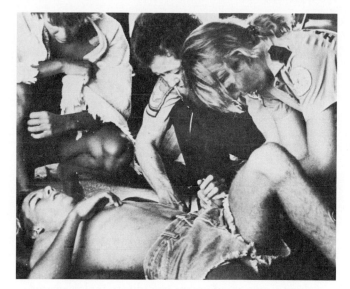

1.5-mile run performance. In general, the better the physical fitness, the better tolerance to a given heat stress.

In earlier studies, investigators found that female subjects tolerated exercise in the heat less well than males. These findings may have been related to the generally lower level of physical fitness of women at that time. More recent studies using subjects with comparable levels of physical fitness found that female responses to heat stress are similar to those found in males. On the other hand, a recent review by Stephenson and Kolka suggested that thermoregulation may be more impaired during the luteal phase of the menstrual cycle, possibly because of the elevated body temperature associated with increased progesterone levels. Also, postmenopausal women experience more favorable thermoregulatory responses during exercise after estrogen replacement therapy than they did before therapy.

Figure 9.12 Heat stroke may be caused by exercising in the heat without taking proper precautions.

Table 9.10 Heat injuries: causes, clinical findings, and treatment

Heat injury	Causes	Clinical findings	Treatment*
Heat syncope	Excessive vasodilation; pooling of blood in the skin	Fainting Weakness Fatigue	Place on back in cool environment; give cool fluids
Heat cramps	Excessive loss of electrolytes in sweat; inadequate salt intake	Cramps	Rest in cool environment; oral ingestion of salt drinks; salt foods daily; medical treatment in severe cases
Salt-depletion heat exhaustion	Excessive loss of electrolytes in sweat; inadequate salt intake	Nausea Fatigue Fainting Cramps	Rest in cool environment; replace fluids and salt by mouth; medical treatment in severe cases
Water-depletion heat exhaustion	Excessive loss of sweat; inadequate fluid intake	Fatigue Nausea Cool, pale skin Active sweating Rectal temperature lower than 104° F	Rest in cool environment; drink cool fluids; cool body with water; medical treatment if serious
Anhidrotic heat exhaustion	Same as water-depletion heat exhaustion	Nausea Sweating stopped Dry skin Rectal temperature lower than 104° F	Same as water-depletion heat exhaustion
Heat stroke	Excessive body temperature	Headache Vomiting Disorientation Unconsciousness Rectal temperature greater than 105.8° F	Cool body immediately to 102° F (38.9° C) with ice packs, ice, or cold water; give cool drinks with glucose if conscious; get medical help immediately

*Begin treatment as soon as possible. In cases of suspected heat stroke, begin immediately.

Individuals at both ends of the age spectrum may have problems exercising in the heat. The American Academy of Pediatrics noted that when compared to adults, young children may produce more metabolic heat during exercise in comparison to their body size, do not have as great a sweating capacity, and have a reduced capacity to convey heat from the core to the skin. These factors would increase the chances of heat injury. At high levels of heat stress, tolerance to the heat is decreased in older individuals, possibly because they sweat less. Reduced heat toleration in the elderly may also be related to fitness levels. As more and more people become and remain physically active throughout middle age and advanced years, we may see the older person tolerating exercise in the heat as well as younger adults.

Obese individuals not only have high amounts of body fat to deter heat losses, but also generate more heat during exercise because of a low level of fitness; thus they are more susceptible to heat injuries. In the Marine Corps study cited above, another major predictor of exertional heat illness was a higher body weight in relation to height.

Individuals who have experienced previous heat injury may be less tolerant to exercise in the heat. Many individuals do regain heat tolerance 8–12 weeks after heat injury. Others lose some of the ability for the circulatory system to adjust to heat stress, possibly because temperature-regulating centers in the brain are irreversibly damaged. The transfer of heat from the core to the skin becomes impaired and the body temperature rises faster.

One of the more important factors determining an individual's response to exercise in the heat is degree of acclimatization, which is discussed on the following pages. Although some individuals may be susceptible to heat illnesses, all individuals who exercise under warm or hot environmental conditions may benefit from the following recommendations.

How can I reduce the hazards associated with exercise in a hot environment?

The following list represents a number of guidelines, which if followed, will reduce considerably your chances of suffering heat injury. For additional information, you may contact the Gatorade Sports Science Institute at (800) 616-4774.

1. Check the temperature and humidity conditions before exercising. Even if the dry temperature is only 65–75° F, a high humidity will increase the heat stress. Warm, humid conditions cause fatigue sooner, so slow your pace or shorten your exercise session.

2. Exercise in the cool of the morning or evening to avoid the heat of the day.

3. Exercise in the shade, if possible, to avoid radiation from the sun. If you run in the sun, wear an appropriate sunscreen to prevent sun damage to the skin.

4. Wear minimal clothing that is loose to allow air circulation, white or a light color to reflect radiant heat, and porous to permit evaporation. Do not wear a hat if running in the shade, but wear a loose hat if running in the sun.

5. If you are running and there is a breeze, plan your route so that you are running into the wind during the last part of your run. The breeze will help cool you more effectively at the time you need it most.

6. Drink cold fluids periodically. For a long training run, plan your route so that it passes some watering holes, such as gas stations or other sources of water. Alternatively, you may purchase a water-bottle belt that will help you carry your own water supply. Take frequent water breaks, consuming about 6–8 ounces of water every 15 minutes or so. During exercise, thirst is not an adequate stimulus to replace water losses, so you should drink before you get thirsty.

7. Replenish your water daily. Keep a record of your body weight. For each pound you lose, drink one pint (16 ounces) of fluid. Your body weight should be back to normal before your next workout.

8. Hyperhydrate if you plan to perform prolonged, strenuous exercise in the heat. In essence, drink about 16–32 ounces of fluid 30–60 minutes prior to exercising.

9. Replenish lost electrolytes (salt) if you have sweated excessively. Put a little extra salt on your meals and eat foods high in potassium, such as bananas and citrus fruits.

10. Avoid excessive intake of protein, as extra heat is produced in the body when protein is metabolized. This may contribute slightly to the heat stress.

11. Avoid consuming beverages with caffeine several hours before exercising. Caffeine may increase the stress in two ways. First, it is a diuretic and may increase body-water losses. Second, caffeine will increase metabolic heat production at rest, which will raise the body temperature prior to exercise.

12. Because alcohol is a diuretic, excess amounts should be avoided the night before competition or prolonged exercise in the heat.

13. If you are sedentary, overweight, or aged, you are less likely to tolerate exercise in the heat and should therefore use extra caution.

14. Be aware of the signs and symptoms of heat exhaustion and heat stroke, as well as the treatment for each. Chills, goose pimples, dizziness, weakness, fatigue, mental disorientation, nausea, and headaches are some symptoms that may signify the onset of heat illness. Stop activity, get to a cool place, and consume some cool fluids.

15. Do not exercise if you have been ill or have had a fever within the last few days.

16. If you plan to compete in a sport held under hot environmental conditions, you must become acclimatized to exercise in the heat.

How can I become acclimatized to exercise in the heat?

It is a well-established fact that **acclimatization** to the heat will help increase performance in warm environments as compared with an unacclimatized state. Simply living in a hot environment confers a small amount of acclimatization. Physical training, in and of itself, provides a significant amount of acclimatization, possibly up to 50 percent of that which can be expected. However, neither of these two adjustments, either singly or together, can prevent the deterioration of exercise performance in the heat by an unacclimatized individual. Thus, a period of active acclimatization is necessary to optimize performance when exercising in the heat.

The technique of acclimatization is relatively simple. Simply cut back on the intensity or duration of your normal activity. When the hot weather begins, moderate your activity. Do not avoid exercise in the heat completely, but after an initial reduction in your activity level, increase it gradually. For example, if you were running five miles a day, cut your distance back to two to three miles in the heat; if you need to do five a day, do the remaining miles in the evening. Eventually build up to three, four, and five miles. The acclimatization process usually takes about one to two weeks to complete. However, even when acclimatized, an athlete's endurance capacity in the heat, particularly with high humidity, still will be less than under cooler conditions.

If you live in a cool climate, like New England, and want to compete in a marathon in Florida in January, how do you become acclimatized? Exercising indoors at a warmer temperature will help. Extra layers of clothes can help prevent evaporation and build a hot, humid micro-climate around your body. Research has shown that this technique can provide a degree of acclimatization. However, this is advisable only in cool weather and should not be attempted under hot conditions. Wearing a sweat suit or rubberized suit while exercising in the heat may precipitate heat illness. Moreover, even in a cool environment this technique may cause heat injury. Again, be wary of the symptoms of impending heat illness.

The body makes the following important adjustments during acclimatization to the heat. Terrados and Maughan indicate that most of the following adjustments occur in 6–8 days, but full acclimatization may take 14 days or more. Bar-Or notes that heat acclimatization in children takes several weeks.

1. The plasma volume expands considerably to increase the total blood volume. This occurs because the blood vessels conserve more protein and sodium, which tend to hold water.

2. The increased blood volume allows the heart to pump more blood per beat, so the stress on the heart is reduced.

3. When volume increases, more blood flows to the muscles and skin. The muscles receive more oxygen and skin cooling increases, improving endurance performance.

4. Less muscle glycogen is used as an energy source at a given rate of exercise, sparing this energy source in endurance events.

5. The sweat glands hypertrophy and secrete about 30 percent more sweat, allowing for greater evaporative heat loss.

6. The amount of salt in the sweat decreases by about 60 percent; evaporation becomes more efficient and electrolytes are conserved.

7. Sweating starts at a lower core temperature, leading to earlier cooling.

8. The core temperature will not rise as high or as rapidly as in the unacclimatized state.

9. The psychological feeling of stress is reduced at a given exercise rate.

In essence, as illustrated in Figure 9.13, these changes increase the ability of the body to dissipate heat with less stress on the cardiovascular system. The end result is a more effective body-temperature control and improved performance when exercising in the heat. These adaptations may be maintained by exercising in the heat several days per week but are lost in about 7–10 days in a cool environment. If you are interested in learning more about acclimatization, consult the review by Maughan and Shirreffs.

What is high blood pressure, or hypertension?

Everybody has blood pressure, for without it we would not be able to sustain body metabolism. Simply speaking, blood pressure is the force that the blood exerts against the blood vessel walls. Although pressure is present in all types of blood vessels, the arterial blood pressure is the one most commonly measured and most important to our health. Blood pressure is usually measured by a sphygmo-manometer, which records the pressure in millimeters of mercury (mmHg). Blood pressure readings are given in two numbers, for example 120/80 mmHg. The higher number represents the *systolic* phase, when the heart is pumping blood through the arteries. The lower number represents the *diastolic* phase, when the heart is resting between beats and blood is flowing back into it. Two important determinants of blood pressure are the volume

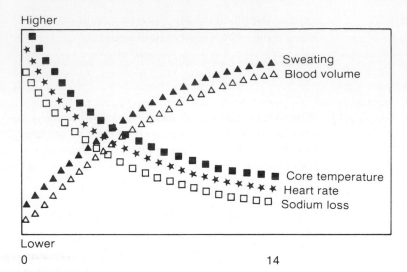

Figure 9.13 Changes with acclimatization. Acclimatization to the heat for 7–14 days will lead to an increase in the blood volume and the ability to sweat. For a standardized exercise task in the heat, these changes will lead to a lower heart rate, less sodium loss, and a lower core temperature. These changes will lead to improved exercise performance in the heat.

Table 9.11	Classification of blood pressure for adults age 18 years and older	
Category	**Systolic (mmHg)**	**Diastolic (mmHg)**
Normal	<130	<85
High normal	130–139	85–89
Hypertension		
Stage 1 (mild)	140–159	90–99
Stage 2 (moderate)	160–179	100–109
Stage 3 (severe)	180–209	110–119
Stage 4 (very severe)	≥210	≥120

Source: The Fifth Report of the Joint National Committee on Detection, Evaluation, and Treatment of High Blood Pressure, National Institutes of Health, National Heart, Lung, and Blood Institute. *NIH Publication No. 93–1088*, January 1993.

of blood in the circulation and the resistance to blood flow, known as peripheral vascular resistance.

High blood pressure, also known as **hypertension** (hyper = high; tension = pressure), is known as a silent disease. The American Heart Association indicates that nearly 60 million Americans have high blood pressure. However, millions do not know they have it because it has no outstanding symptoms. Some general symptoms include headaches, dizziness, and fatigue, but since they can be caused by a multitude of other factors, they may not be recognized as symptoms of high blood pressure. Although a great deal of research about the cause of high blood pressure has been conducted, the exact cause is unknown in about 90 percent of all cases. In these cases, the condition is known as essential hypertension, which cannot be cured, although life-style changes or medications can lower the pressure by reducing the blood volume or decreasing the peripheral vascular resistance.

High blood pressure is dangerous for several reasons. The heart must work much harder to pump the extra blood volume or to overcome the peripheral vascular resistance. This normally leads to an enlarged heart, but over time the increase in heart size becomes excessive and the efficiency of the heart actually decreases, making it more prone to a heart attack. Second, high blood pressure may directly damage the arterial walls. It is thought to be a major contributing factor in the development of atherosclerosis and a predisposing factor to coronary disease and stroke. High blood pressure is itself a disease, but it is also involved in the etiology of other diseases. It is one of the primary risk factors for heart disease.

The National Research Council has noted that any definition of high blood pressure is arbitrary. Traditionally, physicians have used elevations in diastolic blood pressure as the basis for their diagnosis, but the Joint National Committee on Detection, Evaluation, and Treatment of High Blood Pressure (JNCDET) of the National Institutes of Health recently released its classification of blood pressure for adults age 18 years and older. It includes both systolic and diastolic pressures and rates the severity of high blood pressure from mild to very severe. The classification system is presented in Table 9.11.

How is high blood pressure treated?

Many individuals with essential hypertension need to take medications to control their blood pressure. Diuretics are often used to reduce body-water levels—and hence blood volume—and thus reduce blood pressure. Beta-blockers are also used to block the pressure-raising effect of epinephrine and norepinephrine upon the blood vessels and heart. Tanji and Batt provide a detailed discussion of the pharmacological treatment of hypertension in physically active individuals.

Unfortunately, such drugs may exert other adverse effects, so a nonpharmacologic approach is often a first choice of treatment in cases of mild to moderate hypertension. In a recent review, Beilin indicated that a variety of life-style changes may be important in the nonpharmacological treatment of hypertension. One of the most important is to avoid the use of tobacco, but several dietary practices and exercise may also help reduce both systolic and diastolic blood pressure.

What dietary modifications may help reduce or prevent hypertension?

How much and what you eat may influence your blood pressure. The following are the key points to help reduce or prevent hypertension.

1. *Achieve and maintain a healthy body weight.* Numerous studies have shown that reducing body weight, particularly body fat, will reduce blood pressure in hypertensive individuals. Maintaining a healthy body weight may be an effective preventive measure. Thus, restriction of caloric intake to either lose or maintain body weight may be a helpful dietary strategy.

2. *Reduce or moderate sodium intake.* Most health organizations recommend reducing the dietary intake of sodium chloride. Until the late 1980s, most dietary recommendations for the treatment of hypertension focused upon the reduction of dietary sodium, although whether or not reduction of dietary sodium would reduce blood pressure was controversial. However, Einhorn and Landsberg have noted that most of the sodium controversy actually concerns sodium chloride because chloride may also have important effects on blood pressure. The National Research Council, in *Diet and Health*, and the JNCDET report on high blood pressure suggest that while both sodium and chloride may be necessary to produce hypertension, the matter still remains unresolved.

Despite the ongoing controversy about the etiological role of sodium chloride in hypertension, it may be prudent to restrict consumption. It is true that most individuals possess physiological control systems that effectively maintain a proper balance of sodium in the body. It is also true that current medical and scientific evidence does not support the concept that a normal intake of salt in amounts common to the U.S. diet causes hypertension in persons with normal blood pressure. This finding has been supported by a recent meta-analysis—by Midgley and others—of 56 research trials involving dietary sodium intake and blood pressure. However, many individuals are sodium-sensitive, or salt-sensitive, in that their blood pressure may increase with excessive consumption of salt. Possibly because of a defect in excretion, sodium accumulates in the body and holds fluids, particularly blood, thereby raising the blood pressure. In the United States, approximately 20 percent of the adult population, or one in every five individuals, is predisposed to high blood pressure. Of this 20 percent, about one-third to one-half, or 6–10 percent of the entire adult population, appears to be sensitive to salt. Since many individuals do not know their blood pressure, millions of Americans may benefit from a reduced-salt diet.

The current prudent medical recommendation for dietary prevention or treatment of hypertension is to decrease sodium consumption simply by eating a wide variety of foods in their natural state. Avoid highly salted foods, restrict intake of processed foods, and hide your salt shakers. The recommended upper limit is about 6 grams of salt per day, just a little over 1 teaspoon, the equivalent of about 2.4 grams of sodium.

3. *Consume foods rich in potassium, calcium, and magnesium.* In a recent review, Reusser and McCarron suggested that potassium, calcium, and magnesium are involved in the etiology of high blood pressure, for reduced serum levels or low dietary intake of these three minerals have been associated with hypertension. In particular, the JNCDET recommends a high intake of potassium because a potassium deficiency may increase blood pressure. The committee recommends that normal plasma concentrations of potassium be maintained, preferably through food sources and not supplements. Foods rich in calcium and magnesium should also be included in the daily diet.

4. *Consume a diet rich in fruits, vegetables, and low-fat dairy foods and with reduced saturated and total fat.* A recent intervention study by Appel and others found that a diet rich in fruits and vegetables reduced blood pressure in both normotensive and hypertensive adults. When this diet was combined with a low-fat diet, particularly low-fat dairy foods and reduced saturated and total fat, the reductions in blood pressure were even greater. Fruits and vegetables are excellent sources of potassium, while low-fat dairy products provide calcium without fat.

5. *Moderate alcohol consumption.* As noted in Chapter 4, moderate alcohol consumption may actually confer some health benefits, particularly the prevention of cardiovascular disease. However, excess alcohol intake may increase the risk, possibly because it is linked to high blood pressure.

As you probably noticed, all of these recommendations are in accord with the Healthy North American Diet.

Can exercise help prevent or treat hypertension?

Regular mild- to moderate-intensity aerobic exercise such as jogging, brisk walking, swimming, cycling, and aerobic dancing has also been recommended to reduce high blood pressure. Since exercise may be an effective means to lose excess body fat, it may exert a beneficial effect through this avenue. However, the exact role or mechanism of exercise as an independent factor in lowering blood pressure has not been totally resolved. Although a number of studies have shown that exercise training helps decrease resting systolic blood pressure (about 5–25 mmHg) in those who are hypertensive and may even elicit a slight decrease in those with normal blood pressure, not all studies are in agreement. Not all individuals will experience a decrease in blood pressure from an exercise program; they may be exercise-insensitive, or nonresponders, just as some individuals are salt-sensitive. Nevertheless, most investigators find the available information sufficient to justify an aerobic exercise program as a useful adjunct for the treatment of high blood pressure, reporting an average reduction of 10 mmHg in both systolic and diastolic blood pressure in individuals with mild hypertension. Also, in a recent meta-analysis of over 35 human clinical training studies, Kelley and Tran concluded that aerobic exercise training results in small reductions in both resting systolic and diastolic blood pressures in normotensive individuals. The interested student is referred to the excellent reviews by Charles Tipton, James Hagberg, and the recent position stand of the American College of Sports Medicine relative to physical activity, physical fitness, and hypertension. In general, the ACSM recommends aerobic exercise with large muscle groups at an intensity of 50–85 percent of VO_2 max or lower (40–70 percent), 20–60 minutes in duration, and a frequency of 3–5 times per week.

Individuals who have high blood pressure should consult with their physicians about mode and intensity of exercise. Although aerobic exercise may help reduce blood pressure at rest and may evoke a lessened blood pressure rise during exercise, a protective effect, other exercises may be harmful. For example, high-intensity aerobic exercise and activities that require intense straining, lifting, or hanging, such as isometric exercises, weight lifting, or pull-ups, should be avoided. The use of hand-held weights in aerobic exercises may also be a concern. These activities create a physiological response that rapidly raises the blood pressure to rather high levels. This increase may be hazardous to someone whose resting blood pressure is already at an elevated level.

References

Books

Buskirk, E., and Puhl, S. 1996. *Body Fluid Balance: Exercise and Sport.* Boca Raton, FL: CRC Press.

Gisolfi, C., and Lamb, D., eds. 1990. *Perspectives in Exercise Science and Sports Medicine. Fluid Homeostasis During Exercise.* Indianapolis, IN: Benchmark.

Gisolfi, C., et al., eds. 1993. *Perspectives in Exercise Science and Sports Medicine. Exercise, Heat, and Thermoregulation.* Dubuque, IA: WCB Brown and Benchmark.

Haymes, E., and Wells, C. 1986. *Environment and Human Performance.* Champaign, IL: Human Kinetics.

Hunt, S., and Groff, J. 1990. *Advanced Nutrition and Human Metabolism.* St. Paul, MN: West.

National Institutes of Health. 1993. *The Fifth Report of the Joint National Committee on Detection, Evaluation, and Treatment of High Blood Pressure.* National Institutes of Health. National Heart, Lung, and Blood Institute. NIH Publication No. 93–1088. January.

National Research Council. 1989. *Diet and Health: Implications for Reducing Chronic Disease Risk.* Washington, DC: National Academy Press.

National Research Council. 1989. *Recommended Dietary Allowances.* Washington, DC: National Academy Press.

Shils, M., et al. 1994. *Modern Nutrition in Health and Disease.* Philadelphia: Lea and Febiger.

Wolinsky, I., and Hickson, J., eds. 1994. *Nutrition in Exercise and Sport.* Boca Raton, FL: CRC Press.

Reviews

American Academy of Pediatrics. 1982. Climatic heat stress and the exercising child. *Pediatrics* 69: 808–9.

American College of Sports Medicine. 1996. American College of Sports Medicine position stand: Exercise and fluid replacement. *Medicine and Science in Sports and Exercise* 28 (1): i–vii.

American College of Sports Medicine. 1996. American College of Sports Medicine position stand: Heat and cold illnesses during distance running. *Medicine and Science in Sports and Exercise* 28 (12): i–x.

American College of Sports Medicine. 1993. Physical activity, physical fitness, and hypertension. *Medicine and Science in Sports and Exercise* 25 (10): i–x.

American Running and Fitness Association. 1996. Glycerol helps fluid balance. *FitNews* 14 (6): 1.

Applegate, E. 1989. Nutritional concerns of the ultraendurance athlete. *Medicine and Science in Sports and Exercise* 21:S205–S208.

Armstrong, L., et al. 1990. Time course or recovery and heat acclimation ability of prior exertional heatstroke patients. *Medicine and Science in Sports and Exercise* 22:36–48.

Askew, E. 1994. Nutrition and performance at environmental extremes. In *Nutrition in Exercise and Sport,* eds. I. Wolinsky and J. Hickson. Boca Raton, FL: CRC Press.

Bar-Or, O. 1994. Children's responses to exercise in hot climates: Implications for performance and health. *Sports Science Exchange* 7 (2): 1–4.

Bar-Or, O., and Wilk, B. 1996. Water and electrolyte replenishment in the exercising child. *International Journal of Sport Nutrition* 6:93–99.

Beilin, L. 1994. Non-pharmacological management of hypertension: Optimal strategies for reducing cardiovascular risk. *Journal of Hypertension Supplement* 12:S71–S81.

Bennett, B., and Dotson, C. 1990. Effects of carbohydrate solutions on gastric emptying: A meta-analysis. *Medicine and Science in Sports and Exercise* 22:S121.

Bentley, S. 1996. Exercise-induced muscle cramp: Proposed mechanisms and management. *Sports Medicine* 21:409–20.

Brouns, F., and Beckers, E. 1993. Is the gut an athletic organ? Digestion, absorption and exercise. *Sports Medicine* 15:242–57.

Brouns, F., et al. 1992. Rationale for upper limits of electrolyte replacement during exercise. *International Journal of Sport Nutrition* 2:229–38.

Clark, N. 1995. Water: The ultimate nutrient. *Physician and Sportsmedicine* 23 (5): 21–22.

Coggan, A., and Coyle, E. 1991. Carbohydrate ingestion during prolonged exercise: Effects on metabolism and performance. *Exercise and Sport Sciences Reviews* 19: 1–40.

Costill, D. 1990. Gastric emptying of fluids during exercise. In *Perspectives in Exercise Science and Sports Medicine. Fluid Homeostasis During Exercise,* eds. C. Gisolfi and D. Lamb. Indianapolis, IN: Benchmark.

Costill, D. 1977. Sweating: Its composition and effects on body fluids. *Annals of the New York Academy of Sciences* 301:160–74.

Costrini, A. 1990. Emergency treatment of exertional heatstroke and comparison of whole body cooling techniques. *Medicine and Science in Sports and Exercise* 22:15–18.

Coyle, E. 1994. Fluid and carbohydrate replacement during exercise: How much and why? *Sports Science Exchange* 7 (3): 1–6.

Coyle, E., and Montain, S. 1993. Thermal and cardiovascular responses to fluid replacement during exercise. In *Perspectives in Exercise Science and Sports Medicine. Exercise, Heat, and Thermoregulation,* eds. C. Gisolfi, D. Lamb, and E. Nadel. Dubuque, IA: Brown and Benchmark.

Coyle, E., and Montain, S. 1992. Carbohydrate and fluid ingestion during exercise: Are there trade-offs? *Medicine and Science in Sports and Exercise* 24: 671–78.

Dennis, S., et al. 1997. Nutritional strategies to minimize fatigue during prolonged exercise: Fluid, electrolyte and energy replacement. *Journal of Sports Sciences* 15:305–13.

Denton, D., et al. 1996. Hypothalamic integration of body fluid regulation. *Proceedings of the National Academy of Sciences* 93:7397–7404.

Einhorn, D., and Landsberg, L. 1988. Nutrition and diet in hypertension. In *Modern Nutrition in Health and Disease,* eds. M. Shils and V. Young. Philadelphia: Lea and Febiger.

Epstein, Y. 1990. Heat intolerance: Predisposing factor or residual injury. *Medicine and Science in Sports and Exercise* 22:29–35.

Fishbane, S. 1995. Exercise-induced renal and electrolyte changes. *Physician and Sportsmedicine* 23 (8): 39–46.

Galloway, J. 1997. Cool tips for hot running. *Runner's World* 32 (6): 38–39.

Gisolfi, C. 1996. Fluid balance for optimal performance. *Nutrition Reviews* 54:S159–S168.

Gisolfi, C., and Duchman, S. 1992. Guidelines for optimal replacement beverages for different athletic events. *Medicine and Science in Sports and Exercise* 24:679–87.

Greenleaf, J. 1992. Problem: Thirst, drinking behavior, and involuntary dehydration. *Medicine and Science in Sports and Exercise* 24:645–56.

Hagberg, J. 1990. Exercise, fitness and hypertension. In *Exercise, Fitness, and Health,* eds. C. Bouchard, et al. Champaign, IL: Human Kinetics.

Heigenhauser, G., and Jones, N. 1991. Bicarbonate loading. In *Perspectives in Exercise Science and Sports Medicine. Ergogenics: The Enhancement of Sports Performance,* eds. D. Lamb and M. Williams. Dubuque, IA: Brown & Benchmark.

Hickey, M., and Israel, R. 1997. Fluid replacement and exercise-thermal stress: An update. *AMAA Quarterly* 11:10–11.

Hiller, D. 1989. Dehydration and hyponatremia during triathlons. *Medicine and Science in Sports and Exercise* 21:S219–S221.

Horswill, C. 1991. Does rapid weight loss by dehydration adversely affect high-power performance? *Sports Science Exchange* 3 (30): 1–4.

Hubbard, R., and Armstrong, L. 1990. Clinical symposium: Exertional heatstroke: An international perspective. *Medicine and Science in Sports and Exercise* 22:2–48.

Kelley, G., and Tran, Z. 1995. Aerobic exercise and normotensive adults: A meta-analysis. *Medicine and Science in Sports and Exercise* 27:1371–77.

Lefferts, L. 1990. Water: Treat it right. *Nutrition Action Health Letter* 17:5–7.

Linderman, J., and Fahey, T. 1991. Sodium bicarbonate ingestion and exercise performance. *Sports Medicine* 11:71–77.

Macdonald, I. 1992. Food and drink in sport. *British Medical Journal* 48:605–14.

Matson, L., and Tran, S.V. 1993. Effects of sodium bicarbonate ingestion on anaerobic performance: A meta-analytic review. *International Journal of Sport Nutrition* 3:2–28.

Maughan, R. 1996. Rehydration and recovery after exercise. *Sports Science Exchange* 9 (3): 1–5.

Maughan, R. 1991. Carbohydrate-electrolyte solutions during prolonged exercise. In *Perspectives in Exercise Science and Sports Medicine. Ergogenics: Enhancement of Performance in Exercise and Sport,* eds. D. Lamb and M. Williams. Dubuque, IA: Brown & Benchmark.

Maughan, R., and Shirreffs, S. 1997. Preparing athletes for competition in the heat: Developing an effective acclimatization strategy. *Sports Science Exchange* 10 (2): 1–4.

Maughan, R., and Shirreffs, S. 1997. Recovery from prolonged exercise: Restoration of water and electrolyte balance. *Journal of Sports Sciences* 15:297–303.

Maughan, R., et al. 1997. Factors influencing the restoration of fluid and electrolyte balance after exercise in the heat. *British Journal of Sports Medicine* 31:175–82.

Maughan, R., et al. 1993. Fluid replacement in sport and exercise. A consensus statement. *British Journal of Sports Medicine* 27:34–35.

Meyer, F., and Bar-Or, O. 1994. Fluid and electrolyte loss during exercise: The pediatric angle. *Sports Medicine* 18:4–9.

Midgley, J., et al. 1996. Effect of reduced dietary sodium on blood pressure: A meta-analysis of randomized controlled trials. *Journal of the American Medical Association* 275:1590–97.

Millard-Stafford, M. 1992. Fluid replacement during exercise in the heat. *Sports Medicine* 13:223–33.

Morris, C. 1997. Effect of dietary sodium restriction on overall nutrient intake. *American Journal of Clinical Nutrition* 65:687S–691S.

Murray, B. 1996. Fluid replacement: The American College of Sports Medicine position stand. *Sports Science Exchange* 9 (4): 1–4.

Murray, R. 1997. Drink. More! Advice from a world-class expert. *ACSM's Fitness Journal* 1 (1): 19–23.

Murray, R. 1992. Nutrition for the marathon and other endurance sports: Environmental stress and dehydration. *Medicine and Science in Sports and Exercise* 24:S319–S323.

Nadel, E. 1988. Temperature regulation and prolonged exercise. In *Perspectives in Exercise Science and Sports Medicine. Prolonged Exercise,* eds. D. Lamb and R. Murray. Indianapolis, IN: Benchmark.

Noakes, T. 1993. Fluid replacement during exercise. *Exercise and Sport Sciences Reviews* 21:297–330.

Noakes, T. 1992. The hyponatremia of exercise. *International Journal of Sport Nutrition* 2:205–28.

Peters, H., et al. 1995. Gastrointestinal symptoms during exercise: The effect of fluid supplementation. *Sports Medicine* 20:65–76.

Puhl, S., and Buskirk, E. 1994. Nutrient beverages for exercise and sport. In *Nutrition in Exercise and Sports,* eds. I. Wolinsky and J. Hickson. Boca Raton, FL: CRC Press.

Reusser, M., and McCarron, D. 1994. Micronutrient effects on blood pressure regulation. *Nutrition Reviews* 52:367–75.

Roberts, W. 1992. Managing Heatstroke. On-site cooling. *Physician and Sportsmedicine* 20(5):17–28.

Sawka, M. 1992. Physiological consequences of hypohydration: Exercise performance and thermoregulation. *Medicine and Science in Sports and Exercise* 24:657–70.

Sawka, M., and Greenleaf, J. 1992. Current concepts concerning thirst, dehydration, and fluid replacement: Overview. *Medicine and Science in Sports and Exercise* 24:643–44.

Sawka, M., and Pandolf, K. 1990. Effects of body water loss on physiological function and exercise performance. In *Perspectives in Exercise Science and Sports Medicine. Fluid Homeostasis During Exercise,* eds. C. Gisolfi and D. Lamb. Indianapolis, IN: Benchmark.

Schedl, H., et al. 1994. Intestinal absorption during rest and exercise: Implications for formulating an oral rehydration solution (ORS). *Medicine and Science in Sports and Exercise.* 26:267–80.

Spickard, A. 1968. Heat stroke in college football and suggestions for prevention. *Southern Medical Journal* 61:791–96.

Stephenson, L., and Kolka, M. 1993. Thermoregulation in women. *Exercise and Sport Sciences Reviews* 21:231–62.

Tanji, J., and Batt, M. 1995. Management of hypertension: Adapting new guidelines for active patients. *Physician and Sportsmedicine* 23 (2): 47–55.

Taylor, N. 1986. Eccrine sweat glands: Adaptations to physical training and heat acclimation. *Sports Medicine* 3:387–97.

Terrados, N., and Maughan, R. 1995. Exercise in the heat: Strategies to minimize the adverse effects on performance. *Journal of Sports Sciences* 13:S55–S62.

Thadani, U. 1996. Hypertension and cardiovascular disease risk in women. *Medicine and Science in Sports and Exercise* 28:7–8.

Tipton, C. 1988. Exercise and hypertension: Management concepts for coaches and educators. *Sports Science Exchange* 1 (June): 1–4.

Werner, J. 1993. Temperature regulation during exercise: An overview. In *Perspectives in Exercise Science and Sports Medicine. Exercise, Heat, and Thermoregulation,* eds. C. Gisolfi, D. Lamb, and E. Nadel. Dubuque, IA: Brown and Benchmark.

Williams, M. 1992. Bicarbonate loading. *Sports Science Exchange* 4 (January): 1–4.

Young, A. 1990. Energy substrate utilization during exercise in extreme environments. *Exercise and Sport Sciences Reviews* 18:65–118.

Specific Studies

Appel, L., et al. 1997. A clinical trial of the effects of dietary patterns on blood pressure. *New England Journal of Medicine* 336:1117–24.

Armstrong, L., et al. 1993. Symptomatic hyponatremia during prolonged exercise in heat. *Medicine and Science in Sports and Exercise* 25:543–49.

Armstrong, L., et al. 1987. Appearance of ingested H_2O_{18} in plasma and sweat during exercise-heat exposure. *Medicine and Science in Sports and Exercise* 19:S56.

Barr, S., et al. 1991. Fluid replacement during prolonged exercise: Effects of water, saline, and no fluid. *Medicine and Science in Sports and Exercise* 23:811–17.

Below, P., et al. 1995. Fluid and carbohydrate ingestion independently improve performance during 1 h of intense exercise. *Medicine and Science in Sports and Exercise* 27:200–10.

Bergeron, M. 1996. Heat cramps during tennis: A case report. *International Journal of Sport Nutrition* 6:62–68.

Bird, S., et al. 1995. The effect of sodium bicarbonate ingestion on 1500-m racing time. *Journal of Sports Sciences* 13:399–403.

Costill, D., et al. 1982. Dietary potassium and heavy exercise: Effects on muscle water and electrolytes. *American Journal of Clinical Nutrition* 36:266–75.

Davis, J., et al. 1988. Effects of ingesting 6% and 12% glucose/electrolyte beverages during prolonged intermittent cycling in the heat. *European Journal of Applied Physiology* 57:553–59.

DeLuca, J., et al. 1993. Hormonal responses to hyperhydration with glycerol vs water alone. *Medicine and Science in Sports and Exercise* 25:S26.

Freund, B., et al. 1993. Renal responses to hyperhydration using aqueous glycerol vs water alone provide insight to the mechanism for glycerol's effectiveness. *Medicine and Science in Sports and Exercise* 25:S35.

Gardner, J., et al. 1996. Risk factors predicting exertional heat illness in male Marine Corps recruits. *Medicine and Science in Sports and Exercise* 28:939–44.

Hargreaves, M., et al. 1996. Effect of fluid ingestion on muscle metabolism during prolonged exercise. *Journal of Applied Physiology* 80:363–66.

Hargreaves, M., et al. 1994. Influence of sodium on glucose bioavailability during exercise. *Medicine and Science in Sports and Exercise* 26:365–68.

Hausswirth, C., et al. 1995. Sodium citrate ingestion and muscle performance in acute hypobaric hypoxia. *European Journal of Applied Physiology* 71:362–68.

Hiller, W.D., et al. 1987. Medical and physiological considerations in triathlons. *American Journal of Sports Medicine* 15:164–67.

Hinchcliff, K., et al. 1993. Effect of oral sodium loading on acid: base status and athletic capacity of horses. *Medicine and Science in Sports and Exercise* 25:S25.

Kingwell, B., and Jennings, G. 1993. Effects of walking and other exercise programs upon blood pressure in normal subjects. *Medical Journal of Australia* 158:234–38.

Koizumi, T., et al. 1996. Fatal rhabdomyolysis during mountaineering. *Journal of Sports Medicine and Physical Fitness* 36:72–74.

Kozak-Collins, K., et al. 1994. Sodium bicarbonate ingestion does not improve performance in women cyclists. *Medicine and Science in Sports and Exercise* 26:1510–15.

Lamb, D., et al. 1997. Prehydration with glycerol does not improve cycling performance vs 6% CHO-electrolyte drink. *Medicine and Science in Sports and Exercise* 29:S249.

Lambert, G., et al. 1993. Effects of carbonated and noncarbonated beverages at specific intervals during treadmill running in the heat. *International Journal of Sport Nutrition* 3:177–93.

Latzka, W., et al. 1997. Hyperhydration: Thermoregulatory effects during compensable exercise-heat stress. *Medicine and Science in Sports and Exercise* 29:S132.

Lindeman, A. 1991. Nutrient intake of an ultraendurance cyclist. *International Journal of Sport Nutrition* 1:79–85.

Lyons, T., et al. 1990. Effects of glycerol-induced hyperhydration prior to exercise in the heat on sweating and core temperature. *Medicine and Science in Sports and Exercise* 22:477–83.

McNaughton, L., 1992. Sodium bicarbonate ingestion and its effects on anaerobic exercise of various durations. *Journal of Sports Sciences* 10:425–35.

McNaughton, L. 1992. Bicarbonate ingestion: Effects of dosage on 60 s cycle ergometry. *Journal of Sports Sciences* 10:415–23.

McNaughton, L., and Cedaro, R. 1992. Sodium citrate ingestion and its effects on maximal anaerobic exercise of different durations. *European Journal of Applied Physiology* 64:36–41.

Meyer, F., et al. 1992. Sweat electrolyte loss during exercise in the heat: Effects of gender and maturation. *Medicine and Science in Sports and Exercise* 24:776–81.

Millard-Stafford, M. 1997. Water versus carbohydrate-electrolyte ingestion before and during a 15-km run in the heat. *International Journal of Sport Nutrition* 7:26–38.

Mitchell, J., and Voss, K. 1991. The influence of volume on gastric emptying and fluid balance during prolonged exercise. *Medicine and Science in Sports and Exercise* 23:314–19.

Montner, P., et al. 1996. Pre-exercise glycerol hydration improves cycling endurance time. *International Journal of Sports Medicine* 17:27–33.

Noakes, T., et al. 1991. Metabolic rate, not percent dehydration, predicts rectal temperature in marathon runners. *Medicine and Science in Sports and Exercise* 23:443–49.

Peters, H., et al. 1993. Gastrointestinal problems as a function of carbohydrate supplements and mode of exercise. *Medicine and Science in Sports and Exercise* 25:1211–24.

Potteiger, J., et al. 1996. The effects of buffer ingestion on metabolic factors related to distance running performance. *European Journal of Applied Physiology* 72:365–71.

Potteiger, J., et al. 1995. The effects of sodium citrate ingestion on 30 km cycling performance. *Medicine and Science in Sports and Exercise* 27:S148.

Rehrer, N., et al. 1993. Effects of electrolytes in carbohydrate beverages on gastric emptying and secretion. *Medicine and Science in Sports and Exercise* 25:42–51.

Rehrer, N., et al. 1992. Gastrointestinal complaints in relation to dietary intake in triathletes. *International Journal of Sport Nutrition* 2:48–59.

Rico-Sanz, J., et al. 1996. Effects of hyperhydration on total body water, temperature regulation and performance of elite young soccer players in a warm climate. *International Journal of Sports Medicine* 17:85–91.

Rogers, G., et al. 1997. Water budget during ultra-endurance exercise. *Medicine and Science in Sports and Exercise* 29:1477–81.

Rozycki, T. 1984. Oral and rectal temperatures in runners. *Physician and Sportsmedicine* 12:105–8.

Sawka, M., et al. 1997. Hyperhydration: Thermal and cardiovascular effects during uncompensable exercise-heat stress. *Medicine and Science in Sports and Exercise* 29:S132.

Sawka, M., et al. 1993. Total body water (TBW), extracellular fluid (ECF), and plasma responses to hyperhydration with aqueous glycerol. *Medicine and Science in Sports and Exercise* 25:S35.

Sherriffs, S., et al. 1996. Post-exercise rehydration in man: Effects of volume consumed and drink sodium content. *Medicine and Science in Sports and Exercise* 28:1260–71.

Shi, X., et al. 1995. Effects of carbohydrate type and concentration and solution osmolality on water absorption. *Medicine and Science in Sports and Exercise* 27:1607–15.

Verde, T., et al. 1982. Sweat composition in exercise and in heat. *Journal of Applied Physiology* 53:1540–45.

Waller, M., and Haymes, E. 1996. The effects of heat and exercise on sweat loss. *Medicine and Science in Sports and Exercise* 28:197–203.

Webster, M., et al. 1993. Effect of sodium bicarbonate ingestion on exhaustive resistance exercise performance. *Medicine and Science in Sports and Exercise* 25:960–65.

Webster, S., et al. 1990. Physiological effects of a weight loss regimen practiced by college wrestlers. *Medicine and Science in Sports and Exercise* 22:229–34.

Wendtland, C., et al. 1997. Glycerol-induced hyperhydration does not provide cardiovascular or thermoregulatory benefit during prolonged exercise. *Medicine and Science in Sports and Exercise* 29:S133.

Yaspelkis, B., et al. 1993. Carbohydrate metabolism during exercise in hot thermoneutral environments. *International Journal of Sports Medicine* 14:13–19.

Zachwieja, J., et al. 1992. The effects of a carbonated carbohydrate drink on gastric emptying, gastrointestinal distress, and exercise performance. *International Journal of Sport Nutrition* 2:239–50.

Zachwieja, J., et al. 1991. Effects of drink carbonation on the gastric emptying characteristics of water and flavored water. *International Journal of Sport Nutrition* 1:45–51.

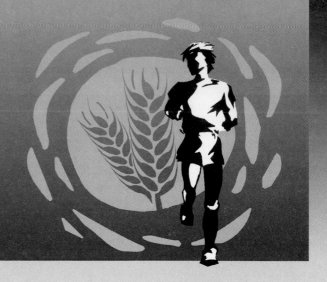

CHAPTER 10

Body Weight and Composition for Health and Sport

KEY TERMS

aminostatic theory
android-type obesity
anorexia athletica
anorexia nervosa
bioelectrical impedance
 analysis (BIA)
body image
Body Mass Index (BMI)
body plethysmography
brown fat
bulimia nervosa
cellulite
Dual Energy X-ray
 Absorptiometry (DXA;
 DEXA)
eating disorder
essential fat
fat-free mass
glucostatic theory
gynoid-type obesity
hunger center
hyperplasia
hypertrophy
lean body mass
leptin
lipostatic theory
metabolic syndrome
morbid obesity
obesity
regional fat distribution
relative-weight method
satiety center
set-point theory
settling-point theory
skinfold technique
storage fat
subcutaneous fat
underwater weighing
very-low-Calorie diets (VLCD)
visceral fat
waist:hip ratio (WHR)
weight cycling

KEY CONCEPTS

• Height-weight charts and the Body Mass Index do not measure body composition but may be useful as a screening device to determine whether one is overweight or obese.

• The body consists of four components: body fat, protein, minerals, and water.

• For practical purposes, body composition may be classified as consisting of two components: fat-free weight, which is about 70 percent water, and body fat.

• The body needs a certain amount of fat content, the so-called essential fat, but excessive body fat may contribute to several major health problems and may also impair athletic performance.

• All techniques that currently are used to measure body composition are prone to error; even the underwater-weighing technique, supposedly the most accurate technique, may be in error by 2–2.5 percent.

• Our present level of knowledge does not provide us with the ability to predict precisely what the optimal body composition should be for health or physical performance.

• The brain's hypothalamus appears to be the central control mechanism in appetite regulation, which involves a complex interaction of physiological and psychological factors.

• Although the ultimate cause of obesity is a positive energy balance, the underlying cause is not known but probably involves the interaction of many genetic and environmental factors.

• Excessive body fat is associated with a variety of chronic diseases and impaired health conditions, including coronary heart disease, diabetes, high blood pressure, and arthritis.

• For children and adolescents, the major adverse health effects of excessive body fat appear to be social and psychological, but in future years, they may be more prone to chronic diseases than their nonobese peers.

• Being physically fit and eating a healthful diet may help reduce some of the health risks associated with being overweight.

• Excessive weight losses, usually associated with behaviors characteristic of eating disorders, may result in health problems ranging from mild to severe and may also have a negative impact upon physical performance.

• Drugs and very-low-Calorie diets may be very effective for weight loss under medical supervision, but they may be associated with a variety of health risks if not used properly.

• Disordered eating in female athletes, usually excessive dieting and exercise to control body weight, may lead to amenorrhea and osteoporosis.

• Although the average body-fat percentages for young men and women are, respectively, 15–18 percent and 22–25 percent, those involved in athletic competition may be advised to reduce these levels.

• Losing excess body weight may impair sport performance. Young athletes who exercise and diet excessively may experience a decrease in growth rate.

INTRODUCTION

The human body is a remarkable machine. In most cases it may consume nearly a ton of food, nearly one million Calories, over a year and not change its weight by a single pound. Individuals are constantly harnessing and expending energy through the intricacies of their bodily metabolism in order to remain in energy balance. To maintain a given body weight, energy input must balance energy output. However, sometimes the energy-balance equation becomes unbalanced, and the normal body weight will either increase or decrease.

The term **body image** refers to the mental image we have of our own physical appearance, and it can be influenced by a variety of factors, including how much we weigh or how that weight is distributed. Body weight appears to be a major concern of many Americans. Research has revealed that about 40 percent of adult men and 55 percent of adult women are dissatisfied with their current body weight. Similar findings have also been reported at the high school and even the elementary school level, primarily with female students, and some research has found that 85 percent of both male and female first-year college students desired to change their body weight. The primary cause of this concern is the value that American society, in general, assigns to physical appearance. Being overweight is viewed by many as a handicap to both personal and professional fulfillment, and the term "fattism" has been coined to reflect society's prejudice toward the obese. Thinness is currently an attribute that females desire highly. Males generally desire muscularity, which is also becoming increasingly popular among women. Most individuals who are dissatisfied with their physical appearance feel that they are overweight, and federal surveys have shown that approximately 35–40 percent of adult women and 20–25 percent of adult men are currently attempting to lose weight.

According to a recent national survey, nearly 60 percent of American men and 50 percent of American women are overweight. Being overweight also may have a significant effect upon health and physical performance. Excessive body weight, particularly in the form of body fat, has been associated with a wide variety of health problems. Obesity is one of the most prominent medical concerns in industrialized societies today, and the Public Health Service has stated in *Healthy People 2000* that one of the major health objectives for the year 2000 is to decrease the proportion of adults and children who are significantly overweight or obese. For some athletes, simply being a little overweight may prove to be detrimental to physical performance because it costs energy to move the extra body mass. On the other hand, increased body weight, provided it is of the right composition, may be advantageous to other athletes.

At the other end of the body-weight continuum, weight losses leading to excessive thinness also may have an impact upon health and physical performance. Anorexia nervosa and bulimia are two serious health disorders associated with obsessive concern about body weight. Although losing excess body fat may improve performance in some sports, excessive weight losses may have a negative impact upon athletic performance.

The major focus of this chapter is on the basic nature of body composition and its effect on health and physical performance. The following two chapters deal with weight-control methods used to maintain or modify body composition.

Body Weight and Composition

What is the ideal body weight?

We all have heard at one time or another that there is an ideal body weight for our particular height. But ideal in terms of what? Health? Appearance? Physical performance? There appears to be no sound evidence to suggest a specific ideal weight for a given individual, but some general guidelines have been proposed relative to health and physical performance, the major focus of this chapter.

Most of us have our own images of how we would like to look, and indeed most individuals who attempt to attain an ideal body weight do so to enhance their appearance. An enhanced physical appearance may improve one's body image and self-esteem, factors important to psychological health. An enhanced physical appearance may also influence performance in certain sports that involve judging of aesthetic movements, such as gymnastics and diving. Although society may create a perception of an ideal body weight for appearance, this ideal body weight may or may not be in accord with optimal health and physical performance.

Most research efforts have attempted to find an ideal body weight for good health. For example, data collected during the past century, mainly by life insurance companies, have been compiled into normal or desirable ranges of body weight for a given height and age. These height-weight charts represent the ideal weights at which Americans can expect to live the longest. The terminology of ideal weight has changed over the years, today being referred to as a healthy body weight.

Tables 2 and 3 in Appendix E represent two of the more popular desirable height-weight charts developed for adults by the Metropolitan Life Insurance Company. The height is measured without shoes and weight is measured with no or very light clothing. Body-weight ranges are given for three body frames—small, medium, and large. Table 1 in Appendix E provides a procedure for estimating your body frame size.

Although the Metropolitan Life Insurance Company released new height-weight tables for Americans in 1983, the data in Tables 1 through 3 in Appendix E represent figures generated in 1959. Unfortunately the 1983 report has been challenged by several major health groups, including the American Heart Association, because the average body weights are generally higher than the 1959 figures. In general, other health factors that have changed in American society may have biased the new tables. For example, there is an increasing death rate among heavy smokers, who are usually underweight, which would increase the average weights in the 1983 tables because they are based on mortality.

Tables 2 and 3 in Appendix E have been developed for females and males 25 years of age and over. For women under the ages of 18 and 25, one pound should be subtracted for each year under 25. As an example, a 5-foot 8-inch, 20-year-old woman with a medium frame would have a weight range of 127–142, or 5 pounds below the desirable level at age 25 (132–147). Although different age levels are not built into this scale, the range of values for each height and body frame helps account for this. You may use Method A in Appendix E to determine your height-weight relationship. In general, as we get older our body weight usually increases, although nutrition scientists recommend that it remain stable or decrease slightly.

Another commonly used height-weight relationship is the **Body Mass Index (BMI),** also known as Quetelet's Index. The BMI is a weight:height ratio using the metric system. The formula is

$$\frac{\text{Body weight in kilograms}}{(\text{Height in meters})^2}$$

An individual who weighs 70 kg (154 pounds) and is 1.78 meters (70 inches) in height would have a BMI of 22.1 ($70 \div [1.78^2]$). If you want to use pounds and inches, the formula is

$$\frac{(\text{Body weight in pounds}) \times 705}{(\text{Height in inches})^2}$$

For the same example using pounds and inches, the BMI is also 22.1 ($154 \times 705 \div [70^2]$). In general, a BMI range of 20–25 is considered to be normal. You may calculate your BMI using Method B in Appendix E.

What are the values and limitations of height-weight charts and the BMI?

Height-weight charts are based on measurements obtained from large populations of people. The data obtained are then treated statistically, and the values that tend to cluster toward the midpoint (the median) are considered to be normal, average, or desirable, at least as related to a lower rate of mortality. The Metropolitan Life Insurance Company tables have been criticized because they are based upon a selective population, insurance policy holders, which may not represent the average American population. Noncaucasians are underrepresented in these tables. Moreover, data from the National Institute of Aging (NIA) suggest that age was not taken into account. Although the tables reflect data for the ages 25–59, the NIA report suggests that the recorded desirable weights are too high for the younger age groups, just right for the 40s, and too low for older age groups.

Nevertheless, in relation to determining whether an individual possesses normal body weight for a given age and sex, these tables may have some value as a screening device. If you are more than 10 percent below the average you may be considered to be underweight. Ten percent over the normal value may be classified as overweight, and 20 percent above normal is often used as a criterion for obesity.

Comparable to height-weight charts, the BMI may be a useful screening device for health problems. The Consumers Union indicates that a low BMI may be a symptom of a serious disease, while a high BMI may be indicative of obesity.

However, height-weight tables and the BMI reveal nothing to us about our body composition. Two individuals may be exactly the same height and weight; however, the distribution of their body weight might be so different that one individual could possibly be considered obese while the other might be considered very muscular. For example, 20 percent additional weight could represent muscle mass developed through a strength training program or it could be body fat resulting from a sedentary life-style.

What is the composition of the body?

The human body contains many of the elements of the earth, twenty-five of which appear to be essential for normal physiological functioning. The vast majority of the human body, about 96 percent, consists of four elements (carbon, hydrogen, oxygen, and nitrogen) in various combinations. These four elements are the structural basis for body protein, carbohydrate, fat, and water. The remaining 4 percent of our body is composed of minerals, primarily calcium and phosphorus in the bones, but also including others such as iron, potassium, sodium, chloride, and magnesium. Figure 10.1 illustrates some normal percentages for carbohydrate, fat, protein, water, and bone minerals.

Because body composition may have a significant impact on health and physical performance, scientists have developed a variety of techniques to measure various body components. Depending on the purpose, Wang and others noted that body composition may be evaluated at the atomic, molecular, cellular, tissue-system, and whole-body levels. Although measurement of carbohydrate stores, as liver and muscle glycogen, is important for sport performance research, carbohydrates contribute little to

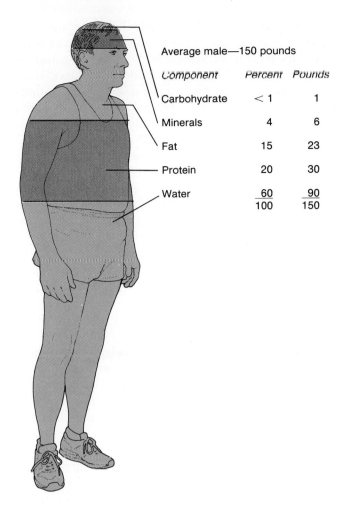

Average male—150 pounds		
Component	Percent	Pounds
Carbohydrate	< 1	1
Minerals	4	6
Fat	15	23
Protein	20	30
Water	60	90
	100	150

Figure 10.1 The majority of body weight is water, while varying amounts of fat, protein, minerals, and carbohydrate make up the solid tissues. Body-weight losses or gains may be related to changes in any of these components.

body weight or composition. Of major interest to body composition scientists are four major body components: total body fat, fat-free mass, bone mineral, and body water. Each of these components has a different density. Density represents mass divided by volume, and in body composition analysis is usually expressed as grams per milliliter (g/ml) or grams per cubic centimeter (g/cc^3). The standard for comparison is water, which has a density of 1.0, or 1 g/ml. Corresponding densities for the other components are approximately 1.3–1.4 for bone, 1.1 for fat-free protein tissue, and 0.9 for fat. The density of the human body as a whole may have a wide range, approximately 1.020 to 1.100. The body-density value may be used to determine the body-fat percentage; a higher density represents a greater amount of fat-free mass and a lower amount of body fat.

Depending on the purpose, body composition may be analyzed as two, three, or all four components. The two components most commonly measured are total body fat and fat-free mass; bone mineral content and body water may be measured with more elaborate techniques.

Total Body Fat   The total body fat in the body consists of both essential fat and storage fat. **Essential fat** is necessary for proper functioning of certain body structures such as the brain, nerve tissue, bone marrow, heart tissue, and cell membranes. Essential fat in adult males represents about 3 percent of the body weight. Adult females also have additional essential fat associated with their reproductive processes. This additional 9–12 percent of sex-specific fat gives them a total of 12–15 percent essential fat, although this amount may vary considerably among individuals. **Storage fat** is simply a depot for excess energy, and the quantity of body fat in this form may vary considerably.

Some storage fat is found around body organs for protection, but over 50 percent of total body fat is found just under the skin and is known as **subcutaneous fat.** When this latter type of fat is separated by connective tissue into small compartments, it gives a dimpled, quilt-like look to the skin and is popularly known as **cellulite.** Cellulite is primarily fat, but may contain high concentrations of glycoproteins, particles that can attract water and possibly give cellulite skin that waffle-like appearance. Other storage fat is located deep in the body, particularly in the abdominal area. This deep fat is referred to as **visceral fat,** which as noted below is associated with increased health risks.

Fat-Free Mass   **Fat-free mass** primarily consists of protein and water, with smaller amounts of minerals and glycogen. The tissue of skeletal muscles is the main component of fat-free mass, but the heart, liver, kidneys, and other organs are included also. A more common term often used interchangeably with fat-free mass is **lean body mass;** technically, however, lean body mass includes essential fat. In a two-component body composition analysis, fat-free or lean body mass complements total body fat. An individual who has 20 percent body fat has 80 percent fat-free mass.

Bone Mineral   Bone gives structure to our body, but it is also involved in a variety of metabolic processes. Bone consists of about 50 percent water and 50 percent solid matter, including protein and minerals. Although total bone weight, including water and protein, may be 12–15 percent of the total body weight, the mineral content is only 3–4 percent of total body weight.

Body Water   The average adult body weight is approximately 60 percent water, the remaining 40 percent consisting of dry weight materials that exist in this internal water environment. Some tissues, like the blood, have a high water content, whereas others, like bone tissue, are relatively dry. The fat-free mass is about 70 percent water, while adipose fat tissue is less than 10 percent. Under normal conditions the water concentration of a given tissue is regulated quite nicely relative to its needs. When we look at the percentage of the body weight that may be attributed to a given body tissue, the weight of that tissue includes its normal water content.

Although the amount of fat, lean tissue, bone and water may vary widely in individuals, the following might represent a normal distribution in a young adult male: 60 percent body water and 40 percent solid matter subdivided into 14 percent fat, 22 percent protein, and 4 percent bone minerals.

Body composition may be influenced by a number of factors such as age, sex, diet, and level of physical activity. Age effects are significant during the developmental years as muscle and other body tissues are being formed. Also, during adulthood, muscle mass may decrease, probably because the level of physical activity declines. There are some minor differences in body composition between boys and girls up to the age of puberty, but at this age the differences become fairly great. In general, girls deposit more fat beginning with puberty, while boys develop more muscle tissue. Diet can affect body composition over the short haul, such as during acute water restriction and starvation, but the main effects are seen over the long haul. For example, chronic overeating, particularly with high-fat diets, may lead to increased body-fat stores. Physical activity may also be very influential, with a sound exercise program helping to build muscle and lose fat.

What techniques are available to measure body composition and how accurate are they?

The measurement of body fat has become very popular in recent years. Many high school and university athletic departments routinely analyze the body composition of their athletes in attempts to predict an optimal weight for competition. Fitness and wellness centers also usually include a body-fat analysis as one of their services. Unfortunately, some of the individuals who analyze body composition in these situations are unaware of the limitations of the tests they employ.

The only direct, accurate method to analyze body composition is by chemical extraction of all fat from body tissues, obviously not appropriate with living humans. Thus, a variety of indirect methods have been developed to assess body composition. Some are relatively simple, such as visual observation by an experienced judge, and others are rather complex, such as nuclear magnetic resonance imaging, using multimillion dollar machines. Indirect methods are used to measure body fat, lean body mass, bone mineral content, and body water. Some techniques are also used to measure fat in specific locations of the body.

Before continuing this discussion, it must be emphasized that measurement of body composition is not an exact science. All techniques currently used to predict body density or percentage of body fat are only estimates and are prone to error, particularly when used to determine the body fat of a given individual. Such errors usually are expressed statistically as standard errors of measurement or estimate, which can be used to show the accuracy of the body-fat measurement. Without going into the statistics of standard errors, look at the following example. Let us suppose that a formula using skinfold techniques predicts your body fat at 17 percent, yet the formula has a standard error of 3 percent. What this means is that your true body fat percentage is probably (about 70 percent probability) somewhere between one standard error of the predicted value, or somewhere between 14–20 percent. It may even be lower than 14 and higher than 20 percent, but less likely so. Thus, you should not think of body-fat determinations as precise measures, but consider them as a possible range associated with the error of measurement. A number of body composition measurement techniques are highlighted in Table 10.1, but only the more commonly used or promising techniques will be discussed.

Underwater Weighing   One of the most common research techniques for determining body density is **underwater weighing,** also known as hydrodensitometry. The technique is based on Archimedes' principle that a body immersed in a fluid is acted upon by a buoyancy force in relation to the amount of fluid the body displaces (see Figure 10.2). Since fat is less dense and bone and muscle tissue are more dense than water, a given weight of fat will displace a larger volume of water and exhibit a greater buoyant effect than the corresponding weight of bone and muscle tissue. Different formulas are recommended for determination of body density, depending upon the age and sex of the individual. Although this technique is often referred to as the "gold standard" in body-composition analysis and is still one of the most commonly used methods for research purposes, it has its weaknesses. For example, the assumption that the density of the fat-free protein tissue is 1.10 g/cc^3 may not be valid for all individuals, such as athletes and older persons. The standard error is still about 2–2.5 percent. Thus, Heyward recently noted that underwater weighing should not be regarded as the "gold standard" because of these errors. Because the underwater-weighing technique is rather time consuming and difficult for some individuals, other techniques have been developed either for research purposes or practical applications.

Body Plethysmography   A new technique is **body plethysmography.** Subjects enter a dual-chamber plethysmograph designed to measure the amount of air they displace, somewhat comparable to the water displacement technique of underwater weighing. One commercial product available is called the Bod Pod (see Figure 10.3). It is portable, easy to operate, requires little time, and eliminates the necessity of going underwater, several clear advantages compared to underwater weighing. A recent study by McCrory and others indicated that body plethysmograph measurements correlate highly with underwater

Table 10.1 Methods used to determine body composition

Anthropometry	Measures body segment girths to predict body fat
Bioelectrical impedance analysis (BIA)	Measures resistance to electric current to predict body-water content, lean body mass, and body fat
Body plethysmography	Whole-body plethysmograph measures air displacement and calculates body density. Comparable to water displacement protocol used in underwater weighing
Computed tomography (CT)	X-ray scanning technique to image body tissues. Useful in determining subcutaneous and deep fat to predict body-fat percentage. Used to calculate bone mass
Dual energy X-ray absorptiometry (DEXA; DXA)	X-ray technique at two energy levels to image body fat. Used to calculate bone mass
Dual photon absorptiometry (DPA)	Beam of photons passes through tissues, differentiating soft tissues and bone tissues. Used to predict body fat and calculate bone mass
Infrared interactance	Infrared light passes through tissues, and interaction with tissue components used to predict body fat
Magnetic resonance imaging (MRI)	Magnetic-field and radio-frequency waves are used to image body tissues similar to CT scan. Very useful for imaging deep abdominal fat
Neutron activation analysis	Beam of neutrons passes through the tissues, permitting analysis of nitrogen and other mineral content in the body. Used to predict lean body mass
Skinfold thicknesses	Measures subcutaneous fat folds to predict body-fat content and lean body mass
Total body electrical conductivity (TOBEC)	Measures total electrical conductivity in the body, predicting water and electrolyte content to estimate body fat and lean body mass
Total body potassium	Measures total body potassium, the main intracellular ion, to predict lean body mass and body fat
Total body water	Measures total body water by dilution techniques to predict lean body mass and body fat
Ultrasound	High frequency ultrasound waves pass through tissues to image subcutaneous fat and predict body-fat content
Underwater weighing (Hydrodensitometry)	Underwater-weighing technique based on Archimedes' principle to predict body density, body fat, and lean body mass

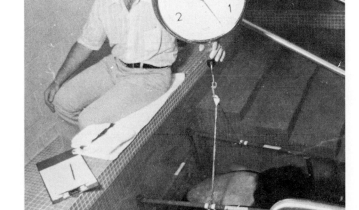

Figure 10.2   Underwater weighing is one of the more accurate means for determining body composition. However, all current techniques for estimating percent body fat are subject to error. See text for discussion.

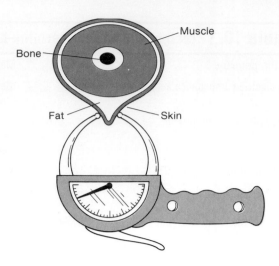

Figure 10.4 A schematic drawing showing the skinfold of fat that is pinched up away from the underlying muscle tissue.

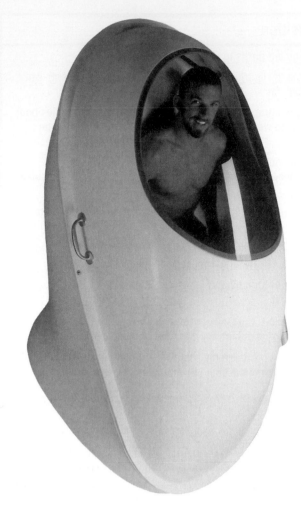

Figure 10.3 The Bod Pod. A new application of total body plethysmography, an air displacement technique, to evaluate body composition.

Photo courtesy of Life Measurement Instruments.

weighing. If these preliminary data are confirmed, the use of body plethysmography could replace underwater weighing as a technique to measure body fat and lean body mass.

Skinfolds The **skinfold technique** is designed to measure the subcutaneous fat (see Figure 10.4). It appears to be the most common procedure for nonresearch purposes. The values obtained are inserted into an appropriate formula to calculate the body-fat percentage. The formula chosen should be specific to the sex and age of the individual. Some formulas also have been developed for specific athletic groups. To improve the accuracy of this technique, skinfold measures should be obtained from a variety of body sites, because using a single skinfold site may be unrepresentative of total storage fat. The test also should be administered with an acceptable pair of skinfold calipers by an experienced tester. Ultrasound techniques are also available to assess skinfold thicknesses, but these are more

expensive than calipers. Orphanidou and others found that measurements of subcutaneous body fat with skinfold techniques were comparable to those obtained by ultrasound and computed tomography, suggesting the use of skinfold calipers in the clinical setting is appropriate.

Because this method involves some measurement error, and because the formulas usually are based upon the underwater-weighing technique, the standard error for the skinfold technique is about 3–4 percent, which should be kept in mind when using this method to estimate body fat. Nevertheless, Lohman and others indicated the skinfold technique is one of the best practical methods to measure body composition. For those who have access to a good skinfold caliper, generalized equations for the calculation of body fat may be found in Appendix E for males and females of several ages.

Body Impedance Analysis (BIA) A more expensive, practical technique is **bioelectrical impedance analysis (BIA).** BIA is based on the principle of resistance to an electrical current that is applied to the body. The less the recorded resistance, the greater the water content, and hence the greater the body density. Early research with BIA revealed large standard errors in predicting lean body mass, so it was not considered to be very valid. However, body composition researchers have developed newer techniques and prediction equations with lower standard errors (3–4 percent), comparable to skinfold techniques. Lohman and others recently noted that BIA is a good practical method to assess body composition. Nevertheless, several problems still appear to exist, including the application to the very obese, the lean athlete, and the elderly. BIA may not accurately predict lean body mass in those with abnormal body-water supplies; it may underestimate lean body mass in athletes and overestimate it in the obese. Pichard and others recently reported valid BIA formulas for female runners, but recommended research to validate formulas for other athletes.

Dual Energy X-Ray Absorptiometry (DXA; DEXA)
Dual energy X-ray absorptiometry (DXA or DEXA) is a computerized X-ray technique used to image body tissues and has been used to assess bone mineral content, fat-free mass, and body fat concurrently. DEXA may also be used to assess deep visceral fat, as can other sophisticated techniques such as magnetic resonance imaging (MRI) and computed tomography (CT).

However, Kohrt recently indicated that although DEXA is the method of choice for measuring bone mass, its use has been associated with errors in measuring fat content. There are different DEXA models, data collection modes, and software, and each may be a source of error. For example, Van Loan and others reported differences in body composition measurements when two different software packages were used. Although DEXA, and other sophisticated techniques such as MRI and CT, may provide us with valuable information on specific tissues in the body, overall they do not appear to be any more effective than underwater weighing to predict body-fat percentage.

Nevertheless, DEXA is a valuable technique because it uses only one measurement session to evaluate body fat, fat-free mass, and bone tissue. As new DEXA techniques are developed and validated, it may become the method of choice for body composition evaluations that include bone density. Although expensive, mass utilization may decrease the cost of DEXA analysis.

Infrared Interactance
Another device marketed commercially is based upon infrared interactance. In essence, infrared light passes through the tissues, and its interaction with tissue components is used to predict body fat. One commercial model is the Futrex 5000, and Dotson and others recently completed a study with the Futrex 6000. Studies have shown somewhat higher standard errors of measurement with infrared interactance, approximately 4–5 percent.

Anthropometry
Anthropometry, or measurement of body parts, is an inexpensive, practical method to assess body composition. Body measurements include girths such as the neck and abdomen, and bone diameters such as the hip, shoulders, elbow, and wrist. Girth and bone diameter measurements may be incorporated into various formulas to predict body fat and lean body mass.

Girth measurements of the abdomen, hips, buttocks, thigh, and other body parts, may be important indicators of **regional fat distribution,** which is a concept representing the anatomical distribution of fat over the body. As noted below, regional fat distribution may be associated with several major health problems. A measure of regional fat distribution is the **waist:hip ratio (WHR),** which is the abdominal or waist circumference (measured by a flexible tape at the narrowest section of the waist as seen from the front) divided by the gluteal or hip circumference (measured at the largest circumference including the buttocks). The WHR, sometimes referred to as the gut:butt ratio, is a good screening technique for regional fat distribution, but it does not provide an accurate measure of deep visceral fat, such as provided by CT or MRI techniques.

What problems may be associated with rigid adherence to body fat percentages in sport?

Table 10.1 lists most of the methods used to estimate body composition. Several recent studies have attempted to validate these techniques, usually against the underwater-weighing method, and have shown some significant differences. In one study comparing four different methods, some individuals were estimated to have body-fat percentages that ranged as much as 10 percent depending on the method used, while another study using four different prediction equations with the BIA reported predicted body-fat percentages ranging from 12.2 to 22.8 in gymnasts. In addition, Stout and others cross-validated sixteen skinfold formulas for prediction of body fat in wrestlers, and reported error values of almost 5 percent. Given the fact that the wrestlers in this study averaged 10.8 percent fat, they concluded that this level of accuracy is not acceptable. Some formulas overestimated body-fat percentage, while others underestimated it. Currently, given the problems with assumptions underlying the various methods of body composition determination, estimates of body-fat percentages are approximations only.

The rigid use of body-fat percentages in weight-control sports, such as gymnastics and wrestling, may lead to excessive weight loss. For example, suppose you are a wrestler and your coach requires you to reach a 5 percent body-fat level. Using a skinfold caliper technique, he finds that you are at 8 percent body fat, and suggests that you lose 3 percent more body fat. However, given the standard error of 3–4 percent, you may already be at 5 percent. Losing extra weight may be very difficult because you are already near minimal body-fat levels, so additional weight loss may include muscle tissue that may lead to possible decreases in performance. In young athletes, such practices may also lead to disordered eating, and possibly clinical eating disorders.

For one of the best resources to select a body composition formula for individuals of different ages, ranging from children to the aged, and with varying physical activity levels, the interested reader is referred to the book by Heyward and Stolarzyk. The review by Heyward is also very informative. Keep in mind, however, that all body fat prediction methods have some error.

Gilbert Forbes, probably the leading expert in body composition analysis over several decades, has noted that each technique used to assess body fat is prone to errors, so the goal of developing a highly precise method for estimating body composition may never be achieved. In any case, most of us do not need a highly accurate assessment of body composition. The critical question probably should be, "How can I tell if I am too fat?" Jean Mayer, an internationally renowned nutritionist, has suggested the use of the mirror test to answer this question. He suggests you look at yourself, nude, from the front and from the side in a full-length mirror. This is usually all the evidence we need if we study ourselves objectively. We probably have a pretty good idea of how we would like our bodies to look, and this test offers us a guide to our desirable physical appearance, at least as far as body-weight distribution is concerned. Exceptions to this suggestion are individuals who are obsessed with thinness and believe they are always too fat, no matter how thin they get. This topic is covered later in this chapter.

How much should I weigh or how much body fat should I have?

That is a complex question, and the response depends on whether you are concerned primarily about appearance, health, or physical performance. From the perspective of physical appearance, you are the best judge of how you wish to look. However, a distorted image may lead to serious health problems or impairment in physical performance.

The effect of body weight and body fat on physical performance is discussed in a later section, although some general guidelines are presented below. The effect of body weight and fat on health has received considerable research attention. Although being underweight may impair health, most of the focus has been on excess body weight and fat, particularly the relationship of obesity to health. By medical definition, **obesity** is simply an accumulation of fat in the adipose tissue. Obesity is also referred to as a disease or disorder, and is the most common nutritional health problem in North America. The actual measurement and determination of clinical obesity is a controversial issue. Several approaches have been used to define the point at which a person is classified as clinically obese.

Unfortunately, our present level of knowledge does not provide us with the ability to predict precisely what the optimal weight or percent body fat should be for health. However, some general guidelines have been developed by various professional and health organizations.

As a screening method for health you may use the height-weight tables and BMI, discussed previously, to assess your body weight. Consult the tables in Appendix E to see if you are in the healthful weight range for your height. The **relative-weight method** (weight to height ratio) is based upon the height-weight tables. As an example, suppose you are a young male and your desirable weight for your height (5′10″) is 143–158. If you weigh 176 pounds, and if we use the midpoint (150 pounds) of

the weight range, then you are about 117 percent of your desirable weight (176/150 × 100). Thus, you are 17 percent above the desirable weight and could be considered to be overweight.

Although various investigators have used values ranging from 115–130 percent of the desirable weight as the determining point of obesity, the National Institute of Health uses a value of 120 percent, which is 20 percent above the desirable weight. Thus, an individual who has a desirable weight of 150 would be classified as obese at a weight of 180 (150 × 1.20). Similar logic could be used for the determination of underweight.

You can also calculate your BMI in Appendix E. The Consumers Union presented the following interpretation of the BMI as related to health risks:

Below 19: May signal malnutrition or serious disease

19–25: Healthy weight range

25–27: Over your healthy body weight

27–30: At increased risk for health problems, especially if you have a weight-related medical condition

Above 30: Obesity, more than 20 percent over healthy body weight

These values are in accordance with figures presented by the National Research Council. Additionally, the Food and Agriculture Organization has proposed the use of a BMI less than 18.5 as a criterion for starvation. Other investigators indicate that a BMI greater than 35 or 40 is classified as severe, or **morbid obesity.**

As noted previously, the use of these height-weight relationships do not evaluate body composition. Thus, the Consumers Union notes that there are exceptions to their BMI classifications, indicating that a low BMI may be a symptom of a serious disease, not a cause, and that muscular people may have a high BMI and not be obese.

For health purposes, the body has a need for the essential fat described previously. At a minimum essential fat approximates 3 percent for males and 12–15 percent for females. Several authorities have included additional levels of storage fat and suggested that minimal levels of total body fat for health range from 5–10 percent for males and 15–18 percent for females. The average percentages of body fat for U.S. males and females are, respectively, approximately 15–18 and 22–25 percent.

Lower levels of body fat may be required for optimal performance in certain types of athletic events. Certain male athletes such as wrestlers and gymnasts may function effectively at 5–7 percent body fat. Recommendations have been made for females who compete in distance running to have no more than 10 percent body fat. However, some athletes have performed very successfully even though their body-fat percentage was higher than the recommended values.

Table 10.2	Ratings of body-fat percentage levels for males and females age 18–30	
Rating	**Males**	**Females**
Excellent	6–10	10–15
Good	11–14	16–19
Acceptable	15–18	20–25
Too fat	19–24	26–29
Obese	25 or over	30 or over

Note: Keep in mind that these are approximate values. The excellent category may apply particularly to athletes who compete in events where excess body fat may be a disadvantage.

Table 10.3	Waist:hip ratio health-risk rating scale	
Health risk	**Men**	**Women**
Higher risk	>.95	>.85
Moderately high risk	.90–.95	.80–.85
Lower risk	<.90	<.80

Source: Based on data from T. B. Van Itallie, "Topography of body fat: Relationship to risk of cardiovascular and other diseases" in *Anthropometric Standardization Reference Manual*, edited by T. G. Lohman, A.F. Roche, and R. Martorell, Human Kinetics Press, Champaign, IL. Copyright 1988 by Timothy Lohman, Alex Roche, and Reynaldo Martorell. Reprinted by permission.

Body Composition and Health

How does the human body normally control its own weight?

As noted previously, you may eat over a ton of food—nearly a million Calories—a year and yet not gain one pound of body weight. For this to occur, your body must possess an intricate regulatory system that helps to balance energy intake and output. The regulation of human energy balance is complex. At the present time we do not know all the exact physiological mechanisms whereby body weight is maintained relatively constant over long periods, but some information is available relative to both energy intake and energy expenditure.

Energy Intake Appetite regulation in relation to energy needs involves a complex interaction of numerous physiological factors including the appetite centers in the brain, feedback from peripheral centers outside the brain such as the liver and intestines, metabolism of ingested foods, and hormone actions. Environmental conditions, such as the home environment, also influence food intake. These factors may interact to regulate the appetite on a short-term basis (daily basis), or on a long-term basis, as in keeping the body weight constant for a year.

The control of the appetite appears to be centered in the hypothalamus, a small substructure in the brain. You may recall from the last chapter that the hypothalamus is also involved in body temperature control. A **hunger center** may stimulate eating behavior. A **satiety center,** when stimulated, will inhibit the hunger center. No single specific biochemical mechanism has been identified, but a number of factors have been theorized to influence the function of these centers to control food intake, as indicated in Figure 10.5. The following may be involved in one way or another.

Although different levels of body-fat percentages have been cited as the criterion for clinical obesity, the American Dietetic Association and the National Research Council set the value at 25 percent for males and 30 percent for females. A proposed rating scale is presented in Table 10.2, keeping in mind that the excellent category is associated with athletes competing in weight-control sports or sports where excess body fat may be a disadvantage. Also, as noted below, although obesity generally increases health risks, some individuals with higher body-fat percentages may not develop obesity-related health problems if they are otherwise physically fit and consume a healthful diet. For example, Lohman and his colleagues recently presented new percent-fat fitness standards for physically active men and women, suggesting a slight increase in fat content as we age. For example, their recommended body-fat ranges are 5–15 percent for active young men, 7–18 percent for middle-aged men, and 9–18 percent for elderly men; female ranges are 16–28 percent for young women, 20–33 percent for middle-aged women, and 20–33 percent for elderly women.

In this regard, it may not be how much fat you have that affects your health, but where that fat is located. The health implications of regional fat distribution are discussed below, but you may use Method D in Appendix E to calculate your waist circumference or your waist:hip ratio (WHR). As a screening measure for deep visceral fat, increased health risks are associated with waist circumferences greater than 39 inches in females and 35 inches in males, and with a WHR greater than 0.90 in males and greater than 0.80 in females. Table 10.3 provides a useful guide for the WHR.

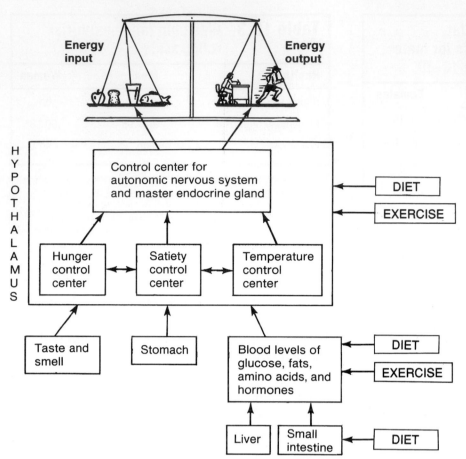

Figure 10.5 Basic control mechanisms for body weight. The control of food intake (energy intake) and resting metabolism (energy output) is governed primarily by the hypothalamus in the brain. The numerous control centers in the hypothalamus are influenced by feedback from the body, such as the blood concentrations of glucose and other nutrients. In turn, food intake and energy expenditure may influence the hypothalamus. For example, exercise will stimulate the hypothalamus, leading to the secretion of several hormones by the endocrine glands in the body. The effects of exercise will also influence the temperature control center and the blood levels of several nutrients, which will in turn influence the hypothalamus. See the text for an expanded discussion.

Stimulation of several senses like sight, taste, and smell. These senses may influence neural or hormonal activity to stimulate or depress our appetites.

An empty or full stomach. An empty stomach may stimulate the hunger center by various neural pathways, whereas a full stomach may stimulate the satiety center.

Receptors in the hypothalamus, liver, or elsewhere that may be able to monitor blood levels of various nutrients. In regard to this, three theories center on the three energy nutrients. The **glucostatic theory** suggests that food intake is related to changes in the levels of blood glucose. A fall will stimulate appetite whereas an increased blood glucose level will decrease appetite. The **lipostatic theory** suggests a similar mechanism for fats as does the **aminostatic theory** for amino acids, or protein. In essence, by-products of carbohydrate, fat, and protein metabolism may influence production of neurotransmitters that influence appetite, such as serotonin, in the hypothalamus.

Changes in body temperature. A thermostat in the hypothalamus may respond to an increase in body temperature and inhibit the feeding center.

Secretion of hormones. A number of different hormones in the body have been shown to affect feeding behavior, including insulin, thyroxine, and several others, particularly a number of peptides produced in the intestines that can function as hormones or neurotransmitters.

Energy Expenditure Although all of the above may be involved in the physiological regulation of food intake, the other side of the energy-balance equation is energy expenditure, or metabolism. Although exercise is one way to increase energy expenditure, the vast majority of the energy that is expended by the body on a daily basis is accounted for by the basal metabolic rate (BMR) or resting energy expenditure (REE), as was detailed in Chapter 3. Changes in the REE may be involved in the regulation of body weight. Several mechanisms of body-weight regulation have been proposed.

Brown fat. **Brown fat,** which is distinct from the white fat that comprises most fat tissue in the body, is found in small amounts around the neck, back, and chest areas. It has a high rate of metabolism and releases energy in the form of heat without ATP production. Activity of the brown fat tissue may be increased or decreased under certain conditions, such as after a meal or exposure to the cold. This activity is referred to as nonshivering thermogenesis. Research with rats has indicated low levels of brown fat are associated with a higher incidence of dietary-induced obesity. The amount of brown fat in humans appears to be small (about 1 percent of body fat or less) but Stock indicates that as little as 50 grams (about 2 ounces) could make a contribution of 10–15 percent energy turnover in humans. Its role in the etiology of human obesity is being researched.

White fat tissue and muscle tissue. In a recent review, Melby and others noted that both white adipose tissue and muscle tissue may also experience thermogenesis without ATP production under conditions of high energy intake, particularly as dietary fat.

Hormones. Levels of hormones from the thyroid and adrenal glands may rise or fall and affect energy metabolism accordingly. Triiodothyronine and thyroxine, hormones from the thyroid gland, may be involved in the stimulation of brown adipose tissue. Hormones, such as epinephrine, also may increase the activity of certain enzymes resulting in increased energy expenditure. Decreases in such hormonal activity may depress energy metabolism. Other hormones may stimulate or depress thermogenesis in adipose or muscle tissues.

Feedback Control of Energy Intake and Expenditure

As noted in an earlier chapter, the human body has developed a number of physiological systems, called feedback systems, to regulate most body processes. Temperature control is a good example. Feedback systems controlling body weight may operate on both a short-term and long-term basis.

On a short-term basis, for example, as the stomach expands while eating a meal, nerve impulses are sent from receptors in the stomach wall to the hypothalamus to help suppress food intake, helping to maintain overall energy balance. Body stores of carbohydrate, protein, and fat are also regulated on a short-term basis. The human body has a limited capacity to store excess carbohydrate and protein, so changes in blood glucose and amino acid levels help regulate carbohydrate and protein intake. Although the human body possesses a high capacity to store fat, blood lipids and other factors help maintain body-fat balance on a short-term basis.

On a long-term basis, the **set-point theory** of weight control is a proposed feedback mechanism. This theory proposes that your body is programmed to be a certain weight, or a set point, something comparable to a set body temperature of 98.6° F. If you begin to deviate from this set point, your body will make metabolic adjustments to return you to normal. This is often referred to as adaptive thermogenesis. Although developed primarily with rats and still only a theory, the set-point concept does involve the interaction of those factors cited above, particularly the lipostatic theory, which may influence energy intake and expenditure in humans.

In a recent review, Schwartz and Seeley noted the hypothalamus contains several redundant systems to regulate energy balance. In long-term control of body weight, imbalances in energy intake are usually reflected by changes in body-fat stores, and Schwartz and Seeley discuss one hypothalamic mechanism whereby body weight is regulated via a hormone in the blood that is derived from body fat. In brief, the regulating hormone is called **leptin,** which is encoded by the OB gene in the adipose cells. The more body fat you have, the more leptin you produce; conversely, less leptin is produced when body-fat stores are low. When leptin is released into the blood, it circulates to the hypothalamus and is believed to inhibit the production of a neuropeptide, specifically neuropeptide Y (NPY) (see Figure 10.6). NPY is a potent stimulant of food intake and also acts to reduce energy expenditure by decreasing the REE. Thus, as you begin to accumulate body fat your fat cells produce more leptin, which then circulates to the hypothalamus and depresses the formation of NPY. Because NPY stimulates food intake and depresses energy expenditure, decreased levels of NPY will suppress hunger and reduce voluntary food intake, and may also stimulate increases in REE by activating thermogenesis in adipose and muscle tissues. Thus, your body reacts to the increased body fat by decreasing energy intake and increasing energy expenditure. Conversely, if you decrease body fat rapidly via dieting, leptin production is decreased, reducing the inhibitory effect on NPY production. Increased levels of NPY stimulate hunger and reduce energy expenditure, thus resisting the effect of the diet and promoting restoration of the lost weight. NPY belongs to a family of hypothalamic neuropeptides, labeled orexins by Sakurai and others, involved in appetite control.

Although the set point is a theory, it may help explain why many people maintain a normal body weight throughout life.

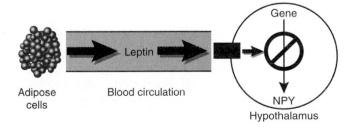

Figure 10.6 One possible mechanism of the set-point theory. Leptin is produced in proportion to body-fat stores. When body fat increases, more leptin is released into the bloodstream, circulates to the hypothalamus, and inhibits the formation or release of neuropeptide Y (NPY). NPY is a potent stimulator of food intake and may also decrease energy expenditure.

What is the cause of obesity?

Energy processes in the human body, like those of other machines, are governed by the laws of thermodynamics. If the human body consumes less energy in the form of food Calories than it expends in metabolic processes, then a negative energy balance will occur and the individual will lose body weight. Conversely, a greater caloric intake in comparison to energy expenditure will result in a positive energy balance and a gain in body weight. In simple terms, obesity is caused by this latter condition of energy imbalance.

Claude Bouchard, a prominent international authority on obesity and weight control, noted that at this time there is no common agreement on the specific determinants of obesity, stressing that numerous factors are correlated with body fat content. In general, most obesity scientists support a multicausal theory involving the interaction of a number of genetic and environmental factors.

Genetic Factors Heredity appears to be a very important factor in the etiology of obesity, particularly morbid obesity. For example, several genetic diseases result in clinical obesity. Also, studies of adopted children, including both fraternal and identical twins who were separated and adopted by different families, have shown a greater relationship of the body composition between the children and their biological parents as compared to the adoptive parents. For a review of two meticulous studies of the genetic role in obesity, the interested reader is referred to the reports by Bouchard and others on long-term overfeeding of identical twins, and by Stunkard and others on the Body Mass Index of twins who were raised apart. It appears heredity may determine those internal factors in the body that may predispose one to gain weight.

Research into the genetics of obesity has been progressing at a rapid pace. Delivering the Wolffe lecture at a recent meeting of the American College of Sports Medicine, Bouchard noted that seventy putative obesity genes have been identified, and strong evidence supports a linkage of eight of these genes with obesity. Bouchard indicated that genetic heritability of obesity approximates 25–40 percent. In essence, obesity genes influence appetite to increase energy intake or affect metabolism to decrease energy expenditure. For example, genes in the hypothalamus may decrease the number of protein receptors for leptin, thus preventing leptin from inhibiting the formation of NPY. NPY may then stimulate the appetite. Also, a protein known as the uncoupling protein (UCP) is believed to activate thermogenesis; UCP1 activates thermogenesis in brown fat, whereas UCP2 activates thermogenesis in white fat and muscle tissue. Defects in UCP genes may decrease resting energy expenditure.

Genetic factors that have been implicated in the development of obesity include a predisposition to sweet, high-fat foods; impaired functions of hormones such as insulin and cortisol; a lower REE; a decreased TEF; an inability of nutrients or hormones in the blood to suppress the appetite control center; an enhanced metabolic efficiency in storing fat; a greater number of fat cells; a smaller percentage of slow-twitch muscle fibers; decreased levels of human growth hormone; lower levels of spontaneous physical activity during the day; and lower levels of energy expenditure during light exercise. Some scientists have coined the term the "thrifty gene" to indicate an increased efficiency in the obese to conserve energy, and they consider obesity a metabolic disease.

Environmental Factors Although heredity may predispose one to obesity, environmental factors, such as drinking alcohol and smoking cessation, are also highly involved. For example, Tremblay and others reported that concurrent alcohol intake does not suppress the appetite nor does it suppress fat intake; thus, the Calories in alcohol are additive and may lead to an energy surplus and weight gain. Nicotine in cigarettes is a stimulant that may inhibit the appetite and increase REE. Flegal and others reported that smokers who quit gained weight over a 10-year period as compared to those who continued smoking. Other environmental factors may be involved in the etiology of obesity but the two key factors that contribute to the development of obesity are excessive intake of Calories, particularly as dietary fat, and physical inactivity.

Excess Calories, or overfeeding, may lead to obesity. Although an excess of caloric input over output will lead to a weight gain, researchers suggest that the main culprit in the diet that leads to obesity is dietary fat. Epidemiological research has supported a positive association between dietary fat and obesity, and there may be a number of possible explanations for this relationship. First, dietary fat is highly palatable to most individuals, stimulating hedonistic responses and encouraging overconsumption. Dietary fat contains more Calories per gram, and may not provide the same satiety as carbohydrate and protein. Gibbs noted that the body systems respond quickly to protein and carbohydrates but slowly to fat, too slowly to stop ingestion of a high-fat meal before the body has had too much. Green and Blundell also note that high-fat foods give rise to higher energy intake during a meal than do carbohydrate foods, and Calorie for Calorie are less effective in suppressing subsequent food intake. In support of this point, Shah and Garg reported that spontaneous energy intake is higher on an unrestricted high-fat diet compared to a high-carbohydrate diet. Second, dietary fat may be stored as fat more efficiently compared to carbohydrate and protein. It takes some energy to synthesize fat and store it in the adipose tissue, but Dattilo noted that in comparison to dietary fat, it may cost up to three or four times more energy to convert carbohydrate and protein to body fat. Third, Behme indicates that chronic intake of a high-fat diet will lead to leptin resistance in the hypothalamus and physiological changes in the body, discussed previously, that may lead to increased body-fat deposition. The interested student is referred to the reviews by Dattilo, and Rolls and Shide regarding the relationship of dietary fat to body weight.

Physical inactivity may also be involved in the etiology of obesity, but the evidence is less clear compared to that available for diet. In a recent review, DiPietro noted that the influence of regular physical activity on body composition is complex. However, although there are some methodological problems with the epidemiological research, DiPietro indicated that several cross-sectional studies have reported an inverse relationship between physical activity and body weight; that is, those who were physically inactive weighed more. DiPietro and other reviewers, such as Saris, noted that physical activity and exercise is an important factor in the prevention of overweight or obesity. Furthermore, de Groot and van Staveren indicate that once an individual becomes obese, physical activity decreases, setting up a vicious cycle of increasing body weight and even less physical activity.

Interaction of Genetics and Environment Many individuals who have maintained a normal body weight during childhood and adolescence begin to put on weight gradually in young adulthood (ages 20–40). The basic cause of this creeping obesity, as depicted in Figure 10.7, is usually an increased consumption of Calories, particularly fat Calories, and a decreased level of physical activity, or a combination of the two. In a major epidemiologic study, Simoes and others reported that dietary fat intake and physical activity were strongly and inversely associated, meaning those who ate the most fat had the least physical activity. For young college students, weight gain may be more rapid due to life-style changes (i.e., a high-fat, high-Calorie diet and decreased physical activity) during the first year of college life, with some students gaining 10–15 pounds, the proverbial "freshman fifteen." Also, several studies have shown that the risk of developing obesity is directly related to the amount of time spent watching television, a sedentary activity usually accompanied by consumption of high-Calorie snack foods.

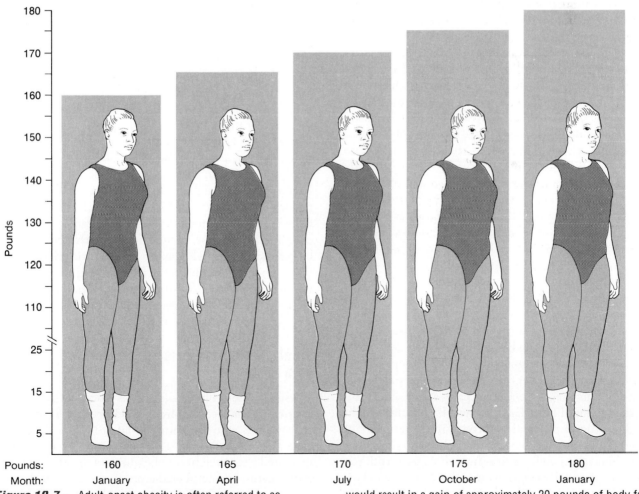

Figure 10.7 Adult-onset obesity is often referred to as creeping obesity, for it creeps up on adults slowly. As little as 200 additional Calories per day above normal requirements would result in a gain of approximately 20 pounds of body fat in 1 year.

If the set-point theory is valid, why do some people attain and maintain body weights higher than their set point? Some investigators have proposed a new theory, the "settling-point" theory. The **settling-point theory** suggests that the set point may be modified, and in the case of weight gain, set at a higher level. Gibbs indicates that whatever genes we have that make us susceptible to obesity settle into a happy equilibrium with our environment. For example, a chronic high-fat diet may modify our genes, possibly increasing leptin resistance, and our body weight rises to a new level. Gibbs provides an example of the Pima Indians living in the United States and Mexico. Both groups have similar genetic backgrounds, yet the Pima Indians living in the United States who consume a high-fat diet are generally obese, while the Pima Indians living in Mexico who consume a grain/vegetable-based diet are generally normal weight. Clearly, genetics and environment interact to influence body weight and composition.

Once an individual is obese, treatment is not very effective. Most scientists agree that prevention of obesity is of prime importance, particularly in childhood. Gibbs speculates that there must be a window of opportunity in childhood where the environment influences the set point. However, the role of diet and physical activity in the development of obesity during childhood, when the most severe cases of obesity begin to develop, is not totally clear. Of the two, an improper diet appears to be the major problem. There may be a familial factor involved here, as the child may be raised in a family where high-fat meals and overeating are common, as suggested in a recent study by Fisher and Birch. Also, the supermarket diet of today makes it easy for children to consume large amounts of Calories. Sugar and fat are found in a wide variety of foods that we eat and constitute about 50 percent of our daily caloric intake. Although some studies have shown that obese children do not consume more Calories than their nonobese peers, the data were not collected during the period when the obese children were gaining weight. Studies in which the investigators actually lived with the children suggest that the obese child does eat more, and also eats faster.

Physical inactivity may also be involved in the etiology of childhood obesity. In children, studies have shown that body weight and the amount of time spent watching television are directly related; that is, the more television is watched the greater the body weight. However, watching television per se may not contribute to obesity because any sedentary activity over the same amount of time would produce similar effects. Being physically active during this time frame would burn Calories and help deter weight gain. The role of physical inactivity in the etiology of childhood obesity does not appear to be as important as that of diet. In general, studies show that obese children are just as physically active as nonobese children. This may not be surprising in that typical nonobese American children are not very physically active either. These comments should not be construed as suggesting that exercise is unimportant in the prevention and treatment of obesity, for Pate recently noted the true potential for preventing obesity through physical activity is not known, and some data suggest physical activity and body fatness are moderately and inversely related in youngsters. Recent research by Bernard Gutin has shown that exercise, independent of diet, may lead to weight loss in obese children. Exercise is important for weight control, as will be documented in the next chapter.

Individuals with a genetic tendency to obesity do not necessarily have to become obese. Individuals with a weak predisposition to obesity may become obese. Although genetics plays an important role in the etiology of obesity, a desirable body weight may be achieved and maintained in those individuals so predisposed. It may be more difficult and may involve a lifetime of vigilance, but it can be done with an appropriate program of diet and exercise.

How is fat deposited in the body?

The actual deposition of fat in the human body may occur in two ways: **hyperplasia** (an increase in the number of fat cells), or **hypertrophy** (an increase in the amount of fat in each cell). Earlier research appeared to support the theory that hyperplasia is a major cause in the development of childhood obesity whereas hypertrophy is the primary cause in adulthood. However, Widdowson has criticized the research upon which these theories are based and recently noted that the assumptions and limitations in calculating the number of adipocytes (fat cells) in an individual are so great that the concepts of a hyperplastic or hypertrophic obesity have largely been abandoned. Moreover, Forbes noted that there are not two types of obesity but rather a gradual increase in both size and number of adipocytes. Existing fat cells apparently have a maximal size potential, which when exceeded stimulates the formation of new fat cells or the accumulation of fat in preadipocytes, small cells in the adipose tissue that have the potential to become adipocytes. Thus, although a genetic predisposition to inherit a greater number of fat cells, thereby facilitating the development of obesity, may exist, individuals without this genetic predisposition may still become obese with a positive energy balance stored as fat.

What health problems are associated with obesity?

Obesity shortens life, possibly by as much as 4 years. Even in ancient Greece, the physician Hippocrates recognized that persons who are naturally fat are apt to die sooner than slender individuals. Kushner noted that carefully measured body weight and height, as a measure of nutritional status, are useful predictors of mortality for the general population. Reports from the National Institute of Health conclude that being overweight contributes to serious health consequences and that obesity is a killer disease. One report has noted that obesity is associated with twenty-six known health conditions and accounts for 15–20 percent of deaths annually. Assessing composite data from various reports, Gibbs indicated a 60 percent increase in all-cause mortality with a BMI of 27–29, a 110 percent increase with a BMI of 29–32, and a 120 percent increase with a BMI of 32–35. Some health problems associated with obesity are kidney disease, cirrhosis of the liver, arthritis, and cancer of the colon and rectum.

The primary health condition associated with excess body fat is coronary heart disease (CHD). Excess body fat increases the risk of developing high blood pressure, hypercholesterolemia, and diabetes, all of which are risk factors leading to the development of CHD. In particular, Gibbs reports that obesity increases the risk of Type II diabetes by an astonishing 1,480 percent with a BMI of 27–29, 2,660 percent with a BMI of 29–31, 3,930 percent with a BMI of 31–33, and 5,300 percent with a BMI of 33–35. Data from the renowned Framingham Heart Study also suggest that obesity is an independent risk factor associated with CHD. The National Center for Health Statistics has reported that susceptibility to CHD increases substantially when the BMI exceeds 27.8 for males and 27.3 for females. Gibbs provided more specific data, indicating that obesity increased the risk of CHD by 210 percent with a BMI of 27–29, 360 percent with a BMI of 29–32, and 480 percent with a BMI of 32–35. Manson and others recently reported that body weight and mortality from all causes were directly related among middle-aged women in the ongoing Nurses' Health Study. However, although at increased risk, the overall effect was small because a woman's risk of dying in midlife, particularly of heart disease, is not great. Stevans and others noted recently that a greater BMI was associated with higher mortality from all causes in men and women up to 75 years of age. The detrimental effects of obesity relative to the development of chronic disease occur when it persists for 10 years or more. In general, thinner individuals live longer.

These figures were derived from the general population and indicate that, in general, obesity is associated with increased health risks. However, some investigators have challenged these data, suggesting that a slightly elevated BMI may not be associated with increased health risks. For example, Troiano and others, in a recent meta-analysis of 19 longitudinal studies encompassing over 350,000 subjects and 38,000 deaths, reported a U-shaped relationship between all-cause mortality and the BMI. All-cause mortality was lowest at a BMI of 24 and increased with both smaller and larger BMIs. Mortality increased gradually in both directions, but increased dramatically at BMIs of 29 or larger and 20 or lower. However, the authors noted some limitations to their analysis. For one, the BMI was measured only at the onset of the study, and the authors indicated possible changes in the BMI over time may have influenced the results. For another, subjects with a low BMI may have been of lower socioeconomic status and may not have had adequate access to health care, which could precipitate premature mortality. Also, they noted that BMI does not measure body composition, but a meta-analysis of the relationship between body composition and all-cause mortality may be forthcoming as more studies become available.

It should be noted that although this review reported an increased mortality with lower BMIs, other research does not support this finding. For example, in the study by Manson and others, lean women did not have excess mortality. Moreover, in a recent study, Losonczy and others noted that the inverse association of weight and mortality as one ages appears to reflect illness-related weight loss from heavier weight in middle-age. When they excluded subjects who lost weight due to illness, there was no higher risk of death associated with low weight.

As noted previously, the BMI does not evaluate body composition. Although it may be useful in determining health risks in the general population because a high BMI is usually associated with excess body fat, it does not apply to muscular individuals. A high BMI may be associated with the development of various diseases if it does represent obesity and increases various risk factors, such as high serum cholesterol levels and high blood pressure. Glenn Gaesser, an exercise physiologist at the University of Virginia, in his book *Big Fat Lies*, indicated that being overweight is not necessarily associated with increased health risks. Life-style may be an important moderating factor. For example, research from the Cooper Institute for Aerobics Research indicates that overweight individuals who have moderate and high levels of physical fitness have a lower risk of mortality than their low-fit peers. In general, these scientists suggest that overweight or obesity does not increase mortality unless it is associated with adverse effects on blood pressure, glucose tolerance, serum cholesterol levels, and physical fitness. Thus, some have proposed use of the term "healthy weight" for overweight individuals who are otherwise healthy.

Although there may be some debate regarding the health risks associated with being overweight or slightly obese, most investigators agree that the location of the fat in the body is a major health risk factor.

Regional Fat Classifications of different types of obesity based upon regional fat distribution have been proposed, the most popular differentiation being the android versus the gynoid types. **Android-(male) type obesity** is characterized by accumulation in the abdominal region—particularly the intraabdominal region—of deep, visceral fat, but also of subcutaneous fat. Android-type obesity is also known by other terms, such as abdominal, central, upper body, or lower trunk obesity, and is sometimes referred to as the apple-shape obesity. **Gynoid-type (female) obesity** is characterized by fat accumulation in the gluteal-femoral region—the hips, buttocks, and thighs. It is also known as lower body obesity, and is often referred to as pear-shape obesity (see Figure 10.8). Both types of obesity have a strong genetic component. As

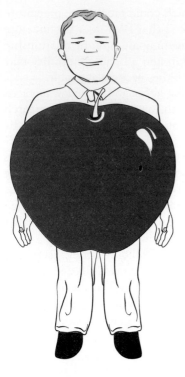

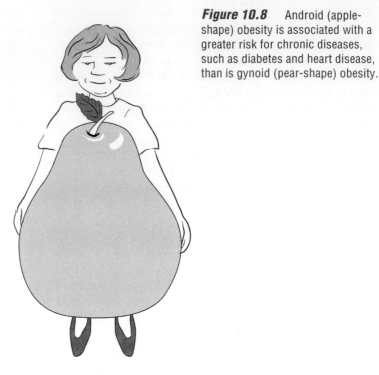

Android
(apple-shape)
obesity

Gynoid
(pear-shape)
obesity

mentioned earlier, either a waist measurement or the waist:hip ratio (WHR) may be an appropriate screening technique for android-type or gynoid-type obesity. The procedure is described in Appendix E.

Android-type obesity is increasingly being recognized as causing a greater health risk than obesity itself. It appears that android-type and gynoid-type fat cells possess dissimilar biochemical functions because of differences in the activity of lipoprotein lipase, an enzyme that regulates fat metabolism. Fat cells in the deep visceral depots are large and highly metabolically active. They readily release free fatty acids into the blood when stimulated by epinephrine, and thus may contribute to abnormalities in glucose and lipid metabolism, particularly in individuals under psychological stress. Data from animal studies have provided direct evidence that the interaction of insulin and fat cell metabolism varies in different fat regions. This finding may be related to humans, for epidemiological data have shown that android-type obesity is associated with hyperinsulinemia, insulin resistance, impaired glucose tolerance, hypercholesteremia, hypertriglyceridemia, diabetes, and hypertension. This cluster of symptoms has been referred to as the **metabolic syndrome,** or syndrome X, and all are risk factors for coronary heart disease. Hunter and others found that physically active men may have a lower risk of developing the metabolic syndrome because of lower levels of deep abdominal fat.

Although android-type obesity occurs primarily in males, recent reports by St. Jeor and Folsom and others noted it is also a major risk factor for mortality in women as well.

Gynoid-type fat cells appear to store fat more readily and tend to lose it less readily, and thus the health risks do not appear to be as great as those associated with android-type obesity. A combined diet-exercise program may help to reduce gynoid-type obesity, but the pear-shape figure appears to be more resistant to change compared to the apple type. Several recent studies in men, women, and adolescents have shown that weight loss via dieting and exercise will preferentially decrease fat from the abdominal area and, concomitantly, improve the serum lipid profile.

Health Risks in Youth Obesity also increases the risk factors associated with CHD in children and adolescents, and although youngsters do not normally die of cardiovascular disease, epidemiological research has shown recently that obese adolescents are at greater risk for chronic disease in adulthood and all-cause mortality compared to their nonobese peers. However, some of the major adverse health effects of excess body fat during childhood and adolescence appear to be social and psychological rather than medical. Because personality development occurs primarily during childhood and adolescence, excessive body fat may contribute more greatly to social-emotional problems at this time than during adult-onset obesity. The Nutrition Committee of the Canadian Paediatric Society noted that obesity interferes with the development of a satisfying self-image and social status, thereby impairing psychological development. Obese children often are rejected by their peers, superiors, and even parents, resulting in a negative self-image, low self-esteem, and even serious psychological illness. A contributing factor to the development of psychological problems may be the adverse effect of excessive body fat on physical fitness and athletic performance. A child who is unsuccessful in play activities probably will not participate, and thus will miss the socializing aspects of play. It should also be noted that adults are not immune to the adverse psychological consequences of obesity.

Treatment and Prevention of Health Risks Approximately 30 percent of the adult population and 25 percent of adolescents and children in the United States are carrying too much body fat for optimal health, and Kuczmarski and others recently noted that the prevalence of overweight is increasing. Not all who are overweight or obese develop medical or psychosocial problems, just as not all cigarette smokers contract lung cancer. However, excessive body fat, particularly abdominal fat, increases the risk of developing such problems and should be corrected as early as possible. Individuals who are morbidly obese, defined as being at least 70 percent over the ideal body weight or having a BMI greater than 40, are in dire need of prompt medical attention.

Treatment of obesity helps reduce risk factors associated with several chronic diseases. Stern and others note that losing even a relatively small amount of weight is likely to decrease blood pressure, reduce abnormally high levels of glucose, improve serum lipid status, decrease depression, and increase self-esteem, improving overall physiological and psychological health.

For children, and adults, prevention is the key because once individuals become obese, treatment is difficult. Researchers are looking for clues such as genetic, metabolic, or anthropometric markers that can predict which children will become obese. In the meantime, some successful programs for the prevention and treatment of obesity have been developed, and appropriate guidelines are presented in the next chapter.

What health problems are associated with excessive weight losses?

Losing excess body fat and attaining a desirable body weight may confer some significant health benefits by counteracting the adverse effects of obesity. However, many individuals attempt to lose weight for other reasons. Slimness is currently very fashionable, particularly among females of all ages. It is desired not only for attractiveness but also for psychological undertones of independence, achievement, and self-control. Also, both male and female athletes, such as distance runners, gymnasts, wrestlers, jockeys, and dancers, practice weight control to improve

their performance. Losing body weight for improved performance may also provide some health benefits, for Paul Williams theorized that the elevated HDL cholesterol concentrations of long-distance runners are primarily a result of reduced adiposity. However, excessive weight loss may actually lead to deterioration of health.

As shall be noted in the next chapter, a well-designed diet and proper exercise are the cornerstones of a sound weight-control program. However, some individuals may establish unrealistically low body-weight goals, which may lead to pathogenic weight-control behaviors. Such techniques as complete starvation, self-induced vomiting, or the use of drugs, diet pills, laxatives, and diuretics may initially be employed to achieve rapid weight losses but may evolve into serious medical disorders, even death, if prolonged. The general effects of excessive rapid and long-term weight losses on health are highlighted below. Rapid weight losses over a week or two usually are achieved by dehydration techniques, drugs, or by starvation-type diets characterized by very low energy intake, whereas long-term weight losses may be associated with eating disorders or problems in young athletes.

Dehydration Dehydration may be induced by exercise, exposure to the heat (as with a sauna), or the use of diuretics and laxatives. The effect of dehydration upon one's health, particularly in relation to heat illnesses, was detailed in the previous chapter. The use of diuretics and laxatives may increase potassium losses from the body, which may lead to electrolyte imbalances and disturbed neurological function, including heart function. For example, in a recent case study Sturmi and Rutecki reported life-threatening hyperkalemia associated with ECG changes and indicators of muscle and kidney damage in a bodybuilder who used diuretics and potassium supplements, along with dietary restrictions, in preparation for competition. Vigorous potassium-lowering maneuvers helped resolve these problems, but the patient's symptoms resembled those of another professional bodybuilder who died after employing similar drug and diet strategies. Disturbed kidney function has also been observed following severe dehydration. The recent deaths of three young collegiate wrestlers have been associated with excessive dehydration.

Weight-Loss Drugs Various drugs are used to stimulate weight loss and generally are prescribed for the obese, not for those individuals who want to lose a few pounds. Nevertheless, it appears that individuals across the weight spectrum, including physically active individuals and athletes are using drugs for weight-control purposes. Some drugs are available without prescription, while others need to be used with medical supervision.

In general, drugs are used to suppress the appetite by increasing the secretion or decreasing the reuptake of various neurotransmitters in the hypothalamus—such as the depressant serotonin, the adrenergic stimulant norepinephrine, or neuropeptide Y (NPY)—involved in appetite

Table 10.4 Some common and proposed weight-control drugs

Adrenergic agents

Amphetamines: Increase norepinephrine activity to help suppress the appetite

Ephedrine: Inhibits appetite via adrenergic effects comparable to norepinephrine; may also elicit thermogenic effect and increase resting energy expenditure

Ephedrine/caffeine: Caffeine may potentiate the effect of ephedrine

Phentermine: Increases adrenergic activity to help suppress the appetite via its amphetamine-like effects

Serotonin agents

Dexfenfluramine: Increases serotonin to help suppress the appetite, a trade name is Redux

Fenfluramine: Increases serotonin to help suppress the appetite.

Fluoxetine (Prozac): Blocks reuptake of serotonin in nerve endings, prescribed for antidepressant effects, but some individuals may use it for weight control

Combined agents

Phen-Fen: Combines effects of both phentermine and fenfluramine to influence serotonin (depressant) and norepinephrine (stimulant) effects to suppress appetite; need to take both pills

Sibutramine: Increases levels of both serotonin and noradrenaline to help suppress appetite; the brand name Meridia has recently been approved by the FDA

Others

Neuropeptide Y inhibitors: inhibit activity of NPY to help suppress appetite and increase energy expenditure

Leptin: Inhibits activity of NPY to help suppress appetite and increase energy expenditure

CCK promoters: Increase activity of cholecystokinin (CCK) at neural receptors to help suppress appetite

Orlistat: Inhibits pancreatic lipase in the intestines, decreasing the digestion and absorption of fat

Beta-3 agonists: Increase response to Beta-3 receptor stimulation in fat tissues and possibly muscle tissue, increasing resting energy expenditure

---

control. Increasing serotonin and norepinephrine and decreasing NPY will suppress the appetite. Other drugs may be used to increase energy expenditure in the peripheral tissues, particularly agents designed to increase resting energy expenditure (REE) by stimulating special receptors (Beta-3 receptors) in brown fat and abdominal adipose tissue, and possibly muscle tissue. Table 10.4 highlights some common or proposed weight-control drugs.

Research shows that many of these drugs may be effective, but the lost weight is regained upon cessation of use of the drug if life-style is not changed. The Food and Drug Administration (FDA) recommends that weight-control drugs only be used on a short-term basis in conjunction with an education program stressing proper diet, exercise, and behavior modification. Long-term use of such drugs has been associated with adverse side effects in some individuals, including tremor, seizures, psychoses, heart arrhythmias, pulmonary hypertension, habituation, addiction, and death. Recently, at the urging of the FDA, manufacturers of dexfenfluramine (Redux) and fenflur-

amine pulled these drugs from the market because their use has been associated with heart valve problems, some requiring surgery. Over-the-counter weight-loss products—such as herbal phen-fen—contain ephedrine, whose use also has been associated with adverse health effects. Individuals should consult appropriate health professionals regarding the use of drugs for weight control, including both prescription and non-prescription agents.

However, some scientists contend that obesity is an incurable disease, somewhat comparable to Type I diabetes. Type I diabetics need to take insulin daily to control their disease. Thus, the search for an effective, safe drug with few or no side effects that will help promote fat loss and maintain a healthful body weight continues.

Very-Low-Calorie Diets Starvation-type diets may involve either complete fasting or **very-low-Calorie diets (VLCD)** (< 800 Calories/day), often referred to as modified fasts. These diet plans are most often used with inpatient programs in hospitals. The National Task Force on the

Prevention and Treatment of Obesity indicated such diets, under proper medical supervision, are generally regarded as safe and have been effective in inducing rapid weight loss in very obese patients. Apparently little or no harm is caused by a 1- or 2-day fast, and some authorities have reported that a healthy man or woman can fast completely for 2 weeks and suffer no permanent ill effect. Although VLCD may be safe and effective for promoting short-term weight loss, they are not very satisfactory in long-term maintenance of weight loss and fare no better than other dietary approaches. Atkinson notes, moreover, that there may be some contraindications to their use and they should be used only after a thorough medical examination. A variety of complications may arise with the use of VLCD, including fatigue, weakness, headaches, nausea, constipation, loss of libido, kidney stones, gallbladder disease, decreased HDL cholesterol, impaired phagocytic function of the white blood cells, inflammation of the intestines and pancreas, decreases in blood volume, decreases in heart muscle tissue, low blood pressure, cardiac arrhythmias, and even death.

Weight Cycling

Grodner suggested that the chronic dieting syndrome, characterized by intervals of high-Calorie diets and VLCD, may be counterproductive as it may lead to **weight cycling** (yo-yo syndrome), a vicious cycle involving repeated bouts of weight loss followed by weight gain. Research has revealed that VLCD may lead to a decreased thermic effect of food (TEF), a decreased resting energy expenditure (REE), and an enhanced food efficiency (less energy wasted in processing dietary Calories). In essence, your body recognizes that it is being starved and will attempt to conserve body stores of energy by reducing energy output. When you resume normal eating, these energy-conservation mechanisms may continue to function for some time, so you actually gain more weight. It is possible that a good proportion of the weight lost during the fasting state is protein, primarily from muscle tissue, which is used to produce glucose for the central nervous system. When you resume eating, the protein tissue is not readily replaced, so the extra Calories may be converted to fat. Moreover, resumption of normal dietary habits may lead to binge eating, episodes in which large amounts of Calories are consumed. Earlier research had suggested that weight cycling would lead to increased amounts of body fat at the same body weight. For example, an individual who started out at 200 pounds with 30 percent body fat would, after several cycles, eventually return to the same weight, but at 35 percent fat. Judith Rodin and her associates at Yale found that weight-cycling women are more prone to deposit fat in the abdominal area, thereby developing an android-type obesity and increased health risks.

However, more current research with both animals and humans suggests that weight cycling may not be associated with any adverse effects on body composition or health. Recent studies by McCargar and others reported that chronic dieting does not result in a sustained reduction in REE, while Bartlett and others found no adverse psychological effects in women who had a history of weight cycling. Moreover, a recent detailed meta-analysis by the National Task Force on the Prevention and Treatment of Obesity revealed that weight cycling does not exert any adverse effect on body composition, metabolism, risk factors for cardiovascular disease, or on the effectiveness of future efforts to lose weight. The Task Force noted that although the evidence currently available indicates weight cycling does not affect morbidity and mortality, conclusive data regarding its long-term health effects are lacking. Currently, the Task Force indicates that obese individuals should not allow any perceived risks of weight cycling deter them from attempts to lose weight, but the Task Force also notes such individuals should commit to lifelong changes in behavior, diet, and exercise.

Some investigators believe the issue of weight cycling and health is still open for debate. Brownell and Rodin have suggested that while there has been no consistent demonstration that, as was first thought, weight cycling makes subsequent weight loss more difficult or regain more rapid, it is possible that this does occur under some conditions or in particular individuals. Although the mechanisms are not clear at present, they also note stronger and more consistent links between body-weight variability and negative health outcomes, particularly all-cause mortality and mortality from coronary heart disease. They indicate there is a clear need for further research on the effects of weight cycling on behavior, metabolism, and health.

Young Athletes

One of the major medical concerns is the effect that severe weight restriction over a longer period may have upon children who are still in the growth and development stages of life. For example, young athletes are at a critical age as far as nutritional needs are concerned, yet the importance of making weight for certain sports often outweighs consideration of a balanced diet, adequate fluid intake, and a minimum caloric requirement. Hence they may go for months without adequate intake of essential nutrients like protein, iron, zinc, and calcium. Although numerous studies have revealed nutrient deficiencies and pathogenic weight-control behaviors in young athletes such as wrestlers and ballet dancers, unfortunately we have very few data on the long-range effects of such practices. Benardot and Czerwinski, comparing the height:age and weight:age percentiles for female gymnasts between the ages of 7 and 10 versus 11 and 14, suggested that the decreased percentiles in the older gymnasts could be attributed to nutritional deficits, sport-specific selection factors favoring retention of small muscular gymnasts, or a combination of the two. In a recent prospective study, Theintz and others studied the growth rate of adolescent female gymnasts and swimmers over a 2- to 3-year period and observed that the growth velocity of the gymnasts was lower than the swimmers. They theorized growth rate was impaired by heavy training (> 18 hours/week), possibly combined with the metabolic effects of dieting, leading to inhibition of the hypothalamus and pituitary gland with resultant suppression of proper sexual development.

Within the past 15 years there has been increasing concern over the development of chronic dieting problems, that is, eating disorders in children, adolescents, and young adults that could have serious adverse health consequences.

What are the major eating disorders?

An obsession with having a low body weight may lead to a number of different **eating disorders,** which may become serious health problems. Currently, the American Psychiatric Association, in their *Diagnostic and Statistical Manual of Mental Disorders*, recognizes two clinical eating disorders, anorexia nervosa and bulimia nervosa. In a recent review, Neumark-Sztainer indicated that dieting itself is not necessarily a harmless behavior and has been shown to be a risk for developing an eating disorder. Weltzin and others indicated that women with eating disorders, particularly bulimia nervosa, may show signs of reduced serotonin activity, which may be related to other psychopathology seen with eating disorders, such as depression, anxiety, and thoughts of suicide, as noted by Buddeberg-Fischer and others.

Anorexia nervosa is a complex disorder that is not completely understood but is thought to be a sign of other psychological problems. Research has suggested that anorexics possess characteristics that underlie compulsive personality disorders, and the prevalence of anorexia nervosa is greatest in groups that abuse psychoactive substances. The diagnostic criteria for anorexia nervosa, as developed by the American Psychiatric Association, are summarized below:

1. Refusal to maintain the body weight over a minimal normal weight for age and height. A weight loss leading to maintenance of body weight less than 85 percent of that expected, including the expected weight gain during the period of growth.

2. An intense fear of gaining weight or becoming fat, even though underweight.

3. A disturbance in the way one's body weight or shape is perceived.

4. Amenorrhea, or the absence of at least three consecutive menstrual cycles in normally menstruating females.

Individuals with anorexia nervosa may be the binge-eating/purging type, engaging in binge eating or purging behavior, such as self-induced vomiting or the misuse of laxatives, diuretics, and enemas. The restricting type does not engage in such behaviors.

The prevalence of anorexia nervosa is relatively low, about 1 percent or less in the general population, but reported to be as high as 2 percent in college underclassmen. Anorexia nervosa is generally found in adolescent women, and about 85–95 percent of those affected are young females, usually under the age of 25. Multiple factors underlie the development of anorexia nervosa, but it prevails more in societies that savor the thin physique and consider dieting normal behavior. It appears that the person with the highest probability of developing anorexia nervosa is a perfectionistic and self-critical individual who comes from an upper-middle socioeconomic status, possibly being raised in an overprotective home environment. Chronic low self-esteem has been identified as a strong risk factor. Although most anorexics are female, male anorexics possess similar characteristics.

Medical consequences of anorexia nervosa can be very serious, including anemia, decreased heart muscle mass, heart beat arrhythmias attributed to electrolyte imbalances, and even death. Treatment is generally prolonged for several years and primarily involves psychological therapy.

The term **bulimia nervosa** means *morbid hunger*, and the disorder involves a loss of control over the impulse to binge. The bulimic individual repeatedly ingests large quantities of food within a discrete period of time, such as 2 hours, but follows this by self-induced vomiting and other measures to avoid weight gain; this is the binge-purge syndrome. However, not all bulimics are the purging type, but may use other techniques, such as fasting or excessive exercise, to compensate for the binge. The American Psychiatric Association criteria for bulimia nervosa include the following:

1. Recurrent episodes of binge eating, at least two per week for 3 months.

2. Lack of control over eating during the binge.

3. Regular use of self-induced vomiting, laxatives, diuretics, fasting, or excessive exercise to control body weight.

4. Persistent concern with body weight and body shape.

Bulimia nervosa is more common than anorexia nervosa, the prevalence in the general population being about 2–3 percent. However, the prevalence among college students may be much higher. In a recent review, Haller indicated up to 10 percent of college students may be bulimic. As with anorexia nervosa, similar characteristics may underlie the development of bulimia nervosa, including the desire for thinness and chronic low self-esteem.

Adverse health effects of bulimia nervosa include erosion of tooth enamel, tears in the esophagus, aspiration pneumonia, and heart failure, all of which may be vomiting-induced. As with anorexics, bulimics are in need of psychological counseling by qualified medical professionals. Prozac, a drug that helps increase serotonin levels, has recently been approved for use in treating bulimia nervosa.

In a recent review, Wilson and Eldredge noted that although an estimated 30–60 percent of young females in the United States currently diet to influence body weight and shape, the prevalence of full-blown eating disorders, such as anorexia nervosa and bulimia nervosa, in the general population is only about 1–3 percent. However, Brownell and Rodin reported that the number of people who experience eating problems associated with body-weight concerns, but do not meet the strict criteria of the American Psychiatric Association for an eating disorder, is much higher. Research has also suggested that such eating problems may be more prevalent in certain professions or personal pursuits, one in particular being sports.

What eating problems are associated with sports?

Depending on the nature of the sport, the loss of excess body weight may improve appearance and/or biomechanics and enhance the potential for success. Examples of such sports include wrestling, gymnastics, ballet, bodybuilding, figure skating, diving, lightweight football, lightweight rowing, and distance running. To lose weight, athletes in these sports may exhibit some, but not all, of the characteristics associated with eating disorders. Because they may not have a fully diagnosed eating disorder, a more appropriate term may be "disordered eating."

The American Psychiatric Association lists a category, Eating Disorders not Otherwise Specified, for individuals who do not meet the criteria for anorexia nervosa or bulimia nervosa. In recent years the term **anorexia athletica** has been applied to those athletes who become overly concerned with their weight and exhibit some of the diagnostic criteria associated with anorexia nervosa or bulimia nervosa. According to Jorunn Sundgot-Borgen, an international authority on eating disorders in athletes, individuals must meet five criteria for anorexia athletica:

1. Excessive fear of becoming obese
2. Restriction of caloric intake
3. Weight loss
4. No medical disorder to explain leanness
5. Gastrointestinal complaints

In addition, they must meet one or more of these related criteria:

1. Disturbance in body image
2. Compulsive exercising

3. Binge eating
4. Use of purging methods
5. Delayed puberty
6. Menstrual dysfunction

In a recent study conducted by the National Collegiate Athletic Association (NCAA), Dick indicated that at least one documented case of an eating disorder in athletes was reported in 70 percent of the member institutions surveyed. Studies have revealed that approximately 20–40 percent of female athletes may exhibit such criteria, and rates from 50–74 percent have been reported for certain sports, such as gymnastics, distance running, and competitive bodybuilding, sports that emphasize leanness or a specific body weight. In general, this condition improves when the athletic season is completed and the athlete resumes normal dietary habits. For example, O'Conner, and others reported that symptoms of eating disorders in female college gymnasts abated after their retirement from the sport. However, what begins as a means to control weight for athletic competition on a short-term basis may develop into a long-term medical problem. Anderson proposed the notion that the development of an eating disorder is analogous to the process whereby an individual gets into a canoe some distance above Niagara Falls. When paddling downstream, the person is in control, but there reaches a point where the current of the falls takes over and the individual loses control. Several investigators have suggested that special attention should be devoted to young female athletes, particularly those involved in such sports as gymnastics and ballet, because they may meet the age, sex, and socioeconomic-status criteria that may predispose to anorexia nervosa. Coaches and others should look for unexplained weight losses, frequent weight fluctuations, sudden increases in training volume, obsession with exercise, excessive concern with body weight and appearance, and evidence of bizarre eating practices. A summary of warning signs is presented in Table 10.5.

Female Athlete Triad The female athlete triad—disordered eating, amenorrhea, and osteoporosis—was introduced in Chapter 8, with the primary focus being on calcium balance and osteoporosis. In this section, we shall consider the role of disordered eating and negative energy balance in the etiology of amenorrhea in female athletes. For a more detailed discussion, the interested reader is referred to the American College of Sports Medicine position stand on the female athlete triad.

The second component of the female athlete triad is amenorrhea, and when it occurs in athletes or those who exercise, it is often known as athletic amenorrhea. Benson and others noted female athletes may go without menstruation for 3–6 months. Although the precise cause of this form of secondary amenorrhea has not been identified, a number of theories have been proposed. Those related to

Table 10.5	**National Collegiate Athletic Association warning signs for anorexia nervosa and bulimia nervosa**

Warning Signs for Anorexia Nervosa

Dramatic loss in weight

A preoccupation with food, Calories, and weight

Wearing baggy or layered clothing

Relentless, excessive exercise

Mood swings

Avoiding food-related social activities

Warning Signs for Bulimia Nervosa

A noticeable weight loss or gain

Excessive concern about weight

Bathroom visits after meals

Depressive moods

Strict dieting followed by eating binges

Increasing criticism of one's body

National Collegiate Athletic Association. Reprinted by permission.

disordered eating include a vegetarian diet with decreased intake of Calories, protein and fat, and excessive losses of body weight. In several recent reviews, Benson and Dueck, and their colleagues, indicated that amenorrhea involves the interaction of diet and exercise, leading to a negative energy balance and possibly overtraining. Other theories involve increased intensity and duration of exercise and increased levels of psychological stress. The current focus of research is upon how these factors, primarily the hypothalamus-pituitary-gonad axis, may affect hormonal activity that governs menstruation. The hypothalamus may be influenced by all of these factors, and since the hypothalamus helps to regulate the pituitary gland, it may affect pituitary hormone secretions. The pituitary hormones, in turn, affect the gonadal secretion of sex hormones, such as the estrogens. Other hormones may also be involved, such as cortisol and epinephrine.

One of the prominent hypotheses underlying the development of athletic amenorrhea is related to excessive loss of body fat. Although no specific body-fat percentage has been associated with the development of athletic amenorrhea, the available evidence suggests that decreased fat levels may lead to a decreased production of one form of estrogen. As noted in Chapter 8, estrogen helps to reg-

ulate bone metabolism. During estrogen deficiency, the bone is more sensitive to parathyroid hormone, which gradually extracts calcium from the bone. In essence, decreased estrogen levels will impair bone tissue formation, leading to loss of bone mass and the development of osteoporosis. Although exercise is generally advocated as a means to prevent osteoporosis, it does not appear to counteract the adverse effects associated with decreased estrogen levels in athletic amenorrhea. A number of studies have shown that amenorrheic athletes have lower bone-density levels in nonweight-bearing bones such as the spine. Recent research by Myburgh and others also revealed decreased density in appendicular bones, such as the femur, although other research indicates that athletes involved in high-impact sports, such as gymnastics, may have increased bone mass. Amenorrheic athletes are more prone to musculoskeletal injuries, such as stress fractures, than athletes who have normal menstruation. Other hormonal changes in athletic amenorrhea may reduce the resting metabolic rate. These problems are currently the focus of some extensive research, but unfortunately, studies with humans are difficult to control since the cause of athletic amenorrhea itself is not known.

Unfortunately, imprecise measurement of body composition may be a predisposing factor to the development of eating disorders in athletes. As noted previously, prediction of body fat may vary considerably, so an athlete who may predict to be 10 percent by one method or prediction equation may predict to be 15–20 percent by others. If, for some reason, a coach believed that an athlete should achieve a set body-fat percentage (e.g., 8 percent), it would be wise to use a variety of techniques to predict body-fat percentages and use the lowest value predicted. This might be the safest approach to help prevent an excessive target loss of body fat that might lead to disordered eating.

Local dieticians and psychologists are excellent contacts if assistance is needed in dealing with eating disorders and may provide addresses for national help groups, such as the American Anorexia/Bulimia Association, whose website is listed in Appendix N. Many hospitals have eating disorder programs and may be able to provide questionnaires to help detect an eating disorder. The NCAA also offers brochures and videotapes to help develop awareness among athletes of the potential health risks associated with these disorders. A local college or university athletic department should be able to provide information about how to contact the NCAA.

The treatment of athletic amenorrhea involves two simple moves, exercise somewhat less and eat a little more. In some athletes, simply decreasing the amount of weekly exercise by 10 percent or so will help return normal menses, while others may resolve the problem by gaining several pounds, usually less than five. Dietary changes should include additional Calories and increased amounts of animal protein, including small amounts of meat several times per week. Increased protein and calcium from milk and other dairy products are also recommended.

Prevention of eating disorders in young athletes should receive more attention, and some state athletic associations have initiated programs for wrestling. Oppliger and others discuss the Wisconsin wrestling minimum weight project, which includes new rules and an education program to curtail "weight cutting" among high school wrestlers. This project involves skinfold estimates of fatness to determine a minimum competitive weight, a limit on weekly weight loss, and presentation of nutrition education information to help wrestlers diet effectively. The project has been very successful and provides a model for others facing similar problems with weight-control practices in sports.

Body Composition and Physical Performance

What effect does excess body weight have on physical performance?

In some sports, extra body weight might prove to be an advantage, especially in football, ice hockey, sumo wrestling, and other sports in which body contact may occur or in which maintaining body stability is important. The effect of the extra weight may be neutralized, however, if the individual loses a corresponding amount of speed. Hence, increases in body weight for sports competition should maximize muscle mass and minimize body-fat gains. In rare instances, such as long-distance swimming in cold water, extra body fat may be helpful for its insulation and buoyancy effects.

On the other hand, there are a variety of sports where excess body weight may be disadvantageous. Whenever the body has to be moved rapidly or efficiently, excess weight in the form of body fat only serves as a burden. Take a good look at high jumpers, long jumpers, ballet dancers, gymnasts, sprinters, and long-distance runners. The amount of musculature may vary in each, but the body-fat percentage is extremely low. Research has also shown that even professional football players have relatively low percentages of body fat.

According to basic principles of physics, body fat in excess of the amount necessary for optimal functioning will impair physical performance. Body fat increases the mass, or inertia, of the individual but does not contribute directly to energy production, so excess fat will detract from performance in events in which the body must be moved. For example, a high jumper can develop only so much power through muscular force when taking off. Basic laws of physics tell us that an extra 5 pounds of body fat would decrease the height to which the body center of gravity could be raised, thus decreasing the height that could probably be cleared. Extra poundage on a distance runner could add a considerable energy cost. Adding body fat would slow the running pace. In essence, the body becomes a less efficient machine when it must transport extra weight that has no useful purpose. That extra weight is usually excess body fat. Losing excess fat will not influence the total VO_2 max, but will increase VO_2 max when expressed in milliliters per kilogram body weight. For example, Craig Dean, a physician writing for *Running Times*, indicates there is a 1 percent increase in running-speed capacity for every 1 percent reduction in total body weight, provided it is primarily fat loss and not lean muscle mass. Thus, if your current running speed for a 10-kilometer (6.2-mile) race is 8:00 per mile and you lose 5 percent of your body weight as fat, your running speed would then approximate 7:36 per mile (8:00 min × 0.05 = 0:24 sec; 8:00 − 0:24 = 7:36). Similar percentage time savings are associated with other running distances, such as the marathon.

For a number of reasons it is difficult to predict with certainty a precise percentage of body fat for a given athlete that will result in optimal performance. Nevertheless, studies with elite athletes have given us some general guidelines. Male sprinters, long-distance runners, wrestlers, gymnasts, basketball players, soccer players, swimmers, bodybuilders, and football backs have functioned effectively with 5–10 percent body fat. Other male athletes such as baseball players, football linemen, tennis players, weight lifters, and weight men in track and field may average 11–15 percent, or just below the average for the nonathletic individual. Several authorities have suggested that female athletes should carry no more than 20 percent fat while others note it should be below 15 percent. Female gymnasts and distance runners have been recorded well below 15 percent; some gymnasts were even below 10 percent. Most other female athletes range between 15 and 20 percent, with some of the strength-type athletes, such as discus throwers, recording values of 25 percent or greater. Although these are some general guidelines, it should be noted that body-fat percentage is only one of many factors that may influence physical performance, and athletes may perform well even though their body fat is above these levels. However, everything else being equal, excess body fat is a disadvantage.

Care should be taken in advising athletes to lose body weight to achieve an arbitrary predetermined goal, that is, 5 percent body fat. First, recall that the measurement techniques for body composition have a 2–4 percent error rate or higher for estimating body fat. Second, the nature of the athlete's body composition may make it impossible to achieve that low level. And third, excessive weight losses may actually lead to a decrease in physical performance, just the opposite of the desired goal.

Does excessive weight loss impair physical performance?

Weight-reduction programs used by wrestlers and other athletes have been condemned by sports medicine groups, not only for health reasons but also because these practices may impair physical performance. In its recent position stand on weight loss in wrestlers, the American College of Sports Medicine noted that the practice of "weight cutting" involving food restriction, fluid deprivation, and dehydration could not only affect physical health and growth and development, but also impair competitive performance. This impairment in performance may be attributed to decreased blood volume, decreased testosterone levels, impaired cardiovascular function, decreased ability to regulate body temperature, hypoglycemia, or depletion of muscle and liver glycogen stores. However, the ultimate effect upon performance may be dependent upon the technique used—dehydration or starvation—and the time over which the weight is lost.

The effect of rapid weight loss by voluntary dehydration upon physical performance was covered in Chapter 9. In general, events characterized by power, strength, and speed may not be adversely affected by short-term dehydration, whereas performance in aerobic and anaerobic endurance events is likely to deteriorate, particularly if exercising under warm environmental conditions.

Starvation and semistarvation studies have been conducted over periods ranging from 1 day to 1 year. Short-term starvation, involving rapid weight loss, may impair physical performance if blood glucose and muscle glycogen levels are lowered substantially. Although strength and VO$_2$ max generally are not affected by acute starvation, recent studies using a 24-hour fast have shown that anaerobic and aerobic endurance performance will suffer if dependent upon muscle glycogen or normal blood glucose levels. Long-term semistarvation may lead to significant losses of lean muscle tissue and decreased performance in almost all fitness components. For example, Roemmich and Sinning compared body composition and strength measures of adolescent wrestlers with controls over the course of a wrestling season, and found that the wrestlers decreased body weight, body fat, and various measures of strength and power from pre-season to late-season. The wrestlers failed to gain lean tissue during this time frame, which the authors associated with the decrease in strength and power. However, body weight, strength, and power returned to normal during the post-season. Also, wrestlers who weight cycle during the competitive season do not experience sustained decreases in resting energy expenditure, according to a recent study by Schmidt and others who followed wrestlers over two seasons.

It was interesting to note that in some semistarvation studies in which fewer than 1,000 Calories were consumed daily, vigorous exercise programs were maintained even though the subjects were losing substantial amounts of body weight. In general, the authors noted that the key point was to prevent hypoglycemia, dehydration, and excessive loss of lean muscle mass. If these goals could be achieved, physical performance need not deteriorate on weight-loss programs. Nevertheless, Horswill and others recently found that performance on a high-intensity arm exercise task decreased significantly after subjects lost 6 percent of their body weight by either a hypocaloric low-carbohydrate diet or a hypocaloric high-carbohydrate diet. However, the impairment was less with the high-carbohydrate diet, suggesting that athletes undergoing weight loss for competition should increase the carbohydrate proportion of the hypocaloric diet. Walberg-Rankin and others also reported that although weight loss by Calorie restriction significantly reduced anaerobic performance in wrestlers, those on a high-carbohydrate refeeding diet tended to recover their performance while those on a moderate carbohydrate diet did not. Maffulli, in a case study of two elite Sumo wrestlers, noted that an 8 percent loss of body weight over a 22-day period had no effect on aerobic power (VO$_2$ max) and maximal isometric strength, but prolonged anaerobic exercise performance was impaired. Conversely, Fogelholm and others found that body-weight losses approximating 5 percent of body weight, either done rapidly in about 2 days or gradually over 3 weeks, did not impair anaerobic performance in experienced wrestlers and judo athletes.

In a unique study of the NCAA wrestlers, Scott and Horswill and their associates found that on the average, wrestlers gained approximately 10 pounds between the time of the weigh-in and NCAA championship competition 20 hours later, and that the average difference in weight between opponents on the mat was only about 3 pounds. They also reported that neither acute weight gain after the weigh-in or the weight discrepancy between opponents in the first round influenced success in this national tournament. It appears that all wrestlers are employing similar weight loss and weight regain protocols eliminating any potential competitive advantage on the mat.

It is difficult to predict the specific body weight at which physical performance will begin to deteriorate for a given individual. For those athletes who are on a weight-loss program, it may be wise to monitor performance through certain standardized tests appropriate for their sport. Some examples include basic fitness tests with measures of strength, local muscular endurance, and cardiovascular endurance. A decrease in performance may be indicative that the weight loss is excessive. Personality changes, excessive tiredness, weakness, and lack of enthusiasm may also be telltale clues.

In a recent review, Fogelholm indicated that although various forms of physical performance were adversely affected by rapid weight loss, a gradual weight loss was less likely to impair performance, and might actually improve it. Weight losses may either improve or diminish performance. The key is to lose weight properly, primarily body fat. The basic guidelines for the development of such a program to improve physical performance, or health, are presented in the next chapter.

References

Books

American Psychiatric Association. 1994. *Diagnostic and Statistical Manual of Mental Disorders DSM IV.* Washington, DC: American Psychiatric Association.

Brownell, K., Rodin, J., and Wilmore, J., eds. 1992. *Eating, Body Weight and Performance in Athletes: Disorders of Modern Society.* Philadelphia, PA: Lea and Febiger.

Heyward, V., and Stolarzyk, L. 1996. *Applied Body Composition Assessment.* Champaign, IL: Human Kinetics.

Lamb, D., and Murray, R., eds. 1998. *Exercise, Nutrition, and Weight Control.* Carmel, IN: Cooper Publishing Group.

Lee, R., and Nieman, D. 1993. *Nutritional Assessment.* Madison, WI: Brown and Benchmark.

National Research Council. 1989. *Diet and Health: Implications for Reducing Chronic Disease Risk.* Washington, DC: National Academy Press.

Shils, M., et al., eds. 1994. *Modern Nutrition in Health and Disease.* Philadelphia: Lea and Febiger.

Simopoulos, A., ed. 1992. *Metabolic Control of Eating, Energy Expenditure and the Bioenergetics of Obesity.* Basel, Switzerland: Karger.

U.S. Department of Health and Human Services Public Health Service. 1991. *Healthy People 2000.* Washington, DC: U.S. Government Printing Office.

Reviews

Ailhaud, G., et al. 1992. A molecular view of adipose tissue. *International Journal of Obesity* 16 (2): S17–S21.

American College of Sports Medicine. 1997. Position stand: The female athlete triad. *Medicine and Science in Sports and Exercise.* 29 (5): i–ix.

American College of Sports Medicine. 1996. American College of Sports Medicine Position Stand: Weight loss in wrestlers. *Medicine and Science in Sports and Exercise* 28 (6): ix–xii.

American Dietetic Association. 1989. Position of the American Dietetic Association: Optimal weight as a health promotion strategy. *Journal of the American Dietetic Association* 89:1814–17.

American Dietetic Association. 1990. Position of the American Dietetic Association: Very-low-calorie weight loss diets. *Journal of the American Dietetic Association* 90:722–26.

Anderson, A. 1990. A proposed mechanism underlying eating disorders and other disorders of motivated behavior. In *Males with Eating Disorders,* ed. A. Anderson. New York: Brunners/Mazel.

Anderson, G. 1994. Regulation of food intake. In *Modern Nutrition in Health and Disease,* eds. M.Shils, et al. Philadelphia: Lea and Febiger.

Atkinson, R. 1992. Treatment of obesity. *Nutrition Reviews* 50:338–45.

Atkinson, R. 1989. Low and very low calorie diets. *Medical Clinics of North America* 73:203–16.

Atkinson, R., and Walberg-Rankin, J. 1994. Physical activity, fitness, and severe obesity. In *Physical Activity, Fitness, and Health,* eds. C. Bouchard, et al. Champaign, IL: Human Kinetics.

Baumgartner, R., et al. 1990. Bioelectric impedance for body composition. *Exercise and Sport Sciences Reviews* 18:193–224.

Beals, K., and Manore, M. 1994. The prevalence and consequences of subclinical eating disorders in female athletes. *International Journal of Sport Nutrition* 4:175–95.

Behme, M. 1996. Leptin: Product of the obese gene. *Nutrition Today* 31:138–41.

Benson, J., et al. 1996. Nutritional aspects of amenorrhea in the female athlete triad. *International Journal of Sport Nutrition* 6:134–45.

Blundell, J., et al. 1996. Control of human appetite: Implications for intake of dietary fat. *Annual Reviews in Nutrition* 16:285–319.

Blundell, J., and King, N. 1996. Overconsumption as a cause of weight gain: Behavioural-physiological interactions in the control of food intake. CIBA Foundations Symposium. 201:138–54.

Bouchard, C. 1997. The current obesity epidemic: Chaos, gluttony, sloth, or nature? American College of Sports Medicine National Convention. Denver, CO, May 28.

Bouchard, C. 1996. Can obesity be prevented? *Nutrition Reviews* 54:S125–S130.

Bouchard, C. 1991. Heredity and the path to overweight and obesity. *Medicine and Science in Sports and Exercise* 23:285–91.

Bray, G. 1993. The nutrient balance approach to obesity. *Nutrition Today* 28 (May/June): 13–18.

Brownell, K., and Rodin, J. 1994. Medical, metabolic, and psychological effects of weight cycling. *Archives of Internal Medicine* 154:1325–29.

Brownell, K., and Rodin, J. 1992. Prevalence of eating disorders in athletes. In *Eating, Body Weight and Performance in Athletes: Disorders of Modern Society,* eds. K. Brownell, et al. Philadelphia: Lea and Febiger.

Campaigne, B. 1990. Body fat distribution in females: Metabolic consequences and implications for weight loss. *Medicine and Science in Sports and Exercise* 22:291–97.

Clarkson, P. 1998. Dietary supplements and pharmaceutical agents for weight loss and gain. In *Exercise, Nutrition, and Weight Control,* eds. D. Lamb and R. Murray. Carmel, IN: Cooper Publishing Group.

Consumers Union. 1997. What's your BMI? *Consumer Reports on Health* 9:37.

Czajka-Narins, D., and Parham, E. 1990. Fear of fat: Attitudes towards obesity. *Nutrition Today* 25 (January/February): 26–32.

Dattilo, A. 1992. Dietary fat and its relationship to body weight. *Nutrition Today* 27 (January/February): 13–19.

Dattilo, A., and Kris-Etherton, P. M. 1992. Effects of weight reduction on blood lipids and lipoproteins: A meta-analysis. *American Journal of Clinical Nutrition* 56:320–28.

Dean, C. 1994. Less weight, more speed. *Running Times* (April): 18–19.

de Groot, L., and van Staveren, W. 1995. Reduced physical activity and its association with obesity. *Nutrition Reviews* 53:11–12.

Despres, J. P. 1998. Exercise, nutrition and body fat distribution. In *Exercise, Nutrition, and Weight Control,* eds. D. Lamb and R. Murray. Carmel, IN: Cooper Publishing Group.

Despres, J. P. 1997. Visceral obesity, insulin resistance, and dyslipidemia: Contribution of endurance exercise training to the treatment of the plurimetabolic syndrome. *Exercise and Sport Sciences Reviews* 25:271–300.

DiPietro, L. 1995. Physical activity, overweight, and adiposity: An epidemiologic perspective. *Exercise and Sport Sciences Reviews* 23:275–303.

Drinkwater, B. 1992. Amenorrhea, body weight, and osteoporosis. In *Eating, Body Weight and Performance in Athletes: Disorders of Modern Society,* eds. K. Brownell, et al. Philadelphia: Lea and Febiger.

Dueck, C., et al. 1996. Role of energy balance in athletic menstrual dysfunction. *International Journal of Sport Nutrition* 6:165–90.

Eichner, E., 1992. General health issues of low body weight and undereating in athletes. In *Eating, Body Weight and Performance in Athletes: Disorders of Modern Society,* eds. K. Brownell, et al. Philadelphia: Lea and Febiger.

Fiatarone, M. Body composition and weight control in older adults. In *Exercise, Nutrition, and Weight Control,* eds. D. Lamb and R. Murray. Carmel, IN: Cooper Publishing Group.

Fogelholm, M. 1994. Effects of bodyweight reduction on sports performance. *Sports Medicine* 18:249–67.

Forbes, G. 1994. Body composition: Influence of nutrition, disease, growth, and aging. In *Modern Nutrition in Health and Disease,* eds. M.Shils, et al. Philadelphia: Lea and Febiger.

Forbes, G. 1993. Diet and exercise in obese subjects: Self-report versus controlled measurements. *Nutrition Reviews* 51:296–300.

Foster, K., and Lukaski, H. 1996. Whole-body impedance: What does it measure? *American Journal of Clinical Nutrition* 64:388S–396S.

Fraser, L. 1997. Say good-bye to dieting. *Health* (April): 57–60.

Gibbs, W. 1996. Gaining on fat. *Scientific American* 275 (August): 88–94.

Grodner, M. 1992. "Forever dieting": Chronic dieting syndrome. *Journal of Nutrition Education* 24:207–10.

Gutin, B., and Humphries, M. 1998. Exercise, body composition, and health in children. In *Exercise, Nutrition, and Weight Control,* eds. D. Lamb and R. Murray. Carmel, IN: Cooper Publishing Group.

Haller, E. 1992. Eating disorders. A review and update. *Western Journal of Medicine* 157:658–62.

Heyward, V. 1996. Evaluation of body composition: Current issues. *Sports Medicine* 22:146–56.

Hill, J., and Commerford, R. 1996. Physical activity, fat balance, and energy balance. *International Journal of Sport Nutrition* 6:80–92.

Hoffer, L. 1994. Starvation. In *Modern Nutrition in Health and Disease,* eds. M. Shils, et al. Philadelphia: Lea and Febiger.

Horswill, C. 1993. Weight loss and weight cycling in amateur wrestlers: Implications for performance and resting metabolic rate. *International Journal of Sport Nutrition* 3:245–60.

Houtkooper, L. 1998. Exercise and eating disorders. In *Exercise, Nutrition, and Weight Control,* eds. D. Lamb and R. Murray. Carmel, IN: Cooper Publishing Group.

Houtkooper, L. 1996. Assessment of body composition in youths and relation to sport. *International Journal of Sport Nutrition* 6:146–64.

Houtkooper, L., and Going, S. 1994. Body composition: How should it be measured? Does it affect sport performance? *Sports Science Exchange* 7 (5): 1–8.

Institute of Food Technologists Expert Panel on Food Safety and Nutrition. 1994. Human obesity. *Contemporary Nutrition* 18 (7, 8): 1–4.

Kinney, J. 1995. Influence of altered body weight on energy expenditure. *Nutrition Reviews* 53:265–68.

Kohrt, W. 1995. Body composition by DXA: Tried and true? *Medicine and Science in Sports and Exercise* 27:1349–53.

Kreipe, R., and Harris, J. 1992. Myocardial impairment resulting from eating disorders. *Pediatric Annals* 21:760–68.

Kushner, R. 1993. Body weight and mortality. *Nutrition Reviews* 51:127–36.

Leibel, R. 1992. Fat as fuel and metabolic signal. *Nutrition Reviews* 50:12–16.

Lindeman, A. 1994. Self-esteem: Its application to eating disorders and athletes. *International Journal of Sport Nutrition* 4:237–52.

Lohman, T., et al. 1997. Body fat measurement goes high-tech: Not all are created equal. *ACSM's Health & Fitness Journal* 1 (1): 30–35.

Lohman, T., and Going, S. 1998. Assessment of body composition and energy balance. In *Exercise, Nutrition, and Weight Control,* eds. D. Lamb and R. Murray. Carmel, IN: Cooper Publishing Group.

Melby, C., et al. 1998. Exercise, macronutrient balance, and weight control. In *Exercise, Nutrition, and Weight Control,* eds. D. Lamb and R. Murray. Carmel, IN: Cooper Publishing Group.

Miller, W. 1991. Clinical symposium: Obesity: Diet composition, energy expenditure, and treatment of the obese patient. *Medicine and Science in Sports and Exercise* 23:273–97.

Moore, M. 1983. New height-weight tables gain pounds, lose status. *Physician and Sportsmedicine* 11 (May): 25.

National Task Force on the Prevention and Treatment of Obesity. 1996. Long-term pharmacotherapy in the management of obesity. *Journal of the American Medical Association* 276:1907–15.

National Task Force on the Prevention and Treatment of Obesity. 1994. Weight cycling. *Journal of the American Medical Association* 272:1196–1202.

National Task Force on the Prevention and Treatment of Obesity. 1993. Very-low-Calorie diets. *Journal of the American Medical Association* 270:967–74.

Neumark-Sztainer, D. 1995. Excessive weight preoccupation: Normative but not harmless. *Nutrition Today* 30 (2): 68–74.

Nielsen, F. 1996. Controversial chromium: Does the superstar mineral of the mountebanks receive appropriate attention from clinicians and nutritionists? *Nutrition Today* 31:226–33.

Oppliger, R., et al. 1995. The Wisconsin wrestling minimum weight project: A model for weight control among high school wrestlers. *Medicine and Science in Sports and Exercise* 27:1220–24.

Pate, R. 1993. Physical activity in children and youth: Relation to obesity. *Contemporary Nutrition* 18 (2): 1–2.

Pi-Sunyer, F. X. 1994. The fattening of America. *Journal of the American Medical Association* 272:238.

Pi-Sunyer, F.X. 1991. Health implications of obesity. *American Journal of Clinical Nutrition* 53:S1595–S1603.

Raithel, K. 1988. Are American children really unfit? *Physician and Sportsmedicine* 16:146–53.

Robinson, J., et al. 1993. Obesity, weight loss and health. *Journal of the American Dietetic Association* 93:445–49.

Rodin, J., et al. 1989. Psychological features of obesity. *Medical Clinics of North America* 73:47–66.

Rolls, B., and Shide, D. 1992. The influence of dietary fat on food intake and body weight. *Nutrition Reviews* 50:283–90.

Saris, W. 1996. Physical inactivity and metabolic factors as predictors of weight gain. *Nutrition Reviews* 54:S110–S115.

Schwartz, M., and Seeley, R. 1997. The new biology of body weight regulation. *Journal of the American Dietetic Association* 97:54–58.

Shah, M., and Garg, A. 1996. High-fat and high-carbohydrate diets and energy balance. *Diabetes Care* 19:1142–52.

Silverstone, P. 1992. Is chronic low self-esteem the cause of eating disorders? *Medical Hypotheses* 39:311–15.

Smith, T. 1997. Fat or total Calories? Fat still dominates weight control. *Running & FitNews* 15 (5): 4–5.

Stern, J., et al. 1995. Weighing the options: Criteria for evaluating weight-management programs. *Obesity Research* 3:589–90.

St. Jeor, S. 1993. The role of weight management in the health of women. *Journal of the American Dietetic Association* 93:1007–12.

Stock, M. 1989. Thermogenesis and brown fat: Relevance to human obesity. *Infusiontherapie* 16:282–84.

Thornton, J. 1990. How can you tell when an athlete is too thin? *Physician and Sportsmedicine* 18:124–33.

Trials of Hypertension Prevention Collaborative Research Group. 1997. Effects of weight loss and sodium reduction intervention on blood pressure and hypertension incidence in overweight people with high-normal blood pressure. *Archives of Internal Medicine* 157:667 67.

Van Itallie, T., and Simopoulos, A. 1993. Summary of the National Obesity and Weight Control Symposium. *Nutrition Today* 28 (July/August): 33–35.

Vogel, J., and Friedl, K. 1992. Body fat assessment in women. *Sports Medicine* 13:245–69.

Walberg-Rankin, J. Changing body weight and composition in athletes. In *Exercise, Nutrition, and Weight Control,* eds. D. Lamb and R. Murray. Carmel, IN: Cooper Publishing Group.

Wang, L., et al. 1992. The five-level model: A new approach to organizing body-composition research. *American Journal of Clinical Nutrition* 56:19–28.

Weltzin, T., et al. 1994. Serotonin and bulimia nervosa. *Nutrition Reviews* 52:399–408.

White, J. 1992. Women and eating disorders, Part I: Significance and sociocultural risk factors. *Health Care for Women International* 13:351–62.

White, J. 1992. Women and eating disorders, Part II: Developmental, familial, and biological risk factors. *Health Care for Women International* 13:363–73.

Widdowson, E. 1988. Nutrition and cell and organ growth. In *Modern Nutrition in Health and Disease,* eds. M. Shils and V. Young. Philadelphia: Lea and Febiger.

Wilmore, J. 1991. Eating and weight disorders in the female athlete. *International Journal of Sport Nutrition* 1:104–17.

Wilson, G., and Eldredge, K. 1992. Pathology and development of eating disorders: Implications for athletes. In *Eating, Body Weight and Performance in Athletes: Disorders of Modern Society,* eds. K. Brownell, et al. Philadelphia: Lea and Febiger.

Wolf, G. 1996. Leptin: The weight-reducing plasma protein encoded by the obese gene. *Nutrition Reviews* 54:91–93.

York, D. 1990. Metabolic regulation of food intake. *Nutrition Reviews* 48:64–70.

Specific Studies

Barrow, G., and Saha, S. 1988. Menstrual irregularity and stress fractures in collegiate female distance runners. *American Journal of Sports Medicine* 16:209–16.

Bartlett, S., et al. 1996. Psychosocial consequences of weight cycling. *Journal of Consulting and Clinical Psychology* 64:587–92.

Bemben, M., et al. 1995. Age-related patterns in body composition for men aged 20–79 yr. *Medicine and Science in Sports and Exercise* 27:264–69.

Benardot, D., and Czerwinski, C. 1991. Selected body composition and growth measures of junior elite gymnasts. *Journal of the American Dietetic Association* 91:29–33.

Bergh, V., et al. 1991. The relationship between body mass and oxygen uptake during running in humans. *Medicine and Science in Sports and Exercise* 23:205–11.

Bouchard, C., et al. 1990. The response to long-term overfeeding in identical twins. *New England Journal of Medicine* 322:1477–82.

Bouten, C., et al. 1996. Body mass index and daily physical activity in anorexia nervosa. *Medicine and Science in Sports and Exercise* 28:967–73.

Buddeberg-Fischer, B., et al. 1996. Relationship between disturbed eating behavior and other psychosomatic symptoms in adolescents. *Psychotherapy and Psychosomatics* 65:319–26.

Busetto, L., et al. 1992. Assessment of abdominal fat distribution in obese patients: Anthropometry versus computerized tomography. *International Journal of Obesity* 16:731–36.

Christakis, G., and Miller-Kovach, K. 1996. Maintenance of weight goal among Weight Watchers lifetime members. *Nutrition Today* 31 (1): 29–31.

Clasey, J., et al. 1997. Body composition by DEXA in older adults: Accuracy and influence of scan mode. *Medicine and Science in Sports and Exercise* 29:560–67.

Clement, K., et al. 1995. Genetic variation in the β3-adrenergic receptor and an increased capacity to gain weight in patients with morbid obesity. *New England Journal of Medicine* 333:352–54.

Dahlstrom, M., et al. 1995. Do highly physically active females have a lowered basal metabolic rate? *Scandinavian Journal of Medicine & Science in Sports* 5:81–87.

Davis, C. 1992. Body image, dieting behaviours, and personality factors: A study of high-performance female athletes. *International Journal of Sport Psychology* 23:179–92.

DePalma, M. T., et al. 1993. Weight control practices of lightweight football players. *Medicine and Science in Sports and Exercise* 25:694–701.

Dick, R. 1993. Eating disorders in NCAA athletics programs: Replication of a 1990 study. *NCAA Sports Sciences* 3 (Spring).

Dotson, C., et al. 1997. Calibration and validation of the Futrex 6000 body composition analyzer. *Medicine and Science in Sports and Exercise* 29:S56.

Dueck, C., et al. 1996. Treatment of athletic amenorrhea with a diet and training intervention program. *International Journal of Sport Nutrition* 6:24–40.

Eckerson, J., et al. 1992. Validity of bioelectrical impedance equations for estimating fat-free weight in lean males. *Medicine and Science in Sports and Exercise* 24:1298–1302.

Fisher, J., and Birch, L. 1995. Fat preferences and fat consumption of 3- to 5-year-old children are related to parental adiposity. *Journal of the American Dietetic Association* 95:759 64.

Flegal, K., et al. 1995. The influence of smoking cessation on the prevalence of overweight in the United States. *New England Journal of Medicine* 333:1165–70.

Fogelholm, G. M., et al. 1993. Gradual and rapid weight loss: Effects on nutrition and performance in male athletes. *Medicine and Science in Sports and Exercise* 25:371–77.

Folsom, A., et al. 1993. Body fat distribution and 5-year risk of death in older women. *Journal of the American Medical Association* 269:483 87.

Frisch, R., et al. 1989. Lower prevalence of nonreproductive system cancers among female former college athletes. *Medicine and Science in Sports and Exercise* 21:250–53.

Frusztajer, N., et al. 1990. Nutrition and the incidence of stress fractures in ballet dancers. *American Journal of Clinical Nutrition* 51:779–83.

Gleeson, M., et al. 1988. Influence of a 24 h fast on high intensity cycle exercise performance in man. *European Journal of Applied Physiology* 57:553–59.

Green, S., and Blundell, J. 1996. Effect of fat- and sucrose-containing foods on the size of eating episodes and energy intake in lean dietary restrained and unrestrained females: Potential for causing overconsumption. *European Journal of Clinical Nutrition* 50:625–35.

Hahn, R., et al. 1990. Excess deaths from nine chronic diseases in the United States, 1986. *Journal of the American Medical Association* 264:2654–59.

Horswill, C., et al. 1994. Influence of rapid weight gain after the weigh-in on success in collegiate wrestlers. *Medicine and Science in Sports and Exercise* 26:1290–94.

Horswill, C., et al. 1990. Weight loss, dietary carbohydrate modifications, and high intensity, physical performance. *Medicine and Science in Sports and Exercise* 22:470–76.

Hunter, G., et al. 1997. Fat distribution, physical activity, and cardiovascular risk factors. *Medicine and Science in Sports and Exercise* 29:362–69.

Iwao, S., et al. 1996. Effects of meal frequency on body composition during weight control in boxers. *Scandinavian Journal of Medicine & Science in Sports* 6:265–72.

Kaats, G., et al. 1996. Effects of chromium picolinate supplementation on body composition: A randomized, double-masked, placebo-controlled study. *Current Therapeutic Research: Clinical and Experimental* 57:747–56.

Kaminsky, L., and Whaley, M. 1993. Differences in estimates of percent body fat using bioelectrical impedance. *Journal of Sports Medicine and Physical Fitness* 33:172–77.

Kanaley, J., et al. 1993. Differential health benefits of weight loss in upper-body and lower-body obese women. *American Journal of Clinical Nutrition* 57:20–26.

Katzel, L., et al. 1995. Effects of weight loss vs aerobic exercise training on risk factors for coronary disease in healthy, obese, middle-aged and older men. *Journal of the American Medical Association* 274:1915–21.

Kirchner, E., et al. 1996. Effect of past gymnastics participation on adult bone mass. *Journal of Applied Physiology* 80:226–32.

Kiriike, N., et al. 1992. Reduced bone density and major hormones regulating calcium metabolism in anorexia nervosa. *Acta Psychiatrica Scandinavica* 86:358–63.

Kirkwood, S., et al. 1990. Spontaneous physical activity is a major determinant of 24-hour sedentary energy expenditure. *Medicine and Science in Sports and Exercise* 22:S49.

Klein, S., et al. 1996. Adipose tissue leptin production and plasma leptin kinetics in humans. *Diabetes* 45:984–87.

Klesges, R., et al. 1993. Effects of television on metabolic rate: Potential implications for childhood obesity. *Pediatrics* 91:281–86.

Kono, I., et al. 1988. Weight reduction in athletes may adversely affect the phagocytic function of monocytes. *Physician and Sports Medicine* 16 (July): 56–65.

Kuczmarski, R., et al. 1994. Increasing prevalence of overweight among U.S. adults. *Journal of the American Medical Association* 272:205–11.

Liebel, R., et al. 1995. Changes in energy expenditure resulting from altered body weight. *New England Journal of Medicine* 332:621–28.

Losonczy, K., et al. 1995. Does weight loss from middle age to old age explain the inverse weight mortality relation in old age? *American Journal of Epidemiology* 141:312–21.

Lotti, T., et al. 1990. Proteoglycans in so-called cellulite. *International Journal of Dermatology* 29:272–74.

Lukaski, H. 1993. Soft tissue composition and bone mineral status: Evaluation by dual-energy x-ray absorptiometry. *Journal of Nutrition* 123 (2): 438–43.

Maffulli, N. 1992. Making weight: A case study of two elite wrestlers. *British Journal of Sports Medicine* 26:107–10.

Manson, J., et al. 1995. Body weight and mortality among women. *New England Journal of Medicine* 333:677–85.

Marin, P., et al. 1992. The effects of testosterone treatment on body composition and metabolism in middle-aged obese men. *International Journal of Obesity* 16:991–97.

Marin, P., et al. 1992. The morphology and metabolism of intraabdominal adipose tissue in men. *Metabolism* 41:1242–48.

Mattes, R. 1993. Fat preference and adherence to a reduced-fat diet. *American Journal of Clinical Nutrition* 57:373–81.

McCargar, L., et al. 1996. Chronic dieting does not result in a sustained reduction in resting metabolic rate in overweight women. *Journal of the American Dietetic Association* 96:1175–77.

McCrory, M., et al. 1995. Evaluation of a new air displacement plethysmograph for measuring human body composition. *Medicine and Science in Sports and Exercise* 27:1686–91.

McLean, K., and Skinner, J. 1992. Validity of Futrex-5000 for body composition determination. *Medicine and Science in Sports and Exercise* 24:253–58.

Must, A., et al. 1992. Long-term morbidity and mortality of overweight adolescents. *New England Journal of Medicine* 327:1350–55.

Myburgh, K., et al. 1993. Low bone mineral density at axial and appendicular sites in amenorrheic athletes. *Medicine and Science in Sports and Exercise* 25:1197–1202.

Nelson, M., et al. 1996. Analysis of body-composition techniques and models for detecting change in soft tissue with strength training. *American Journal of Clinical Nutrition* 63:678–86.

O'Conner, P., et al. 1996. Eating disorder symptoms in former female college gymnasts: Relations with body composition. *American Journal of Clinical Nutrition* 64:840–43.

Orphanidou, C., et al. 1994. Accuracy of subcutaneous fat measurement: Comparison of skinfold calipers, ultrasound, and computed tomography. *Journal of the American Dietetic Association* 94:855–58.

Pate, R., et al. 1989. Relationship between skinfold thickness and performance of health related fitness test items. *Research Quarterly for Exercise and Sport* 60:183–88.

Pichard, C., et al. 1997. Body composition by x-ray absorptiometry and bioelectrical impedence in female runners. *Medicine and Science in Sports and Exercise* 29:1527–34.

Rodin, J., et al. 1990. Weight cycling and fat distribution. *International Journal of Obesity* 14:303–10.

Roemmich, J., and Sinning, W. 1996. Sport-seasonal changes in body composition, growth, power and strength of adolescent wrestlers. *International Journal of Sports Medicine* 17:92–99.

Rogol, A., et al. 1992. Long-term endurance training alters the hypothalamic-pituitary axes for gonadotropins and growth hormone. *Endocrinology and Metabolism Clinics of North America* 21:817–32.

Sakurai, T., et al. 1998. Orexins and orexin receptors: A family of hypothalamic neuropeptides and G protein-coupled receptors that regulate feeding behavior. *Cell* 92:573–85.

Schmidt, W., et al. 1993. Two seasons of weight cycling does not lower resting metabolic rate in collegiate wrestlers. *Medicine and Science in Sports and Exercise* 25:613–19.

Scott, J., et al. 1994. Acute weight gain in collegiate wrestlers following a tournament weigh-in. *Medicine and Science in Sports and Exercise* 26:1181–85.

Shake, C., et al. 1993. Predicting percent body fat from circumference measurements. *Military Medicine* 158:26–31.

Simoes, E., et al. 1995. The association between leisure-time physical activity and dietary fat in American adults. *American Journal of Public Health* 85:240–44.

Stevens, J., et al. 1998. The effect of age on the association between body-mass index and mortality. *New England Journal of Medicine* 338:1–7.

Stout, J., et al. 1995. Validity of skinfold equations for estimating body density in youth wrestlers. *Medicine and Science in Sports and Exercise* 27:1321–25.

Stout, J., et al. 1994. Validity of percent body fat estimations in males. *Medicine and Science in Sports and Exercise* 26:632–36.

Strauss, R., et al. 1993. Decreased testosterone and libido with severe weight loss. *Physician and Sportsmedicine* 21 (December): 64–71.

Stunkard, A., et al. 1990. The body-mass index of twins who have been reared apart. *New England Journal of Medicine* 322:1483–87.

Sturmi, J., and Rutecki, G. 1995. When competitive body builders collapse. *Physician and Sportsmedicine* 23 (11): 49–53.

Sundgot-Borgen, J. 1994. Risk and trigger factors for the development of eating disorders in female elite athletes. *Medicine and Science in Sports and Exercise* 26:414–19.

Sundgot-Borgen, S. 1996. Eating disorders, energy intake, training volume, and menstrual function in high-level modern rhythmic gymnasts. *International Journal of Sport Nutrition* 6:100–109.

Sykora, C., et al. 1993. Eating, weight and dietary disturbances in male and female lightweight and heavyweight rowers. *International Journal of Eating Disorders* 14:203–11.

Telch, C., and Agras, W. 1993. The effects of a very low Calorie diet on binge eating. *Behavior Therapy* 24:177–93.

Theintz, G., et al. 1993. Evidence for a reduction of growth potential in adolescent female gymnasts. *Journal of Pediatrics* 122:306–13.

Tremblay, A., et al. 1995. Alcohol and a high-fat diet: A combination favoring overfeeding. *American Journal of Clinical Nutrition* 62:639–44.

Tremblay, A., et al. 1991. Nutritional determinants of the increase in energy intake associated with a high fat diet. *American Journal of Clinical Nutrition* 53:1134–37.

Trent, L., and Thieding-Cancel, D. 1995. Effects of chromium picolinate on body composition. *Journal of Sports Medicine and Physical Fitness* 35:273–80.

Troiano, R., et al. 1996. The relationship between body weight and mortality: A quantitative analysis of combined information from existing studies. *International Journal of Obesity* 20:63–75.

Tucker, L., and Friedman, G. 1989. Television viewing and obesity in adult males. *American Journal of Public Health* 79:516–18.

van der Kooy, K., et al. 1993. Waist-hip ratio is a poor predictor of changes in visceral fat. *American Journal of Clinical Nutrition* 57:327–33.

Van Loan, M., et al. 1995. Evaluation of body composition by dual energy x-ray absorptiometry and two different software packages. *Medicine and Science in Sports and Exercise* 27:587–91.

Walberg-Rankin, J., et al. 1996. Effect of weight loss and refeeding diet composition on anaerobic performance in wrestlers. *Medicine and Science in Sports and Exercise* 28:1292–99.

Webster, B., and Barr, S. 1993. Body composition analysis of female adolescent athletes: Comparing six regression equations. *Medicine and Science in Sports and Exercise* 25:648–53.

Williams, D., et al. 1995. Practical techniques for assessing body composition in middle-aged and older adults. *Medicine and Science in Sports and Exercise* 27:776–83.

Williams, N., et al. 1995. Strenuous exercise with caloric restriction: Effect on luteinizing hormone secretion. *Medicine and Science in Sports and Exercise* 27:1390–98.

Williams, P. 1990. Weight set-point theory and the high-density lipoprotein concentrations of long-distance runners. *Metabolism* 39:460–67.

Withers, R., et al. 1992. A comparison of four methods of estimating the body composition of male endurance athletes. *European Journal of Clinical Nutrition* 46:773–84.

CHAPTER 11

Weight Maintenance and Loss Through Proper Nutrition and Exercise

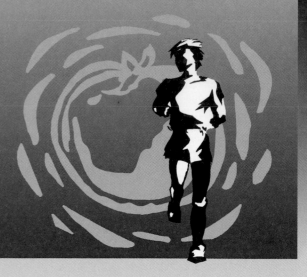

KEY CONCEPTS

• A comprehensive weight-control program involves a balanced low-Calorie diet, an aerobic exercise program, and appropriate behavior modification.

• The caloric deficit, which represents caloric intake minus caloric expenditure, may be useful as a means to predict body-weight losses on a long-term basis, because 3,500 Calories equals approximately 1 pound of body fat.

• The average adult female should be able to maintain her body weight with a daily average of approximately 14–17 Calories per pound of body weight, while males need about 15–18 Calories per pound of body weight. Slightly higher amounts of Calories are needed by children, adolescents, and physically active individuals.

• For the overweight individual who desires to lose weight without the guidance of a physician, the recommended maximal weight loss is 2 pounds per week.

• Keeping a record of your daily eating habits will help you identify behavioral patterns relative to overeating and may be used as a basis for the elimination of cues that trigger eating.

• Rapid loss of body weight, which may occur during the early stages of dieting, is due primarily to body-water changes. The rate at which weight loss occurs will slow down as your body weight decreases, for then body-fat stores are the prime source of weight loss.

• The key principle of dieting is to select low-Calorie, high-nutrient foods from among the six food exchanges that appeal to your taste and are easily incorporated into your daily life-style.

• Counting Calories and grams of fat may be a useful technique during the early stages of a diet, for the more knowledge you have about the caloric and nutrient content of foods, the better equipped you are to make wise selections.

• Very-low-Calorie diets (VLCD) may be effective for weight loss under strict medical supervision but are not recommended for the average individual trying to lose excess pounds.

• Exercise can increase energy expenditure considerably, but in order to lose body fat through exercise one should think in terms of months, not days.

• Weight-reduction exercises need to involve large muscle masses, such as the legs in jogging or bicycling or the arms and legs in swimming. Brisk walking is a highly recommended exercise program.

• The general design of the weight-reduction exercise program involves three phases: warm-up, exercise stimulus, and warm-down.

• An effective means of monitoring exercise intensity is the exercise heart rate (HR), but the exercise target HR varies depending upon age and level of conditioning. Ratings of perceived exertion (RPE) may also be used to gauge exercise intensity.

- A slow, steady progression in exercise intensity is important in preventing excess stress and injuries.
- The minimum exercise goals for losing weight are an intensity of 50–85 percent maximal HR reserve, a duration of 20–60 minutes, and a frequency of 3–5 times per week; however, duration and frequency of exercise are more important than intensity for losing weight.
- For several reasons weight loss may not occur in the early stages of an exercise program; however, the body composition changes are favorable, that is, a decrease in body fat and increase in fat-free mass.
- The rapid weight loss observed after a single bout of exercise is due to water loss through sweating.
- Although diet and exercise may each be effective in losing body weight, a combination of the two would be even more beneficial.
- Prevention of obesity is more effective than treatment, and appropriate programs should be developed early for children and adolescents.

INTRODUCTION

Given the obsession we have with slimness in the United States and the fact that millions of Americans are overweight, it is no wonder that a multibillion-dollar weight-control industry has developed. Weight-loss centers and health and fitness spas cater to this obsession and promise us new bodies just in time for the swimsuit season. Pharmaceutical companies produce drugs, both prescription and over-the-counter types, to help us lose fat the easy way. Food manufacturers market convenient, low-Calorie, prepackaged—but expensive—meals. Newspaper and magazine advertisements claim you can "Lose weight while you sleep" or "Lose 30 pounds in just 30 days." Each year at least one diet book on the best-seller list is advertised as the last diet we will ever need. One of the latest is *The Zone*.

A variety of techniques, some useful and some not, are used in attempts to stimulate weight loss. Drugs are used to depress the appetite or increase metabolism. Creams are applied to specific body parts to shrink local fat deposits. Surgical techniques include intestinal bypasses, removal of or stapling part of the stomach, excision or suction removal of subcutaneous fat tissue, and wiring the jaw shut. Weight-loss diets involve almost every possible manipulation, including the high-fat diet, the high-protein diet, the chocolate diet, the grapefruit diet, the starvation diet, and even the "no diet" diet. Advertisements claim specially designed clothing worn during exercise can help you lose inches of fat in hours. Psychological techniques such as hypnosis or behavior modification are designed to change your eating habits.

In a recent report, the Committee to Develop Criteria for Evaluating the Outcomes of Approaches to Prevent and Treat Obesity identified three types of programs and approaches to treat obesity or overweight: clinical programs, nonclinical programs, and do-it-yourself programs. No matter which program an individual selects to lose weight, the Committee recommended consultation with one's primary health care provider before engaging in a weight-loss program.

In severe cases of clinical obesity, treatment usually is administered in a clinical program under medical supervision and may involve a combination of many techniques, including surgery, hormone therapy, drugs, and starvation-type diets. An individualized, medically supervised weight-control program is very important for the clinically obese because so many health risks are related to obesity. Unfortunately, clinical obesity is very resistant to treatment and over 95 percent of those individuals who lose weight regain it within 1–5 years and may do this repeatedly. As noted in Chapter 10, these fluctuations in body weight, known as weight cycling, may not exert deleterious effects on metabolism and health and should not deter obese individuals from attempts to lose weight. The National Institute of Health notes that other groups may need medically supervised weight-loss programs, including children, pregnant women, persons over the age of 65, and individuals with medical conditions that could be exacerbated by weight loss.

Nonclinical programs for the treatment of obesity are primarily commercial franchises, using packaged materials provided by counselors who are not professional health care providers. Do-it-yourself programs include any effort by the individual to lose weight by himself or herself or through community-based and work-site programs. These treatment programs may be well-suited for individuals who have accumulated excess body fat through environmental conditions, such as excessive eating and decreased physical activity. Such programs may be beneficial to the typical adult, for substantial amounts of body fat appear to accumulate between the ages of 25 and 35. The prevalence of overweight individuals, as measured by the Body Mass Index (BMI), in the United States has increased in the past quarter-century in both children and adults. The latest government report, using a BMI of 25 as the criterion, indicated that the majority of American adults were overweight.

Because the majority of obese people who lose weight put it back on, most weight-control experts indicate the focus should be on prevention and maintenance. Prevention of excess weight gain is more effective than treatment. Prevention should be a lifelong life-style, beginning in childhood and continuing through adulthood. Preventive techniques may be especially helpful during the first 2 years of college, when young females typically gain 10–15 pounds. As noted in a twin study by Newman and others, prevention may also curtail the weight gain in those genetically predisposed. Many overweight individuals often note that the hard part is not losing weight, it's keeping it off, but that may not necessarily be so. Maintenance of a healthy body weight is a simple form of prevention; preventing weight regain is comparable to preventing weight gain in the first place.

This chapter centers on some basic questions relative to the construction, implementation, and maintenance of a sound weight-control program using the do-it-yourself approach. The principles and suggestions advanced here apply to the overweight individual who wants to lose excess body fat and also to the person with normal body weight who may want to maintain that weight level or even lose additional poundage in order to improve physical performance. For individuals interested in participating in nonclinical or clinical programs, some guidelines are offered later in this chapter.

A comprehensive weight-control program involves three components: (1) a dietary regimen stressing balanced nutrition but with reduced caloric intake; (2) an aerobic exercise program to increase caloric expenditure; and (3) a behavior modification program to facilitate the implementation of the first two components. These components are emphasized in this chapter.

Basics of Weight Control

How many Calories are in a pound of body fat?

One pound is equivalent to 454 grams. Because we know that 1 gram of fat is equal to 9 Calories, it would appear that a pound of fat would equal about 4,086 Calories (9 × 454). However, the fat stored in adipose tissue contains small amounts of protein, minerals, and water, which reduces the caloric content of 1 pound of body fat to approximately 3,500 Calories.

Is the caloric concept of weight control valid?

The caloric concept of weight control is relatively simple. As illustrated in Figure 11.1, if you take in more Calories than you expend, you will gain weight, a positive energy balance. If you expend more than you take in, you lose weight, a negative energy balance. To maintain your body weight, caloric input and output must be equal. As far as we know, human energy systems are governed by the same laws of physics that rule all energy transformations. The First Law of Thermodynamics is as pertinent to us in the conservation and expenditure of our energy sources as it is to any other machine. Because a Calorie is a unit of energy, and because energy can neither be created nor destroyed, those Calories that we eat must either be expended in some way or conserved in the body. No substantial evidence is available to disprove the caloric theory. It is still the physical basis for body-weight control.

Keep in mind, however, that the total body weight is made up of different components, those notable in weight-control programs being body water, protein in the fat-free mass, small amounts of carbohydrate, and fat stores. Changes in these components may bring about body-weight fluctuations that would appear to be contrary to the caloric concept since protein and carbohydrate contain only

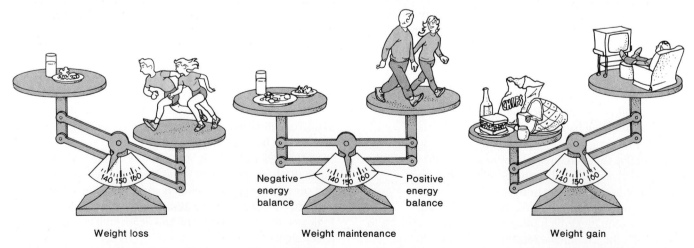

Weight loss   Weight maintenance   Weight gain

Negative energy balance   Positive energy balance

Figure 11.1 Weight control is based upon energy balance. Too much food input or too little exercise output can result in a positive energy balance or weight gain. Decreased food intake or increased physical activity can result in a negative caloric balance or weight loss.

4 Calories per gram and water contains no Calories. You may lose 5 pounds in an hour, but it will be mostly water weight. Starvation techniques may lead to rapid weight losses, but some of the weight loss will be in glycogen stores, body-protein stores such as muscle mass, and the water associated with glycogen and protein stores. In programs to lose body weight, we usually desire to lose excess body fat, and certain dietary and exercise techniques may help to maximize fat losses while minimizing protein losses.

The metabolism of human energy sources is complex, and although the caloric theory is valid relative to body-weight control, one must be aware that weight changes will not always be exactly in line with caloric input and output, and that weight losses may not be due to body fat loss alone. Also keep in mind one of the concepts advanced in the last chapter relative to individual variability in metabolic rates; two individuals may consume the same amount of Calories, yet one may gain while the other may maintain or even lose weight. Other than differences in metabolism, this possibility also may be related to the type of Calories in the diet; research has suggested that the body may store dietary fat Calories in the adipose tissue more efficiently than carbohydrate or protein Calories. In essence, compared to dietary fat, it may take more energy to convert dietary carbohydrate and protein into body fat. These concepts are explored further in this chapter.

How many Calories do I need per day to maintain my body weight?

This depends on a number of factors, notably age, body weight, sex, resting energy expenditure (REE), the thermic effect of feeding (TEF), and physical activity levels.

The caloric requirement per kilogram of body weight is very high during the early years of life when a child is developing and adding large amounts of body tissue. The Calorie/kilogram requirement decreases throughout the years from birth to old age, with exceptions during pregnancy and lactation.

Body weight influences the total amount of daily Calories you need, but not the Calorie/kilogram level. The large individual simply needs more total Calories to maintain body weight. Body weight is the most significant factor determining daily caloric intake necessary to maintain weight, although body composition also may be important.

Up to the age of 11 or 12, the caloric needs of boys and girls are similar in terms of Calories/kilogram body weight. After puberty, however, males need more Calories/kilogram, probably because of their greater percentage of muscle tissue in comparison to females.

Individual variations in REE may either increase or decrease daily caloric needs, depending on whether the REE is above or below normal. Individual variations may vary 10–20 percent from normal. An extended discussion of the REE was presented in Chapter 3.

The TEF effect may also vary among individuals. The TEF is also covered in more detail in Chapter 3.

Physical activity levels above resting may have a very significant impact upon caloric needs. Some sports, like bowling, may increase energy needs only slightly, while high-energy sports may add 1,000–1,500 or more Calories to the daily energy requirement. You may wish to review Chapter 3 regarding the caloric cost of exercise.

All of these factors make it difficult to make an exact recommendation relative to daily caloric needs. The Food and Nutrition Board of the National Research Council, for example, notes a 20 percent variation in daily caloric needs for those who engage in light to moderate physical activity. Using the data presented in Appendix A, the calculated range of caloric needs for the average adult male and female, aged 19–24, would be, respectively, 2,320–3,480 and 1,760–2,640 Calories per day. Additional ranges for other age levels may be calculated from Appendix A.

For children involved in normal activities and for adults involved in light work, Table 11.1 presents caloric needs based on body weight, expressed in both kilograms and pounds. These data are derived from the National Research Council recommendations in Appendix A, and they represent the average daily caloric intake. To calculate your average caloric needs, simply multiply your body weight by the appropriate figure in the table. For example, a 25-year-old woman who weighs 55 kg or 121 lbs would need approximately 1,925 Calories/day (55×35).

Table 11.2 represents some figures from the American Heart Association. It may be a more appropriate guide for those who want to lose some extra body fat because it provides information relative to activity level. The Calories

Table 11.1 Recommended dietary allowances for energy

	Males		Females	
Age	C/lb	C/kg	C/lb	C/kg
11–14	25	55	21	47
15–18	20	45	18	40
19–24	18	40	17	38
25–50	17	37	16	35
51 and over	14	31	14	31

Keep in mind that the values in this table are approximations. They are based on National Research Council data and represent caloric needs for children involved in normal activities and adults in light, sedentary occupations. These values may be increased significantly in those individuals who are physically active.

Table 11.2 Approximate daily caloric intake needed to maintain desirable body weight

Activity level	Calories per pound	Calories per kilogram
1. Very sedentary (movement restricted such as patient confined to house)	13	29
2. Sedentary (most Americans, office job, light work)	14	31
3. Moderate activity (weekend recreation)	15	33
4. Very active (meet ACSM standards for vigorous exercise three times/week)	16	35
5. Competitive athlete (daily vigorous activity in high-energy sport)	17 +	38 +

allocated per pound are somewhat less than those advocated by the National Research Council. For example, a sedentary individual who weighs 170 pounds needs approximately 2,380 Calories per day (170×14) simply to maintain body weight. To lose or gain weight, the caloric intake must be adjusted downward or upward. Keep in mind that the figures in both tables are approximations, and actual daily caloric needs may vary somewhat. However, these tables do offer an estimate of daily caloric needs and may be useful in starting a weight-control program.

How much weight can I lose safely per week?

If you decide to lose weight without medical supervision, the recommended maximal weight loss is 2 pounds per week. Because there are 3,500 Calories in a pound of body fat, this would necessitate a deficit of 7,000 Calories for the week, or 1,000 Calories per day. For growing children who carry excess fat, the general recommendation is about 1 pound per week, or a daily 500-Calorie deficit. Keep in mind that these are *maximal* recommended weight-loss values for medically unsupervised programs. Lower weight-loss goals, such as 1 pound per week for adults and one-half pound per week for children and adolescents, may be more appropriate, realizable goals.

As we shall see later in this chapter, weight losses may not parallel the caloric deficit we incur during early stages of a weight-reduction program, and the 2-pound limit may be adjusted during this time period. In addition, as mentioned previously, we want our weight loss to be body-fat tissue, not lean body mass. A loss of 10 pounds of body weight may help improve physical performance, but if 5 pounds is muscle tissue, then performance could possibly deteriorate. Thus, you should monitor your weight loss not only with a scale but also with skinfolds and girth measures to help ensure that you are losing body fat, hopefully in the right places.

How can I determine the amount of body weight I need to lose?

As noted in the last chapter, individuals desire to lose weight for one of three reasons—to improve appearance, health, or physical performance. As for your appearance, you are the judge, but consult with your physician or other health professional. You do not want your weight-loss program to induce an eating disorder. Losing excess body fat for health is a good reason. Check with your physician, who can also monitor health risks, such as blood pressure, serum lipids, blood glucose, and regional adiposity, associated with excess body weight. Losing weight in attempts to enhance physical performance should involve interactions between the athlete, coach, and team physician, and in the case of young athletes parents should be involved. In a recent review, Brownell and Rodin indicated that weight-loss goals should account for how much weight an individual can reasonably lose and should not be determined solely by health standards. The same reasoning applies for appearance and physical performance standards. They note that pursuit of an unrealistic ideal may lead to various health problems.

If you want to attain a body weight consistent with the Metropolitan Life Insurance Company height-weight standards presented in Appendix E, simply consult the appropriate table for your gender, height, and frame size, and set your goal to reach the appropriate weight range, preferably the midpoint. For example, if you are a 5′10″ medium-frame male, the recommended weight range is 143–158 pounds, with the midpoint about 150 pounds. If you weigh 180 pounds, you may need to develop a plan to lose 30 pounds.

If you want to use the body mass index (BMI) as a guide, you will need to calculate your current BMI and determine your target BMI. Calculation of the BMI was presented on page 316, and a healthy BMI range is approximately 19–25. The formula to calculate your desired body weight in kilograms is

Target body weight (kg) = Target BMI × height in meters^2

As an example, if you are 5′8″ (1.72 meters) tall and weigh 196 pounds (89.4 kilograms), then you have a BMI of 30 (89.4/1.72^2). If you want to achieve a healthier BMI of 22, simply multiply 22 by 1.72^2 to determine your body-weight goal; 22 by 2.96 equals 65.1 kilograms, or 143 pounds. The desired weight loss would be 53 pounds (196–143).

If you want to use body-fat percentage as the guide to weight loss, you will need to measure your current body-fat percentage and determine your target goal. Methods of determining body-fat percentage are presented on pages 318–321 and in Appendix E. If you are an athlete with 20 percent body fat but desire to get down to 15 percent, you may use the following formula:

$$\text{Target body weight} = \frac{\text{Lean body mass in pounds}}{1.00 - \text{desired body-fat percentage}}$$

As an example, an athlete who weighs 150 pounds and is 20 percent body fat has 30 pounds of body fat, and the remaining 120 pounds (150 – 30) is lean body mass. Substituting in the formula provides the following data:

$$\frac{120}{1.00 - 0.15} = \frac{120}{0.85} = 141 \text{ pounds}$$

Thus, this athlete would need to lose 9 pounds of body fat (150 – 141) to achieve a 15 percent body-fat percentage. If proper methods of weight loss are used as discussed later in this chapter, the losses will be in body fat, not lean body mass.

Behavior Modification

What is behavior modification?

One of the key components of a successful weight-control program is the need to identify and modify those behaviors that contribute to the weight problem. The subject of human behavior development and change is very complex, but psychologists note that three factors are generally involved—the physical environment, the social environment, and the personal environment. For the person with a weight problem, a refrigerator brimming with food (physical environment), a family that consumes high-Calorie snack foods around the house (social environment), and an acquired taste for high-fat or sweet foods (personal environment) may trigger behaviors that make it very difficult to maintain a proper body weight.

A model often used to explain the development or modification of health behaviors, such as a proper diet and exercise program for weight control, involves three steps—knowledge, values, and behavior. First, proper knowledge

is essential. A considerable amount of misinformation relative to the roles of nutrition and exercise in weight control exists, so you need to possess accurate information. Second, the health implications of this knowledge may help you develop a set of personal values, or attitudes, toward a specific health behavior. If you perceive excess body fat as a threat to your personal physical or psychological health, you are more likely to initiate behavioral changes. Third, your health behavior should then reflect the knowledge you acquired and the values you developed.

Behavior modification is a technique often used in psychological therapy to elicit desirable behavioral changes. The rationale underlying behavior modification is that many behavioral patterns are learned via stimulus-response conditioning; for example, a stimulus in your environment such as a commercial break in a television program elicits a response of a mad dash to the refrigerator. Because such responses are learned, they also may be unlearned. For a discussion of a comprehensive program conducted by a behavioral psychologist, the reader is referred to the review by Brownell and Kramer. Relative to a self-designed program of weight control, behavior modification is used primarily to reduce or eliminate physical or social stimuli that may lead to excessive caloric intake or decreased physical activity. George Bray, an international authority on obesity treatment, noted that the most important component of any weight-control program is the associated behavior modification through which the individual learns new ways to deal with old problems. In a recent study stressing the importance of behavior modification, Haus and others recommended that potential weight program participants should learn and practice the weight maintenance behavior of reduced dietary fat and regular exercise, independent of and before any weight reduction attempts.

How do I apply behavior-modification techniques in my weight-control program?

When breaking any well-established habit, self-discipline, or will power, is the key. The most important component of a weight-control program is you. You must want to lose weight, and you must take the major responsibility for achieving your goals. You must be convinced that reduced body weight will enhance your life, and you must establish this goal as a high priority. You must be able to tolerate some discomfort as you make life-style changes.

Both long-range and short-range realistic goals need to be established. A long-range goal may be to lose 40 pounds over 6 months, whereas a short-range goal would be to lose about 1–2 pounds per week. Losing 40 pounds may seem like a daunting task, but setting small goals, a few pounds at a time, is one of the keys to success indicated by the National Weight Control Registry, which consists of individuals who have lost at least 30 pounds and have kept it off for a year or more. A long-range goal

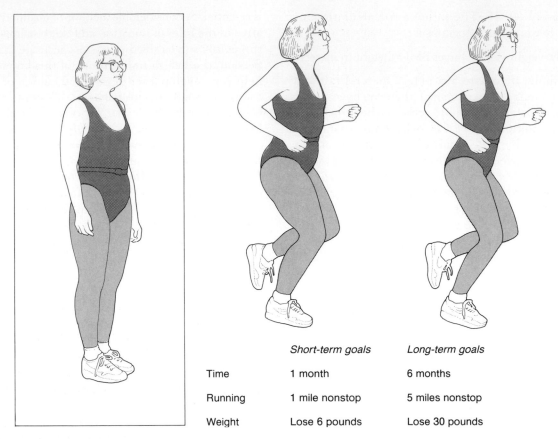

	Short-term goals	Long-term goals
Time	1 month	6 months
Running	1 mile nonstop	5 miles nonstop
Weight	Lose 6 pounds	Lose 30 pounds

Figure 11.2 Goal setting is an important factor in an exercise program.

may also include a large number of behavioral changes to achieve the 40-pound weight loss, but the number of changes would be phased in gradually on a short-term basis. Do not expect to make all recommended behavioral changes overnight. (See Figure 11.2.)

As the saying goes, nothing breeds success like success, so it is extremely important to set short-term goals that may be attainable in a reasonable length of time so that you may experience multiple successes in pursuit of your long-term goal. When you achieve your first short-term goal, a new short-term goal should be established as you progress toward your long-term goal. It is also important to remember that no initial short-term goal is too small, nor is any new short-term goal too small in the progress towards your long-term goal. As you achieve each short-term goal, you should reward yourself with something appropriate to the occasion; a reward will provide you with positive feedback to your commitment to your weight-loss program.

One of the first steps in a behavior modification program is to identify those physical and social environmental factors that may lead to problem behaviors. Keeping a diary of your daily activities for a week or two may help you identify some behavioral patterns that may contribute to overeating and extra body weight. The following are some of the factors that might be recorded each time you eat, along with a brief explanation of their possible importance. You should also record your daily physical activity.

Type of food and amount This may be related to the other factors. For example, do you eat a high-Calorie food during your snacks?

Meal or snack You may find yourself snacking four or five times a day.

Time of day Do you eat at regular hours or have a full meal just before retiring at night?

Degree of hunger How hungry were you when you ate—very hungry or not hungry at all? You may be snacking when not hungry.

Activity What were you doing while eating? You may find TV watching and eating snack foods are related.

Location Where do you eat? The office or school cafeteria may be the place you eat a high-Calorie meal.

Persons involved Whom do you eat with? Do you eat more when alone or with others? Being with certain people may trigger overeating.

Emotional feelings   How do you feel when eating? You might eat more when depressed than when happy, or vice versa.

Exercise   How much walking, stair climbing, or regular exercise do you get? Do you ride when you could possibly walk? How much time do you just sit?

Recording this information may make you aware of the physical and social circumstances under which you tend to overeat or be physically inactive. This awareness may be useful to help implement behavioral changes that may make weight control easier. The following suggestions are often helpful:

Foods to eat:
1. Use low-Calorie foods for snacks.
2. Plan low-Calorie, high-nutrient meals.
3. Plan your food intake for the entire day.
4. Eat only foods that have had minimal or no processing.
5. Allow yourself very small amounts of high-Calorie foods that you like, but stay within daily caloric limitations.
6. Know the Food Exchange System, particularly high-fat foods.

Food purchasing:
1. Do not shop when hungry.
2. Prepare a shopping list and do not deviate from it.
3. Buy only foods that are low in Calories and high in nutrient value. Read food labels.
4. Buy natural foods as much as possible.

Food storage:
1. Keep high-Calorie food out of sight and in sealed containers or cupboards.
2. Have low-Calorie snacks like carrots and radishes readily available.

Food preparation and serving:
1. Only buy foods that need preparation of some type.
2. Do not add fats or sugar in preparation, if possible.
3. Prepare only small amounts.
4. Do not use serving bowls on the table.
5. Put the food on the plate, preferably a small one.

Location:
1. Eat only in one place, such as the kitchen or dining area.
2. Avoid food areas such as the kitchen or snack table at a party.
3. Avoid restaurants where you are most likely to buy high-Calorie items.

Restaurant eating:
1. When eating out, select the low-Calorie items.
2. Request your meals be prepared without fat.

3. Have condiments like butter, mayonnaise, and salad dressing served on the side.

Methods of eating:
1. Eat slowly; chew food thoroughly or drink water between bites.
2. Eat with someone, for conversation can slow down the eating process.
3. Cut food into small pieces.
4. Do not do anything else while eating, such as watching TV.
5. Relax and enjoy the meal.
6. Eat only at specified times.
7. Eat only until pleasantly satisfied, not stuffed.
8. Spread your Calories over the day, eating small amounts more often.

Activity:
1. Walk more. Park the car or get off the bus some distance from work. Briskly walk the dog.
2. Use the stairs instead of the elevator when possible.
3. Take a brisk walk instead of a coffee-donut break.
4. Get involved in activities with other people, preferably physical activities that will burn Calories.
5. Avoid sedentary night routines.
6. Start a regular aerobic exercise program including both aerobic and resistance exercises.

Mental attitude:
1. Recognize that you are not perfect and lapses may occur.
2. Deal positively with your lapse; put it behind you and get back on your program.
3. Put reminders on the refrigerator door at home or on your telephone at work.
4. Reward yourself for sticking to your plans.

Self-discipline and self-control:
1. Establish weight loss as a high priority.
2. Think about this priority before eating.

For the interested reader, the books by Dusek and Miller provide an in-depth coverage of behavior modification for weight-control purposes. Many of the commercial, medically oriented weight-loss centers as well as organizations such as Weight Watchers International also may be sources of information. Self-taught, self-administered weight-loss programs may also be very effective, as indicated in the study by Wayne Miller and his associates.

Individuals with clinical obesity may need professional assistance from health counselors to implement a behavior modification program for weight control. However, others with less severe weight problems may be able to initiate their own program if they have adequate accurate information.

In a recent position statement, the American Dietetic Association resolved that successful weight management requires a lifelong commitment to healthful lifestyle behaviors emphasizing eating practices and daily physical activities that are attainable and enjoyable. The remainder of this chapter focuses on the development of a proper diet and exercise program for losing weight safely.

Dietary Modifications

How can I determine the number of Calories needed in a diet to lose weight?

To determine the number of Calories you may consume daily on your diet, you need to estimate your current daily energy expenditure, which includes your basal metabolic rate and your normal daily activities. One way to do this would be to keep track of your daily caloric intake (some guidelines are presented later) for 3–7 days when your body weight is stable. Computerized dietary analyses facilitate this task and many programs will also calculate the number of Calories you may consume to reach a desired body weight.

Other methods to estimate your daily energy expenditure are also available. For example, you may refer to Table 11.2 on page 348 to determine the approximate number of Calories per day you need to maintain your current body weight. Next, you need to decide how much weight you want to lose per week. One pound is a preferable goal, but you may lose up to 2 pounds safely.

For our purposes, we will use the value of 3,500 Calories to represent 1 pound of body-fat, or body-weight, loss. To lose 1 pound of body fat, you must create a 3,500 Calorie deficit. To lose 1 pound per week your daily caloric deficit should be 500 (3,500/7). To lose 2 pounds per week, the recommended maximum unless under medical supervision, the daily caloric deficit should be 1,000 (7,000/7).

Once you calculate your daily energy expenditure, simply subtract your daily caloric deficit from it; the result will be your recommended daily caloric intake. An example is presented below:

Example: 35-year-old sedentary woman who weighs 140 pounds desires to lose 1 pound per week.

1. From Table 11.2, Calories/lb needed to maintain body weight: 14

2. Predicted total number of Calories to maintain body weight:

$$14 \times 140 = 1,960 \text{ Calories/day}$$

3. Recommended daily caloric deficit = 500 Calories/day

4. Recommended daily caloric intake = 1,460 Calories

$$(1,960 - 500 = 1,460 \text{ Calories/day})$$

Another technique that has been recommended simply multiplies the body weight in pounds by 10 Calories. This technique is based upon the premise that the body weight may not be maintained at this level of caloric intake. For our example above, the recommended daily caloric intake would be 1,400 (10×140).

However, it is important to note that most health professionals do not recommend weight-loss diets lower than 1,000 Calories unless medically supervised.

How can I predict my body-weight loss through dieting?

As mentioned in the last chapter, the human body is composed of different components, most commonly compartmentalized into body fat and lean body mass; lean body mass is about 70 percent water. On a dietary program, weight loss may reflect decreases in body fat, body water, or muscle mass, all of which present different caloric values. For example, 1 pound of body fat equals about 3,500 Calories, while an equivalent weight of water contains no Calories. Because of this fact, it is difficult to predict exactly how much body weight one will lose on any given diet, but an approximate value of the time it will take to lose excess body fat may be obtained.

The key point is the caloric deficit. The number of days it takes for this daily deficit to reach 3,500 is how long it will take you to lose 1 pound.

Table 11.3 illustrates the importance of the caloric deficit in determining the rapidity of weight loss by dieting. The higher the deficit, the faster you lose weight. However, rapid weight-loss programs are not usually desirable, and the dieter should realize that a moderate caloric deficit, say 500 Calories/day, may effectively reduce weight in time and yet provide a satisfying diet.

This table is based upon the value of 3,500 Calories for a pound of body fat. There is one precaution, however. Once you lose 5 pounds and every succeeding 5 pounds thereafter, you must adjust the number of Calories it takes to maintain your body weight, for now you are 5 pounds lighter. In our example above, for every 5-pound loss the woman would need to reduce about 70 Calories ($5 \times 14 = 70$ Calories) from her diet to keep the caloric deficit at 500 Calories/day.

Although these prediction methods are good for the long run, daily body-weight changes may not coincide with daily caloric deficits.

Why does a person usually lose the most weight during the first week on a reducing diet?

If you start a diet with a significant caloric deficit, say 1,000 Calories/day, it would normally take you about 3.5 days to lose 1 pound of body fat. However, body-weight loss would be more rapid than this during the first several days, possibly totaling as much as 3–4 pounds. A large percentage of this weight loss would be due to a decrease

Table 11.3 Approximate number of days required to lose weight for a given caloric deficit

Daily caloric deficit	To lose 5 pounds	To lose 10 pounds	To lose 15 pounds	To lose 20 pounds	To lose 25 pounds
100	175	350	525	700	875
200	87	175	262	350	438
300	58	116	175	232	292
400	44	88	131	176	219
500	35	70	105	140	175
600	29	58	87	116	146
700	25	50	75	100	125
800	22	44	66	88	109
900	19	39	58	78	97
1,000	17	35	52	70	88
1,250	14	28	42	56	70
1,500	12	23	35	46	58

See text for explanation.

in body carbohydrate and associated water stores. When you restrict your food intake, the body would then draw on its reserves to meet its energy needs. These reserves consist of both fat and carbohydrate stores, but much of the carbohydrate, stored as liver and muscle glycogen, could be used up in several days. Because 1 gram of glycogen is stored with about 3 grams of water, a significant weight loss could occur. For example, 300 grams of glycogen, along with 900 grams of water stored with it, would account for a loss of 1,200 grams, or 1.2 kilograms; this would equal over 2.5 pounds alone. About 70 percent of the weight loss during the first few days of a reduced Caloric diet is due to body-water losses. About 25 percent comes from body-fat stores and 5 percent from protein tissue. It should be noted that loss of body protein is also accompanied by body-water losses, about 4–5 grams of water per gram of protein. As noted later, very-low-Calorie diets may lead to greater protein losses.

If you desired to lose a maximal amount of weight during a 2- to 3-day period, water restriction would cause an even greater weight loss. However, this practice is not recommended, as you would only be decreasing body-water levels. They would return to normal when you returned to normal water intake. There is one additional point relative to body water. At the conclusion of your diet, if you return to a normal caloric diet to maintain your new body weight, you may experience a rapid weight gain of 2 or 3 pounds. This may represent a replenishment of your body glycogen

stores with the accompanying water weight. It is important to keep in mind that rather large fluctuations in daily body weight, say in the order of 2 to 3 pounds, are not due to rapid changes in body fat or lean body mass; these fluctuations are due primarily to body-water changes accompanying carbohydrate and protein losses.

Why does it become more difficult to lose weight after several weeks or months on a diet program?

Weight loss is rapid during the first few days on a diet, primarily because of water loss. Because water contains no Calories, our caloric loss does not need to total 3,500 in order to lose 1 pound of weight. We may lose 1 pound of body weight with a deficit of only about 1,200 Calories, because 70 percent of the weight loss is water. The 1,200 Calories are mostly from fat with a small amount of protein. However, by the end of the second week of dieting, water loss may account for only about 20 percent of body-weight loss; one pound of weight loss will now cost us approximately 2,800 Calories. At the end of the third week, water losses are minimal. The energy deficit to lose 1 pound of body weight now approximates 3,500 Calories. In essence, as you continue your diet, weight losses cost you more Calories because less body water is being lost. At the end of three weeks, you still can be losing weight, but at a much slower rate than during the early stages.

Another factor also slows down the rate of weight loss. As you lose weight, you need fewer Calories to maintain your new body weight. Let's take an example. Suppose you are an athlete who weighs 200 pounds and from Table 11.2 you see that you need 17 Calories/pound body weight to maintain your weight. At 200 pounds this would represent 3,400 Calories/day (200 × 17). However, if your weight drops to 180 pounds after dieting for 10 weeks, you now need only 3,060 Calories, a difference of 340 Calories per day. If you want to continue to have a standard caloric deficit, then you will have to adjust your caloric intake as you lose weight. Suppose our 200-pounder wanted to have a daily caloric deficit of 1,000 Calories. His initial diet should then contain about 2,400 Calories/day (3,400–1,000). However, once he is down to 180 pounds, his diet should now include only 2,060 Calories/day (3,060–1,000). If he did not adjust his diet from 2,400 Calories, then the daily deficit would only be 660 Calories/day (3,060–2,400), not the standard 1,000 he wanted. Weight loss would continue, but at a slower rate.

You should realize that the rate of weight loss will slow as a natural consequence of your diet, but the weight you are losing at that point is primarily body fat. Keeping a standard caloric deficit may also require an additional reduction in caloric intake as you progress on your diet. Knowledge of these factors may help you through the latter stages of a diet designed to attain a set weight goal. Other factors associated with very-low-Calorie diets and exercise, discussed later, may also influence the magnitude of the caloric intake necessary to sustain a given rate of weight loss.

What are the major characteristics of a sound diet for weight control?

As you probably are aware, literally hundreds of different diet plans are available to help you lose weight. Hardly a month goes by without a new miracle diet being revealed in a leading magazine or Sunday newspaper supplement. Some of these plans may be highly recommended, for they satisfy the criteria for a safe and effective weight-reduction diet. On the other hand, many of these diets may be nutritionally deficient or even potentially hazardous to your health. For example, an analysis of eleven popular diets revealed deficiencies in one or more of several key nutrients, containing less than 70 percent of the Reference Daily Intake (RDI) for several of the B vitamins, calcium, iron, or zinc. Moreover, one of the diets contained 70 percent of the Calories as fat, and such a high content of fat and/or cholesterol may increase cardiovascular disease risk factors in certain individuals.

Certain types of diets should be avoided, including one-food diets such as the rice diet or the bananas-and-milk diet, for they may be deficient in certain key nutrients. Avoid diets that are advertised to contain a special weight-reducing formula or fat-burning enzymes, for such compounds simply do not exist or are not effective. In general, you should avoid diets that promise fast and easy weight losses. There is no fast and easy dietary method to lose excess body fat.

Highly recommended diets are based upon sound nutritional principles and also are designed to satisfy the individual's personal food tastes. Research with dieters has shown that any weight reduction diet, to be safe, effective, and realistic, should adhere to the following principles:

1. It should be low in Calories and yet supply all nutrients essential to normal body functions.

2. It should contain a wide variety of foods that appeal to your taste and help prevent hunger sensations between meals.

3. It should be suited to your current life-style, being easily obtainable whether you eat most of your meals at home or you dine out frequently.

4. It should provide for a slow rate of weight loss, about 1–2 pounds per week.

5. It should be a lifelong diet, one that will satisfy the first three principles once you attain your desired weight.

In addition, foods that adhere to the principles of healthful eating should be selected. This information was summarized in Chapter 2, but for now the major concern is with Calories.

Is it a good idea to count Calories when attempting to lose body weight?

There are both pros and cons to counting Calories. On the con side, counting Calories may not be practical for many who are too busy to plan a daily menu designed around a caloric limit. How many Calories are in the lunch or dinner you eat out daily? And how about serving sizes? Can you picture 3 ounces of roast beef or an ounce of cheese? Also, it may be difficult to calculate the exact amount of Calories consumed, as the caloric content in foods may vary somewhat. For example, certain slices of bread are larger than others and may have a correspondingly higher caloric content. Although these problems are not difficult to solve, it does take some effort.

On the pro side, counting Calories may be very helpful during the early stages of a diet. Knowledge of the food exchange lists and use of Nutrition Facts on food labels will enable you to substitute one low-Calorie food for another in your daily menu. As you become familiar with the caloric content of various foods it becomes easier to select those that are low in Calories but high in nutrient value, and to avoid those foods just the opposite, high in

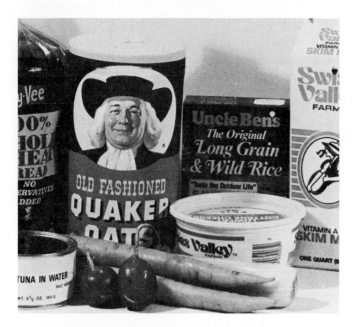

Figure 11.3 A key dietary principle is to select foods high in nutrients but low in Calories.

Calories and low in nutrients. It will require a little effort in the beginning phases of a diet to learn the Calories in a given quantity of a certain food, but once learned and incorporated into your life-style this knowledge is a valuable asset to possess not only when trying to lose weight, but also when maintaining a healthy weight over a lifetime. As you incorporate low-Calorie, high-nutrient foods into your diet, as depicted in Figure 11.3, it will eventually become second nature to you, and you may eliminate the need to count Calories.

The key to keeping track of Calories is to keep track of dietary fat. With knowledge of the Food Exchange System and the new food labels, you should be able to determine the grams of fat that you consume daily. Less than 30 percent of your dietary Calories should be derived from fat. On a diet of 1,800 Calories per day, less than 540 Calories should come from fat (1,800 × 0.30), which is the equivalent of 60 grams of fat because 1 gram of fat contains 9 Calories (540/9). Diets containing only 10–20 percent fat Calories may also be recommended.

Once you have attained your desired weight, a good set of scales would be most helpful. Keeping track of your weight on a day-to-day basis will enable you to decrease your caloric intake for several days once you notice your weight beginning to increase again. Individuals in the National Weight Control Registry who have lost weight and kept it off weigh themselves daily once their weight goal is reached, noting it is easier to deal with a gain of a few pounds rather than 10 or 20. Short-term prevention is more effective than long-term treatment. The dietary habits you acquire during the Calorie-counting phase of your diet will help you during these short-term prevention periods.

What is the Food Exchange System?

At this time it is important to expand our discussion of the Food Exchange System, which was introduced in Chapter 2. The **Food Exchange System** was developed by a group of health organizations, including the American Dietetic Association, as a means to advise patients about healthy eating. In essence, six food groups were established, and foods were assigned to these groups on the basis of similar caloric content and nutritional value. For our purposes at this time, we will concentrate upon the caloric value, but you may also want to refresh your memory on the grams of fat per food exchange.

The six food exchange lists may be found in Appendix F. You should study these lists and get an idea of the types and amounts of foods in each that constitute one exchange. Memorizing the caloric value of each food exchange is instrumental in determining the number of Calories you consume daily and also in planning a healthful, low-Calorie diet. The caloric content of one serving from each of the six exchanges is listed below and expressed in Figure 11.4.

1 vegetable exchange	= 25 Calories
1 fruit exchange	= 60 Calories
1 fat exchange	= 45 Calories
1 starch exchange	= 80 Calories
1 meat exchange	= 35–100 Calories
Very lean	= 35 Calories
Lean	= 55 Calories
Medium fat	= 75 Calories
High fat	= 100 Calories
1 milk exchange	= 90–150 Calories
Skim	= 90 Calories
Low fat	= 120 Calories
Whole	= 150 Calories

Table 11.4 presents a breakdown of the carbohydrate, fat, protein, and Calorie content of each food exchange.

How can I determine the number of Calories I eat daily?

Simply keep an accurate daily record of what you eat and then determine the caloric value from Appendix F. Food intake should be recorded over a 3–7 day period, as one single day may give a biased value. Experiments have shown that this method may provide relatively accurate accounts of caloric intake if the amounts of food ingested are measured accurately. The main problem for most

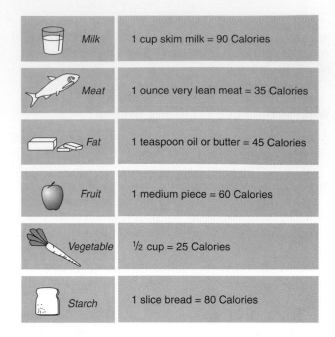

Figure 11.4 Knowledge of the various food exchanges and their caloric values can be very helpful in planning a diet. With a little effort, you can learn to estimate the caloric value of most basic foods. See Appendix F for other food examples and serving sizes.

people is determining what and how much has been eaten. An 8-ounce glass of skim milk is easy to record, and the caloric value in Appendix F is rather precise. However, how many Calories are in a slice of pizza at your favorite Italian restaurant? How big was the piece? What is the caloric content of the cheese, green peppers, pepperoni, and mushrooms? When we deal with complex food combinations such as this, our estimates of caloric content are not as precise. However, some estimates are presented in Appendix F in the section on combination foods. For example, one-quarter of a 10-inch cheese pizza with thin crust contains two starch, two medium-fat meat, and one fat exchange, or the equivalent of 355 Calories.

Although you may wish to use a ruler, a small measuring scale, and a measuring cup at home to accurately record the amount of food you eat, they are not practical for many dining situations. The following may serve as guidelines for you to record the type and amount of food you eat:

1. Keep a small notepad with you. Record the foods you have eaten as soon as possible, noting the kind of food and the amount.

2. Check the labels of the foods you eat. Most commercial products today have nutritional

Table 11.4 Carbohydrate, fat, protein, and Calories in the six food exchanges

Food exchange	Carbohydrate	Fat	Protein	Calories	Average serving size*
Vegetables	5	0	2	25	1/2 cup cooked; 1 cup raw
Fruits	15	0	0	60	1/2 cup fresh fruit or juice
Fat	0	5	0	45	1 teaspoon (5 grams)
Meat and meat substitutes					1 ounce
Very lean	0	0–1	7	35	
Lean	0	3	7	55	
Medium fat	0	5	7	75	
High fat	0	8	7	100	
Starch	15	0–1	3	80	1/3–1/2 cup cereal or pasta; 1 slice of bread
Milk					1 cup (8 fluid ounces)
Skim and very low fat	12	0–3	8	90–110	
Low fat	12	5	8	120	
Whole	12	8	8	150	

Carbohydrate, fat, and protein in grams.

1 g carbohydrate = 4 Calories
1 g fat = 9 Calories
1 g protein = 4 Calories

*See Appendix F for specific foods.

Source: *Exchange Lists for Meal Planning*, American Diabetes Association and American Dietetic Association, Chicago, ADA, 1995.

information listed, including the number of Calories per serving. Record these data when available.

3. Calories for most fluids are given in relationship to ounces. For fluids, remember that 1 cup or regular glass is about 8 ounces. Most regular canned drinks contain 12 ounces, although smaller and larger sizes are available.

4. Calories for meat, poultry, fish, and other related products are usually given by ounces. To get an idea of how many ounces are in these products, you could purchase a set weight of meat, say 16 ounces, and cut it into four equal pieces. Each would weigh approximately 4 ounces, or about the visual size of a deck of playing cards. Get a mental picture of this size and use it as a guide to portion sizes.

5. For fruits and vegetables the caloric values are usually expressed relative to 1/2 cup or a small-sized piece. At home, measure 1/2 cup of vegetables or fruit and place it in a bowl or on a plate. Again, make a mental picture of this serving size and use it as a reference. Compare the sizes of different fruits and notice the difference between a small, medium, and large piece.

6. For starch products, the Calories are most often expressed per serving, such as an average-size slice of bread or a dinner roll. In these cases it is relatively easy to determine quantity. Depending on the type of cereal, pasta, grain, or starchy vegetable, the measure for one exchange is usually 1/3 or 1/2 cup, but some serving sizes are larger, such as puffed cereals. See Appendix F. Use the mental picture concept again to estimate quantities.

7. For substances such as sugar, jams, jellies, nondairy creamers, and related products, make a mental picture of a teaspoon and tablespoon. These are common means whereby Calories are given. One level teaspoon of sugar is about 20 Calories; jams and jellies contain similar amounts. Caloric values of other products may be obtained from nutrition labels.

8. Some combination foods, such as a homemade casserole, are included in Appendix F. However, for combination foods not listed, you will need to list the ingredients separately to calculate the caloric content. Labels on most food products list caloric content per serving.

9. Caloric values for many fast-food restaurant items may be found in Appendix G. Most fast-food restaurants provide information on the nutrient content of their products, but you need to ask for it.

Through experience you should be able to readily identify, within a small error range, the quantities of food you eat. This is not only helpful for determining your caloric intake but may also serve as a motivational device to restrict portion sizes when you are on a weight-loss diet.

The following represents an example of how you might record one meal and calculate the caloric intake from Appendix F or food labels.

Breakfast Food	Quantity	Calories
Milk, skim	1 glass, 8 ounces	90
Eggs	2, poached	150
Toast, whole wheat	2 slices	160
with butter	2 pats	90
with jelly	1 tablespoon	60
Orange juice	1 glass, 8 ounces	120
Coffee	1 cup, 8 ounces	0
with sugar	1 teaspoon	20
TOTAL		690

Computer programs are available to calculate caloric intake as well as nutrient content. Local hospitals or universities should be able to direct you to a source. Moreover, nutritional analysis software programs are available from many software retailers or on the Internet for personal home computers.

Knowledge, however, is not the total answer; your behavior should reflect your knowledge. For example, you may know that whole milk contains about 60 more Calories per glass than skim milk, but if you cannot develop a taste for skim milk then the advantage of your knowledge is lost in this instance.

What are some general guidelines I can use in the selection and preparation of foods to reduce caloric intake?

As for the diet itself, there are a variety of helpful suggestions in the battle against Calories.

1. The key principle is to select foods with **quality Calories**—low-Calorie, high-nutrient foods from across the six food exchanges or the food groups in the Food Guide Pyramid. Avoid refined, processed foods as much as possible and include more natural, unrefined products in your diet. If you do buy convenience meals, select those that are low in Calories and fat. Check the label for total fat and total Calories from fat. Review the technique presented in Table 5.2 on page 141.

2. Reduce the amount of fat in the diet. Dietary fat appears to play several roles in the development of obesity. First, it is rich in Calories—more than double the amount of Calories per gram as compared to carbohydrate and protein. Second, dietary fat is appetizing and does not appear to rapidly suppress the appetite, leading to a greater intake of Calories as recently suggested by Blundell and Green. Third, dietary fat appears to be stored as

fat more efficiently than either carbohydrate or protein, even if the caloric intake is similar; this is especially true in individuals who have lost weight and may be one of the most important reasons why they regain weight so readily. Fourth, dietary fat may also be stored preferentially in the abdominal region, which may increase health risks. In a recent study, Wayne Miller and his colleagues found that lean subjects obtained a lower percentage of their dietary Calories from fat compared with obese subjects, and other research has shown that obese subjects maintain their weight by consuming foods of high-caloric density.

To reduce the amount of fat in your diet, you may wish to count the total grams of fat you eat each day. As mentioned above, a general recommendation is to keep your daily total fat intake to 30 percent or less of your total caloric intake. To calculate the total grams of fat you may eat per day, simply multiply your caloric intake by 30 percent and divide by 9 (the Calories per gram of fat). You may wish to get the fat content to a lower percentage, such as 20 percent. Table 11.5 presents the formula and some calculations for different caloric intake levels and percentages of dietary fat intake.

The recent development of fat substitutes may be helpful in reducing fat intake. Many fat-free products are currently available and may decrease total fat and caloric intake if used judiciously within a healthful diet. However, Miller and Groziak noted that although fat substitutes may help decrease dietary fat intake and percentage of caloric intake from fat, many individuals will compensate by increasing their consumption of other macronutrients, primarily carbohydrate. Research by Shide and Rolls supports this point, indicating individuals eat more food at a given meal if they know some of the meal consists of low-fat items. Cotton and others suggest you gradually blend fat substitutes into your diet; making many changes at one time may lead to overconsumption of other foods, and hence your overall caloric intake may remain the same, or even increase. Fat substitutes can be part of an overall healthful diet for weight loss, provided you do not compensate for the saved Calories by ingesting other Calorie-rich foods. Remember that you need some fat in your diet for essential fatty acids and fat-soluble vitamins, which you may be able to obtain in a diet containing 10 percent fat Calories. Do not eliminate all fat from your diet.

Additional suggestions for reducing dietary fat are included in the following guidelines, but you may wish to review Chapter 5 for additional information. Once individuals adapt to a low-fat diet, they may prefer it because high-fat meals are

Table 11.5 Calculation of daily fat intake in grams

To use this table, determine the number of Calories per day in your diet and the percent of dietary Calories you want from fat, and then find the grams of fat you may consume daily. For example, if your diet contains 2,200 Calories and you desire to consume only 20 percent of your daily Calories as fat, then you could consume 49 grams of fat.

Daily caloric intake	30% fat Calories (maximal grams)	20% fat Calories (maximal grams)	10% fat Calories (maximal grams)
1,000	33	22	11
1,200	40	26	13
1,500	50	33	16
1,800	60	40	20
2,000	66	44	22
2,200	73	49	24
2,500	83	55	28

digested more slowly, possibly leading to indigestion and some gastrointestinal distress.

3. Reduce the amount of simple refined sugars in the diet. This may be accomplished by restricting the amount of sugar added directly to foods and limiting the consumption of highly processed foods that may add substantial amounts of sweeteners. Artificial sweeteners may be helpful. In a recent review, F. Xavier Pi-Sunyer noted that substitution of artificial sweeteners, such as aspartame, for sugar has been shown to reduce caloric intake without leading to an increased consumption of other foods. Drewnowski also reported that some short-term studies and one long-term study have shown that artificial sweeteners could decrease caloric intake and increase weight loss, but more long-term research is recommended. Again, like fat substitutes, sugar substitutes may be an effective part of a healthful weight-loss diet.

4. In many cases, simply reducing the fat and sugar content in the diet will save substantial numbers of Calories and may be all that is needed. Did you know that fat and sugar together account for nearly 50 percent of the Calories in the average American diet? That represents 5 out of every 10 Calories. Table 11.6 provides some examples of how to save Calories via simple substitutions for comparable foods containing fat or sugar.

Table 11.6 Simple food substitutions to save Calories

Instead of	Select	To save this many Calories
1 croissant	1 plain bagel	35
1 whole egg	2 egg whites	50
1 ounce cheddar cheese	1 ounce mozzarella (skim)	30
1 ounce regular bacon	1 ounce Canadian bacon	100
3 ounces tuna in oil	3 ounces tuna in water	60
1 cup regular ice cream	1 cup fat-free frozen dessert	150
1 ounce turkey bologna	1 ounce turkey breast	50
1 McDonald's Big Mac	1 McDonald's grilled chicken	120
1 cup whole milk	1 cup skim milk	60
1 ounce potato chips	1 ounce pretzels	90
1 tablespoon mayonnaise	1 tablespoon fat-free mayonnaise	90
1 can regular cola	1 can diet cola	150

5. Milk exchange products are excellent sources of protein but may contain excessive Calories unless the fat is removed. Use skim milk, low-fat cottage cheese, low-fat yogurt, and nonfat dried milk instead of their high-fat counterparts like whole milk, sour cream, and powdered creamers.

6. The meat and meat substitute exchange products are sources of high-quality protein and many other nutrients but also may contain excessive fat Calories. Select very-lean and lean meat exchanges. Per one ounce serving, very-lean meat and meat substitutes contain only 35 Calories and less than 1 gram of fat. Examples include the white meat of chicken and turkey, tuna fresh or canned in water, shrimp, fat-free cheese, egg whites, and egg substitutes. See Appendix F for other sources. If you enjoy beef and pork, use leaner cuts such as beef eye of round, flank steak, pork tenderloin, and 96 percent fat-free hamburger. Trim away excess fat; broil or bake your meats to let the fat drip away. If you eat in fast-food restaurants, select foods that are low in fat, such as grilled chicken, lean meats, and

salads. Avoid the high-fat foods, which normally contain 40–60 percent fat Calories. Also be aware that serving sizes have increased dramatically in recent years. That large hamburger deluxe may have triple or more the Calories of a regular hamburger.

7. The starch exchange is high in vitamins, minerals, and fiber. Eating a high-fiber diet increases the gastric volume, which might help suppress appetite. Use whole-grain breads and cereals, brown rice, oatmeal, beans, bran products, and starchy vegetables for dietary fiber. Limit the use of processed grain products that add fat and sugar. Substitute products low in fat, such as bagels, for those high in fat, like croissants.

8. Foods in the fruit exchange are high in vitamins and fiber. Select fresh, whole fruits or those canned or frozen in their own juices. Avoid those in heavy sugar syrups. Limit the intake of dried fruits, which are high in Calories. Eat at least one citrus fruit daily.

9. The vegetable exchange foods are low in Calories yet high in vitamins, minerals, and fiber. Select dark-green leafy and yellow-orange vegetables daily. Low-Calorie items like carrots, radishes, and celery are highly nutritious snacks for munching. Many of these vegetables are listed as free exchanges in Appendix F because they contain fewer than 20 Calories per serving. Fruits and vegetables may provide bulk to the diet and a sensation of fullness without excessive amounts of Calories.

10. Use lesser amounts of high-Calorie fat exchanges like salad dressings, butter, margarine, and cooking oil. If necessary, substitute low-Calorie or fat-free dietary versions instead. Fat-free mayonnaise tastes good and has 90 fewer Calories than a serving of regular mayonnaise. Do not prepare foods in fats, such as with frying. Use nonstick cooking utensils.

11. Beverages other than milk and juices should have no Calories. Fluid intake should remain high, for it helps create a sensation of satiety during a meal. Water is the recommended fluid, although diet drinks and unsweetened coffee and tea may be used. Consult the free-food list in Appendix F.

12. Limit your intake of alcohol. It is high in Calories and zero in nutrient value. One gram of alcohol is equal to 7 Calories, almost twice the value of protein and carbohydrate. For 100 Calories in a shot of gin you receive zero nutrient value, but for the same amount of Calories in approximately 2 ounces of chicken breast you get nearly one-third of your RDA in protein plus substantial amounts of iron, zinc, niacin, and other vitamins. Research indicates that consuming alcohol with a meal does not substitute for other foods, so the total caloric

intake of the meal is increased. If you desire alcohol, select the light varieties of wine and beer. Substitution of a light beer for a regular beer will save about 50 Calories. You may wish to try the nonalcoholic beers, which may contain even fewer Calories.

13. Salt intake should be limited to that which occurs naturally in foods. Try to use dry herbs, spices, and other nonsalt seasonings as substitutes to flavor your food. Salt may increase the appetite or thirst for Calorie-containing beverages.

14. Instead of gorging on two or three large meals a day, eat five or six smaller ones. Although Bellisle and others reported no difference between gorging and nibbling on daily energy expenditure, they indicated that any effects of nibbling on the regulation of body weight is likely to be mediated through effects on food intake. Use low-Calorie, nutrient-dense foods for snacks. Research has shown that nibbling may help control sensations of hunger between meals and may help in other ways, possibly by minimizing the release of insulin, which assists in the storage of fat in the body.

15. Cook and serve small portions of food for meals. The temptation to overeat may be removed.

16. Learn what foods are low in Calories in each of the six food exchanges and incorporate those palatable to you in your diet. Learn to substitute low-Calorie foods for high-Calorie ones. The key to a lifelong weight-maintenance diet is your knowledge of sound nutritional principles and the application of this knowledge to the design of your personal diet.

How can I plan a nutritionally balanced, low-Calorie diet?

The key to a sound diet for weight loss is nutrient density, or the selection of low-Calorie, high-nutrient foods. The sixteen points addressed in the previous section represent important guidelines to implement such a diet. Table 11.7 presents a suggested meal pattern based upon the Food Exchange System. The foods should be selected from the food exchange lists found in Appendix F. You may use the adjacent form as a guide.

The total caloric values are close approximations for a three-meal pattern. If you decide to include snacks in your diet, such as a fruit or vegetable, then remove each snack from one of the main meals. The salads should contain vegetables with negligible Calories, such as lettuce and radishes. Note that under the exchange system, starchy vegetables such as potatoes are included in the starch group because their caloric content is similar. The beverages, other than milk and fruit juice, should contain no Calories. Although you may drink as many noncaloric bev-

Calories: _____

Meal	Number of servings	Calories per serving	Total Calories	Foods selected
Breakfast				
Milk, skim		90		
Meat, very lean		35		
Fruit		60		
Vegetable		25		
Starch		80		
Fat		45		
Beverage		0		
Lunch				
Milk, skim		90		
Meat, very lean		35		
Fruit		60		
Vegetable		25		
Salad		20		
Starch		80		
Fat		45		
Beverage		0		
Dinner				
Milk, skim		90		
Meat, very lean		35		
Fruit		60		
Vegetable		25		
Salad		20		
Starch		80		
Fat		45		
Beverage		0		

erages as you wish over the course of the day, drinking at least one at each meal will help provide a feeling of satiation and may help suppress the appetite somewhat.

Although only seven levels of caloric intake are presented in Table 11.7, you may adjust it according to your needs by simply adding or subtracting appropriate food

Table 11.7 Suggested daily meal pattern based on the Food Exchange System

	Approximate daily caloric intake						
	1,000	**1,200**	**1,500**	**1,800**	**2,000**	**2,200**	**2,500**
Breakfast							
Milk, skim	1	1	1	1	1	1	1
Meat, very lean	1	1	2	2	2	3	3
Starch	1	2	2	3	3	3	3
Fruit	1	1	1	1	2	2	2
Fat	0	0	1	1	1	2	2
Beverage	1	1	1	1	1	1	1
Lunch							
Milk, skim	1	1	1	1	1	1	2
Meat, very lean	2	2	2	3	3	3	4
Starch	2	2	2	2	2	3	3
Vegetable	1	1	2	2	2	2	2
Salad	1	1	1	1	1	1	1
Fruit	1	2	2	2	2	2	2
Fat	1/2	1/2	1	2	2	2	2
Beverage	1	1	1	1	1	1	1
Dinner							
Milk, skim	0	0	0	1	1	1	1
Meat, very lean	2	2	3	3	3	4	4
Starch	2	2	3	3	4	4	5
Vegetable	1	2	2	2	2	2	3
Salad	1	1	1	1	1	1	1
Fruit	0	0	1	2	2	2	3
Fat	1/2	1	1	1	2	2	2
Beverage	1	1	1	1	1	1	1
Totals							
Milk, skim	2	2	2	3	3	3	4
Meat, very lean	5	5	7	8	8	10	11
Starch	5	6	7	8	9	10	11
Vegetable	2	3	4	4	4	4	5
Salad	2	2	2	2	2	2	2
Fruit	2	3	4	5	6	6	7
Fat	1	2	3	4	5	6	6
Beverage	3	3	3	3	3	3	3

Key points

1. Caloric values:

Milk exchange, skim	= 90
Meat exchange, very lean	= 35
Fruit exchange	= 60
Vegetable exchange	= 25
Starch exchange	= 80
Fat exchange	= 45
Beverage	= 0
Salad	= 20

2. See Appendix F for a listing of foods in each exchange. Note the following:
   a. Foods other than milk, such as yogurt, are included in the milk exchange.
   b. The meat list includes foods such as eggs, cheese, fish, and poultry; low-fat legumes, like beans and peas, may be considered as meat substitutes.
   c. Some starchy vegetables are included in the bread list.
3. Foods should not be fried or prepared in fat unless you count the added fat as a fat exchange. Broil or bake foods instead.
4. Low-Calorie vegetables like lettuce and radishes should be used in the salads. Use only small amounts of very-low-Calorie salad dressing.
5. Beverages should contain no Calories.

exchanges. For example, if you wanted a 1,700-Calorie diet, you could subtract one starch exchange and one-half fat exchange (about 100 Calories) from the 1,800-Calorie diet.

After you have determined the number of Calories you need daily, select the appropriate diet plan from Table 11.7. To help implement your diet plan and to keep day-to-day track of the food exchanges you eat, you should design a 3″ × 5″ card similar to the model below for the number of food exchanges in your daily diet. As you consume an exchange at each meal, simply cross it off on the card. Make a new card for each day. The model shown is for 1,500 Calories. The total exchanges are summed from Table 11.7.

Daily meal plan		1,500 Calories
Milk exchange, skim	(2)	1 2
Meat exchange, very lean	(7)	1 2 3 4 5 6 7
Starch exchange	(6)	1 2 3 4 5 6
Vegetable exchange	(3)	1 2 3
Salads	(2)	1 2
Fruit exchange	(4)	1 2 3 4
Fat exchange	(2)	1 2
Beverages	(3)	1 2 3

Keep in mind that this is not a rigid diet plan. At a minimum you should have 2 skim milk exchanges, 5 very lean meat exchanges, 5 starch exchanges, 2 vegetable exchanges and 2 fruit exchanges. Once you have guaranteed these minimum requirements, you may do some substitution between the various exchanges so long as you keep the total caloric content within range of your goals. For example, you may delete 2 starch exchanges (160 Calories) in the model and substitute 1 skim milk and 2 very lean meat exchanges (160 Calories). You may also shift a limited number of the exchanges from one meal to another. If you prefer a more substantial breakfast and a lighter lunch, simply shift some of the exchanges from lunch to breakfast.

It may be a good idea to take a little time and construct a diet for yourself, using the following guidelines for your calculations. Use the form on page 360.

1. Calculate the number of Calories you want per day. See pages 347–348 for guidelines.

2. Use Table 11.7 to determine how many servings you need from each food exchange.

3. Multiply the number of servings by the Calories per serving to get the total Calories. Add the total Calories column to get total daily intake.

4. Select appropriate foods from the exchange list in Appendix F.

One final point: If your diet contains less than 1,600 Calories, it would be wise to take a daily vitamin/mineral supplement with the RDA for all essential vitamins and key minerals such as iron and zinc.

Table 11.8 presents an example of a 1,500-Calorie diet based on the Food Exchange System.

Are very-low-Calorie diets effective and desirable means to lose body weight?

As noted in Chapter 10, very-low-Calorie diets (VLCD) are defined technically as containing less than 800 Calories per day and are often referred to as modified fasts. In some medical institutions, total fasting programs are used. Under proper medical supervision, such diets are generally regarded as safe and have been effective in inducing rapid weight losses in very obese patients. However, VLCD are not recommended for the individual who wants to lose 10–20 pounds or for the individual who is not under medical supervision, not only because of the possible adverse health consequences noted in Chapter 10, but also because VLCD may be counterproductive to the ultimate goal of long-term weight loss. They do not satisfy the criteria for a recommended weight-loss program for individuals who are not medically supervised and often lead to weight cycling.

It is recommended that any individual contemplating the use of VLCD should consult a physician and a dietitian.

Is it harmful to overeat occasionally?

Most of us occasionally overindulge in food, particularly on holidays and other festive occasions or when we dine at all-you-can-eat restaurants. Eating is a pleasurable activity, and an occasional pig-out is not harmful, as long as it does not become a habit. After a very large meal you may step on the scale and find that you have gained 5 pounds or more. Not to worry. Most of that weight is water, which may be bound to the increased carbohydrate (glycogen) stores in your body. Additionally, if the meal was high in sodium, your extracellular water stores will also increase. Going back to your regular diet and exercise program will reduce these water stores in a day or so, and your body weight will return to normal.

Exercise Programs

What role does exercise play in weight reduction and weight maintenance?

Humans are meticulously designed for physical activity, and yet our modern mechanical age has eliminated many of the opportunities our ancient ancestors once had to incorporate moderate physical activity as a natural part of daily living. The regulation of our food intake has not adapted to the highly mechanized conditions in today's society. As discussed in Chapter 10, whether or not physical inactivity is a cause of obesity is debatable. However, experts on obesity note that in reality inactivity may be a consequence of obesity and can also help maintain it. For

Table 11.8 A 1,500-Calorie diet based on the Food Exchange System

Exchange	Number of servings	Calories per exchange	Total Calories	Foods selected
Breakfast				
Meat, very lean	2	35	70	1 ounce very lean ham and
Fat	1	45	45	1 ounce low-fat cheese melted on
Starch	2	80	160	2 pieces whole-grain toasted bread
Fruit	1	60	60	4 ounces orange juice
Beverage	1	0	0	1 cup coffee with noncaloric sweetener
Lunch				
Milk, low-fat	1	120	120	8 ounces plain, low-fat yogurt
Fruit	1	60	60	with cut-up fresh fruit (1/2 banana)
Meat, very lean	2	35	70	2 ounces turkey breast on
Starch	2	80	160	whole-grain bun
Vegetable	1	25	25	1 carrot
Salad	1	20	20	lettuce with
Fat	1	45	45	low-Calorie dressing
Beverage	1	0	0	diet cola
Dinner				
Milk, skim	1	90	90	1/2 cup ice milk
Meat, very lean	3	35	105	3 ounces broiled fish
Starch	3	80	240	1 baked potato and 1 slice whole wheat bread
Vegetable	3	25	75	1 1/2 cups steamed broccoli and cauliflower
Salad	1	20	20	cucumbers
Fat	1	45	45	small amount of margarine for potato and low-Calorie dressing for salad
Fruit	2	60	120	1 banana cut up on ice milk
Beverage	1	0	0	iced tea
TOTAL			1,530	

example, a sedentary life-style, principally TV watching, has been significantly associated with obesity in adolescents and adults. Indeed, the late Dr. Jean Mayer, an international authority on weight control, reported that no single factor is more frequently responsible for obesity than lack of physical exercise.

Wim Saris, an internationally respected authority on obesity, noted that although there is some uncertainty regarding the role of exercise in the treatment of obesity, a considerable amount of knowledge substantiates the point that exercise can help reduce and control body weight and should be included in a weight-loss or maintenance program. Indeed the Consumers Union recently noted that

to slim down permanently, you need to make a lifelong commitment to regular exercise, including not only aerobic exercise to burn Calories, but strength training to build or at least preserve muscle. In addition to the physiological effects upon energy expenditure, exercise may also confer significant psychological and medical benefits.

Exercise burns Calories (Figure 11.5). The primary function of exercise in a weight-control program is simply to increase the level of energy expenditure and help tip the caloric equation so that energy output is greater than energy input. As mentioned in Chapter 3, the metabolic rate may be increased tremendously during exercise. For example, while the average person may expend only 60–70

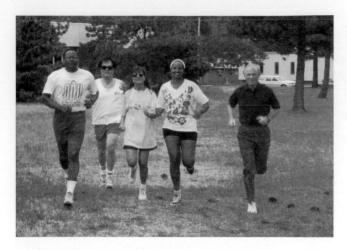

Figure 11.5 Exercise can be an effective means of increasing energy expenditure and losing excess Calories.

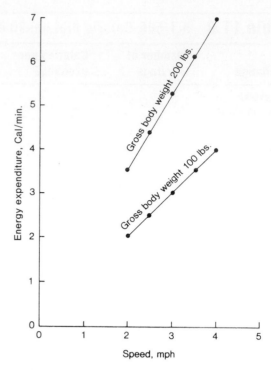

Figure 11.6 Effect of speed (mph) and gross body weight (lbs) on energy expenditure (Calories/minute) of walking. The heavier the individual, the greater the expenditure of Calories for any given speed of walking. The same would be true for running and other physical activities in which the body must be moved by foot.

From *Textbook of Work Physiology* by P.O. Astrand and K. Rodahl. Copyright © 1977 McGraw-Hill Book Company. Used with the permission of McGraw-Hill Book Company.

Calories per hour during rest, this value may approach 1,000 Calories per hour during a sustained high-level activity such as rapid walking, running, swimming, or bicycling. Athletes involved in endurance events, such as the Tour de France, and ultradistance runners, such as Yannis Kouros, have been reported to consume between 6,000 and 13,000 Calories per day.

If you are overweight, the same amount of exercise will cost you more Calories than your leaner counterpart. Because you have more weight to move, you will expend more energy and lose more body fat in the long run. For example, the energy cost of jogging 1 mile would be 70 Calories for the 100-pound individual and 140 Calories for someone twice that weight. Figure 11.6 depicts this concept graphically for one type of exercise—walking.

One major misconception may deter many individuals from initiating an exercise program for weight control. They believe that exercise is a poor means to lose body weight because it expends so few Calories. For example, they have heard that you have to jog about 35 miles to lose a pound of body fat. Because the average-sized male uses approximately 100 Calories per mile of jogging, and because 1 pound of body fat contains about 3,500 Calories, there is some truth to that statement. However, you must look at the **long-haul concept** of weight control (Figure 11.7). Jogging about 2 miles a day will expend about 6,000 Calories in a month, accounting for almost 2 pounds of body fat. Over 6 to 8 months or longer, the weight loss may be substantial provided the individual does not compensate by consuming more Calories.

In addition to the direct effect of increased energy output during exercise, exercise has been theorized to facilitate weight loss by other means. As noted in Chapter 3, exercise may increase the REE during the period immediately following the exercise bout and may also increase the thermic effect of food (TEF) if you exercise after eating a meal. Unfortunately, the magnitude of this increased

energy expenditure is relatively minor and not considered to be of any practical importance in a weight-loss program. Thus, it does not matter if you exercise before or after a light meal, although as noted below, exercise before a meal may help curb the appetite.

However, exercise may have a beneficial effect on the REE in other ways. As noted previously, very-low-Calorie diets (VLCD) may reduce the REE, and this effect may be counterproductive in a weight-loss program. Less severe caloric restriction also may reduce the REE. Although exercise will not totally prevent the decrease in the REE normally seen with weight loss, particularly with large weight losses, some studies suggest that it may help minimize the decrease, thereby helping maintain energy expenditure near normal levels during rest. However, not all research supports this finding. The interested reader is referred to the review articles by Donnelly and others, Hill and others, and Forbes.

Moreover, during exercise, the body mobilizes its fat cells to supply energy to the muscle cells. Hence, body-fat stores are reduced. Exercise, partically resistance exercise, may also stimulate the development of muscle tissue and thus increase lean body mass. In the long run, this change in body composition may actually favor a slight

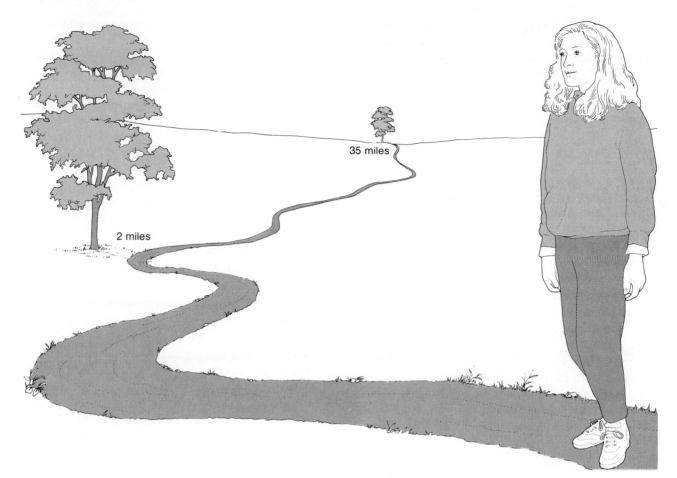

Figure 11.7 To lose body fat by exercising, you must look at the long-haul concept of weight control. The average-weight individual needs to jog about 35 miles to burn off 1 pound of body fat. This would be nearly impossible for most of us to do in 1 day. At 2 miles per day, however, it could be done in about 2 1/2 weeks—and at 5 miles per day, in only 1 week. Even though it takes time, an exercise program is a very effective approach to reducing excess body fat.

increase in the REE because muscle tissue is more active metabolically than fat tissue. For example, Calles-Escandon and others found that exercise training over a 10-day period increased fat oxidation at rest, suggesting this may be beneficial in weight-loss programs. Recall that in dieting alone, some lean muscle mass may be lost. In a recent study comparing the effects of either dieting or exercise on loss of body fat and lean tissue, Pritchard and others reported that 40 percent of the weight loss in dieters was lean tissue, while exercisers lost only 20 percent.

It should be noted that some research suggests exercise may decrease the REE in individuals who are already lean, suggesting that the body is attempting to preserve its energy reserves. This may be particularly true among elite endurance athletes, as noted by Sjodin and others. Although this does not appear to be of any concern to overweight individuals who desire to lose weight, it may pose a problem to the lean athlete attempting to shed a few additional pounds for competition.

Other than the physiological effects noted above, exercise also may confer some significant psychological benefits to the overweight individual. As the fitness level and body composition improve, the individual may experience improvements in mood, energy levels, body image, and self-esteem. Exercise may also be the psychological catalyst that helps individuals to improve their nutritional habits and other health-related behaviors.

Exercise may render significant health benefits. For example, as documented in the recent *Surgeon General's Report on Physical Activity and Health,* exercise, as a form of physical activity, is becoming increasingly important as a means to help prevent, and even treat, many chronic diseases, such as cardiovascular disease, diabetes, and osteoporosis. Many of the health benefits of exercise are related to weight loss and were discussed in Chapters 1 and 10. Exercise appears to be particularly effective in reducing abdominal fat stores, those most related to increased chronic disease risk.

For individuals with normal body weight, exercise is highly recommended for its preventive role. It is generally recognized that prevention of obesity or excess body weight is more effective than treatment. In a recent review, Epstein and others noted that exercise is an important adjunctive treatment for childhood and adolescent obesity, but indicated it may be of even greater benefit in the prevention of obesity. Moreover, the National Research Council recently noted that the long-term well-being of our children may depend on increased physical activity. Most people do not become overweight overnight, but rather accumulate an extra 75–150 Calories per day, which over time will lead to excessive fat tissue. A daily exercise program could easily counteract the effect of these additional Calories. For those who like to eat but not gain weight, exercise is the intelligent alternative.

Does exercise affect the appetite?

On a long-term basis, in general, increased energy expenditure through physical activity is counterbalanced by an increased food intake. This is one of the major mechanisms whereby normal body weight is controlled in the average individual. However, this may not be universally true for sedentary individuals with excess body fat. Research has shown that sedentary, overweight individuals who begin an exercise program do not necessarily increase food consumption above normal, the caloric intake actually decreasing in some cases.

An important concern for the athletic individual is the fact that the appetite may not normally decrease with a decreased activity level. If you are physically active, but then must curtail your activity because of an injury or some other reason, your appetite may remain elevated above what you need to maintain body weight at your reduced energy levels. Body fat will increase. Hence, you must reduce your food intake to balance the caloric equation or suffer the consequences.

As will be discussed later, a combined diet and exercise program would be most effective as a means to body weight control. In this regard, exercise, particularly intense exercise, may be used to curb the appetite on a short-term basis at an appropriate time. Thompson and others found that low-intensity exercise did not suppress hunger, but high-intensity exercise (68 percent VO_2 max) did. Research has related the appetite-suppressing effect of exercise to increased body temperature. The close anatomical relationship of the temperature and hunger centers in the hypothalamus may provide a rationale for the inhibition of the hunger center. Both exercise and the TEF will increase the core temperature of the body, so the body simply may be attempting to protect itself against an excessive rise in core temperature by suppressing the appetite to avoid the TEF. Exercise also will stimulate the secretion of several hormones in the body, notably epinephrine, which may also depress the appetite by affecting the hypothalamus or by increasing serum levels of both glucose and free fatty acids.

If you exercise before a meal, your food intake may be reduced considerably. Try it and see if it works for you. If you have the facilities available, a good half-hour of intense exercise may be an effective substitute for a large lunch. You may lose Calories two ways, expending them through exercise and replacing the large lunch with a low-Calorie, nutritious snack. However, in a recent review King and others noted that although intense exercise may be an effective means to suppress the appetite, the effects are brief. Thus, while intense exercise may help to curb your appetite at lunch, unless you are cautious you may increase your caloric intake above normal at dinner.

Does exercise affect the set point?

As you may recall from Chapter 10, the set-point theory suggests each individual possesses an inborn mechanism that attempts to maintain a certain level of energy balance, or body weight, by modifying energy intake or energy expenditure. In simple terms, the settling-point theory, another theory, suggests the set point may be adjusted to a new level. In a recent review, James Hill and Renee Commerford indicated that physical activity has a significant impact on the settling point, or that level of body weight and body fatness at which a steady-state is reached. They suggested that physical activity will increase total energy expenditure and fat oxidation, which can lead to an overall energy imbalance if there is not complete compensation in terms of increased energy intake and fat intake, and possibly decreased spontaneous daily activities. In essence, Hill and Commerford indicated that physical activity can help individuals reach fat and energy balances at lower levels of body fatness than would have been achieved with lower levels of physical activity. Body weight and fat should decrease until a new steady-state is achieved.

What types of exercise programs are most effective for losing body fat?

As you are probably well aware, a number of different exercise programs designed to reduce body weight are available. Perusal of the daily newspaper reveals numerous advertisements for weight-reduction programs sponsored by various commercial fitness centers. Weight training with sophisticated equipment, Slimnastics exercises, aerobic dancing, and special exercise apparatus are a few of the approaches often advertised as the best means to lose body fat fast. The truth is that you do not need any special apparatus or any specially designed program. You can design your own program once you know a few basic principles about exercise and energy expenditure.

The best type of exercise program for losing body fat involves aerobic exercises, those that utilize the oxygen

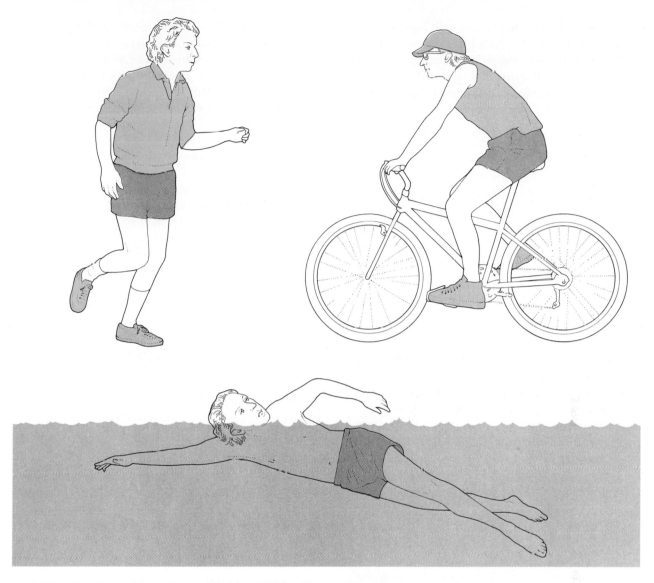

Figure 11.8   Aerobic mode exercises such as running, bicycling, or swimming must involve large muscle groups.

energy system (Figure 11.8). This type of exercise program is also the one that conveys the most significant health benefits. The key points of an aerobic exercise program are as follows:

1. The mode of exercise must involve large muscle groups. The muscles of the legs comprise a good portion of the total body mass, as do the muscles of the arms. Many people do not realize that the major muscles in the chest and back are attached to the upper arm and are actively involved in almost all arm movements. Walking, jogging, hiking, stair climbing, running, and bicycling primarily involve the legs while swimming primarily stress the arms. The use of hand-held weights in walking incorporates arm action with the legs. Cross-country skiing, rowing, and rope jumping use both the arms and legs, as does a good aerobic dance routine. These are good large-muscle activities, although there are a host of others.

2. The second factor is the intensity level. The higher the **exercise intensity,** the more Calories you expend. Per unit of time, normal walking uses fewer Calories than easy jogging, which uses fewer Calories than fast running. Simply put, it costs you more energy to move your body weight at a faster pace. However, there is an optimal intensity level for each person depending on how long the exercise will last. You can run at a very high intensity for 50 yards, but you certainly could not maintain that same fast pace for 2 miles. Intensity and duration are interrelated, but for burning the most total Calories, duration becomes more important, and the intensity must be adapted for the amount of time you plan to exercise.

To get an idea of exercises with high intensity, check Appendix C for Calorie cost per minute relative to your body weight. It is a composite table of a wide variety of individual reports in the literature. When using this appendix, keep these points in mind.

a. The figures are approximate and include the resting metabolic rate. Thus, the total cost of the exercise includes not only the energy expended by the exercise itself, but also the amount you would have used anyway during the same period. Suppose you ran for 1 hour and the calculated energy cost was 800 Calories. During that same time at rest you may have expended 75 Calories, so the net cost of the exercise is 725 Calories.

b. The figures in the table are only for the time you are performing the activity. For example, in an hour of basketball, you may exercise strenuously only for 35–40 minutes, as you may take time-outs and may rest during foul shots. In general, record only the amount of time that you are actually moving during the activity.

c. The figures may give you some guidelines to total energy expenditure, but actual caloric costs might vary somewhat according to such factors as skill level, environmental factors (running against the wind or up hills), and so forth.

d. Not all body weights could be listed, but you can approximate by going to the closest weight listed.

e. There may be small differences between men and women, but not enough to make a marked difference in the total caloric value for most exercises.

Appendix C or Table 3.5 on page 84 may be useful to determine which types of activities may be of the appropriate intensity for your weight-control program. Listing those activities with higher caloric expenditure per minute may suggest several that you could blend into your life-style.

3. Probably the most important factor in total energy expenditure is the duration of the exercise. In swimming, bicycling, running, or walking, distance is the key. For example, running a mile will cost the average-sized individual about 100 Calories. Five miles would approximate 500 Calories. An individual running 1 mile a day would take over 1 month to lose 1 pound of fat, whereas running 5 miles a day would shorten the time span to about 1 week. Thus, if the purpose of the exercise program is to lose weight, the individual should stress the **duration concept.**

One of the key points about the duration concept is the notion of distance traveled rather than time. For example, tennis and running are both good exercises. However, the runner will expend considerably more Calories in an hour than the tennis player because the activity involved in running is continuous. The tennis player has a number of rest periods in which the energy expenditure is lower. Consequently, at the end of an hour's activity, the runner may have expended two to three times as many Calories as the tennis player.

If you cannot find a big block of time, such as 40 minutes, to do your exercise, then try to incorparate more frequent short bouts of exercise throughout the day. In recent research, Jakicic and others reported that exercising in multiple short bouts per day, such as four 10-minute bouts, was just effective as a single 40-minute bout in producing weight loss and improving cardiovascular fitness over a 20-week period. If your day is filled with other activities, try to squeeze in some short exercise bouts, possibly before breakfast, during morning and afternoon work breaks, and before or after lunch and dinner.

A major reason many adults do not use exercise as a weight-loss mechanism is that their level of physical fitness is so low they cannot sustain a moderate level of exercise intensity for very long. However, keep in mind that as you continue to train, your body will begin to adapt so that in time you will be able to exercise for longer and longer periods.

Additionally, intensity and duration are interrelated, and if balanced, will result in equal weight losses. Grediagin and others also found no significant difference in body-fat losses when women engaged in either high-intensity or low-intensity exercise, provided the total caloric expenditure per exercise session was the same. It simply took the low-intensity exercise group longer to expend the same amount of Calories.

4. **Exercise frequency** complements duration and intensity. Frequency of exercise refers to how often each week you participate. As would appear obvious, the more often you exercise, the greater the total weekly caloric expenditure. In general, three to four times per week would be satisfactory, provided duration and intensity were adequate, but six to seven times would just about double your caloric output. A daily exercise program is recommended if weight control is the primary goal.

5. An important factor is enjoyment of the exercise. For an activity to be effective in the long run, it should be one that you enjoy, yet one that will help

expend Calories because it has a recommended intensity level, can be performed for a long time, or both. For example, you may not enjoy jogging or running, so other activities may be substituted. Fast walking with vigorous arm action, golf (pulling a cart), swimming, bicycling, tennis, handball, racquetball, and a variety of other activities may produce a greater feeling of enjoyment and still burn a considerable number of Calories. Even leisure activities and home chores done vigorously such as gardening, yard work, washing the car, and home repairs may be useful in burning Calories and developing fitness. Exercise need not be unpleasant. Enjoy your exercise. Try to make it a lifelong habit by viewing it as play. Next time you vacuum the house or mow the lawn, try to think about it as a good workout rather than work.

6. Practicality is another important factor. You may enjoy swimming, tennis, racquetball, and a variety of other sports, but lack of facilities, poor weather conditions, or high costs may limit your ability to participate. For the active person who travels, this may be a major concern. You probably have noticed by now that an underlying bias toward walking and running exists throughout this book. It is probably because, to me, they satisfy all the previously mentioned criteria necessary for maintaining proper body weight. Moreover, they are very practical activities. All you need is a good pair of shoes and proper clothes for the weather, nothing short of an injury should deter you from your daily exercise routine. Walking, jogging, or running can be very practical substitutes on those days when you cannot participate in your regular physical activity. Peter Wood, an esteemed researcher at Stanford University, indicated brisk walking is perhaps the best single exercise in regard to energy expenditure, feasibility, and acceptability to a large proportion of the population; for those who are physically unfit, overweight, or elderly, it is probably the best choice of exercise.

Indoor exercise equipment is also very practical for a number of reasons. For example it can be used while watching children, avoiding inclement weather, or doing two things at one time such as reading or watching television news. Numerous types of indoor exercise equipment are available, such as bicycling apparatus, cross-country skiing simulators, rowing machines, stair-steppers, and treadmills. All can provide an aerobic workout, but in a recent study Zeni and others reported that the treadmill is the optimal indoor exercise machine for enhancing energy expenditure at a set rating of perceived exertion. Resistance- or strength-training indoor equipment is also

available. For an excellent analysis of indoor exercise equipment, consult the January, 1996 issue of *Consumer Reports*.

7. Versatility is also an important factor. Learn and engage in a variety of physical activities, such as running, cycling, swimming, rowing on stationary machines, stair climbing, and aerobic walking. By cross-training, such as running 3 days per week, cycling 2 days, and swimming 2 days, you are less likely to become bored with exercise or to sustain overuse injuries. Also, if you plan to exercise for an hour daily, one-half hour each of running and cycling, or some other combination of exercises, is also an effective way to cross-train. Moreover, if you become injured and cannot do your favorite type of exercise, you may be able to expend Calories and maintain fitness by using alternative exercises until you heal. For example, if weight-bearing activities such as jogging bother you, do nonweight-bearing activities such as cycling or swimming.

Is resistance training recommended during a weight-loss program?

Resistance-training, or weight-training, programs are detailed in the next chapter in relation to gaining body weight, but such programs may also be very helpful during weight-loss programs. Research by Douglas Ballor and his associates has revealed that weight training may help preserve lean body mass during weight loss. Recall that protein tissue, primarily muscle, may be lost along with body fat during a weight-reduction program. However, weight training may stimulate muscular development and help prevent significant decreases in lean body mass. Such an effect may also help prevent decreases in the REE. Additionally, as is noted in the next chapter, dynamic weight-training programs may also be used to burn additional Calories.

If I am inactive now, should I see a physician before I initiate an exercise program?

Various medical groups, such as the American College of Sports Medicine and the American Heart Association, have developed guidelines to determine who should receive a medical exam prior to initiating an exercise program. A thorough review of these guidelines is not presented here because they are extensive and beyond the scope of this text. However, the following points represent a synthesis of these guidelines.

1. Before initiating any exercise program, you should be aware of any personal medical problems that possibly could be aggravated. If you have concern about any facet of your health, check with your physician before starting an exercise program. This

Table 11.9 Major and predisposing risk factors associated with coronary heart disease

1. High blood pressure

2. Cigarette smoking

3. High blood lipid levels; cholesterol and triglycerides

4. Diabetes

5. Obesity

6. Abnormal resting electrocardiogram (ECG)

7. Family history of coronary heart disease before age fifty

8. Sedentary life-style/physical inactivity

Sources: Data from American College of Sports Medicine, *Guidelines for Graded Exercise Testing and Exercise Prescription*, 5th ed., 1995; and from American Heart Association, *Coronary Risk Factor Statement for the American Public*, 1986.

is especially important in weight-reduction exercise programs where the main stress is placed on the heart and blood vessels, the cardiovascular system.

2. No matter what your age, if you have any of the coronary heart disease risk factors noted in Table 11.9, you should have a medical examination.

3. If you are young (twenties or early thirties), healthy, and have no risk factors, it is probably safe to initiate an exercise program.

4. The older you are, the better the idea to get a medical examination. In fact, it is prudent for those over forty to have an examination.

What other precautions would be advisable before I start an exercise program?

Your initial level of physical fitness is an important determinant of the intensity of exercise during the early stages of the program. If you are completely unconditioned, you should start at a lower intensity level—walk before you jog for example. Keep in mind that it took time for you to gain weight and become unconditioned, so it will also take time to reverse the process. A gradual progression is the key point. Examples are presented later.

Other general precautions involve safety factors, timing of meals, environmental hazards, and equipment. The individual should adhere to safety principles for the activity selected, particularly swimming, bicycling, and pedestrian safety. Strenuous exercise should not be undertaken within 2 or 3 hours of a heavy meal, but may be done earlier with a light meal or just liquids. As noted in Chapter 9, a hot environment poses the most serious threat to the person in training. Be aware of signs of heat

stress such as dizziness, nausea, and weakness. If these occur, stop exercising and find a means to help cool your body. Proper equipment should be selected for the chosen activity. For example, of critical importance to the jogger or walker is a well-designed pair of shoes. They may help prevent certain medical problems, such as tendinitis and shin splints, which may occur during the early stages of training.

What is the general design of exercise programs for weight reduction?

In essence, exercise programs to reduce body fat or to help maintain an optimal weight are based on the same principles that underlie exercise programs to improve the efficiency of the cardiovascular system. The total exercise program is based on a balance of exercise intensity, duration, and frequency. However, each daily exercise bout is usually subdivided into three phases—warm-up, stimulus, and warm-down, in that order (Figure 11.9). A proper warm-up and warm-down are important components of the aerobic exercise prescription. Both may help prevent excessive strain on the heart and may also be helpful in the prevention of muscular soreness or injuries.

The **warm-up** precedes the stimulus period and may be done in several ways. It may be general in nature, such as calisthenics, or specific to the type of exercise you plan to do, such as initially exercising at a lower level of intensity of the actual mode of exercise. Some gentle stretching exercises are also helpful in the warm-up period.

For most aerobic-type exercise, it is probably better to warm up the specific muscles to be used. For example, if you plan to use jogging as your mode of aerobic exercise, you should stretch your leg muscles gently at first and then jog at a slower than normal pace for several minutes. Breaking into a sweat is a good external sign that you have sufficiently elevated your body temperature; by using a specific type of warm-up, the temperature of your exercising muscles will also be increased.

The **warm-down** phase follows the stimulus period and is designed primarily to help restore the cardiovascular system to normal. If one stops exercising abruptly, blood may possibly pool in the exercised body parts, thereby decreasing return of blood to the heart. With less blood to the heart, less will be pumped to the brain and hence dizziness may result. When the warm-down occurs gradually after strenuous exercise—by walking or jogging after a strenuous run, for example—the muscles help massage the blood through the veins back to the heart. Research indicating that abrupt cessation of exercise may increase certain blood hormone levels, which may cause abnormal rhythm of the heart, emphasizes the importance of a gradual warm-down. Complete your warm-down by stretching. Since the muscles are now warm from the exercise they are easier to stretch, which may help prevent muscle stiffness.

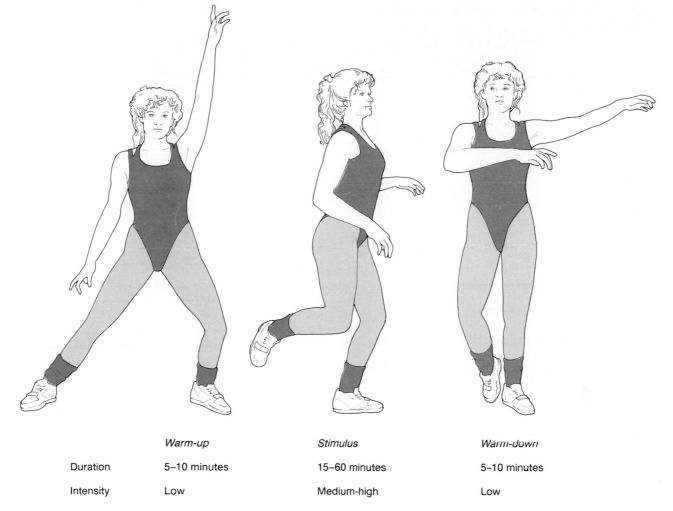

	Warm-up	Stimulus	Warm-down
Duration	5–10 minutes	15–60 minutes	5–10 minutes
Intensity	Low	Medium-high	Low

Figure 11.9 The exercise prescription. The exercise prescription is divided into three phases: warm-up period, stimulus period, and warm-down period. The stimulus period is the key to burning Calories.

The warm-up and warm-down are important components of the daily exercise bout, but most of the Calories are expended during the stimulus period.

What is the stimulus period of exercise?

The **stimulus period** is the most important phase of the daily exercise bout. By modifying the intensity and duration of the exercise, the individual achieves the level of stimulus necessary to elicit a conditioning effect. As illustrated in Figure 11.10, several important physiological and psychological measures increase in proportion to the exercise intensity.

The two major components of the stimulus period are intensity and duration of exercise. In any exercise session, these two components are usually inversely related. In other words, if intensity is high, duration is short, and if intensity is low, duration is long. Frequency (the number of exercise sessions per week) is also an important part of the exercise prescription. A number of medical groups, including the American Heart Association (AHA), the International Fed-

eration of Sports Medicine (FISM), and the American College of Sports Medicine (ACSM), have made specific recommendations concerning the quality and quantity of exercise for developing and maintaining cardiorespiratory fitness in adults. The recommendations from these groups are slightly different, but the differences are very minor.

The recommendations of the ACSM, as presented in their position stand on the recommended quantity and quality of exercise for developing and maintaining cardiorespiratory and muscular fitness in healthy adults, (Appendix J), are based on an exhaustive review of the pertinent research. The most recent ACSM recommendations will be used as the basis for developing an aerobic fitness program here, although they may be modified somewhat under certain circumstances. Such modifications will be noted where appropriate.

1. Intensity of training: 70–90 percent of maximum heart rate (HR max) or 50–85 percent of maximum oxygen uptake reserve (VO_2 max reserve) or HR max reserve (see definition on next page)

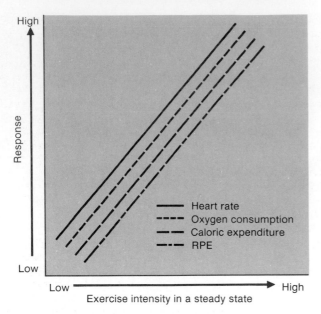

Figure 11.10 The relationship among various measures of energy expenditure. Heart rate, oxygen consumption, caloric expenditure, and RPE are, in general, directly related to the intensity of the exercise under steady-state conditions, i.e., when the oxygen supply is adequate for the energy cost of the exercise.

2. Duration of training: 20–60 minutes of continuous aerobic activity

3. Frequency of training: 3–5 days per week

What is an appropriate level of exercise intensity?

The intensity of exercise is a very important component of the stimulus period; in order to receive the optimal benefits from the exercise program, you must attain a certain **threshold stimulus,** the minimal stimulus intensity that will produce a training effect. The intensity of exercise can be expressed in a number of different ways, such as percentage of VO_2 max, calories/minute, or heart rate. In general, there is a high degree of relationship among these variables during exercise at a steady state. For example, the heart rate may reflect a certain level of oxygen consumption or caloric expenditure. Because the heart rate is easily obtained, it is usually used to determine the threshold level of exercise intensity. Another means to judge exercise intensity is the **rating of perceived exertion (RPE),** your perception of how strenuous the exercise is.

How do you determine your threshold level? Let's look at two ways—the heart rate and RPE. To obtain the heart rate, press lightly with the index and middle fingers on the carotid artery, located just under the jawbone and beside the Adam's apple. Do not use the thumb as it also has a pulse, and do not press hard on the carotid artery, for it may cause a reflex slowing of the beat in some persons. The radial artery pulse is obtained by placing your fingers on the inside of the wrist on the thumb side. These are the two most common locations for monitoring pulse rate, but other locations (the temple, inside the upper arm, and directly over the heart) may be used (see Figure 11.11).

To obtain the heart rate per minute, simply count the pulse rate for 6 seconds and add a zero. Resting and recovery heart rates are easily obtainable, as they may be taken while you are motionless, but it is difficult to manually monitor the heart rate while exercising. Research has shown that the exercise heart rate correlates very highly with the heart rate during the early stages of recovery. Hence, to monitor exercise heart rate, secure the pulse *immediately* upon cessation of exercise and count the beats for 6 seconds. This provides a reliable measure of exercise heart rate, although it may be slightly lower due to the beginning of the recovery effect. If it is difficult for you to monitor your heart rate for 6 seconds, then use a 10-second period and multiply the count by six to obtain your heart rate per minute. You probably should use 30 seconds to determine your resting heart rate; multiply your results by two. It may also be better to measure your resting pulse early in the morning, just after rising. Additionally, for the calculations below, you should take your resting heart rate in the position in which you will exercise, for example lying down if you swim, seated if you cycle, or standing if you walk or run.

One of the most prevalent techniques to determine the threshold stimulus for exercise is based upon the **maximal heart rate reserve (HR max reserve),** the difference between the resting heart rate and the maximum heart rate. You may determine your resting heart rate shortly after you arise in the morning. If you have not been physically active in some time, it may not be advisable for you to engage in strenuous physical activity in order to determine your actual maximal heart rate (HR max), but there are ways to predict it based upon your age. Although there are individual variations, a general guide for the prediction of HR max in women and untrained men is 220 minus the person's age. For physically trained men, the formula 205 minus one-half the person's age may be more appropriate, while for obese individuals, the formula 200 minus one-half the person's age may be best. Based upon the first formula, a 40-year-old untrained individual would have a predicted HR max of 180. Using the second formula, a trained 40-year-old male would have a predicted HR max of 185. Keep in mind, however, that there is considerable

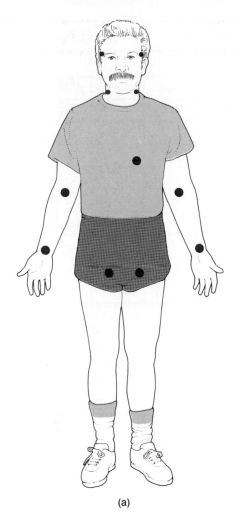

(a)

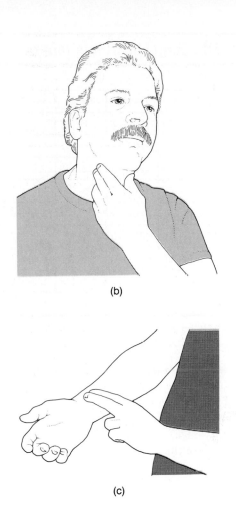

(b)

(c)

Figure 11.11 Palpation of the heart rate. The pulse rate may be taken at a variety of body locations (a), but the two most common locations are (b) the neck (carotid artery) and (c) the wrist (radial artery).

individual variation relative to predicted HR max. For example, a 40-year-old man may predict a HR max of 180, yet it may be 200, 160, or much lower if he was a victim of coronary heart disease.

There is rather widespread general agreement that, in order to obtain a training effect, the heart rate response should be increased above the resting level by about 50–85 percent of the HR max reserve. Recent research has revealed that lower levels, 45 percent, may also be effective, particularly in individuals with poor levels of physical fitness.

Continuing with our example of the 40-year-old man, we can calculate the heart rate range needed to elicit a training effect. This is called the **target heart rate range,** or **target HR.** To complete the calculations, we need to know the age-predicted HR max and the resting heart rate (RHR); the latter should be determined under relaxed circumstances. If we assume a RHR of 70 and a HR max of 180, the following formula would give us the target range:

$$\text{Target HR} = X\% \ (\text{HR max} - \text{RHR}) + \text{RHR}$$

For the 50 percent threshold level, the target heart rate for our example would be calculated as follows:

$$.5 \ (180 - 70) + 70 =$$

$$.5(110) + 70 = 55 + 70 = 125$$

For the 85 percent level, the target heart rate would be

$$.85(180 - 70) + 70 =$$

$$.85(110) + 70 = 93 + 70 = 163$$

Thus, in order to achieve a training effect, our 40-year-old man needs to train within a target HR range of 125–163.

If you wish to bypass the calculations, Table 11.10 presents the target HR ranges for various age groups with RHR between 45 and 90 beats/minute. Simply find your age group and RHR in the headings and locate your target HR range. The table is based on a predicted HR max of 220 − age.

In general, this table is a useful guide to the threshold heart rate and target HR range. However, there is considerable

Table 11.10 Target heart rate zones

RHR	Age											
	15–19	20–24	25–29	30–34	35–39	40–44	45–49	50–54	55–59	60–64	65–69	70–74
45–49	125–180	123–175	120–171	118–167	115–163	113–158	110–154	108–150	105–146	103–141	100–137	98–133
50–54	127–181	125–176	122–172	120–168	117–164	115–159	112–155	110–151	107–147	105–142	102–138	100–134
55–59	130–181	128–176	125–172	123–168	120–164	118–159	115–155	113–151	110–147	108–142	105–138	103–134
60–64	132–182	130–177	127–173	125–169	122–165	120–160	117–156	115–152	112–148	110–143	107–139	105–135
65–69	135–183	133–178	130–174	128–170	125–166	123–161	120–157	118–153	115–149	113–144	110–140	107–136
70–74	137–184	135–179	132–175	130–171	127–167	125–162	122–158	120–154	117–150	115–145	112–141	110–137
75–79	140–184	138–180	135–176	133–172	130–168	128–163	125–159	123–155	120–151	118–146	115–142	113–138
80–84	142–185	140–181	137–177	135–173	132–169	130–164	127–160	125–156	122–152	120–147	117–143	115–139
85–89	145–186	143–181	140–177	138–173	135–169	133–164	130–160	128–156	125–152	123–147	120–143	118–139

The target zone (50–85 percent threshold) is based upon the median figure for each age range and resting heart rate range.

variability in HR max among individuals, particularly in the older age groups. If your true HR max is below the predicted value (220 − age), the target HR range in the table would be higher than the recommended level. If your true HR max is higher than the predicted value, the target HR range in the table is lower than the recommended level. Although the target HR range might vary by a few beats, if your actual HR max is slightly higher or lower than the predicted value, you will still receive a good training effect—assuming you are in the middle of the range.

Once you have been training for a month or so, you may desire to determine your HR max in the specific activity you do. You may use the procedures described below, that is, running on a track at different speeds until you reach your maximal level, modifying the test dependent upon your aerobic exercise. For example, research has revealed that HR max is lower in swimming, possibly as much as ten to fifteen beats per minute, so the target heart rate may be slightly lower if this mode of exercise is used. William McArdle of Queens College recommends use of the formula 205 minus age to predict maximal heart rate while swimming.

Although the target heart rate approach is a sound means for monitoring exercise intensity, you may also wish to use the RPE scale developed by Gunnar Borg. This scale was originally designed to reflect heart rate responses by adding a zero to the rating. You simply rate the perceived difficulty or strenuousness of the exercise task according to the scale in Table 11.11. If you are running, how do your legs feel? Do they feel light and easy to move, or are they heavy, or possibly beginning to ache or burn? How is your breathing? Are you breathing easily and able to carry on a conversation, or are your sentences shortened to a few

Table 11.11 The RPE scale

6	14
7 very, very light	15 hard
8	16
9 very light	17 very hard
10	18
11 fairly light	19 very, very hard
12	20
13 somewhat hard	

words? In general, how does your total body feel? Is the exercise too easy, or are you working too hard? A new ten-point rating scale has been developed by Borg, but the American College of Sports Medicine notes that the original one is still useful because it is based on the heart rate response to exercise.

When you determine your exercise heart rate, it is a good idea to associate an appropriate RPE value with it. For example, at an exercise heart rate of 150 you might make a mental note of the exercise difficulty and assign a value of 15, or hard, to that level of exercise intensity. Research has shown that the RPE can be an effective means to measure exercise intensity in healthy individuals, particularly at heart rates above 150 beats/minute. A general rule of thumb is: If you cannot maintain a conversation while exercising, you are probably exercising too hard, unless you are training for sports competition.

How can I determine the exercise intensity needed to achieve my target HR range?

To determine the exercise intensity necessary to reach your target HR range, all you need is a stopwatch. Where distances are involved, such as with running, swimming, or cycling, an accurate measure is needed. An ideal situation for walking or running would be a quarter-mile (400 meters) high school or college track.

A steady-state HR response may be obtained in 3 to 5 minutes of evenly paced activity. A sound method for walking, jogging, or running follows, but this system may be adapted easily to other activities such as swimming, cycling, calisthenics, and aerobic dance.

Mark a one-half mile course. Two laps on a quarter-mile track would be ideal, but you can pace out a quarter-mile on the sidewalks near your home. Measure your resting HR. Walk until you have an even pace and then time yourself for the one-half mile. Immediately record your HR at the conclusion of the exercise. During your walk, mentally record the RPE. Did you reach the target HR? Was your RPE related to your HR? If the HR response was in the target range or the RPE was not too strenuous, you are at a level to begin your training program. If the HR response was not in the target range, rest until your HR returns close to normal and then take the test at a faster pace. Repeat this procedure until you have a plot of the HR, RPE, and time for the one-half mile. Keep a record of this as it will be useful in evaluating the effects of your conditioning program.

For example, suppose you recorded the following data on the one-half mile test on four trials (Figure 11.12).

Test	Time	RPE	HR	Minutes/Mile
1	8:00	11	108	16:00
2	7:10	13	132	14:20
3	6:30	15	156	13:00
4	6:00	18	180	12:00

As your speed increases, both RPE and HR naturally increase. If your predicted HR max is 200, and your resting HR is 70, the 50–85 percent target range approximates 135–180. Test 1 does not provide adequate stimulus intensity, Test 2 is just below the minimum target HR, Test 3 is in the middle of the range, while Test 4 is at your upper limit. Thus, your training intensity should be between 12 and 14 minutes per mile. The RPE may offer a means of judging the intensity of the exercise when you do not have a set distance and watch.

To determine your speed for these tests, simply double the time for the half-mile and you have the time per mile. The last trial was 12 minutes per mile. The caloric expenditure could be obtained from Appendix C.

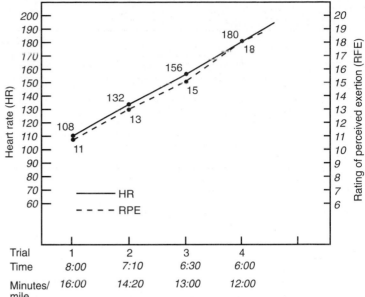

Trial	1	2	3	4
Time	8:00	7:10	6:30	6:00
Minutes/mile	16:00	14:20	13:00	12:00

Figure 11.12 Plot of heart rate and RPE following a half-mile walk in determination of the threshold heart rate.

Another simple way to monitor your exercise effort is to listen to your breathing. Adam Bean, an editor for *Runner's World*, cited research indicating that when you can first hear yourself breathing during exercise, you are entering the lower range of your heart-rate zone. When you have difficulty talking, you are near the upper range.

How can I design my own exercise program?

The exercise program that you design should not only be safe and effective, but it should be one to which you will adhere for a lifetime. Unfortunately, over 50 percent of the individuals who begin an exercise program to lose excess body weight drop out within a short time. Research with successful exercisers has revealed several clues that increase the likelihood of staying with an exercise program.

1. Do not exceed your abilities during the early stages of the program. Start slowly and progress gradually.

2. Set both short-term and long-term goals. A short-term goal may be to walk a mile in 15 minutes, while a long-term goal may be the completion of a local 10-kilometer (6.2-mile) road race.

3. Keep a record of your exercise. This will allow you to evaluate your progress toward your goals.

4. You must have time available to exercise. Most of us are busy with work, school, family, and friends, so finding the time to exercise is often difficult. You need to incorporate exercise into your daily schedule just as you do for other activities.

5. A place to exercise must be convenient. You are more likely to find an excuse not to exercise if you

have to travel 5 miles in heavy traffic to a health club. Find a convenient location.

6. Self-motivation is probably the most important determinant of adherence to an exercise program. Enjoying your exercise program, being capable at the exercise task, and knowing that it will help you attain your goals will improve your motivation and hopefully make daily exercise a lifetime habit.

Although diverse modes of aerobic exercise may be used to lose body weight and to help condition the cardiovascular system, the major focus here will be on walk-jog-run programs. This is because they satisfy many of the criteria that may encourage adherence to an exercise program.

Former U. S. Surgeon General C. Everett Koop indicated that walking for exercise should be elevated to a national priority. Walking may be the ideal exercise program for many individuals. Compared to jogging and running there is less stress on the legs due to impact because one foot is always on the ground supporting the body weight. However, leisurely walking usually will not provide an adequate stimulus to achieve the target HR, so the walking pace must be brisk. Walking at a faster-than-normal pace is often called **aerobic walking,** and if done properly can expend Calories at about the same rate as jogging or running. Vigorous arm action is needed, and the length of the stride as well as the step rate must be increased. Also, using hand weights will increase the energy expenditure by about 5–10 percent and also will help tone the arm muscles if used vigorously. Adding 3 pounds to each wrist will increase energy output about 1 Calorie per minute. Carrying the weights in the hands tends to increase the blood pressure more, so it may be helpful to use weights that strap around the wrist. However, you may expend similar amounts of Calories by simply walking faster or longer without hand weights.

A wide variety of methods may be used to initiate an aerobic exercise program of walking, jogging, or running. The key is to begin slowly, gradually increasing the exercise intensity as you become better conditioned. Once you determine the intensity of exercise necessary to achieve the target HR, it becomes a relatively simple matter to individualize the exercise program. The two tables presented below include exercise programs for individuals who have been sedentary and have low levels of physical fitness. Use your target HR guidelines throughout the 12- to 15-week program.

In the early weeks you should only attempt to exercise at the 50–60 percent target HR range. However, if you find that the exercise intensity needed to achieve this level is too strenuous, reduce it to 40 percent of your calculated heart-rate reserve. As you become more fit, gradually increase your target HR to the 50–85 percent level.

Table 11.12 presents a sample aerobic walking program. It is designed to progress you gradually through 12 weeks to a point where the exercise intensity and duration may make a significant contribution to weight loss over time. If you feel fit you may progress more rapidly than the table indicates, but stay within your target HR range and do not become unduly fatigued.

Table 11.13 presents an exercise program with a rapid progression to jogging, using an interval-training approach. **Interval training** alternates periods of rest and exercise. Again, the target HR method should be used during this exercise program.

Whatever mode of exercise you select, the target HR should be maintained for 20–30 minutes. This may be continuous or intermittent. If 20 minutes is the allotted time, the target HR should be achieved for 20 continuous minutes or four 5-minute intervals of exercise with several minutes of rest in between.

The frequency of exercise should be daily or at least three to five times per week. The American College of Sports Medicine has documented a number of studies that support a frequency level of at least three times per week as being necessary to develop and maintain cardiovascular health. During the early stages, however, it may be advisable to exercise daily in order to form sound habits. The exercise intensity at this time may not be too severe, such as walking, and hence daily exercise bouts may be undertaken without serious muscle soreness or related injury patterns. If you switch to jogging or running, decrease the frequency to three or four times per week to avoid overuse injuries. The frequency per week may be increased as you become better physically conditioned.

For weight-control purposes, duration and frequency of exercise are key elements. The longer and more often you exercise, the greater will be the total amount of energy expended. Aerobic walking for 5 miles on a daily basis is the equivalent of approximately 1 pound of body fat per week.

There are a number of other excellent conditioning programs available for the unconditioned individual. Probably the most popular is the aerobics program developed by Dr. Kenneth Cooper. Although dated, his programs may be found in *The Aerobics Program for Total Well Being,* a highly recommended paperback found in most bookstores. Also, books on initiating walking and other aerobic exercise programs are available at your library or local bookstores.

From what parts of the body does the weight loss occur during an exercise weight-reduction program?

As mentioned previously, weight loss may come from any one of three body sources—body water, lean tissue such as muscle, and body-fat stores. A diet program, especially

Table 11.12 Sample aerobic walking program

	Warm-up	Target zone exercising	Warm-down	Total time
Week 1*	Walk slowly 5 minutes	Walk briskly 5 minutes	Walk slowly 5 minutes	15 minutes
Week 2	Walk slowly 5 minutes	Walk briskly 7 minutes	Walk slowly 5 minutes	17 minutes
Week 3	Walk slowly 5 minutes	Walk briskly 9 minutes	Walk slowly 5 minutes	19 minutes
Week 4	Walk slowly 5 minutes	Walk briskly 11 minutes	Walk slowly 5 minutes	21 minutes
Week 5	Walk slowly 5 minutes	Walk briskly 13 minutes	Walk slowly 5 minutes	23 minutes
Week 6	Walk slowly 5 minutes	Walk briskly 15 minutes	Walk slowly 5 minutes	25 minutes
Week 7	Walk slowly 5 minutes	Walk briskly 18 minutes	Walk slowly 5 minutes	28 minutes
Week 8	Walk slowly 5 minutes	Walk briskly 20 minutes	Walk slowly 5 minutes	30 minutes
Week 9	Walk slowly 5 minutes	Walk briskly 23 minutes	Walk slowly 5 minutes	33 minutes
Week 10	Walk slowly 5 minutes	Walk briskly 26 minutes	Walk slowly 5 minutes	36 minutes
Week 11	Walk slowly 5 minutes	Walk briskly 28 minutes	Walk slowly 5 minutes	38 minutes
Week 12	Walk slowly 5 minutes	Walk briskly 30 minutes	Walk slowly 5 minutes	40 minutes

From week 13 on, check your pulse periodically to see if you are exercising within your target heart rate range. As you become more fit, walk faster to increase your heart rate toward the upper levels of your target range. Follow the principle of progression.

Note: If you find a particular week's pattern tiring, repeat it before going on to the next pattern. *You do not have to complete the walking program in 12 weeks.* Remember that your goal is to continue getting the benefits you are seeking and enjoying your activity. Listen to your body and progress less rapidly, if necessary.

*Program should include at *least* three exercise sessions per week.
Source: U.S. Department of Health and Human Services.

one very low in Calories, will cause a rapid weight loss due to decreases in body water and lean tissue. Body-fat losses are moderate at first but may increase in later stages of the diet. On the other hand, weight lost through an exercise program alone is lost at a much slower rate. Body water levels remain relatively normal after replacement of water lost through exercise. The lean tissues, particularly muscle, might actually increase in amount from the stimulating effect of exercise on muscle development. Because a good proportion of the energy demand for exercise is met by the oxidation of fat, most of the body-weight reduction comes from the body-fat stores, particularly in the abdominal area (Figure 11.13). As we learned previously, the caloric cost of 1 pound of fat is much higher than that of water or lean muscle tissue.

Should I do low-intensity exercises to burn more fat?

A myth that is circulating contends that in order to burn fat, you must exercise at a lower percentage of your VO_2 max. As noted in Chapters 3, 4, and 5, the *percentage* of energy obtained from fat is greater at lower exercise intensities (e.g., 50 percent VO_2 max) than at higher exercise intensities (e.g., 70 percent VO_2 max). However, at the higher energy intensity, you will derive a lower percentage of your energy output from fat, but the total energy expenditure will be greater, and you will still burn about the same amount of fat Calories as you would exercising at the lower intensity. If you want to burn Calories to lose body fat, your objective should be to burn the greatest total Calories possible within the time frame you have to exercise. As an example, suppose a female had 30 minutes to exercise and exercised at 50 percent VO_2 max, running 10-minute miles and deriving 50 percent of her energy from fat. She would cover 3 miles, expending 300 total Calories at an energy cost of about 100 Calories per mile, 150 of which would be fat Calories. If she was able to run at 75 percent VO_2 max, running 7.5-minute miles and deriving 33 percent of her energy from fat, she would cover 4.5 miles, expending 450 total Calories, of which 150 would still be fat Calories. However, she has expended a total of 450 versus 300 Calories at the higher exercise intensity, which will lead to a greater weight loss or permit her to consume an additional 150 Calories in her daily diet. But, if she has unlimited time, she may be able to

Table 11.13 Sample aerobic jogging program (interval training)

	Warm-up	Target zone exercising	Warm-down	Total time
Week 1*	Stretch and limber up 5 minutes	Walk (nonstop) 10 minutes	Walk slowly 3 minutes; stretch 2 minutes	20 minutes
Week 2	Stretch and limber up 5 minutes	Walk 5 minutes; jog 1 minute; walk 5 minutes; jog 1 minute	Walk slowly 3 minutes; stretch 2 minutes	22 minutes
Week 3	Stretch and limber up 5 minutes	Walk 5 minutes; jog 3 minutes; walk 5 minutes; jog 3 minutes	Walk slowly 3 minutes; stretch 2 minutes	26 minutes
Week 4	Stretch and limber up 5 minutes	Walk 5 minutes; jog 4 minutes; walk 5 minutes; jog 4 minutes	Walk slowly 3 minutes; stretch 2 minutes	28 minutes
Week 5	Stretch and limber up 5 minutes	Walk 4 minutes; jog 5 minutes; walk 4 minutes; jog 5 minutes	Walk slowly 3 minutes; stretch 2 minutes	28 minutes
Week 6	Stretch and limber up 5 minutes	Walk 4 minutes; jog 6 minutes; walk 4 minutes; jog 6 minutes	Walk slowly 3 minutes; stretch 2 minutes	30 minutes
Week 7	Stretch and limber up 5 minutes	Walk 4 minutes; jog 7 minutes; walk 4 minutes; jog 7 minutes	Walk slowly 3 minutes; stretch 2 minutes	32 minutes
Week 8	Stretch and limber up 5 minutes	Walk 4 minutes; jog 8 minutes; walk 4 minutes; jog 8 minutes	Walk slowly 3 minutes; stretch 2 minutes	34 minutes
Week 9	Stretch and limber up 5 minutes	Walk 4 minutes; jog 9 minutes; walk 4 minutes; jog 9 minutes	Walk slowly 3 minutes; stretch 2 minutes	36 minutes
Week 10	Stretch and limber up 5 minutes	Walk 4 minutes; jog 13 minutes	Walk slowly 3 minutes; stretch 2 minutes	27 minutes
Week 11	Stretch and limber up 5 minutes	Walk 4 minutes; jog 15 minutes	Walk slowly 3 minutes; stretch 2 minutes	29 minutes
Week 12	Stretch and limber up 5 minutes	Walk 4 minutes; jog 17 minutes	Walk slowly 3 minutes; stretch 2 minutes	31 minutes
Week 13	Stretch and limber up 5 minutes	Walk 2 minutes; jog slowly 2 minutes; jog 17 minutes	Walk slowly 3 minutes; stretch 2 minutes	31 minutes
Week 14	Stretch and limber up 5 minutes	Walk 1 minute; jog slowly 3 minutes; jog 17 minutes	Walk slowly 3 minutes; stretch 2 minutes	31 minutes
Week 15	Stretch and limber up 5 minutes	Jog slowly 3 minutes; jog 17 minutes	Walk slowly 3 minutes; stretch 2 minutes	30 minutes

From week 16 on, check your pulse periodically to see if you are exercising within your target zone. As you become more fit, try exercising within the upper range of your target zone.

Note: If you find a particular week's pattern tiring, repeat it before going on to the next pattern. *You do not have to complete the jogging program in 15 weeks.* Remember that your goal is to continue getting the benefits you are seeking and enjoying your activity.

*Program should include at *least* three exercise sessions per week.
Source: U.S. Department of Health and Human Services.

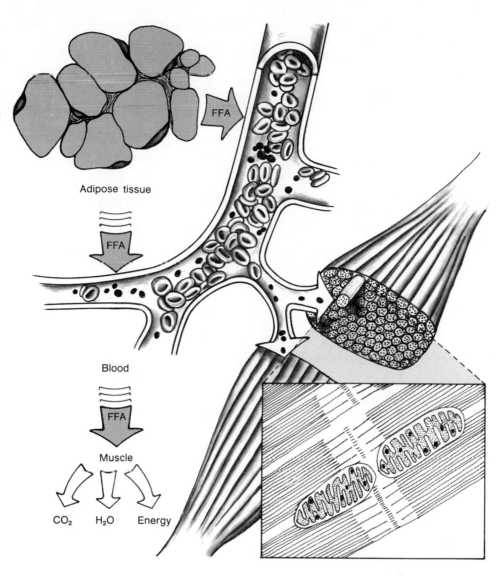

Figure 11.13 Exercise helps to release fat (free fatty acids) from the adipose tissues. The fat then travels by way of the bloodstream to the muscles where the free fatty acids are oxidized to provide the energy for exercise. Thus, exercise is an effective measure of reducing body fat.

Adipose tissue

FFA

FFA

Blood

FFA

Muscle

CO_2 H_2O Energy

exercise longer at the lower exercise intensity and eventually burn more total Calories. If you want to burn 500 Calories per day by running 5 miles, it does not matter how fast you run. The total distance covered is the key point. As noted in Chapter 3, you may calculate the energy it costs you to run 1 mile by simply multiplying your body weight in pounds by 0.73 Calories.

Is spot reducing effective?

Spot reducing uses isolated exercises in an attempt to deplete local fat deposits in specific body areas. These techniques do not appear to be effective. In one study the fat tissue was biopsied to determine whether sit-ups would reduce fat in the abdominal area. Subjects did a total of 5,000 sit-ups over a 27-day period, but this localized exercise did not preferentially reduce the adipose cell size in the abdominal area.

The current view suggests that the reduction of fat in body areas is most likely to occur where fat deposits

are the most conspicuous (usually the abdominal area), regardless of the exercise format. However, some areas of the body are somewhat resistant to change, particularly the gynoid-type fat distribution around the hips and thighs. Although both large-muscle activities and local isolated-muscle exercises may both be beneficial in reducing fat stores, the former are recommended because the total caloric expenditure will be larger.

Is it possible to exercise and still not lose body weight?

Many individuals are disappointed during the early stages of an exercise program because they do not lose weight very rapidly. Unless they understand what is happening in their bodies, the results on the scale may convince them that exercise is not an effective means to reduce weight, and they may quit exercising altogether. There are several reasons why an individual may not lose weight during the early stages of a weight-reduction program,

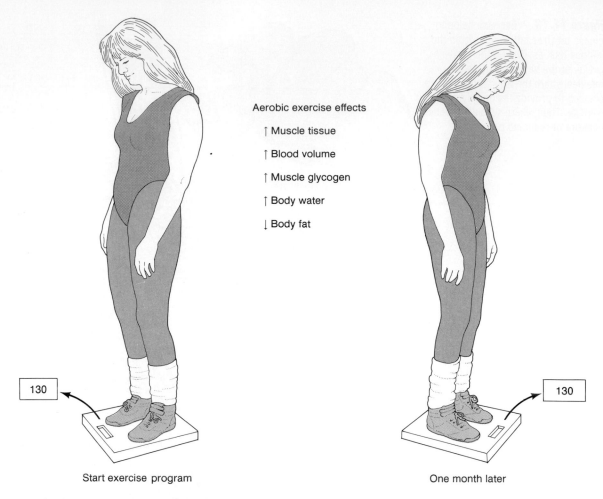

Aerobic exercise effects

↑ Muscle tissue

↑ Blood volume

↑ Muscle glycogen

↑ Body water

↓ Body fat

130

Start exercise program

130

One month later

Figure 11.14 Body weight may not change much during the beginning phases of an aerobic exercise program. However, body composition may change. The exercise stimulates an increase in muscle tissue, blood volume, and muscle glycogen stores, which tend to increase weight. Body fat is reduced, but the increases in the other components can balance out the fat losses with no net loss of body weight. Eventually, body weight begins to drop as the exercise program is continued.

and also why losing weight becomes more difficult after weight loss has occurred.

When a sedentary individual begins a daily exercise program, the body reacts to the exercise stress and changes so it can more easily handle the demands of exercise (Figure 11.14):

1. The muscles may increase in size because of hypertrophy of the muscle cells. The increased protein will hold water.

2. Certain structures within the muscle cell that process oxygen, along with numerous enzymes involved in oxygen use, will increase in quantity.

3. Energy substances in the cell will increase, particularly glycogen, which binds water.

4. The connective tissue will toughen and thicken.

5. The total blood volume may increase. An increase of approximately 500 milliliters, or about a pound, has been recorded in 1 week.

At the same time, however, body-fat stores will begin to diminish somewhat as fat is used as a source of energy for exercise. Overall, there may be an increase in body water and lean body mass, particularly the muscle tissues, and a decrease in body fat. These changes may counterbalance each other, and the individual may not lose any weight. However, although little or no weight is lost during those early phases, the body composition changes are favorable. Body fat is being lost.

Once these adaptive changes have occurred, which may take about a month, body weight should decrease in relationship to the number of Calories lost through exercise. Keep in mind that weight loss will be slow on an exercise program, but if you can build up to an exercise energy expenditure of about 300 Calories per day, then about 3 pounds per month will be exercised away provided you do not compensate by eating more.

After several months you may begin to notice that your body weight has stabilized even though you continue to exercise and have not reached your weight goal. Part of the reason may be your lower body weight. If you look at Appendix C, you can see that the less you weigh, the fewer Calories you burn for any given exercise. If you have been doing the same amount of exercise all along, you may now be at the body weight where your energy output is matched by your energy input in food and your body weight has stabilized. In theory, you have reached your settling point. In addition you may become more skilled, and hence more efficient, in your physical activity. Fewer Calories may then be expended for any given amount of time. However, this is usually only true of activities that involve a skill factor. It can be highly significant in swimming, but not as great in jogging.

In summary, your body weight may not change during the early stages of an exercise program; it may then begin to drop during a second stage, and then plateau at the third stage. If you are aware of these possible stages, your adherence to an exercise program may be enhanced. Also, during the third stage, if you desire to lose more weight by exercise, then the amount of exercise will need to be increased.

What about the five or six pounds a person may lose during an hour of exercise?

A rapid weight loss may occur during exercise. Some individuals have lost as much as 10–12 pounds in an hour or so. As you probably suspect, this weight loss may be attributed to body-water losses. This is particularly evident while exercising in warm or hot weather. The weight loss is temporary, and under normal food and water intake the body-water content will return to normal. Each pound of weight lost this way is 1 pint of fluid, or 16 ounces. A 2.2-pound weight loss would be the equivalent of 1 liter.

In the heat of summer, you may occasionally see an individual training with heavy sweat clothes or a rubberized suit. The reason often given is to lose more body weight. The individual will lose more body weight, but again it will be body water which will be regained as soon as he or she drinks fluids. In this regard, the technique is worthless. Moreover, it may predispose the individual to an unusually high heat stress, causing severe medical problems. Remember, only sweat that actually evaporates will help reduce the heat stress on the body.

Any water lost through dehydration should be replaced before the next exercise session, especially when exercising in warm environments. The importance of rehydration and problems associated with exercise in the heat were covered in Chapter 9.

Comprehensive Weight-Control Programs

In a recent conference relative to methods for voluntary weight loss and control, the National Institutes of Health indicated that the most important feature of a successful weight-loss or weight-control program is maintenance of the stable or reduced body weight. Accordingly, the NIH noted that the fundamental principle of weight loss and control is a commitment to a change in life-style. Behavioral modification incorporating properly designed diets and exercise programs, as detailed in this chapter, may be sufficient to induce and sustain weight losses in the individual with mild obesity, but those with more severe cases may need additional education and skills, social support, and continued professional assistance in order to maintain a stable, healthy body weight.

Which is more effective for weight control—dieting or exercise?

Dieting alone or exercise alone may be effective means to reduce body fat, but both techniques have certain advantages and disadvantages. However, it appears that the advantages of one technique help counterbalance the disadvantages of the other. Dieting will contribute to a negative caloric balance and may help bring about a rapid weight reduction early in the program, but may lead to decreases in lean body mass and REE. Exercise usually results in a slower rate of weight loss but may help develop and maintain the lean body mass and prevent the decrease in REE. Thompson and others used a meta-analysis of twenty-two studies to compare the effect of diet and diet-plus-exercise programs on the resting metabolic rate, and concluded that the addition of exercise to dietary restriction appears to prevent some of the decrease in the REE. Garfinkel and Coscina noted that weight lost by dieting is about 75 percent fat and 25 percent protein, but combining exercise and dieting reduces the protein loss to only 5 percent. Other studies have reported that dieting alone may result in lean tissue loss as high as 40 percent of the total weight loss. Resistance training (covered in the next chapter) added to a weight-reduction program may also be very effective in helping to maintain lean body mass. In a recent excellent review, Hill and others noted that the benefits of exercise alone on body weight, body composition, and energy expenditure are preserved when added to a weight-loss diet.

Hence, a comprehensive weight-reduction program involving both a dietary and an exercise regimen, along with supportive behavioral modification techniques, is highly recommended by major health-related organizations such as the American Dietetic Association and the American College of Sports Medicine. The principles of developing such a program have been presented in the preceding three sections of this chapter. A number of research studies with men, women, and children have supported the value of this type of program. In a recent review, Toth and Poehlman indicated that although more research data is needed regarding the mode, intensity, duration, and amount of exercise to define the most efficacious programs of exercise and diet to promote weight loss, exercise may be a beneficial adjunct to dietary restriction programs. In a recent study comparing the effectiveness of diet with various forms of exercise, Marks and others noted that a moderate diet combined with both aerobic and resistance exercise was effective in decreasing body fat.

Research also has been conducted with individuals who have successfully lost weight and maintained their desired level. In essence, they assumed responsibility for their need to lose weight and planned their own program. They did not necessarily diet per se, but simply decreased the amount of fat and sugar in their diet, ate less between meals, and often skipped meals. They also initiated a reasonable exercise program.

Consider the following. A dietary reduction of 500 Calories per day, along with an exercise energy expenditure of 500 Calories per day, could lead to approximately 2 pounds of weight loss per week, about the maximal amount recommended unless under medical supervision (Figure 11.15). The removal of 500 Calories from the diet could be done immediately by simply reducing the amount of sugar and fat in the daily diet and using some of the behavioral modification techniques cited earlier. You should review those suggestions given earlier relative to the substitution of nutrient-dense foods for high-Caloric ones. Relative to exercise it may take a month or more before you may be able to use 500 Calories daily, but by following the progressive plans outlined earlier in this chapter you should be able to reach that level safely. In the meantime, change your usual behavior by climbing stairs and walking more to add to your caloric expenditure.

Once the excess body fat has been lost, continued exercise appears to be important for maintenance of a stable, healthy body weight. Some preliminary reports from the National Weight Control Registry of individuals who have lost at least 30 pounds and have kept it off indicate that exercise is very important; walking was the most popular activity and the average weekly energy expenditure was 2,667 Calories for women and 3,489 Calories for men.

Schoeller and others recently reported that daily exercise of approximately 5 Calories per pound body weight helped to optimize weight maintenance after weight loss. In three reviews, King and Tribble, Phinney, and Safer all indicated that exercise exerted a strong influence on long-term preservation of weight loss, a finding also echoed by the Consumers Union.

If I want to lose weight through a national or local weight-loss program, what should I look for?

The weight-loss industry is a billion dollar business. National programs, such as Weight Watchers and the Jenny Craig plan, may charge about $100 per week or more for their comprehensive programs. Unfortunately, there is little governmental control over many of these programs, and while the national programs may be well-designed, others may not provide appropriate programs for safe and effective long-term weight loss.

If you want to enroll in a commercial weight-loss program, what do authorities recommend you should receive for your money? The following points are summarized from the report of a task force to establish weight-loss guidelines for the state of Michigan.

1. The staff should be well trained in their specialty, preferably having appropriate educational backgrounds, such as a physician, nurse, dietician, or exercise physiologist.

2. You should receive a medical screening, verifying you have no medical or psychological condition that might be exacerbated by weight loss through dieting or exercise.

3. A reasonable weight goal should be established given your weight history.

4. The rate of weight loss, after the first 2 weeks, should not exceed 2 pounds per week.

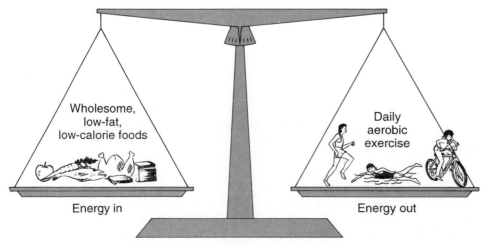

Figure 11.15 The most effective weight-reduction program involves both dieting and exercise. Mild caloric restriction and an aerobic exercise program can be combined effectively to lose one or two pounds per week.

Wholesome, low-fat, low-calorie foods

Energy in

Daily aerobic exercise

Energy out

5. You should receive an individualized treatment plan based on your weight-loss goal.

6. The program should disclose in writing all health risks and benefits associated with the program, and you should have the opportunity to read them and sign an informed consent form.

7. The diet should be one that
   a. contains no less than 1,000 Calories per day
   b. is between 10–30 percent fat Calories
   c. has at least 100 grams of carbohydrate per day
   d. provides at least 100 percent of the RDA; supplements, if used, should not exceed 100 percent of the RDA
   e. if under medical supervision, 600 Calories and 50 grams of carbohydrate per day are minimal levels

8. The program should have a nutrition-education component that stresses permanent life-style changes in your eating habits.

9. Exercise should be a component in the program. The focus should be on aerobic exercise, following the standards relative to mode, intensity, duration, and frequency discussed earlier in this chapter. It should be an exercise program you can live with for a lifetime.

10. Behavior-modification techniques should be individualized to help you incorporate sound dietary and exercise habits into your personal life-style.

11. There should be a weight-maintenance phase in the program once you have achieved your weight-loss goal. This should be a high priority to help you maintain your healthy body weight.

Similar guidelines should be used if you want to join a health or fitness club facility, particularly the qualifications of the staff and the availability of a variety of safe exercise equipment. You may consult the January 1996 issue of *Consumer Reports* for guidelines in selecting a health club.

Although some individuals may need the structure of such programs, many successful individuals have lost excess body fat and kept it off with programs they designed by themselves.

What type of weight-reduction program is advisable for young athletes?

In sports in which athletes compete in weight classes, such as wrestling, or in those where excess body fat may hinder performance, such as gymnastics, most competitors and their coaches believe that it is best to attain the lowest weight possible to increase chances of success. Although most of the concern in the past was devoted to the sport of wrestling, there is increasing concern about this practice in a variety of other sports.

As noted in the preceding chapter, potentially acute health problems may arise when the youngster sets an unrealistically low body-weight goal and uses nonrecommended techniques, such as starvation, diuretics, laxatives, appetite-suppressing drugs, and dehydration. Suzanne Steen and her associates have found that athletes, such as wrestlers, who lose and gain weight repeatedly throughout the season may find it more difficult to lose weight because their metabolism may slow down to conserve energy. However, four recent studies by Schmidt, Loprinzi, Melby, and McCargar and Crawford noted that the decrease in the RMR is transient or returns to normal pre-season values following completion of the competitive wrestling season. There is also some concern by medical personnel that weight loss during the growth and development years may have adverse long-term effects. For example, as noted in Chapter 10, some preliminary research suggests that dieting may retard the growth rate in young gymnasts. On the other hand, many coaches and athletes still remain unconvinced that current weight-control practices pose any immediate or future health hazard. In a questionnaire survey comparing former college wrestlers with other nonwrestling athletes who attended the University of Wisconsin–Madison between 1950 and 1988, Nitzke and others reported no significant differences between the wrestlers and other athletes in the Body Mass Index, weight gained, current exercise practices, or incidence of chronic diseases, even when comparisons were made for all those athletes over the age of 40. Unfortunately, the available scientific data are very limited, and this general area is in dire need of long-term research.

Nevertheless, on the basis of the data that are available, organizations such as the National Collegiate Athletic Association, the American Medical Association, and the American College of Sports Medicine have made some general recommendations to help alleviate potential problems and make weight-control practices in sports as safe as possible.

1. Weight should be lost gradually. A comprehensive program involving a balanced diet of 1,500–2,400 Calories and exercise should be used in the pre-season to lose most of the body weight. With appropriate carbohydrate, protein, minerals, and vitamins in the diet, a limited number of Calories possibly may enable a wrestler or other athlete to lose body weight effectively and yet still maintain high levels of aerobic and anaerobic activity in training.

2. Dehydration techniques such as rubber suits, saunas, steam baths, hot rooms, laxatives, and diuretics should be prohibited.

3. In the sport of wrestling, having the weigh-in immediately prior to performance may discourage rapid dehydration and weight-gain techniques. Also, suggestions have been made to allow more intermediate weight classes because there are more boys at these weight levels.

4. Encourage methods to predict a minimum body-fat percentage or body weight. Although used in

several states, these methods generally have not been applied extensively. Suggestions have been made to have a physician certify a minimum weight for each wrestler, but again this has not been used extensively. As mentioned in Chapter 10, the state of Wisconsin has developed an effective program for weight control in wrestling, which may serve as a model for other such programs.

What is the importance of prevention in a weight-control program?

Health practices designed to prevent the development of chronic diseases currently are being promoted heavily by several major health organizations. Katzel and others found that simply losing weight was effective in reducing the risk of coronary heart disease in obese men, but Haz-zard recommends physicians focus on both exercise and weight control. Exercise may confer some benefits in addition to weight loss. Changing your diet by reducing caloric intake, saturated fats, and cholesterol, and eating more nutritious foods (quality Calories), and concurrently initiating and continuing a good aerobic- and resistance-type exercise program are considered to be two steps toward positive health and the possible prevention of certain health problems. These two steps are also the key elements of a sound weight-control program, for exercise can balance food energy intake (Figure 11.16).

Although most of this chapter has focused on treatment programs for the reduction of excess body fat, the same guidelines may be applied to a prevention program. Obesity in our society is a serious medical problem of epidemic proportions. Although treatment programs for the clinically obese may be successful on a short-term basis,

Figure 11.16   It is very easy to consume 200 additional Calories per day, which can lead to an increase of about 2 pounds of body fat per month. However, increased physical activity may help to expend these Calories.

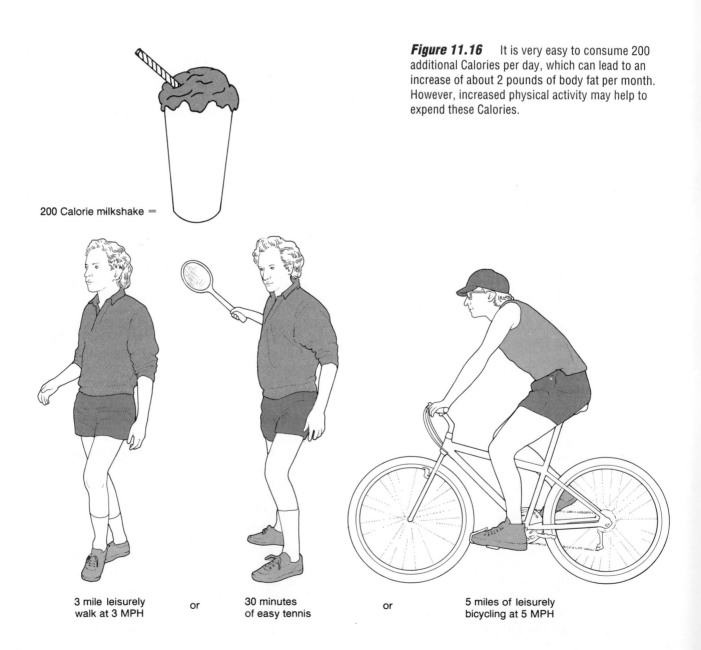

200 Calorie milkshake =

3 mile leisurely walk at 3 MPH   or   30 minutes of easy tennis   or   5 miles of leisurely bicycling at 5 MPH

unfortunately much of the weight loss is regained by the vast majority of those treated. We need to have strong prevention programs in our schools and communities, particularly for children and adolescents, for this appears to be the time of life when chronic cases of obesity develop. It is incumbent upon those involved with the food habits and physical activity of our youth, notably parents and health and physical educators, to instruct and motivate them toward sound health habits. According to the American Medical Association, prevention is the treatment of choice in dealing with obesity.

References

Books

American Diabetes Association and American Dietetic Association. 1995. *Exchange Lists for Meal Planning.* Chicago: American Dietetic Association and American Diabetes Association.

Cooper, K. 1982. *The Aerobics Program for Total Well-Being.* New York: M. Evans.

Dusek, D. 1989. *Weight Management: The Fitness Way.* Boston: Jones and Bartlett.

Mayer, J. 1968. *Overweight: Causes, Cost and Control.* Englewood Cliffs, NJ: Prentice-Hall.

Miller, W. 1998. *Negotiated Peace. How to Win the War Over Weight.* Boston: Allyn and Bacon.

National Research Council. 1989. *Recommended Dietary Allowances.* Washington, DC: National Academy Press.

National Research Council. 1989. *Diet and Health: Implications for Reducing Chronic Disease Risk.* Washington, DC: National Academy Press.

Shils, M., et al. 1994. *Modern Nutrition in Health and Disease.* Philadelphia: Lea and Febiger.

Stamford, B., and Shimer, P. 1990. *Fitness without Exercise.* New York: Warner Books.

U.S. Department of Health and Human Services. Public Health Service. 1996. *The Surgeon General's Report on Physical Activity and Health.* Washington, DC: U.S. Government Printing Office.

Williams, M. 1996. *Lifetime Fitness and Wellness: A Personal Choice.* Dubuque, IA: Wm. C. Brown.

Reviews

American College of Sports Medicine. 1996. American College of Sports Medicine position stand: Weight loss in wrestlers. *Medicine and Science in Sports and Exercise* 28 (2): i–iv.

American College of Sports Medicine. 1990. The recommended quantity and quality of exercise for developing and maintaining cardiorespiratory and muscular fitness in healthy adults. *Medicine and Science in Sports and Exercise* 22:265–74.

American College of Sports Medicine. 1983. Proper and improper weight loss programs. *Medicine and Science in Sports and Exercise* 15:ix–xiii.

American Dietetic Association. 1997. Position of the American Dietetic Association: Weight management. *Journal of the American Dietetic Association* 97:71–4.

American Dietetic Association. 1992. Position of the American Dietetic Association: Fat replacements. *ADA Reports* 91:1285–88.

American Dietetic Association. 1990. Position of the American Dietetic Association: Very-low-Calorie weight loss diets. *Journal of the American Dietetic Association* 90:722–26.

American Heart Association Scientific Council. 1992. Position statement on exercise. Benefits and recommendations for physical activity programs for all Americans. *Circulation* 86:340–44.

Atkinson, R. 1989. Low and very low calorie diets. *Medical Clinics of North America* 73:203–16.

Bean, A. 1997. A new way to monitor effort. *Runners World* 32 (9):22.

Bellisle, F., et al. 1997. Meal frequency and energy balance. *British Journal of Nutrition* 77 (Supplement): S57–S70.

Berggren, R. 1990. Liposuction. What it will and won't do. *Postgraduate Medicine* 87 (May): 187–95.

Birk, T., and Birk, C. 1987. Use of ratings of perceived exertion for exercise prescription. *Sports Medicine* 4:1–8.

Blair, S. 1995. Diet and activity: The synergistic merger. *Nutrition Today* 30 (3): 108–12.

Blundell, J., and Green, S. 1997. Effect of sucrose and sweeteners on appetite and energy intake. *International Journal of Obesity and Related Metabolic Disorders* 20 (Supplement 2): S12–17.

Borg, G. 1973. Perceived exertion: A note on "history" and methods. *Medicine and Science in Sports* 5:90–93.

Bray, G. 1990. Exercise and obesity. In *Exercise, Fitness and Health,* eds. C. Bouchard, et al. Champaign, IL: Human Kinetics.

Brownell, K., and Kramer, F. 1989. Behavioral management of obesity. *Medical Clinics of North America* 73:185–202.

Brownell, K., and Rodin, J. 1994. The dieting maelstrom: Is it possible and advisable to lose weight? *American Psychologist* 49:781–91.

Calles-Escandon, J., and Horton, E. 1992. The thermogenic role of exercise in the treatment of morbid obesity: A critical evaluation. *American Journal of Clinical Nutrition* 55:S533–S537.

Committee to Develop Criteria for Evaluating the Outcomes of Approaches to Prevent and Treat Obesity. 1995. Summary: Weighing the options—Criteria for evaluating weight-management programs. *Journal of the American Dietetic Association* 95:96–105.

Consumers Union. 1998. Exercise: Special section. *Consumer Reports* 63:20–29.

Consumers Union. 1996. Fitness fiction: Working out the facts. *Consumer Reports on Health* 8:114–15.

Consumers Union. 1996. Health clubs: The right choice for you. *Consumer Reports* 61:27–30.

Consumers Union. 1996. Getting in shape: It's more important than ever. *Consumer Reports* 61:14–25.

Consumers Union. 1995. Weight: What have you got to lose? *Consumers Report on Health* 7:97–100.

Convertino, V. 1991. Blood volume: Its adaptation to endurance training. *Medicine and Science in Sports and Exercise* 23:1338–48.

Despres, J. 1994. Physical activity and adipose tissue. In *Physical Activity, Fitness, and Health,* eds. C. Bouchard, et al. Champaign, IL: Human Kinetics.

Donnelly, J., et al. 1991. Diet and body composition: Effect of very low calorie diets and exercise. *Sports Medicine* 12:237–49.

Drewnowski, A. 1995. Intense sweeteners and the control of appetite. *Nutrition Reviews* 53:1–7.

Elrick, H. 1996. Exercise: The best prescription. *Physician and Sportsmedicine* 24 (2): 79–80.

Epstein, L., et al. 1996. Exercise in treating obesity in children and adolescents. *Medicine and Science in Sports and Exercise* 28:428–435.

Fisher, M., and Lachance, P. 1985. Nutrition evaluation of published weight-reducing diets. *Journal of the American Dietetic Association* 85:450–54.

Forbes, G. 1992. Exercise and lean weight: The influence of body weight. *Nutrition Reviews* 50:157–61.

Foreyt, J., and Goodrick, G. 1993. Weight management without dieting. *Nutrition Today* 28:4–9.

Garfinkel, P., and Coscina, D. 1990. Discussion: Exercise and obesity. In *Exercise, Fitness, and Health,* eds. C. Bouchard, et al. Champaign, IL: Human Kinetics.

Gibbs, W. 1996. Gaining on fat. *Scientific American* 275 (August):88–94.

Hazzard, W. 1995. Weight control and exercise: Cardinal features of successful preventive gerontology. *Journal of the American Medical Association* 274:1964–65.

Hill, J., and Commerford, R. 1996. Physical activity, fat balance, and energy balance. *International Journal of Sport Nutrition* 6:80–92.

Hill, J., et al. 1994. Physical activity, fitness, and moderate obesity. In *Physical Activity, Fitness, and Health,* eds. C. Bouchard, et al. Champaign, IL: Human Kinetics.

Hoffer, L. 1994. Starvation. In *Modern Nutrition in Health and Disease,* eds. M. Shils, et al. Philadelphia: Lea and Febiger.

Horswill, C. 1992. When wrestlers slim to win. What's a safe minimum weight? *Physician and Sportsmedicine* 20 (September): 91–101.

King, A., and Tribble, D. 1991. The role of exercise in weight regulation in nonathletes. *Sports Medicine* 11:331–49.

King, N., et al. 1997. Effects of exercise on appetite control: Implications for energy balance. *Medicine and Science in Sports and Exercise* 29:1076–89.

Kromhout, D. 1992. Dietary fats: Long-term implications for health. *Nutrition Reviews* 50:49–53.

Mela, D. 1992. Nutritional implications of fat substitutes. *Journal of the American Dietetic Association* 92:472–76.

Melby, C., et al. 1998. Exercise, macronutrient balance, and weight control. In *Exercise, Nutrition, and Weight Control,* eds. D. Lamb and R. Murray. Carmel, IN: Cooper Publishing.

Miller, G., and Groziak, S. 1996. Impact of fat substitutes on fat intake. *Lipids* 31:S293–S296.

Miller, W. 1991. Diet composition, energy intake, and nutritional status in relation to obesity in men and women. *Medicine and Science in Sports and Exercise* 23:280–84.

National Institutes of Health. 1992. Methods for voluntary weight loss and control. Technology Assessment Conference Statement. *Nutrition Today* 50 (July/August): 27–33.

Nichlas, B. 1997. Effects of endurance exercise on adipose tissue metabolism. *Exercise and Sport Sciences Reviews* 25:77–103.

Parker, D., et al. 1991. Juvenile obesity: The importance of exercise and getting children to do it. *Physician and Sportsmedicine* 19 (June): 113–25.

Parr, R. 1996. Exercising when you're overweight. *Physician and Sportsmedicine* 24 (10): 81–82.

Pera, V., et al. 1992. Current treatment of obesity: A behavioral medicine perspective. *Rhode Island Medicine* 75:477–81.

Perri, M., et al. 1993. Strategies for improving maintenance of weight loss. Toward a continuous care model of obesity management. *Diabetes Care* 16:200–209.

Petersmarck, K. 1992. Building consensus for safe weight loss. *Journal of the American Dietetic Association* 92:679–80.

Phinney, S. 1992. Exercise during and after very-low-calorie dieting. *American Journal of Clinical Nutrition* 56:S190–S194.

Pi-Sunyer, F.X. 1994. Obesity. In *Modern Nutrition in Health and Disease,* eds. M. Shils, et al. Philadelphia: Lea and Febiger.

Pi-Sunyer, F.X. 1990. Effect of the composition of the diet on energy intake. *Nutrition Reviews* 48:94–105.

Robison, J., et al. 1995. Redefining success in obesity intervention: The new paradigm. *Journal of the American Dietetic Association* 95:422–23.

Safer, D. 1991. Diet, behavior modification, and exercise: A review of obesity treatments from a long-term perspective. *Southern Medical Journal* 84:1470–74.

Saris, W. 1993. The role of exercise in the dietary treatment of obesity. *International Journal of Obesity* 17(1): S17–S21.

Schelkun, P. 1993. Treating overweight patients. Don't weigh success in pounds. *Physician and Sportsmedicine* 21 (February): 148–53.

Shaw, J., and Snow-Harter, C. 1995. Osteoporosis and physical activity. *Physical Activity and Fitness Research Digest* 2 (3): 1–8.

Smith, T. 1997. Fat or total Calories? Fat still dominates weight control. *Running & FitNews* 15 (5): 4–5.

Stamford, B. 1993. Tracking your heart rate for fitness. *Physician and Sportsmedicine* 21 (March): 227–28.

Thompson, J., et al. 1996. Effects of diet and diet-plus-exercise programs on resting metabolic rate: A meta-analysis. *International Journal of Sport Nutrition* 6:41–61.

Toth, M., and Poehlman, E. 1996. Effects of exercise on daily energy expenditure. *Nutrition Reviews* 54:S140–S148.

Wood, P. 1996. Clinical applications of diet and physical activity in weight loss. *Nutrition Reviews* 54:S131–S135.

Young, J., and Ruderman, N. 1993. Exercise and metabolic disorders. In *Principles of Exercise Biochemistry,* ed. J. Poortmans. Basel, Switzerland: Karger.

Specific Studies

Abadie, B. 1990. Physiological responses to grade walking with wrist and hand-held weights. *Research Quarterly for Exercise and Sport* 61:93–95.

Ballor, D., et al. 1988. Resistance weight training during caloric restriction enhances lean body weight maintenance. *American Journal of Clinical Nutrition* 47:19–25.

Bengtsson, B., et al. 1993. Treatment of adults with growth hormone (GH) deficiency with recombinant human GH. *Journal of Clinical Endocrinology and Metabolism* 76:309–17.

Bushman, B., et al. 1997. Effect of 4 wk of deep water training on running performance. *Medicine and Science in Sports and Exercise* 29:694–99.

Cabanac, M., and Morrissette, J. 1992. Acute, but not chronic, exercise lowers body weight set-point in male rats. *Physiology and Behavior* 52:1173–77.

Colvin, R., and Olson, S. 1983. A descriptive analysis of men and women who have lost significant weight and are highly successful at maintaining the loss. *Addictive Behaviors* 8:287–95.

Cotton, J., et al. 1996. Replacement of dietary fat with sucrose polyester: Effects on energy intake and appetite control in nonobese males. *American Journal of Clinical Nutrition* 63:891–96.

Eston, R., et al. 1992. Effect of very low calorie diet on body composition and exercise response in sedentary women. *European Journal of Applied Physiology* 65:452–58.

Field, R., et al. 1992. Vertical banded gastroplasty: Is obesity worth it? *Journal of Mississippi State Medical Association* 33:423–32.

Forbes, G., and Brown, M. 1989. Energy need for weight maintenance in human beings: Effect of body size and composition. *Journal of the American Dietetic Association* 89:499–502.

Gillette, C., et al. 1994. Postexercise energy expenditure in response to acute aerobic or resistive exercise. *International Journal of Sport Nutrition* 4:347–60.

Glass, S., et al. 1992. Accuracy of RPE from graded exercise to establish exercise training intensity. *Medicine and Science in Sports and Exercise* 24:1303–7.

Grodiagin, M., ot al. 1005. Exorcico intoncity doob not offect body composition change in untrained, moderately overfat women. *Journal of the American Dietetic Association* 95:661–65.

Haus, G., et al. 1994. Key modifiable factors in weight maintenance: Fat intake, exercise, and weight cycling. *Journal of the American Dietetic Association* 94:409–13.

Jakicic, J., et al. 1995. Prescribing exercise in multiple short bouts versus one continuous bout: Effects on adherence, cardiorespiratory fitness, and weight loss in overweight women. *International Journal of Obesity and Related Metabolic Disorders* 19:893–901.

Jeffrey, R., et al. 1995. A randomized trial of counseling for fat restriction versus calorie restriction in the treatment of obesity. *International Journal of Obesity* 19:132–37.

Katch, F., et al. 1980. Preferential effects of abdominal exercise training on regional adipose cell size. *Medicine and Science in Sports and Exercise* 12:96.

Katzel, L., et al. 1995. Effects of weight loss vs aerobic exercise training on risk factors for coronary disease in healthy, obese, middle-aged and older men: A randomized controlled trial. *Journal of the American Medical Association* 274:1915–21.

Leutholtz, B., et al. 1995. Exercise training and severe caloric restriction: Effect on lean body mass in the obese. *Archives of Physical and Mental Rehabilitation* 76:65–70.

Loprinzi, M., et al. 1991. Resting metabolic rates of wrestlers: Effects of repetitive weight loss. *Medicine and Science in Sports and Exercise* 23:S75.

Makalous, S., et al. 1988. Energy expenditure during walking with hand weights. *Physician and Sportsmedicine* 16:139–48.

Marks, B., et al. 1995. Fat-free mass is maintained in women following a moderate diet and exercise program. *Medicine and Science in Sports and Exercise* 27:1243–51.

McCargar, L., and Crawford, S. 1992. Metabolic and anthropometric changes with weight cycling in wrestlers. *Medicine and Science in Sports and Exercise* 24:1270–75.

Melanson, E., et al. 1996. Exercise responses to running and in-line skating at self-selected paces. *Medicine and Science in Sports and Exercise* 28:247–50.

Melby, C., et al. 1990. Resting metabolic rate in weight-cycling collegiate wrestlers compared with physically active, noncycling control subjects. *American Journal of Clinical Nutrition* 52:409–14.

Miller, W., et al. 1993. Cardiovascular risk reduction in a self-taught, self-administered weight loss program called the nondiet diet. *Medicine and Science in Sports and Exercise* 25:218–23.

Miller, W., ct al. 1990. Dict composition, cnergy intakc, and cxercise in relation to body fat in men and women. *American Journal of Clinical Nutrition* 52:426–30.

Mole, P., et al. 1989. Exercise reverses depressed metabolic rate produced by severe caloric restriction. *Medicine and Science in Sports and Exercise* 21:29–33.

Newman, B., et al. 1990. Nongenetic influences of obesity on other cardiovascular disease risk factors: An analysis of identical twins. *American Journal of Public Health* 80:675–78.

Nitzke, S., et al. 1992. Weight cycling practices and long-term health conditions in a sample of former wrestlers and other collegiate athletes. *Journal of Athletic Training* 27:257–61.

Pamuk, E., et al. 1992. Weight loss and mortality in a national cohort of adults, 1971–1987. *American Journal of Epidemiology* 136:686–97.

Peters, P., et al. 1996. Questionable dieting behaviors are used by young adults regardless of sex or student status. *Journal of the American Dietetic Association* 96:709–11.

Pritchard, J., ot al. 1007. A workcito program for overwoight middle-aged men achieves lesser weight loss with exercise than with dietary change. *Journal of the American Dietetic Association* 97:37–42.

Rumpler, W., et al. 1996. Energy value of moderate alcohol consumption by humans. *American Journal of Clinical Nutrition* 64:108–14.

Saris, W., et al. 1989. Study of food intake and energy expenditure during extreme sustained exercise. The Tour de France. *International Journal of Sports Medicine* 10:S26–S31.

Schmidt, W., et al. 1993. Two competitive seasons of weight cycling does not lower resting metabolic rate in college wrestlers. *Medicine and Science in Sports and Exercise* 25:613–19.

Schoeller, D., et al. 1997. How much physical activity is needed to minimize weight gain in previously obese women? *American Journal of Clinical Nutrition* 66:551–6.

Sedlock, D., et al. 1989. Effect of exercise intensity and duration on postexercise energy expenditure. *Medicine and Science in Sports and Exercise* 21:662–66.

Shide, D., and Rolls, B. 1995. Information about the fat content of preloads influences energy intake in healthy women. *Journal of the American Dietetic Association* 95:993–98.

Sjodin, A., et al. 1996. The influence of physical activity on BMR. *Medicine and Science in Sports and Exercise* 28:85–91.

Steen, S., et al. 1988. Metabolic effects of repeated weight loss and regain in adolescent wrestlers. *Journal of the American Medical Association* 260:47–50.

Suter, P., et al. 1992. The effect of ethanol on fat storage in healthy subjects. *New England Journal of Medicine* 326:983–87.

Sweeney, M., et al. 1993. Severe vs moderate energy restriction with and without exercise in the treatment of obesity: Efficiency of weight loss. *American Journal of Clinical Nutrition* 57:127–34.

Thompson, D., et al. 1988. Acute effects of exercise intensity on appetite in young men. *Medicine and Science in Sports and Exercise* 20:222–27.

Thompson, J., et al. 1995. Daily energy expenditure in male endurance athletes with differing energy intakes. *Medicine and Science in Sports and Exercise* 27:347–54.

Tremblay, A., et al. 1990. Effect of intensity of physical activity on body fatness and fat distribution. *American Journal of Clinical Nutrition* 51:153–57.

Webb, P. 1985. Direct calorimetry and the energetics of exercise and weight loss. *Medicine and Science in Sports and Exercise* 18:3–5.

Westerterp, K., et al. 1992. Long-term effect of physical activity on cnergy balancc and body composition. *British Journal of Nutrition* 68:21–30.

Widerman, P., and Hagan, R. 1982. Body weight loss in a wrestler preparing for competition. A case report. *Medicine and Science in Sports and Exercise* 14:413–18.

Yost, T., and Eckel, R. 1988. Fat calories may be preferentially stored in reduced-obese women: A permissive pathway for resumption of the obese state. *Journal of Clinical and Endocrinological Metabolism* 67:259–63.

Zeni, A., et al. 1996. Energy expenditure with indoor exercise machines. *Journal of the American Medical Association* 275: 1424–27.

CHAPTER 12

Weight Gaining through Proper Nutrition and Exercise

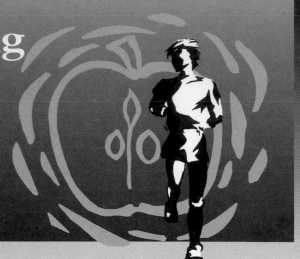

KEY TERMS

anabolic/androgenic
  steroids (AAS)
bulk-up method
circuit aerobics
circuit weight training
concentric method
eccentric method
isokinetic method
isometric method
isotonic method
muscle hypertrophy
principle of exercise
  sequence
principle of overload
principle of recuperation
principle of specificity
principle of progressive
  resistance exercise (PRE)
repetition maximum (RM)
strength-endurance
  continuum
Valsalva phenomenon

KEY CONCEPTS

• There may be a variety of reasons why an individual is underweight, and the cause should be determined before a treatment is prescribed.

• For those who want to gain weight, a weekly increase of 0.5–1 pound is a sound approach, but the weight gain should be primarily muscle tissue and not body fat.

• In essence, adequate rest and sleep, increased caloric intake, and a proper resistance-training program should be effective in helping to increase lean body mass.

• The use of drugs or hormones to increase body weight may be effective, but may also lead to a variety of health problems.

• A basic principle underlying all resistance-training programs is the overload principle, which simply means the muscles should be stressed beyond normal daily levels.

• Progressive resistance is also a basic principle of resistance training, for as you get stronger through use of the overload principle, you must progressively increase the resistance.

• To increase muscle mass and body weight, you should exercise near the strength end of the strength-endurance continuum.

• Your resistance-training program should exercise all major muscle groups in the body.

• A variety of methods and apparatus are available for resistance training, but research suggests that they are equally effective as a means to gain strength and muscle mass if the basic principles of resistance training are followed.

• Resistance training is generally regarded as a safe form of exercise, but it may be contraindicated in some individuals, for example, those with high blood pressure and hernias.

• Although resistance-training programs may confer some significant health benefits, it is also highly recommended that one add an aerobic exercise program to help condition the cardiovascular system.

• The Food Exchange System can serve as the basis for increasing caloric intake to gain body weight if the aspirant eats greater quantities of nutritious foods from each of the six lists in three balanced meals plus several high-Calorie, high-nutrient snacks.

• The individual attempting to gain body weight should obtain necessary protein for muscle synthesis through a well-balanced diet, rather than by consuming expensive protein supplements.

• Most nutrient and dietary supplements marketed to strength-trained individuals are not effective or have not been evaluated by scientific research.

INTRODUCTION

As noted in the previous chapter, there are basically three reasons why individuals attempt to lose excess body weight—to improve appearance, health, or athletic performance. Some individuals may also wish to gain weight for the same three reasons, and may use resistance training, also known as weight training or strength training, as a means to stimulate weight gain.

For those who wish to improve appearance, resistance training will increase muscularity, a desired physical attribute among many males and an increasing number of females. Resistance training is becoming increasingly popular, particularly among women. Recent surveys indicate the number of women who weight train has doubled over the past decade, and the number of males has increased almost 50 percent.

Gaining weight, particularly muscle mass stimulated by resistance training, may also be associated with some health benefits. An increased muscularity that improves physical appearance and body image may help elevate self-esteem, contributing to positive psychological health. Additionally, resistance training is recommended for several health benefits, such as increased bone mineral density, and has been recommended by the American Heart Association and the American College of Sports Medicine as an effective means to promote overall good health. A recent popular book, *Quick Weight-Gain Program* by Dr. David Reuben, is designed to provide sound medical advice for the 26 million Americans who need to gain weight for a variety of medical and cosmetic reasons.

Increased body weight, particularly increased muscle mass, may be associated with improvements in strength and power, two performance factors important for a wide variety of sports. Most colleges and universities, as well as many high schools, have strength-training programs for their athletes, both males and females.

No matter what the reason for gaining body weight, you should be concerned about where the extra pounds will be stored. The energy-balance equation works equally as well for gaining weight as it does for losing weight, but excess body fat in general will not improve physical appearance, health, or athletic performance. On the contrary, it may detract from all three. To put on body weight you have to concentrate on means to increase the fat-free mass, particularly muscle tissue, with little or no increase in body-fat stores.

Numerous approaches are employed in attempts to increase muscle mass. Specialized exercise equipment or exercise techniques are advertised as the most effective methods available to build muscles. Protein supplements have been a favorite among weight lifters for years, but today athletes can buy numerous dietary supplements that are advertised to produce an anabolic, or muscle-building, effect. Some athletes and nonathletes even use drugs to gain weight for enhanced performance or appearance.

Like weight-loss programs, weight-gaining programs may be safe and effective or they can be potentially harmful to your health. Although gaining weight, particularly as muscle mass, is difficult for some individuals, the purpose of this chapter is to present basic information on the type of exercise and diet program that is most likely to be effective as a means to put on weight without compromising your health.

Basic Considerations

Why are some individuals underweight?

Being significantly under a healthy body weight may be due to several factors. Heredity may be an important factor, as genetic factors may predispose some individuals to leanness. For example, a high basal metabolic rate may have been acquired through your parents. Medical problems could adversely affect food intake and digestion, so a physician should be consulted to rule out nutritional problems caused by organic disease, hormonal imbalance, or inadequate absorption of nutrients. Social pressures, such as the strong desire of a teenage girl to have a slender body, could lead to undernutrition; an extreme example is anorexia nervosa, discussed in Chapter 10. Emotional problems also may affect food intake. In many cases, food intake is increased during periods of emotional crisis, but the appetite may also be depressed in some individuals for long periods. Economic hardships may reduce food purchasing power, so some individuals simply may sacrifice food intake for other life necessities.

Being considerably underweight, such as 10 percent below the standard height-weight tables or a Body Mass Index below 19, may be considered a symptom of malnutrition or undernutrition. It is important to determine the cause before prescribing a treatment. Our concern here is the individual who does not have any of these medical, psychological, social, or economic problems, but who simply cannot create a positive energy balance because of excess energy expenditure or insufficient energy (Calorie) intake. Caloric intake has to be increased, and the output has to be modified somewhat.

What steps should I take if I want to gain weight?

The following guidelines may help you develop an effective program to maximize your gains in muscle mass and keep body-fat increases relatively low.

1. Have an acceptable purpose for the weight gain. The desire for an improved physical appearance and body image may be reason enough. For athletes,

increased muscle mass may be important for a variety of sports, particularly if strength and power are improved. However, you do not want to gain weight at the expense of speed if speed is important to your sport.

2. Calculate your average energy needs daily. Use Table 11.1 on page 347 to determine how many Calories you need just to maintain body weight. These values are slightly higher than those in Table 11.2.

3. Keep a 3- to 7-day record of what you normally eat. See pages 355–357 for guidelines to determine your average daily caloric intake. If the obtained value is less than your energy needs calculated under item 2 above, this may be a reason why you are not gaining weight.

4. Check your living habits. Do you get enough rest and sleep? If not, you are burning more energy than the estimate in point 2 above. Smoking increases your metabolic rate almost 10 percent and may account for approximately 200 Calories per day. Caffeine in coffee and soft drinks also increases the metabolic rate for several hours. Getting enough rest and sleep and eliminating smoking and caffeine will help decrease your energy output.

5. Set a reasonable goal within a certain time period. Peter Lemon, an expert in resistance training and protein metabolism, recently indicated that someone starting a resistance-training program may increase body mass by 20 percent in the first year. After that, gains are somewhat less, possibly only 1–3 percent per year. In general, about 0.5–1 pound per week is a sound approach for a novice, but weight gaining is difficult for some individuals and may occur at a slower rate. Specific goals may also include muscular hypertrophy in various parts of the body.

6. Increase your caloric intake. A properly designed diet should include adequate Calories and protein and not violate the principles of healthful nutrition.

7. Start a resistance-training exercise program. This type of exercise program will serve as a stimulus to build muscle tissue.

8. Use a good cloth or steel tape to take body measurements before and during your weight-gaining program. Be sure you measure at the same points about once a week. Those body parts measured should include the neck, upper and lower arm, chest, abdomen, hips, thigh, and calf. This is to ensure that body weight gains are proportionately distributed. You should look for good gains in the chest and limbs; the abdominal and hip girth increase should be kept low because that is where fat is more likely to be stored. If available, skinfold calipers may be used to measure subcutaneous fat skinfolds at multiple sites over the body. Fat skinfold thicknesses should remain the same or decrease to ensure that the weight gain is muscle, not fat.

In summary, adequate rest, increased caloric intake, and a proper resistance-training program may be very effective as a means to gain the right kind of body weight.

What about the use of hormones or drugs to gain body weight?

Several hormones in the body may exert significant anabolic effects on body composition, particularly insulin, human growth hormone (HGH), and testosterone. As noted in previous chapters several nutrient supplements, such as specific amino acids, have been utilized in attempts to increase the secretion of these hormones for anabolic purposes. Two of these hormones, HGH and testosterone, as well as drugs patterned after testosterone, have been used directly to increase muscle mass.

Human Growth Hormone (HGH) HGH is a natural hormone secreted by the anterior pituitary gland in the brain; HGH is an anabolic hormone that stimulates bone growth and the development of muscle tissue through its effects on protein, carbohydrate and fat metabolism. A detailed discussion of the role of HGH is beyond the scope of this text. It is important to note, however, that extensive research into its effects began only recently when genetically engineered versions of the natural body hormone became available. Available data suggest that in elderly men, who normally have reduced levels of HGH, injections of the hormone modify body composition, decreasing body fat and increasing lean body mass. However, MacIntyre, extrapolating from animal data and from studies of adults with acromegaly (a disorder associated with excess secretion of HGH by the pituitary), noted that although the muscles appear larger, they are functionally weaker. He suggested that the increase in muscle bulk may be an enlargement in connective tissue, which does not generate force. In support of these extrapolations, Yarasheski and others recently studied the effect of HGH versus a placebo on adult males who weight-trained for 12 weeks. They reported significant increases in lean body mass in the group receiving HGH, but there were no significant increases in skeletal muscle protein synthesis and size, as measured by magnetic resonance imaging, or in muscular strength, over the effects produced by weight training alone in the placebo group. They suggested that HGH may influence the development of other tissues. Several other well-controlled studies reported similar findings with HGH supplementation to experienced resistance-trained athletes. The interested reader is referred to the review by Yarasheski.

At present, then, there are no data to support an ergogenic effect of HGH on muscle size, strength, or power beyond the effect generated by a proper weight-training program. Moreover, the potential adverse health effects of HGH are substantial, and most researchers caution that the long-term health risks of HGH administration, either as genetically engineered HGH or produced by amino acid supplementation, are unknown. This is particularly distressing as a recent report indicated approximately 5 percent of high school students have used HGH. In some pathological conditions, the pituitary gland secretes excess HGH, which is associated with acromegaly, or thickening of soft tissues in the face, hands, and feet. Excess HGH may also cause enlargement of body organs, such as the liver, and may lead to diabetes.

Additionally, HGH use by athletes is prohibited by the International Olympic Committee.

Testosterone and Anabolic/Androgenic Steroids (AAS)

Testosterone, the male steroid sex hormone produced by the testes, was one of the first anabolic agents used in attempts to enhance physical performance, possibly as early as the 1936 Berlin Olympic Games. As recently documented by Bhasin and others, testosterone is a very effective ergogenic aid, increasing lean muscle mass, decreasing body fat, and increasing strength even without resistance training; these anabolic effects were augmented in subjects who also trained. Testosterone must be injected because ingested testosterone will be catabolized by digestive enzymes. Although injected testosterone use is still prevalent among various athletic groups, oral drug forms of testosterone have been developed, as noted below.

Anabolic/androgenic steroids (AAS) represent a class of synthetic drugs designed to mimic the effects of testosterone. The chemical structure of testosterone may be modified in attempts to maximize the anabolic muscle-building effects and minimize the androgenic male secondary sex characteristics; both oral and injectable AAS have been developed. AAS are the drugs of choice for many strength athletes and bodybuilders to improve performance and appearance. Potteiger and Stilger noted that recent surveys indicate the use of AAS steroids also is prevalent among adolescent athletes, particularly those in high school. Their use is even common among young male nonathletes, and increasing numbers of teen-age girls according to Yesalis and others, who desire to increase muscle mass for an enhanced self-image.

The effects of AAS on body composition and strength have been studied rather extensively, and although there may be some flaws in the experimental designs used, most reviewers agree that AAS use may increase muscle mass and strength, a judgment supported by a recent review of laboratory studies that included meta-analysis as part of the evaluative criteria.

However, AAS use has been associated with a number of medical problems, as documented in a recent brief review by Petersen and Goldberg. Some are relatively minor such as acne and loss of hair. AAS may also adversely affect psychological processes, leading to increased aggression, hostility, depression and possible suicide attempts, and an increased tendency to commit violent crimes, including homicide. Continued use may predispose adults to coronary heart disease by decreasing HDL cholesterol and increasing blood pressure as documented in both epidemiological and experimental studies, and recently reviewed by Nnakwe. Prolonged steroid use may possibly lead to impaired development of tendons, decreasing their strength and contributing to a potential for rupture. Prolonged use has resulted in severe liver diseases, including cancer. Anabolic steroids may cause premature cessation of bone growth in children and adolescents and may result in the appearance of several male secondary sex characteristics in females, some of which may be irreversible, such as deepening of the voice.

However, many of the adverse health effects of AAS use appear to be reversible. For example, Hartgens and others found that bodybuilders who cycled off AAS steroids for 3 months had similar lipoprotein profiles and liver enzymes as their non-drug-using counterparts. Moreover, Yesalis and Bahrke noted that although the short-term health effects of AAS have been increasingly studied and reviewed, and while AAS use has been associated with adverse and even fatal effects, the incidence of serious effects thus far reported has been extremely low. Unfortunately, as they noted, no good scientific data on long-term health effects of AAS use are available and the effects are generally unknown.

Nevertheless, because of the potential health risks, one of the risk-reduction objectives in *Healthy People 2000* is the reduction of AAS use among high school students. Moreover, the U.S. Congress has passed legislation to classify AAS as controlled substances, thus limiting their production and distribution by pharmaceutical companies. Penalties may be severe. Additionally, most individuals obtain these drugs illegally on the black market where quality is not controlled, and chemical analysis has revealed some potentially hazardous constituents in these "homemade" drugs.

As is obvious, the use of testosterone or AAS for the purpose of gaining body weight and strength is not recommended. Moreover, their use by athletes is grounds for disqualification for future competition. The American College of Sports Medicine has developed a position statement on the use of anabolic steroids in sports. Although an extensive discussion of AAS is beyond the scope of this text, the ACSM report provides a detailed review for the interested reader.

Exercise Considerations

In the last chapter we discussed the design of an aerobic exercise program for the loss of excess body fat but also mentioned that a weight-training program could be helpful, for it might help prevent the loss of lean body mass. In this chapter, the focus is upon resistance training, sometimes called weight training, as a means to increase lean body mass and body weight. Before we discuss the principles underlying the design of a proper resistance-training program, let us introduce some basic terminology.

Repetition simply means the number of times you do a specific exercise. *Intensity* is determined by the weight, or resistance, that is lifted. A term used to describe the interrelationship between repetitions and intensity in weight training is **repetition maximum (RM).** If you perform an exercise such as a bench press and lift 150 pounds once, but you cannot do a second repetition, you have done one repetition maximum, or 1RM. If you bench press a lighter weight, say 120 pounds, for five repetitions but cannot do a sixth, you have done five repetition maximum, or 5RM. A *set* is any particular number of repetitions, such as five or ten. The total volume of work you do in a single workout is the product of sets, repetitions, and resistance. For example, if you bench press three sets of five repetitions with a resistance of 100 pounds, your total volume of work is 1,500 pounds ($3 \times 5 \times 100$). The *recovery period* may represent the rest intervals between sets in a single workout or the rest interval between workouts during the week.

What are the primary purposes of resistance training?

As is probably obvious to you, there is an inverse relationship between the amount of weight you can lift and the number of repetitions you can do. If your 1RM in the bench press is 150 pounds, you can do more repetitions with 100 pounds than you can with 140. The **strength-endurance continuum** is a training concept that focuses upon the interrelationship between resistance and repetitions. As depicted in Figure 12.1, to train for strength you must combine high resistance with a low number of repetitions. Conversely, to train for endurance, you must combine a low resistance with a high number of repetitions.

Resistance-training programs may be designed to train all three of the human energy systems. The ATP-PC energy system predominates in strength and power activities, the lactic acid energy system is primarily involved in anaerobic endurance, and the oxygen system is involved in aerobic endurance activities. Thus, resistance-training programs may be developed for various purposes.

In a recent Gatorade Sports Science Institute review regarding effective training methods for muscle and strength gain, Michael Stone, an internationally-renowned strength-training expert from Appalachian State Univer-

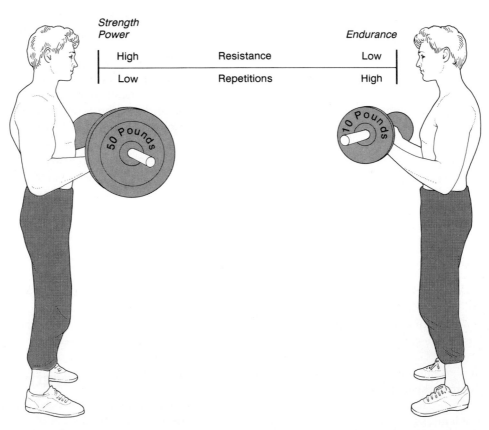

Strength Power			Endurance
High	Resistance		Low
Low	Repetitions		High

Figure 12.1 The strength-endurance continuum. To gain strength, you need to train on the strength end of the continuum; to gain endurance, you need to train on the endurance end of the continuum.

sity, indicated that although this is a complex topic to research, several points may be supported by the available scientific literature, including the following:

1. Appropriate resistance training can result in an increase in lean body mass and muscle hypertrophy

2. Gains in muscle hypertrophy appear to be best accomplished by multiple sets and higher repetitions (8–12) per set

3. Gains in strength/power are better accomplished by using multiple sets with fewer repetitions (4–6) per set.

Let us look at the basic principles of resistance-training programs and how they are related to gains in body weight and muscle mass and possible health benefits as well.

What are the basic principles of resistance training?

The following five principles are not restricted to resistance training but apply to all forms of training, even aerobic exercise training programs as introduced in Chapter 11. For example, intensity of exercise is simply another way of phrasing the overload principle.

The **principle of overload** is the most important principle in all resistance-training programs. The use of weights places a greater than normal stress on the muscle cell. This overload stress stimulates the muscle to grow—to become stronger—in effect to overcome the increased resistance imposed by the weights. (See Figure 12.2.)

To overload the muscle you must increase the volume of work it must do. There are basically two ways to do this. One is to increase the amount of resistance or weight that you use; the other way is to increase the number of repetitions and sets you do. Although there is no single best combination of sets and repetitions, usually two or three sets with 8 to 12 RM provide an adequate stimulus

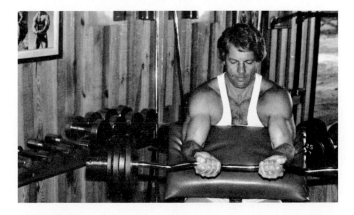

Figure 12.2 The principle of overload in action with weight training. If improvement in strength is to continue, weights must be increased.

for muscle growth. If you know your 1RM, you should be able to do 8 to 12 RM if you use 60 to 80 percent of your 1RM value. For example, if your bench press 1RM is 150 pounds, you should be able to do at least 8RM with 70 percent of that value, or 105 pounds (.70 × 150).

As the muscle continues to get stronger during your training program, you must increase the amount of resistance, the overload, to continue to get the proper stimulus for sustained muscle growth. This is known as **principle of progressive resistance exercise (PRE),** another basic principle of resistance training.

Following a learning period, a recommended program for beginners is three to five sets with 8RM in each set. The first step is to determine the maximum amount of weight that you can lift for eight repetitions. If you can do more than eight repetitions, the weight is too light and you need to add more poundage. As you get stronger during the succeeding weeks, you will be able to lift the original weight more easily. When you can perform twelve repetitions, add more weight to force you back down to eight repetitions; this is the progressive resistance principle. Over several months' time, the weight will probably need to be increased several times as you continue to get stronger. Such a transition is illustrated in Figure 12.3.

The **principle of specificity** is a broad training principle with many implications for resistance training, including specificity for various sports movements, strength gains, endurance gains, and body-weight gains. For example, a swimmer who wants to gain strength and endurance for a stroke should attempt to find a resistance-weight training program that exercises the specific muscles in a way as close as possible to the form used in that stroke. If you want to gain muscle mass in a certain part of the body, those muscles must be exercised.

Your exercise routine should be based upon the **principle of exercise sequence.** This means that if you have ten exercises in your routine, they should be arranged in logical order so that fatigue does not limit your lifting ability. For example, the first exercise in a sequence of ten might stress the biceps muscle, the second the abdominals, the third the quadriceps, and so forth. After you perform one full set of each of the ten exercises, you then do a complete second set, followed by the third set. This approach may be best for beginners.

Another popular option is to do three sets of the same exercise with a rest between sets; then do three sets of the second exercise, and so on. This approach may be a little more fatiguing because you are using the same muscle group in three successive sets, but it appears to be very effective.

Resistance training, if done properly to achieve the greatest gains, imposes a rather severe stress on the muscles, requiring a period of recovery both during the workout and between workouts. Research has shown that high-intensity resistance exercise can lead to rapid depletion of ATP and PC, the high energy phosphates stored in the muscles;

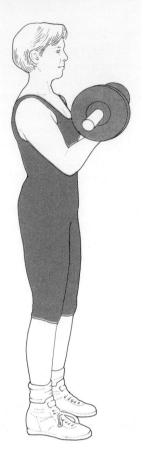

Week:	1	4	7	10	13	16
Weight:	50	50	60	60	70	70
Repetitions:	5	10	5	10	5	10
Sets:	4	4	4	4	4	4

Figure 12.3 The principle of progressive resistance exercise (PRE) states that as you get stronger, you need to progressively increase the resistance in order to continue to gain strength and muscle. In this example, the individual increases the resistance when she can complete ten repetitions with a given weight, but then only doing five repetitions with the increased weight.

however, most of these high energy compounds may be restored in about 2 to 3 minutes of recovery. This is the **principle of recuperation.** Thus, several minutes should intervene between sets if you are using the same exercise. Additionally, for beginners, resistance training should generally be done about 3 days per week, with a rest or recuperation day in between. This day of rest allows sufficient time for your muscle to repair itself and to synthesize new protein as it continues to grow, for research has shown that muscle protein synthesis occurs for up to 24 hours after a single bout of heavy resistance exercise.

These general principles should serve as guidelines during the beginning phase of your resistance-training program and should be used to guide your progress during the first 3 months of the basic resistance-training program described below.

What is an example of a resistance-training program that may help me to gain body weight as lean muscle mass?

If your goal is to gain significant amounts of muscle mass, you may wish to use the **bulk-up method.** This method involves the use of six to ten different exercises that stress the major muscle groups of the body. About three to five sets of each exercise are done. For those with limited time, one set may also provide significant increases in strength and muscle mass, as recently documented by Starkey and others. You should work up to 8–12 repetitions. The PRE concept is used, starting with resistance you can handle for eight repetitions and progressively increasing the repetitions to twelve. After you reach twelve repetitions, increase the resistance until you must come back to eight repetitions.

The bulk-up method should be used for several months to increase your weight. You may then wish to shape that bulk, a technique that bodybuilders call razoring or "cutting up." This technique uses a wide variety of exercises done with lighter weights and many repetitions at high speed; you are exercising on the endurance end of the continuum. Once you have achieved your desired body weight, you may alternate the bulk-up and razoring techniques to maintain your weight and shape.

The beginner should adhere to the following procedure using the basic resistance-training program.

1. Learn the proper technique for each exercise with a light weight, possibly only the bar itself, for 2 weeks. Do eight to twelve repetitions of each exercise to develop form. Do not strain during this initial learning phase.

2. For each exercise, determine the maximum weight that you can lift for eight repetitions after the 2-week learning phase.

3. Do one set of the eight exercises shown in Figures 12.4 to 12.11. The sequence of exercises should be
   a. Bench press: chest muscles
   b. Lat machine pulldown or bent-arm pullover: back muscles
   c. Half squat: thigh muscles
   d. Standing lateral raise: shoulder muscles
   e. Heel raise: calf muscles
   f. Standing curl: front upper arm muscles
   g. Seated overhead press: back upper arm muscles
   h. Curl-up: abdominal muscles

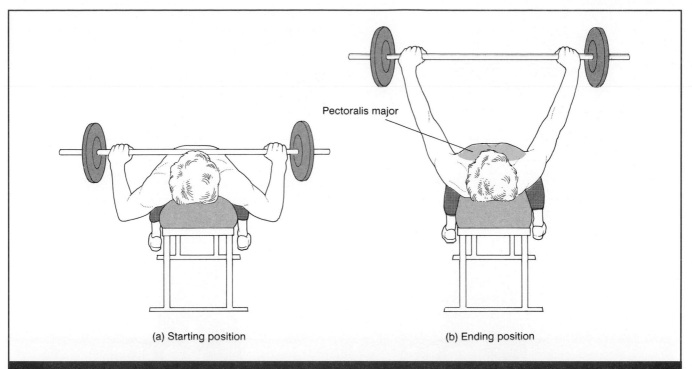

(a) Starting position   (b) Ending position

Figure 12.4 The bench press. The bench press primarily develops the pectoralis major muscle group in the chest; it also develops the deltoids in the shoulder and the triceps at the back of the arm.

Chest

Exercise	Bench press
Chest muscles	Pectoralis major
Other muscles	Deltoid, triceps
Sets	3–5
Repetitions	8–12, PRE concept
Safety	Have spotter stand behind bar to assist as fatigue sets in.
Equipment	Bench with support for weight, or two spotters to hand weight to you.
Description	Lie supine on bench. Use wide grip for chest development. Secure bar and lower *slowly* to chest. Press bar straight up to full extension. Do not arch back.

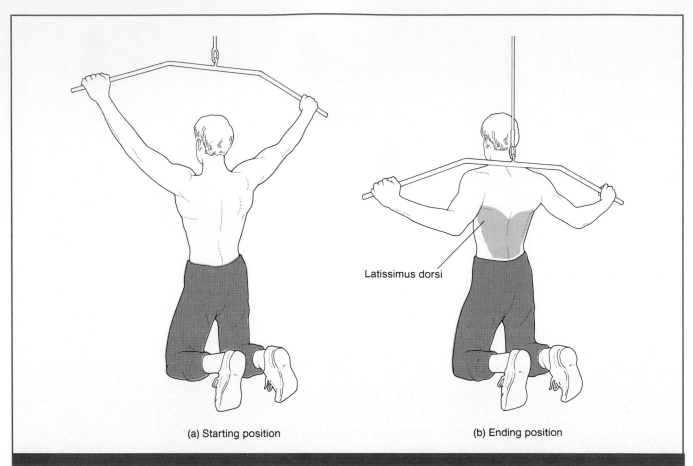

(a) Starting position   (b) Ending position

Latissimus dorsi

Figure 12.5A The lat machine pulldown. The lat machine pulldown trains the latissimus dorsi in the back and side of the upper body, but it also develops the biceps on the front of the upper arm and the pectoralis major in the chest.

Back

Exercise	Lat machine pulldown
Back muscles	Latissimus dorsi
Other muscles	Biceps, pectoralis major
Sets	3–5
Repetitions	8–12, PRE concept
Safety	A very safe exercise
Equipment	Lat machine
Description	From seated or kneeling position, take a wide grip at arm's length on the bar overhead. Pull bar down until it reaches back of the neck. Return slowly to starting position.

Note: If a lat machine is not available, the bent-arm pullover may be substituted.

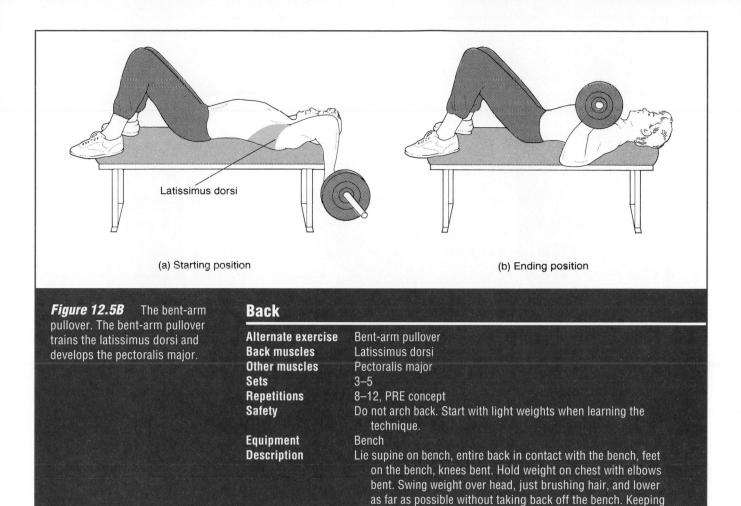

(a) Starting position

(b) Ending position

Latissimus dorsi

Figure 12.5B The bent-arm pullover. The bent-arm pullover trains the latissimus dorsi and develops the pectoralis major.

Back

Alternate exercise	Bent-arm pullover
Back muscles	Latissimus dorsi
Other muscles	Pectoralis major
Sets	3–5
Repetitions	8–12, PRE concept
Safety	Do not arch back. Start with light weights when learning the technique.
Equipment	Bench
Description	Lie supine on bench, entire back in contact with the bench, feet on the bench, knees bent. Hold weight on chest with elbows bent. Swing weight over head, just brushing hair, and lower as far as possible without taking back off the bench. Keeping elbows in, return the weight to the chest.

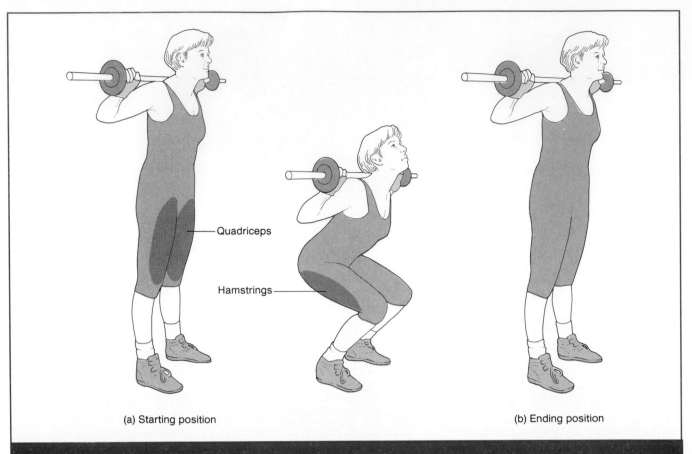

(a) Starting position   (b) Ending position

Quadriceps

Hamstrings

Figure 12.6 The half-squat or parallel squat. The half-squat develops the quadriceps muscle group on the front of the thigh and the hamstrings on the back of the thigh.

Thigh

Exercise	Half-squat or parallel squat
Thigh muscles	Quadriceps (front), hamstrings (back)
Other muscles	Gluteus maximus
Sets	3–5
Repetitions	8–12, PRE concept
Safety	Have two spotters to assist if using free weights. Keep back straight. Drop weight behind you if you lose balance. Do not squat more than halfway down.
Equipment	Squat rack if available. Pad the bar with towels if necessary.
Description	In standing position, take bar from squat rack or spotters and rest on the shoulders behind the head. Squat until thighs are parallel to ground or until buttocks touch a chair at this parallel position. Do not squat beyond halfway. Keep back as straight as possible. Return to standing position.

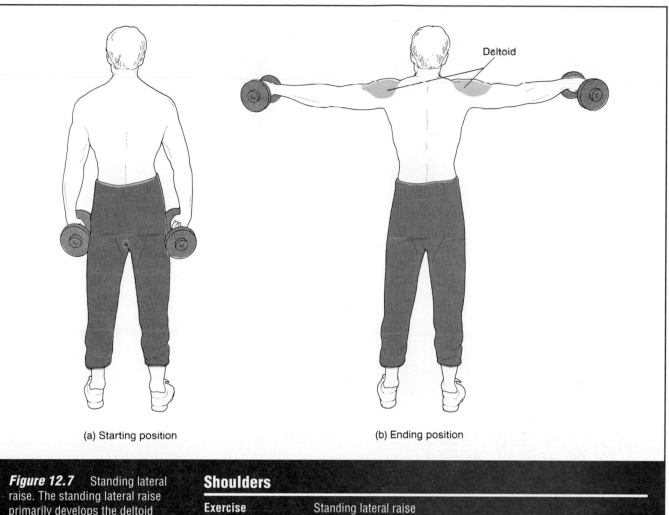

(a) Starting position   (b) Ending position

Figure 12.7 Standing lateral raise. The standing lateral raise primarily develops the deltoid muscles in the shoulder; the trapezius in the upper back and neck area is also trained.

Shoulders

Exercise	Standing lateral raise
Shoulder muscles	Deltoid
Other muscles	Trapezius
Sets	3–5
Repetitions	8–12, PRE concept
Safety	Do not arch back
Equipment	Dumbbells
Description	Stand with dumbbells in hands at sides. With palms down, raise straight arms sideways to shoulder level. Bend elbows slightly. Return slowly to starting position.

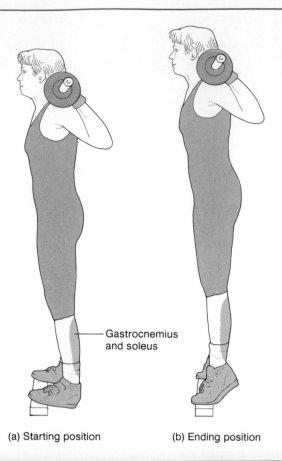

Gastrocnemius
and soleus

(a) Starting position   (b) Ending position

Figure 12.8   Heel raise. The heel raise develops the two major calf muscles—the gastrocnemius and the soleus.

Calf

Exercise	Heel raise
Calf muscles	Gastrocnemius, soleus
Other muscles	Deep calf muscles
Sets	3–5
Repetitions	8–12, PRE concept
Safety	Have two spotters if you use free weights.
Equipment	Squat rack, if available. Pad the bar with a towel if necessary.
Description	Place bar on back of shoulders as in squat exercise. Raise up on your toes as high as possible and then return to standing position. Place the toes on a board so heels can drop down lower than normal. Point toes in, out, and straight ahead during different sets to work the muscles from different angles.

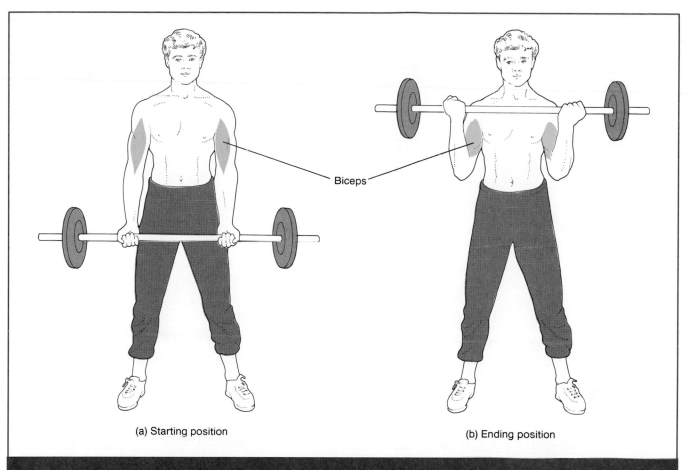

(a) Starting position

(b) Ending position

Biceps

Figure 12.9 The standing curl. The standing curl strengthens the biceps muscle in the front of the upper arm as well as several other muscles in the region that bend the elbow.

Front of arm

Exercise	Standing curl
Arm muscle	Biceps
Other muscles	Several elbow flexors
Sets	3–5
Repetitions	8–12, PRE concept
Safety	Do not arch back. Place back against wall to control arching motion.
Equipment	Curl bar if available
Description	Stand with weight held in front of body, palms forward. Place back against wall. Bend the elbows and bring the weight to the chest. Lower it slowly.

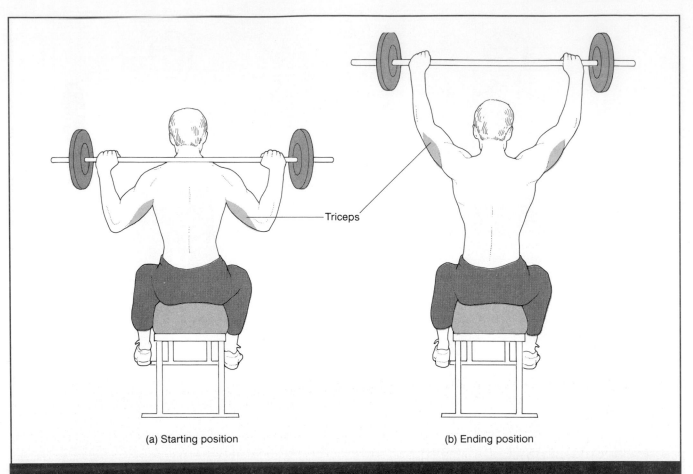

(a) Starting position   (b) Ending position

Triceps

Figure 12.10 The seated overhead press. The seated overhead press primarily develops the triceps muscle on the back of the upper arm; the exercise also trains the trapezius in the upper back and neck and the deltoids in the shoulder.

Back of arm

Exercise	Seated overhead press
Arm muscle	Triceps
Other muscles	Trapezius, deltoids
Sets	3–5
Repetitions	8–12, PRE concept
Safety	Do not arch back excessively. Have spotter available as fatigue sets in.
Equipment	Bench or chair
Description	Sit on bench with weight held behind the head near the neck. Hands should be close together, elbows bent. Straighten elbows and press weight over head to arm's length. Lower weight slowly to starting position.

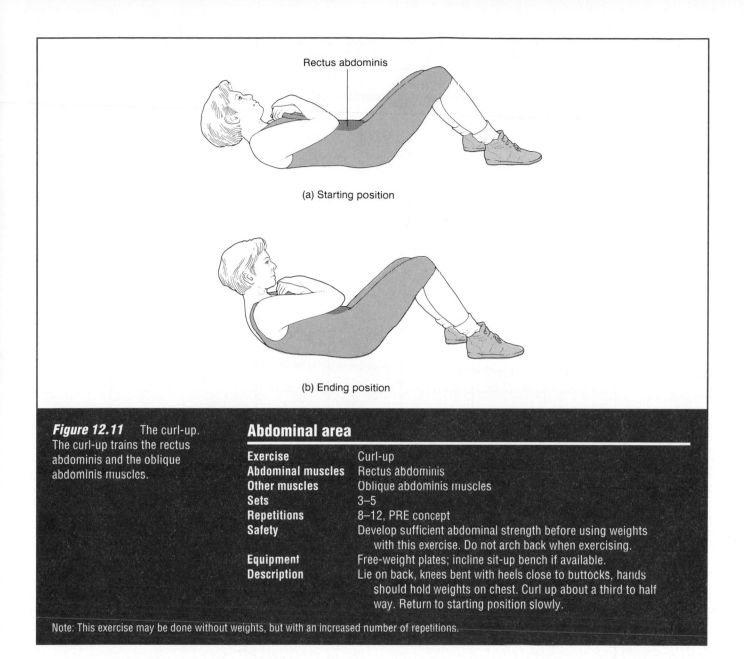

Figure 12.11 The curl-up. The curl-up trains the rectus abdominis and the oblique abdominis muscles.

(a) Starting position

(b) Ending position

Rectus abdominis

Abdominal area

Exercise	Curl-up
Abdominal muscles	Rectus abdominis
Other muscles	Oblique abdominis muscles
Sets	3–5
Repetitions	8–12, PRE concept
Safety	Develop sufficient abdominal strength before using weights with this exercise. Do not arch back when exercising.
Equipment	Free-weight plates; incline sit-up bench if available.
Description	Lie on back, knees bent with heels close to buttocks, hands should hold weights on chest. Curl up about a third to half way. Return to starting position slowly.

Note: This exercise may be done without weights, but with an increased number of repetitions.

4. A weekly record form, similar to the one presented in Table 12.1, should be used to keep track of your progress.

5. Because the exercise sequence is designed to stress different muscle groups in order, not much recuperation is necessary between exercises— possibly only 30 seconds or so.

6. Do three to five complete sets. You may wish to rest 2 to 3 minutes between sets.

7. Exercise 3 days per week; in each succeeding day try to do as many repetitions as possible for each exercise in each set. When you can do twelve repetitions each after a month or so, add more weight so you can do only eight repetitions.

8. Repeat step 7 as you progressively increase your strength.

Because barbells and dumbbells appear to be the most common means of doing resistance training, this is

Table 12.1 Weekly resistance-training record, basic eight exercises

	Chest (Bench Press)		Back (Lat Pulldown)		Thigh (Half Squat)		Shoulder (Lateral Raise)		Calf (Heel Raise)		Front arm (Curls)		Back arm (Seated Press)		Abdominal area (Curl-ups)	
	Wt	Reps	Wt	Reps	Wt	Reps	Wt	Reps	Wt	Reps	Wt	Reps	Wt	Reps	Wt	Reps
Date_____																
Set 1																
Set 2																
Set 3																
Set 4																
Set 5																
Date_____																
Set 1																
Set 2																
Set 3																
Set 4																
Set 5																
Date_____																
Set 1																
Set 2																
Set 3																
Set 4																
Set 5																
Date_____																
Set 1																
Set 2																
Set 3																
Set 4																
Set 5																

the method utilized. However, other apparatus such as the Nautilus, Universal Gym, and others can also be used effectively to gain weight and strength (see Figure 12.12). Most of the exercises described here using barbells or dumbbells have similar counterparts on other apparatus.

Note that muscles seldom operate alone, and that most resistance-training exercises stress more than one muscle group. Thus, keep in mind that although an exer-

cise may be listed specifically for the chest muscles, it may also stress the arm and shoulder muscles. The exercises described in this section generally stress more than one body area, although their main effect is on the area noted.

These eight exercises stress most of the major muscle groups in the body and thus provide an adequate stimulus for gaining body weight and strength through an increase in muscle mass. Literally hundreds of different

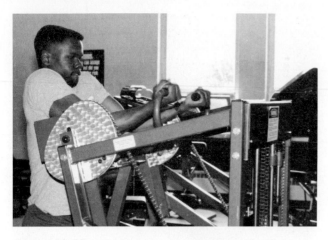

Figure 12.12 Machines such as Nautilus provide an alternative to free weights for development of muscular strength and endurance.

resistance-training exercises and techniques to train are available; if you become interested in diversifying your program (such as using the razoring technique), consult a book specific to resistance training. Several may be found in the reference list at the end of this chapter. For example, nearly thirty different types of programs are presented in the classic text by Fleck and Kraemer, *Designing Resistance Training Programs*.

How does the body gain weight with a resistance-training program?

Muscle hypertrophy simply means increased muscle size. Figure 12.13 depicts the microstructure of muscle tissue. Resistance-training exercises place a heavy overload on the muscle cell, in some way stimulating the DNA within the multiple nuclei found in muscle cells. Carson indicated that the first stage of muscle hypertrophy, at the onset of overload, is associated with increased RNA activity and protein synthesis. Over time the muscle cell tends to adapt to such stress by increasing its size. It may do so in several possible ways. First, the individual muscle cells and myofibrils may simply increase their size by incorporating more protein. Second, the myofibrils in each cell may multiply, which will increase the size of each muscle fiber. Third, the amount of connective tissue around each muscle fiber and around each bundle of muscle may increase and thicken, leading to an overall increase in the size of the total muscle. Fourth, the cell may increase its content of enzymes and energy storage, particularly ATP and glycogen. The increased muscle glycogen, along with increased muscle protein, binds additional water which contributes to an increased body weight. Finally, the muscle fibers themselves may increase in number (hyperplasia), but current evidence suggests this is much less likely to occur compared with the other four means to induce muscle hypertrophy. In addition to the effects on the mus-

cle cell, although not all studies are in agreement, research data indicate that resistance-training exercises may increase bone mineral content, possibly owing to increased muscle tension effects on the bone, which might provide a slight increase in total body weight.

Resistance training may be an effective means to increase muscle size and mass. Such increases help improve muscular strength and endurance and may be important components in weight-control programs. Traditionally, in research studies females did not normally experience the same amount of hypertrophy that males did, although they did experience proportional gains in muscular strength and endurance. However, more recent research revealed a significant increase in muscle cell size when women engaged in an intense, concentrated resistance-training program. Moreover, in a recent study O'Hagan and others found that when exposed to the same short-term resistance training program, muscle size increased similarly in women and men.

Is any one type of resistance-training program or equipment more effective than others for gaining body weight?

There are a variety of methods for resistance training. **Isometric methods** involve a muscle contraction against an immovable object, such as trying to pull a telephone pole out of the ground. However, if you succeed in moving the object, then you are doing an isotonic exercise. **Isotonic methods** are of two types. The **concentric method** means the muscle is shortening, as the biceps does in the up phase of a pull-up. The **eccentric method** means the muscle is lengthening even though it is trying to shorten. In the down phase of the pull-up the biceps is now contracting eccentrically as it slows your rate of descent. Gravity is attempting to pull you down, but your biceps is resisting it. Finally, the **isokinetic method** uses machines or other devices to regulate the speed at which you can shorten your muscles. For example, you may try to move your arm as fast as possible, but you will only be able to move as fast as the setting on the isokinetic machine. Isokinetic exercise is also known as accommodating-resistance exercise because the resistance automatically adjusts to the force exerted, thus controlling the speed of movement.

Several different resistance-training apparatuses are available, such as Nautilus, Universal Gym, Cybex, Hydra-Gym, Soloflex, and other similar machines. Depending upon the model, they are designed to utilize one or more of the training methods cited above.

A number of research studies have been conducted to determine which of these methods or machines is best, particularly in relation to strength and power gains. Research suggests that at the present time it is probably safe to say that isotonic and isokinetic programs are comparable in their ability to produce gains in muscle size and strength. Also, other than possible safety considerations,

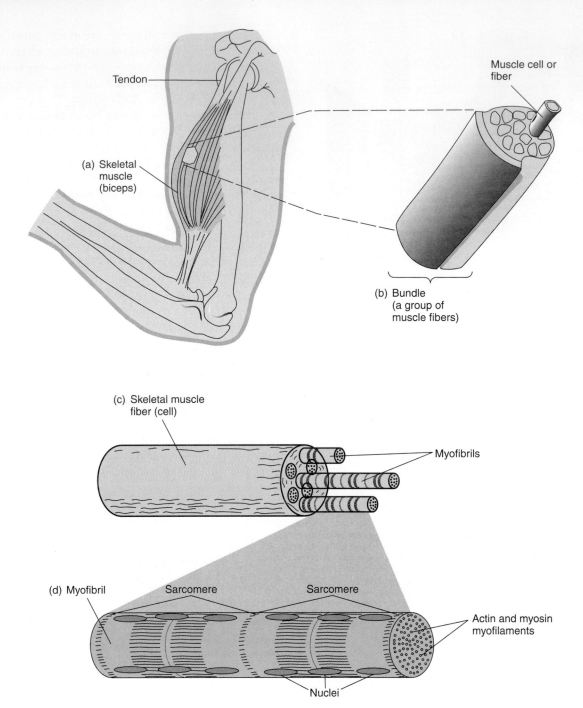

Figure 12.13 Muscle structure. The whole muscle is composed of separate bundles of individual muscle fibers. Each fiber is composed of numerous myofibrils, each of which contains thin protein filaments arranged so that they can slide by each other to cause muscle shortening or lengthening. Several layers of connective tissue surround the muscle fibers, bundles, and whole muscles, which eventually band together to form the tendon.

Source: From John W. Hole, Jr., *Human Anatomy and Physiology,* 3d ed. © 1984 Wm. C. Brown Communications, Inc., Dubuque, Iowa. All Rights Reserved. Reprinted by Permission.

recent research suggests that the use of specialized machines and resistance-training devices does not appear to have any advantage over the use of free weights, such as barbells and dumbbells. All methods may be effective in increasing body weight provided the basic principles of resistance training, particularly the principle of overload, are followed. If you use machines, be sure to exercise all major muscles areas. Free weights are relatively inexpensive and can be used for a wide variety of exercises. They also may be constructed at home, using pipe or solid broomstick handles for the bar and different-sized tin cans filled with cement for the weights.

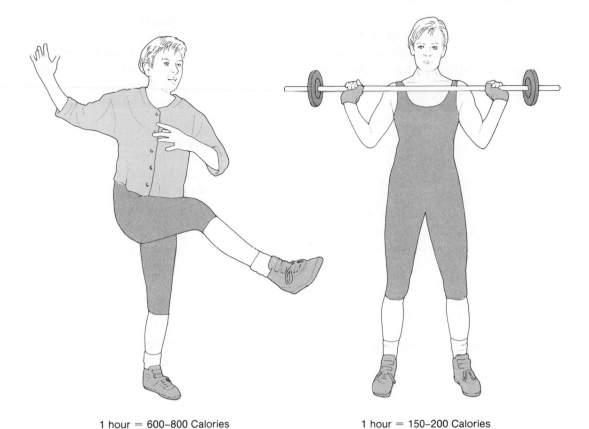

1 hour = 600–800 Calories

1 hour = 150–200 Calories

Figure 12.14 All modes of exercise increase caloric expenditure. However, an hour of regular weight training expends only about one-third to one-fourth as many Calories as vigorous aerobic activity. Combining aerobic exercises with weight training (circuit aerobics) helps burn more Calories than weight training alone; it also provides cardiovascular health benefits while increasing muscular strength and endurance.

There may be some specific training programs that are better suited for specific purposes, such as specific sport performance enhancement or injury rehabilitation. These topics are beyond the scope of this text, so the interested reader is referred to more detailed resources, such as the text by Fleck and Kraemer.

If exercise burns Calories, won't I lose weight on a resistance-training program?

Although exercise does cost Calories, the amount expended during resistance training is relatively small compared to more active aerobic exercise. Resistance training can be a high-intensity exercise, but the time spent actually lifting during a typical workout is usually short, therefore limiting the number of Calories used. For example, in an hour workout, only about 15 minutes may be involved in actual exercise, the remaining time being recovery between each exercise. Based upon metabolic data collected in research studies, the average-sized male uses about 200 Calories in a typical workout, while the average-sized female uses about 150. (See Figure 12.14.)

Are there any contraindications to resistance training?

There are several health conditions that may be aggravated by resistance training, primarily by the increased pressures that occur within the body when you strain to lift heavy weights and hold your breath at the same time. Because the blood pressure can increase rapidly and excessively during weight lifting, to 300 mmHg or higher, individuals with resting blood pressures over 90 mmHg diastolic and 140 mmHg systolic should refrain from heavy lifting, for they may be exposed to an increased risk of blood vessel rupture and a possible stroke. Lifting with the arms and straining exercises also increase the stress on the heart and thus should be avoided by individuals who have heart problems. Individuals with a hernia (a weakness in the musculature of the abdominal wall) also should refrain from strenuous weight lifting because the increased pressure may cause a rupture. Low back problems also may be aggravated by improper weight lifting techniques. Individuals with these types of health problems should seek medical advice before initiating a resistance-training program.

There has been some concern about the advisability of prepubescent youth lifting weights. Damage to the growth plate in the bones may occur when children try to lift weights in excess of their ability. However, the American Academy of Pediatrics endorsed the concept of resistance training for youngsters, provided proper techniques were taught and the program was supervised. In a meta-analysis of twenty-eight studies, Payne and others found that well-designed resistance-training programs appear to enhance muscular endurance and strength in children and youth, including prepubescent children. Although resistance training does not cause drug use, DuRant and others recently noted that adolescent anabolic/androgenic steroid (AAS) users in the United States, both athletes and nonathletes, are more likely to engage in strength training. AAS use is also associated with use of other recreational drugs. Thus, young adolescent athletes and nonathletes engaged in strength training should be educated about the health risks associated with AAS use.

Resistance training may be a very effective means to increase strength in the elderly as well; research has shown that even those in their nineties may experience significant strength gains with appropriately designed resistance-training programs.

Resistance training is generally regarded as a relatively safe sport, particularly if appropriate safety precautions are taken. The following guidelines should be incorporated into all resistance-training programs.

1. Learn to breathe properly. During the most strenuous part of the exercise you are likely to hold your breath. This is a natural response; it helps to stabilize your chest cavity to provide a more stable base for your muscles to function. Usually the breath hold is short and no problems occur. However, if prolonged, it may increase the chances of suffering some of the problems noted previously, such as a hernia.

   Also associated with prolonged breath holding is a response known as the **Valsalva phenomenon** (Valsalva maneuver), which may lead to a possible blackout. Here is what happens. As you reach a sticking point in your lift and strain to overcome it, you normally hold your breath; this causes your glottis to close over your windpipe and the pressure in your chest and abdominal area to rise rapidly. The pressure creates resistance to blood flow, reducing the return of blood to the heart, and eventually leading to decreased blood flow to the brain and a possible blackout. Additionally, the Valsalva maneuver exaggerates the increase in blood pressure during resistance exercises, and although a brief Valsalva maneuver is unavoidable when doing near maximal exercises, its effect may be minimized by proper breathing.

A recommended breathing pattern that will help minimize these adverse effects is to breathe out while lifting the weight and breathe in while lowering it. You should breathe through both your mouth and nose while exercising. Practice proper breathing when you learn new resistance-training exercises.

2. When using free weights, use spotters when doing exercises that may be potentially dangerous, such as the bench press. If you are doing a bench press alone and reach a sticking point in your lift, the Valsalva phenomenon may lead to serious consequences if you lose control of the weight directly above your head. The use of machines such as Nautilus and Universal Gym helps eliminate the need for spotters.

3. If using free weights, place lock collars on the bar ends so the plates do not fall off and cause injury to the feet. Again, the use of machines eliminates this safety hazard. However, do not attempt to change weight plates on machines while they are being used. Your fingers may get caught between the weights.

4. Warm up with proper stretching exercises.

5. Use light weights to learn the proper technique of a given exercise so that you do not strain yourself if you do the exercise incorrectly. When the proper technique is mastered, the weights may be increased.

6. Avoid exercises that may cause or aggravate low back problems. Try to prevent an excessive forward motion or stress in the lower back region. Figure 12.15 illustrates some positions that should be avoided.

7. Lower weights slowly. If you lower them rapidly, your muscles have to contract rapidly to slow the weights down as you reach the starting position. This necessitates the development of a large amount of force that may tear some connective tissue and cause muscle soreness.

Are there any health benefits associated with resistance training?

Although resistance training has been recommended mainly as a means of gaining muscle mass, body weight, and strength, its use normally was not associated with any health benefits. However, increasing research efforts focusing on the health implications of resistance training have suggested several favorable effects. Some of the health benefits are associated with increases in lean body mass and strength. However, Kraemer and others revealed that resistance training affects a number of systems in the body, not

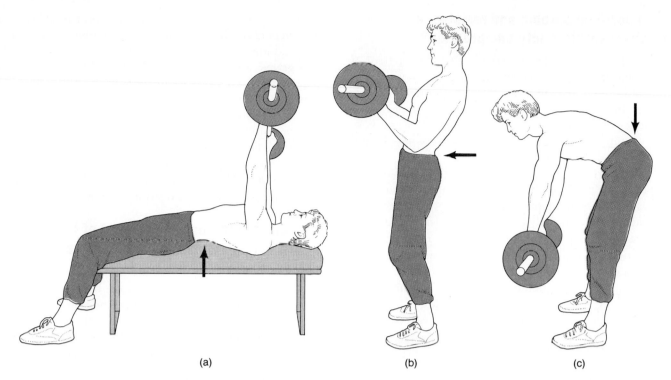

(a)   (b)   (c)

Figure 12.15   Avoid exercises or body positions that place excessive stress on the low-back region. Poor form in exercises like (*a*) the bench press and (*b*) the curl exaggerates the lumbar curve. Be sure to keep the lower back as flat as possible.

Exercises similar to (*c*) the bent-over row place tremendous forces on the lower back because the weight or resistance is so far in front of the body.

only the neuromuscular system, but also the connective tissue, cardiovascular, and endocrine systems. In this regard, resistance training may confer some additional physiological benefits conducive to good health. In a recent review, Pollock and Vincent reported multiple health benefits associated with resistance training which, along with those cited in other reports, include the following:

1. Increased lean body mass to help maintain resting energy expenditure and prevent obesity (The prevention of sarcopenia [loss of muscle mass] as one ages is a major health benefit.)

2. Increased strength to prevent falls and injury as one ages

3. Decreased pain in chronic low-back-pain patients to improve mobility

4. Increased bone mineral density to help prevent osteoporosis, particularly in females

5. Improved glucose metabolism and insulin sensitivity to help prevent diabetes

6. Improved serum lipid profiles, such as increased HDL cholesterol and decreased LDL cholesterol, to help prevent atherosclerosis and coronary heart disease

These findings are contrary to the belief that resistance training does not confer any health benefits comparable to aerobic exercise. It is also notable that many cardiac rehabilitation programs now incorporate resistance-training exercises. Indeed, the American Heart Association, the American College of Sports Medicine, and the recent Surgeon General's report on physical activity and health all have recognized the importance of resistance training as an important component of health.

Nevertheless, it still appears to be prudent health behavior to incorporate some aerobic exercise into your life-style, even when trying to gain body weight. Although the American College of Sports Medicine has recently added resistance training to its recommended exercise program for healthy adults, it is designed to complement aerobic exercise, not to substitute for it. (See Appendix J.) Aerobic exercise programs do consume more Calories, so you would have to balance the expenditure with increased food intake. However, the energy expenditure does not need to be excessive to provide a beneficial training effect. For example, running 2 to 3 miles about 4 days per week would provide you with an adequate training effect for your heart, but it would cost you only about 200–300 Calories a day. This 200- to 300-Calorie expenditure could be replaced easily by consuming two glasses of orange juice or similar small amounts of food.

Can I combine aerobic and resistance training exercises into one program?

Although the principles underlying the development of an aerobic-training program and a resistance-training program are similar, the purposes of each are rather different. An aerobic exercise program is designed to improve the efficiency of the cardiovascular system; the basic purpose of a resistance-training program is to increase muscle size, strength, and body weight.

One form of resistance training that has been used to provide some moderate benefits to the cardiovascular system is **circuit weight training,** a method in which the individual moves rapidly from one exercise to the next. Generally, this type of program uses lighter weights with greater numbers of repetitions, thus increasing the aerobic component of training. Recent research reported energy expenditure of approximately 10 Calories per minute for males and 7 Calories per minute for females.

A newer version of this method is **circuit aerobics.** Circuit aerobics may be done in a variety of ways, but basically it involves an integration of aerobic and resistance-training exercises. It is actually a form of interval aerobic training, but instead of resting or doing a lower level of aerobic activity during the recovery interval, you do resistance-training exercises. Circuit aerobics may offer benefits such as improved cardiovascular fitness, increased caloric expenditure for loss of body fat, improved muscular strength and endurance, and increased muscle tone in body areas not normally stressed by aerobic exercise alone.

However, if the main purpose of your resistance-training program is to gain body weight as muscle mass, then you need to train near the strength end of the strength-endurance continuum. For athletes who need to maximize gains in lean body mass, strength, and especially power, in a recent Gatorade Sports Science Institute review Michael Stone recommends that aerobic training should be markedly reduced if not eliminated, indicating that aerobic endurance training does not create a physiological environment compatible to such gains.

Nutritional Considerations

How many Calories are needed to form one pound of muscle?

Muscle tissue consists of about 70 percent water, 22 percent protein, and the remainder is fat, carbohydrate, and minerals. Because the vast majority of muscle tissue is water, which has no caloric value, the total caloric value is only about 700–800 Calories per pound. However, extra energy is needed to help synthesize the muscle tissue.

It is not known exactly how many additional Calories are necessary to form 1 pound of muscle tissue in human beings, nor is it known in what form these Calories have to be consumed. The National Research Council

notes that 5 Calories are needed to support the addition of 1 gram of tissue during growth, while Forbes cites a value of 8 Calories per gram in adults. Because 1 pound equals 454 grams, a range of 2,300–3,500 additional Calories appears to be a reasonable amount. With a recommended weight gain of 1 pound per week, about 400–500 Calories above your daily needs would provide an amount in the suggested range, 2,800–3,500 Calories per week. One recent study by Robert Bartels and his associates at Ohio State University revealed that an additional 500 Calories per day resulted in nearly a 1 pound increase in lean body weight per week during a resistance-training program.

How can I determine the amount of Calories I need daily to gain one pound per week?

First, use Table 11.1 to determine the number of Calories needed simply to maintain your current body weight. Then add the Calories that you expend during exercise and the additional amount needed to synthesize the muscle tissue. Table 12.2 presents an example of a 150-pound teenage boy who desires to gain a pound per week. You may modify the figures according to your own needs. Remember, a weight gain of 0.5–1.0 pound muscle mass per week is a reasonable goal during the early stages of resistance training.

Increased caloric intake is the key dietary principle, along with adequate protein intake, to gain muscle mass during resistance training, as noted in a recent Gatorade Sports Science Institute review of weight-gain strategies in athletes by leading experts in the area, Gail Butterfield, Susan Kleiner, Peter Lemon, and Michael Stone.

Table 12.2	Caloric intake for a 150-pound teenage boy to gain one pound per week
Energy expenditure	**Daily Calories needed**
Recommended caloric intake to maintain current weight 19 Calories/pound	2,850
Resistance-training 200 Calories per session 4 sessions per week 800/7	115
Aerobic exercise 300 Calories per session 4 sessions per week 1,200/7	170
Muscle tissue synthesis 3,500 Calories per pound 3,500/7	500
Total daily caloric intake	3,635

Is protein supplementation necessary during a weight-gaining program?

Gilbert Forbes indicates we need adequate amounts of protein to support increases in lean body mass, otherwise we would gain body fat. One pound of muscle is equal to 454 grams, but only about 22 percent of this tissue, or about 100 grams, is protein. If we divide 100 grams by 7 days, we would need approximately 14 grams of protein per day above our normal protein requirements if we are in protein balance. However, the average American diet already contains extra protein beyond the RDA, so this need probably is satisfied. Incidentally, 14 grams of protein could be obtained in such small amounts of food as 2 glasses of milk, 2 ounces of cheese, two scrambled eggs, or 2 ounces of meat, fish, or poultry. (See Figure 12.16.)

Although the daily RDA for protein is about 1 gram per kilogram body weight, some authorities in sports nutrition have recommended up to 1.6–1.8 grams per kilogram for the athlete who is training to increase muscle mass. As noted in Chapter 6, a slight increase in the protein content of the typical American daily diet would meet even this recommendation. A brief review of the mathematics in Table 6.6 and the related discussion on pages 190–192 will help substantiate this statement.

Supplementation by expensive protein powders or amino acids is not necessary. The average American diet provides sufficient high-quality protein to meet the needs of a weight-gaining program, even more so if a high-Calorie diet is used as recommended below. It is important to note that dietary protein in excess of needs will be converted to fat unless resistance training is used to stimulate muscle growth.

Are dietary supplements necessary during a weight-gaining program?

Robert Keith, a sport nutrition professor at Auburn University, and his colleagues reported that the nutrient intakes of individuals, such as bodybuilders, attempting to gain muscle mass were well above recommended levels, indicating there probably would not be any advantage for these subjects to take nutrient supplements. However, dietary supplements appear to be very popular among athletes and others attempting to increase muscle mass and strength, if we can use advertisements as evidence to support this contention. For example, in a recent survey of only five magazines targeted to bodybuilding athletes, Grunewald and Bailey reported over 800 performance claims were made for 624 commercially available supplements.

Although there may be some truth underlying the alleged performance-enhancing mechanisms of these supplements, the effectiveness of most has not been evaluated by scientific research. In a review of nutritional supplements for strength-trained athletes, Williams indicated that there is little or no scientific evidence supporting positive effects on muscle growth, body-fat reduction, or strength enhancement in strength-trained athletes for the following: arginine, lysine, and ornithine (amino acids); inosine; choline; yohimbine; glandular products; vitamin B_{12}; carnitine; chromium; boron; magnesium; medium chain triglycerides; omega-3 fatty acids; gamma oryzanol; and Smilax. Most of these nutrients and dietary supplements, and others such as vanadium and HMB, have been discussed in previous chapters and have been found to be ineffective or inadequately researched.

You should be aware that some dietary supplements may contain substances that are prohibited for use in athletic competition. For example, ephedrine in Ma Huang and the steroid hormone dehydroepiandrosterone (DHEA) are prohibited agents even though they are marketed as dietary supplements. Ephedrine is a stimulant that may influence body composition and DHEA is theorized to increase testosterone levels. Incidentally, there are no sound data to support an ergogenic effect from either ephedrine or DHEA.

As noted in Chapter 6, creatine monohydrate supplementation does appear to increase body weight and numerous studies have reported gains in strength, particularly in high-intensity resistance exercises with short-term recovery. Although early increases in body weight may be primarily water, an increased resistance-training capacity may lead to muscle gains over time. Some studies support this finding, but additional confirmatory research is needed. You may wish to review the discussion of creatine supplementation on pages 197–200.

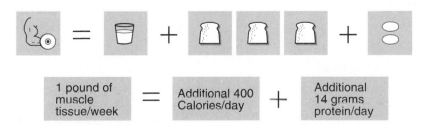

Figure 12.16 To add a pound of muscle tissue per week, you need to consume approximately 400 additional Calories and 14 grams of additional protein per day. A weight-training program is an essential part of a muscle-building program. One glass of skim milk, three slices of whole wheat bread, and two hard-boiled egg whites provide the necessary Calories and about 23 grams of protein.

As indicated in Chapter 1, many of these products are costly and some can have adverse effects on one's health. *Caveat emptor.*

What is an example of a balanced diet that will help me gain weight?

As with losing weight, the Food Exchange System may serve as the basis for a sound weight-gaining diet. Foods must be selected for high nutrient value as well as additional Calories to support the weight gain. In a recent review regarding healthy muscle gains, Susan Kleiner indicated the new school of thought is shifting away from high-meat, high-milk, high-fat diets, and toward high-Calorie, high-carbohydrate, increased-protein diets. Interestingly, research by Tucker and his associates indicated that women who undertook a resistance-training program seemed to modify their diets favorably, reducing the percentage of energy from dietary fat and increasing the percentage of energy from carbohydrate.

The following suggestions may be helpful for those trying to gain weight.

Milk exchange—Drink 1% or 2% milk instead of skim milk, which will add 15–30 Calories per glass. Prepare milk shakes with dry milk powder and supplement with fruit. Add low-fat cheeses to sandwiches or snacks. Eat yogurt supplemented with fruit. The milk exchange is high in protein.

Meat exchange—Increase your intake of lean meats, poultry, and fish. Legumes such as beans and dried peas are high in protein and Calories and low in fat. Use nuts, seeds, and limited amounts of peanut butter for snacks. The meat exchange is also high in protein.

Starch exchange—Increase your consumption of whole-grain products. Pasta and rice are nutritious side dishes that provide adequate Calories. Starchy vegetables like potatoes are also nutritious sources of Calories. Breads and muffins can possibly be supplemented with fruits and nuts. Whole-grain breakfast cereals can provide substantial Calories and even make a tasty dessert or snack with added fruit. The starch exchange is high in complex carbohydrates but also contains about 15 percent of its Calories as protein.

Fruit exchange—Add fruit to other food exchanges. Drink more fruit juices, which are high in both Calories and nutrients. Dried fruits such as apricots, pineapple, dates, and raisins are high in Calories and make excellent snacks.

Vegetable exchange—Use fresh vegetables like broccoli and cauliflower as snacks with melted low-fat cheese or a nutritious dip.

Fat exchange—Try to minimize the intake of saturated fats, using monounsaturated and polyunsaturated fats instead. Salad dressings and soft margarine added to vegetables can increase their caloric content.

Beverages—Milk and juices are nutritious and high in Calories. Those who drink alcohol should obtain only limited amounts of Calories in this way. Some liquid supplements are available commercially and may contain 300–400 Calories with substantial amounts of protein. However, check the label for fat and sugar content.

Snacks—Eat three balanced meals per day supplemented with two or three snacks. Dried fruits, nuts, and seeds are excellent snacks. Some of the high-Calorie, high-nutrient liquid meals on the market also make good snacks.

Table 12.3 presents an example of a high-Calorie diet plan based upon the Food Exchange System. It consists of three main meals and three snacks and totals about 4,000 Calories with 160 grams of protein, which is 16 percent of the Calories. It is also high in carbohydrate, which may increase insulin release, facilitating amino acid transport into the muscle to help promote protein synthesis. Carbohydrate also spares the use of protein as an energy source. Alternative foods may be substituted from the food exchange list presented in Appendix F. This suggested diet provides the necessary nutrients, Calories, and protein essential to increased development of muscle mass and yet fewer than 30 percent of the Calories are derived from fat. The total number of Calories can be adjusted to meet individual needs.

Would such a high-Calorie diet be ill advised for some individuals?

As noted in Chapter 5, one of the general recommendations for an improved diet is to reduce the consumption of fats, particularly saturated fats. Unfortunately, many high-Calorie diets are also high in fats. If there is a history of heart disease in the family or if an individual is known to have high blood lipid levels, then high-fat diets are contraindicated. Individuals with kidney problems also may have difficulty processing high-protein diets because of the increased need to excrete urea. Any person initiating such a weight-gaining program as advised here should be aware of his or her medical history.

Selection of food for a weight-gaining diet, if done wisely, can satisfy the criteria for healthful nutrition. Foods high in complex carbohydrates with moderate amounts of protein and a low fat content are able to provide substantial amounts of Calories and nutrients and yet minimize health risks that have been associated with the typical American diet. To gain weight wisely, you need to continue to eat healthful foods, but just more of them.

Table 12.3	A high-Calorie diet based on the Food Exchange System	
Exchange		**Calories**
Breakfast		
Milk	8 ounces 2% milk	120
Meat	1 poached egg	80
	2 ounces lean ham	110
Starch	2 slices whole wheat toast	160
Fruit	8 ounces orange juice	120
Other	1 tablespoon jelly	50
Mid-morning snack		
Fruit	8 ounces apricot nectar	160
Starch	2 slices whole wheat bread	160
Meat	1 tablespoon peanut butter	100
Lunch		
Milk	8 ounces 2% milk	120
Meat	4 ounces lean sandwich meat	220
Starch	2 slices whole wheat bread	160
	2 granola cookies	100
Fruit	1 banana	120
Vegetable, starchy	1 order french fries	300
Afternoon snack		
Fruit	1/4 cup raisins	120
Dinner		
Milk	8 ounces 2% milk	120
Meat	5 ounces salmon	275
Starch	2 slices whole wheat bread	160
Fruit	1 piece apple pie	350
Vegetable, starchy	1 cup peas	160
	1 sweet potato, candied	300
Evening snack		
Fruit	1/2 cup dried peaches	210
Milk	8 ounces 2% milk with banana	240
TOTAL		4,015

References

Books

Bouchard, C., et al. 1994. *Physical Activity, Fitness, and Health.* Champaign, IL: Human Kinetics.

Fleck, S., and Kraemer, W. 1997. *Designing Resistance Training Programs.* Champaign, IL: Human Kinetics.

Lamb, D., and Williams, M., eds. 1991. *Ergogenics: Enhancement of Performance in Exercise and Sport.* Dubuque, IA: Brown and Benchmark.

National Research Council. 1989. *Recommended Dietary Allowances.* Washington, DC: National Academy of Sciences.

Westcott, W. 1995. *Strength Fitness.* Dubuque, IA: Wm. C. Brown Publishers.

Williams, M. 1998. *The Ergogenics Edge: Pushing the Limits of Sports Performance.* Champaign, IL: Human Kinetics.

Yesalis, C., ed. 1993. *Anabolic Steroids in Sport and Exercise.* Champaign, IL: Human Kinetics.

Zatsiorsky, V. 1995. *Science and Practice of Strength Training.* Champaign, IL: Human Kinetics.

Reviews

American College of Sports Medicine. 1990. Position stand: The recommended quantity and quality of exercise for developing and maintaining cardiorespiratory and muscular fitness in healthy adults. *Medicine and Science in Sports and Exercise* 22:265–74.

American College of Sports Medicine. 1987. American College of Sports Medicine position stand on use of anabolic-androgenic steroids in sports. *Medicine and Science in Sports and Exercise* 19:534–39.

American Academy of Pediatrics. 1983. Weight training and weight lifting: Information for the pediatrician. *Physician and Sportsmedicine* 11 (March): 157–61.

American Medical Association. Council on Scientific Affairs. 1990. Medical and nonmedical uses of anabolic-androgenic steroids. *Journal of the American Medical Association* 264:2923–27.

Bartels, R. 1992. Weight training. How to lift-and eat-for strength and power. *Physician and Sportsmedicine* 20 (March): 223–34.

Blimkie, C. 1992. Resistance training during pre- and early puberty: Efficacy, trainability, mechanisms, and persistence. *Canadian Journal of Sport Sciences* 17:264–79.

Carson, J. 1997. The regulation of gene expression in hypertrophying skeletal muscle. *Exercise and Sport Sciences Reviews* 25:301–20.

Catlin, D., et al. 1993. Assessing the threat of anabolic steroids. *Physician and Sportsmedicine* 21:37–44.

Elashoff, J., et al. 1991. Effects of anabolic-androgenic steroids on muscular strength. *Annals of Internal Medicine* 115:387–93.

Evans, W. 1996. Reversing sarcopenia: How weight training can build strength and vitality. *Geriatrics* 51 (5): 46–54.

Fitts, R., and Widrick, J. 1996. Muscle mechanics: Adaptations with exercise-training. *Exercise and Sport Sciences Reviews* 24:427–73.

Foran, B. 1985. Advantages and disadvantages of isokinetics, variable resistance, and free weights. *National Strength and Conditioning Association Journal* 7:24–25.

Forbes, G. 1994. Body composition: Influence of nutrition, disease, growth and aging. In *Modern Nutrition in Health and Disease,* eds. M. Shils, et al. Philadelphia: Lea and Febiger.

Friedl, K. 1990. Reappraisal of the health risks associated with the use of high doses of oral and injectable androgenic steroids. *NIDA Research Monograph* 102:142–68.

Gatorade Sports Science Institute. 1995. Methods of weight gain in athletes. *Sports Science Exchange Roundtable* 6 (3): 1–4.

Goldberg, A. 1989. Aerobic and resistive exercise modify risk factors for coronary heart disease. *Medicine and Science in Sports and Exercise* 21:669–74.

Kicman, A., and Cowan, D. 1992. Peptide hormones and sport: Misuse and detection. *British Medical Bulletin* 48:496–517.

Kleiner, S. 1995. Healthy muscle gains. *Physician and Sportsmedicine* 23 (4): 21–22.

Kokkinos, P., and Hurley, B. 1990. Strength training and lipoprotein-lipid profiles: A critical analysis and recommendations for further study. *Sports Medicine* 9:266–72.

Kraemer, W., et al. 1996. Strength and power training: Physiological mechanisms of adaptation. *Exercise and Sport Sciences Reviews* 24:363–97.

Laseter, J., and Russell, J. 1991. Anabolic steroid-induced tendon pathology: A review of the literature. *Medicine and Science in Sports and Exercise* 23:1–3.

Lemon, P. 1996. Is increased dietary protein necessary or beneficial for individuals with a physically active lifestyle? *Nutrition Reviews* 54:S169–S175.

Lombardo, J., et al. 1991. Anabolic/androgenic steroids and growth hormone. In *Ergogenics: Enhancement of Performance in Exercise and Sport,* eds. D. Lamb and M. Williams. Dubuque, IA: Brown and Benchmark.

Lukas, S. 1996. CNS effects and abuse liability of anabolic-androgenic steroids. *Annual Reviews of Pharmacology and Toxicology* 36:333–57.

Luke, J., et al. 1990. Sudden cardiac death during exercise in a weight lifter using anabolic androgenic steroids: Pathological and toxicological findings. *Journal of Forensic Sciences* 35:1441–47.

MacIntyre, J. 1987. Growth hormone and athletes. *Sports Medicine* 4:129–42.

National Strength and Conditioning Association. 1987. Breathing during weight training. *National Strength and Conditioning Association Journal* 9:17–24.

Nnakwe, N. 1996. Anabolic steroids and cardiovascular risk in athletes. *Nutrition Today* 31 (5): 206–8.

Pauletto, B. 1986. Choice and order of exercises. *National Strength and Conditioning Association Journal* 8:71–73.

Payne, V., et al. 1997. Resistance training in children and youth: A meta-analysis. *Research Quarterly for Exercise and Sport* 68:80–88.

Pendergast, D. 1989. Cardiovascular, respiratory, and metabolic responses to upper body exercise. *Medicine and Science in Sports and Exercise* 21:S121–S125.

Petersen, R., and Goldberg, L. 1996. Adverse effects of anabolic steroids. *Journal of the American Medical Association* 276:257.

Pollock, M., and Vincent, K. 1996. Resistance training and health. *President's Council on Physical Fitness and Sports Research Digest* 2 (8): 1–6.

Potteiger, J., and Stilger, V. 1994. Anabolic steroid use in the adolescent athlete. *Journal of Athletic Training* 29:60–64.

Stewart, K., and Kelemen, M. 1989. Symposium: Resistive weight training: A new approach to exercise for cardiac and coronary disease prone populations. *Medicine and Science in Sports and Exercise* 21:667–97.

Williams, M. 1993. Nutritional supplements for strength trained athletes. *Sports Science Exchange* 6 (47): 1–6.

Yarasheski, K. 1994. Growth hormone: Effects on metabolism, body composition, muscle mass, and strength. *Exercise and Sport Sciences Reviews* 22:285–312.

Yesalis, C., and Bahrke, M. 1995. Anabolic-androgenic steroids: Current issues. *Sports Medicine* 19:326–40.

Specific Studies

Ballor, D., and Poehlman, E. 1992. Resting metabolic rate and coronary-heart-disease risk factors in aerobically and resistance-trained women. *American Journal of Clinical Nutrition* 56:968–74.

Ballor, D., et al. 1989. Energy output during hydraulic resistance circuit exercise for males and females. *Journal of Applied Sport Science Research* 3:7–12.

Bartels, R., et al. 1989. Effect of chronically increased consumption of energy and carbohydrate on anabolic adaptations to strenuous weight training. In *Report of the Ross Symposium on the Theory and Practice of Athletic Nutrition: Bridging the Gap,* eds. J. Storlie and A. Grandjean. Columbus, OH: Ross Laboratories.

Bhasin, S., et al. 1996. The effects of supraphysiologic doses of testosterone on muscle size and strength in normal men. *New England Journal of Medicine* 335:1–7.

Boyden, T., et al. 1993. Resistance exercise training is associated with decreases in serum low-density lipoprotein cholesterol levels in premenopausal women. *Archives of Internal Medicine* 153:97–100.

Chesley, A., et al. 1992. Changes in human muscle protein synthesis after resistance exercise. *Journal of Applied Physiology* 73:1383–88.

Cohen, L., et al. 1996. Lipoprotein (a) and cholesterol in bodybuilders using anabolic androgenic steroids. *Medicine and Science in Sports and Exercise* 28:176–79.

DuRant, R., et al. 1995. Anabolic-steroid use, strength training, and multiple drug use among adolescents in the United States. *Pediatrics* 96:23–28.

Evans, N. 1997. Gym and tonic: A profile of 100 male steroid users. *British Journal of Sports Medicine* 31:54–58.

Gillette, C., et al. 1994. Postexercise energy expenditure in response to acute aerobic or resistive exercise. *International Journal of Sport Nutrition* 4:347–60.

Grunewald, K., and Bailey, R. 1993. Commercially marketed supplements for bodybuilding athletes. *Sports Medicine* 15:90–103.

Hartgens, F., et al. 1996. Body composition, cardiovascular risk factors and liver function in long term androgenic-anabolic steroids using bodybuilders three months after drug withdrawal. *International Journal of Sports Medicine* 17:429–33.

Heinrich, C., et al. 1990. Bone mineral content of cyclically menstruating female resistance and endurance trained athletes. *Medicine and Science in Sports and Exercise* 22:558–63.

Keith, R., et al. 1996. Nutritional status and lipid profiles of trained steroid-using bodybuilders. *International Journal of Sport Nutrition* 6:247–54.

Koning, M., and Biener, K. 1990. Sport specific injuries in weight lifting. *Schweizerische Zeitschrift für Sport Medizine* 38:25–30.

Kreider, R., et al. 1996. Effects of ingesting supplements designed to promote lean tissue accretion on body composition during resistance training. *International Journal of Sport Nutrition* 6:234–46.

MacDougall, J., et al. 1992. Factors affecting blood pressure during heavy weight lifting and static contractions. *Journal of Applied Physiology* 73:1590–97.

Marin, P., et al. 1992. The effects of testosterone treatment on body composition and metabolism in middle-aged obese men. *International Journal of Obesity* 16:991–97.

Melby, C., et al. 1992. Energy expenditure following a bout of non-steady state resistance exercise. *Journal of Sports Medicine and Physical Fitness* 32:128–35.

Miller, W., et al. 1984. Effect of strength training on glucose tolerance and post-glucose insulin response. *Medicine and Science in Sports and Exercise* 16:539–43.

O'Hagan, F., et al. 1995. Response to resistance training in young women and men. *International Journal of Sports Medicine* 16:314–21.

Peterson, S., et al. 1989. The influence of high-velocity circuit resistance training on VO_2 max and cardiac output. *Canadian Journal of Sport Sciences* 14:158–63.

Poehlman, E., et al. 1992. Resting energy metabolism and cardiovascular disease risk in resistance-trained and aerobically trained males. *Metabolism* 41:1351–60.

Smidt, G., et al. 1992. The effect of high-intensity trunk exercise on bone mineral density of postmenopausal women. *Spine* 17:280–85.

Starkey, D., et al. 1996. Effect of resistance training volume on strength and muscle thickness. *Medicine and Science in Sports and Exercise* 28:1311–20.

Staron, R., et al. 1989. Effects of heavy resistance weight training on muscle fiber size and composition in females. *Medicine and Science in Sports and Exercise* 21:S71.

Sturmi, J., and Rutecki, G. 1995. When competitive bodybuilders collapse. *Physician and Sportsmedicine* 23 (11): 49–53.

Tucker, L., 1987. Effect of weight training on body attitudes: Who benefits most. *Journal of Sports Medicine and Physical Fitness* 27:70–78.

Tucker, L., et al. 1996. Participation in a strength training program leads to improved dietary intake in adult women. *Journal of the American Dietetic Association* 96:388–90.

Wallace, M., et al. 1991. Acute effects of resistance exercise on parameters of lipid metabolism. *Medicine and Science in Sports and Exercise* 23:199–204.

Yarasheski, K., et al. 1993. Short-term growth hormone treatment does not increase muscle protein synthesis in experienced weight lifters. *Journal of Applied Physiology* 74:3073–76.

Yeater, R., et al. 1996. Resistance trained athletes using or not using anabolic steroids compared to runners: Effects on cardiorespiratory variables, body composition, and plasma lipids. *British Journal of Sports Medicine* 30:11–14.

Yesalis, C., et al. 1997. Trends in anabolic-androgenic steroid use among adolescents. *Archives of Pediatric and Adolescent Medicine* 151:1197–1206.

1989 Recommended Dietary Allowances (RDA)

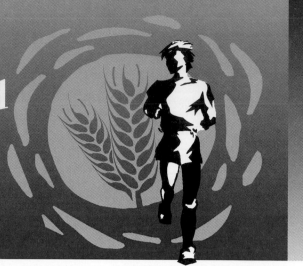

Note: The National Academy of Sciences is currently revising the RDA and releasing the new recommendations (such as those for vitamin D and calcium) in stages. These new values are not incorporated in this table, but are discussed in the text where relevant.

Food and Nutrition Board, National Academy of Sciences—National Research Council Recommended Daily Dietary Allowances,[a] revised 1989. (Designed for the maintenance of good nutrition of practically all healthy people in the United States.)

Category	Age (years) or condition	Weight[b] (kg)	Weight[b] (lb)	Height[b] (cm)	Height[b] (in)	Protein (g)	Vitamin A (μg RE)[c]	Vitamin D (μg)[d]	Vitamin E (mg α-TE)[e]	Vitamin K (μg)
Infants	0.0–0.5	6	13	60	24	13	375	7.5	3	5
	0.5–1.0	9	20	71	28	14	375	10	4	10
Children	1–3	13	29	90	35	16	400	10	6	15
	4–6	20	44	112	44	24	500	10	7	20
	7–10	28	62	132	52	28	700	10	7	30
Males	11–14	45	99	157	62	45	1,000	10	10	45
	15–18	66	145	176	69	59	1,000	10	10	65
	19–24	72	160	177	70	58	1,000	10	10	70
	25–50	79	174	176	70	63	1,000	5	10	80
	51 +	77	170	173	68	63	1,000	5	10	80
Females	11–14	46	101	157	62	46	800	10	8	45
	15–18	55	120	163	64	44	800	10	8	55
	19–24	58	128	164	65	46	800	10	8	60
	25–50	63	138	163	64	50	800	5	8	65
	51 +	65	143	160	63	50	800	5	8	65
Pregnant						60	800	10	10	65
Lactating	1st 6 months					65	1,300	10	12	65
	2nd 6 months					62	1,200	10	11	65

[a]The allowances, expressed as average daily intakes over time, are intended to provide for individual variations among most normal persons as they live in the United States under usual environmental stresses. Diets should be based on a variety of common foods in order to provide other nutrients for which human requirements have been less well defined.

[b]Weights and heights of Reference Adults are actual medians for the U.S. population of the designated age, as reported by NHANES II. The median weights and heights of those under 19 years of age were taken from Hamill et al. (1979). The use of these figures does not imply that the height-to-weight ratios are ideal.

Note: μg = microgram.

Water-soluble vitamins

Minerals

Vitamin C (mg)	Thiamin (mg)	Riboflavin (mg)	Niacin (mg NE)[f]	Vitamin B_6 (mg)	Folate (µg)	Vitamin B_{12} (µg)	Calcium (mg)	Phosphorus (mg)	Magnesium (mg)	Iron (mg)	Zinc (mg)	Iodine (µg)	Selenium (µg)
30	0.3	0.4	5	0.3	25	0.3	400	300	40	6	5	40	10
35	0.4	0.5	6	0.6	35	0.5	600	500	60	10	5	50	15
40	0.7	0.8	9	1.0	50	0.7	800	800	80	10	10	70	20
45	0.9	1.1	12	1.1	75	1.0	800	800	120	10	10	90	20
45	1.0	1.2	13	1.4	100	1.4	800	800	170	10	10	120	30
50	1.3	1.5	17	1.7	150	2.0	1,200	1,200	270	12	15	150	40
60	1.5	1.8	20	2.0	200	2.0	1,200	1,200	400	12	15	150	50
60	1.5	1.7	19	2.0	200	2.0	1,200	1,200	350	10	15	150	70
60	1.5	1.7	19	2.0	200	2.0	800	800	350	10	15	150	70
60	1.2	1.4	15	2.0	200	2.0	800	800	350	10	15	150	70
50	1.1	1.3	15	1.4	150	2.0	1,200	1,200	280	15	12	150	45
60	1.1	1.3	15	1.5	180	2.0	1,200	1,200	300	15	12	150	50
60	1.1	1.3	15	1.6	180	2.0	1,200	1,200	280	15	12	150	55
60	1.1	1.3	15	1.6	180	2.0	800	800	280	15	12	150	55
60	1.0	1.2	13	1.6	180	2.0	800	800	280	10	12	150	55
70	1.5	1.6	17	2.2	400	2.2	1,200	1,200	320	30	15	175	65
95	1.6	1.8	20	2.1	280	2.6	1,200	1,200	355	15	19	200	75
90	1.6	1.7	20	2.1	260	2.6	1,200	1,200	340	15	16	200	75

[c] Retinol equivalents. 1 retinol equivalent = 1 µg retinol or 6 µg β-carotene.

[d] As cholecalciferol. 10 µg cholecalciferol = 400 IU of vitamin D.

[e] α-Tocopherol equivalents. 1 mg d-α tocopherol = 1 α-TE.

[f] 1 NE (niacin equivalent) is equal to 1 mg of niacin or 60 mg of dietary tryptophan.

Estimated safe and adequate daily dietary intakes of selected vitamins and minerals[a]

		Vitamins	
Category	*Age (years)*	*Biotin (μg)*	*Pantothenic acid (mg)*
Infants	0–0.5	10	2
	0.5–1	15	3
Children and adolescents	1–3	20	3
	4–6	25	3–4
	7–10	30	4–5
	11 +	30–100	4–7
Adults		30–100	4–7

		Trace Elements[b]				
Category	*Age (years)*	*Copper (mg)*	*Manganese (mg)*	*Fluoride (mg)*	*Chromium (μg)*	*Molybdenum (μg)*
Infants	0–0.5	0.4–0.6	0.3–0.6	0.1–0.5	10–40	15–30
	0.5–1	0.6–0.7	0.6–1.0	0.2–1.0	20–60	20–40
Children and adolescents	1–3	0.7–1.0	1.0–1.5	0.5–1.5	20–80	25–50
	4–6	1.0–1.5	1.5–2.0	1.0–2.5	30–120	30–75
	7–10	1.0–2.0	2.0–3.0	1.5–2.5	50–200	50–150
	11 +	1.5–2.5	2.0–5.0	1.5–2.5	50–200	75–250
Adults		1.5–3.0	2.0–5.0	1.5–4.0	50–200	75–250

[a]Because there is less information on which to base allowances, these figures are not given in the main table of RDA and are provided here in the form of ranges of recommended intakes.

[b]Since the toxic levels for many trace elements may be only several times usual intakes, the upper levels for the trace elements given in this table should not be habitually exceeded.

Median heights and weights and recommended energy intake

Category	Age (years) or condition	Weight (kg)	Weight (lb)	Height (cm)	Height (in)	REE[a] (kcal/day)	Average energy allowance (kcal)[b] Multiples of REE	Average energy allowance (kcal)[b] Per kg	Average energy allowance (kcal)[b] Per day[c]
Infants	0.0–0.5	6	13	60	24	320		108	650
	0.5–1.0	9	20	71	28	500		98	850
Children	1–3	13	29	90	35	740		102	1,300
	4–6	20	44	112	44	950		90	1,800
	7–10	28	62	132	52	1,130		70	2,000
Males	11–14	45	99	157	62	1,440	1.70	55	2,500
	15–18	66	145	176	69	1,760	1.67	45	3,000
	19–24	72	160	177	70	1,780	1.67	40	2,900
	25–50	79	174	176	70	1,800	1.60	37	2,900
	51 +	77	170	173	68	1,530	1.50	30	2,300
Females	11–14	46	101	157	62	1,310	1.67	47	2,200
	15–18	55	120	163	64	1,370	1.60	40	2,200
	19–24	58	128	164	65	1,350	1.60	38	2,200
	25–50	63	138	163	64	1,380	1.55	36	2,200
	51 +	65	143	160	63	1,280	1.50	30	1,900
Pregnant	1st trimester								+ 0
	2nd trimester								+ 300
	3rd trimester								+ 300
Lactating	1st 6 months								+ 500
	2nd 6 months								+ 500

[a]REE is resting energy expenditure; see Chapter 3 for explanation. Calculation is based on Food and Agriculture Organization equations, then rounded.

[b]In the range of light to moderate activity, the coefficient of variation is ± 20%. Thus, for an individual with an average energy allowance of 2,500 Calories per day, the typical range might be 2,000–3,000, which is plus or minus 500 Calories (.20 × 2,500). See Chapter 3 for expanded discussion of energy requirement based upon physical activity levels.

[c]Figure is rounded.

Recommended Nutrient Intakes for Canadians

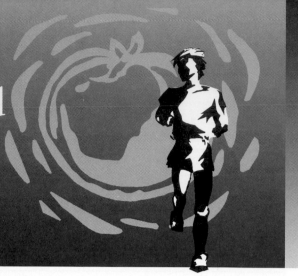

Summary of examples of recommended nutrients based on energy expressed as daily rates

Age	Sex	Energy kcal	Thiamin mg	Riboflavin mg	Niacin NE[b]	n-3 PUFA[a] g	n-6 PUFA g
Months							
0–4	Both	600	0.3	0.3	4	0.5	3
5–12	Both	900	0.4	0.5	7	0.5	3
Years							
1	Both	1,100	0.5	0.6	8	0.6	4
2–3	Both	1,300	0.6	0.7	9	0.7	4
4–6	Both	1,800	0.7	0.9	13	1.0	6
7–9	M	2,200	0.9	1.1	16	1.2	7
	F	1,900	0.8	1.0	14	1.0	6
10–12	M	2,500	1.0	1.3	18	1.4	8
	F	2,200	0.9	1.1	16	1.1	7
13–15	M	2,800	1.1	1.4	20	1.4	9
	F	2,200	0.9	1.1	16	1.2	7
16–18	M	3,200	1.3	1.6	23	1.8	11
	F	2,100	0.8	1.1	15	1.2	7
19–24	M	3,000	1.2	1.5	22	1.6	10
	F	2,100	0.8	1.1	15	1.2	7
25–49	M	2,700	1.1	1.4	19	1.5	9
	F	2,000	0.8	1.0	14	1.1	7
50–74	M	2,300	0.9	1.3	16	1.3	8
	F	1,800	0.8[c]	1.0[c]	14[c]	1.1[c]	7[c]
75 +	M	2,000	0.8	1.0	14	1.0	7
	F[d]	1,700	0.8[c]	1.0[c]	14[c]	1.1[c]	7[c]
Pregnancy (additional)							
1st Trimester		100	0.1	0.1	0.1	0.05	0.3
2nd Trimester		300	0.1	0.3	0.2	0.16	0.9
3rd Trimester		300	0.1	0.3	0.2	0.16	0.9
Lactation (additional)		450	0.2	0.4	0.3	0.25	1.5

[a]PUFA, polyunsaturated fatty acids
[b]Niacin Equivalents
[c]Level below which intake should not fall
[d]Assumes moderate physical activity

From "Nutrition Recommendations," in *Health Canada.* Canada Communication Group, Quebec, Canada. Reproduced with the permission of the Minister of Supply and Services Canada, 1994.

Summary examples of recommended nutrient intake based on age and body weight expressed as daily rates

Age	Sex	Weight kg	Protein g	Vit. A RE[a]	Vit. D μg	Vit. E mg	Vit. C mg	Folate μg	Vit. B$_{12}$ μg	Calcium mg	Phosphorus mg	Magnesium mg	Iron mg	Iodine μg	Zinc mg
Months															
0–4	Both	6.0	12[b]	400	10	3	20	50	0.3	250[c]	150	20	0.3[d]	30	2[d]
5–12	Both	9.0	12	400	10	3	20	50	0.3	400	200	32	7	40	3
Years															
1	Both	11	19	400	10	3	20	65	0.3	500	300	40	6	55	4
2–3	Both	14	22	400	5	4	20	80	0.4	550	350	50	6	65	4
4–6	Both	18	26	500	5	5	25	90	0.5	600	400	65	8	85	5
7–9	M	25	30	700	2.5	7	25	125	0.8	700	500	100	8	110	7
	F	25	30	700	2.5	6	25	125	0.8	700	500	100	8	95	7
10–12	M	34	38	800	2.5	8	25	170	1.0	900	700	130	8	125	9
	F	36	40	800	5	7	25	180	1.0	1,100	800	135	8	110	9
13–15	M	50	50	900	5	9	30	150	1.5	1,100	900	185	10	160	12
	F	48	42	800	5	7	30	145	1.5	1,000	850	180	13	160	9
16–18	M	62	55	1,000	5	10	40[e]	185	1.9	900	1,000	230	10	160	12
	F	53	43	800	2.5	7	30[e]	160	1.9	700	850	200	12	160	9
19–24	M	71	58	1,000	2.5	10	40[e]	210	2.0	800	1,000	240	9	160	12
	F	58	43	800	2.5	7	30[e]	175	2.0	700	850	200	13	160	9
25–49	M	74	61	1,000	2.5	9	40[e]	220	2.0	800	1,000	250	9	160	12
	F	59	44	800	2.5	6	30[e]	175	2.0	700	850	200	13	160	9
50–74	M	73	60	1,000	5	7	40[e]	220	2.0	800	1,000	250	9	160	12
	F	63	47	800	5	6	30[e]	190	2.0	800	850	210	8	160	9
75 +	M	69	57	1,000	5	6	40[e]	205	2.0	800	1,000	230	9	160	12
	F	64	47	800	5	5	30[e]	190	2.0	800	850	210	8	160	9
Pregnancy (additional)															
1st Trimester			5	100	2.5	2	0	300	1.0	500	200	15	0	25	6
2nd Trimester			20	100	2.5	2	10	300	1.0	500	200	45	5	25	6
3rd Trimester			24	100	2.5	2	10	300	1.0	500	200	45	10	25	6
Lactation (additional)			20	400	2.5	3	25	100	0.5	500	200	65	0	50	6

[a]Retinol Equivalents
[b]Protein is assumed to be from breast milk and must be adjusted for infant formula.
[c]Infant formula with high phosphorus should contain 375 mg calcium.
[d]Breast milk is assumed to be the source of the mineral.
[e]Smokers should increase vitamin C by 50%.

Units of Measurement: English System– Metric System Equivalents

The Metric System and Equivalents

To measure ingredients, a standardized system known as the System Internationale (SI) has been established that is interpreted on an international basis. The SI is based on the metric system. However, in the United States we also employ another set of measure and weight, the English system. In the field of dietetics, both systems are employed. The following tables give the quantities of the measures besides stating equivalents. With this information it is possible to calculate in either system of measure and weight.

Household Measures (Approximations)

For easy computing purposes, the cubic centimeter (cc) is considered equivalent to 1 gram:

$$1 \text{ cc} = 1 \text{ gram} = 1 \text{ milliliter (ml)}$$

For easy computing purposes, 1 ounce equals 30 grams or 30 cubic centimeters.

1 quart	=	960 grams
1 pint	=	480 grams
1 cup	=	240 grams
½ cup	=	120 grams
1 glass (8 ounces)	=	240 grams
½ glass (4 ounces)	=	120 grams
1 orange juice glass	=	100–120 grams
1 tablespoon	=	15 grams
1 teaspoon	=	5 grams

Level Measures and Weights

1 teaspoon	=	5 cc or 5 ml
		5 grams
3 teaspoons	=	1 tablespoon
		15 cc
		15 grams
2 tablespoons	=	30 cc
		30 grams
		1 ounce (fluid)
4 tablespoons	=	¼ cup
		60 cc
		60 grams
8 tablespoons	=	½ cup
		120 cc
		120 grams
16 tablespoons	=	1 cup
		240 grams
		240 ml (fluid)
		8 ounces (fluid)
		½ pound
2 cups	=	1 pint
		480 grams
		480 ml (fluid)
		16 ounces (fluid)
		1 pound
4 cups	=	2 pints
		1 quart
		960 cc
		960 ml (fluid)
		2 pounds
4 quarts	=	1 gallon

Units of Weight

		Ounce	Pound	Gram	Kilogram
1 ounce	–	1.0	0.06	28.4	0.028
1 pound	=	16.0	1.0	454	0.454
1 gram	=	0.035	.002	1.0	0.001
1 kilogram	=	35.3	2.2	1,000	1.0

Units of Volume

		Ounce	Pint	Quart	Milliliter	Liter
1 ounce	=	1.0	0.062	0.031	29.57	0.029
1 pint	=	16.0	1.0	0.5	473	.473
1 quart	=	32.0	2.0	1.0	946	.946
1 milliliter	=	0.034	0.002	0.001	1.0	0.001
1 liter	=	33.8	2.112	1.056	1,000	1.0

Units of Length

		Millimeter	Centimeter	Inch	Foot	Yard	Meter
1 millimeter	=	1.0	0.1	0.0394	0.0033	0.0011	0.001
1 centimeter	=	10.0	1.0	0.394	0.033	0.011	0.01
1 inch	=	25.4	2.54	1.0	0.083	0.028	0.025
1 foot	=	304.8	30.48	12.0	1.0	0.333	0.305
1 yard	=	914.4	91.44	36.0	3.0	1.0	0.914
1 meter	=	1,000	100	39.37	3.28	1.094	1.0

1 kilometer	=	1,000 meters	= 0.62 mile
1 mile	=	1,760 yards	= 1.61 kilometers

Units of mechanical, thermal, and chemical energy (approximate equivalents)

	Foot-pounds	Kilogram-meters	Kilojoules	Watts*	Kilocalories	Oxygen**
1 foot-pound	1	0.138	0.00136	0.0226	0.00032	0.000064
1 kilogram-meter	7.23	1	0.0098	0.163	0.0023	0.00046
1 kilojoule	737	102	1	16.66	0.239	0.047
1 watt*	44.27	6.12	0.06	1	0.0143	0.0028
1 kilocalorie	3,088	427	4.18	0.00024	1	0.198
1 liter oxygen**	15,585	2,154	21.1	351.9	5.047	1

Note: Read all tables across, such as 1 watt equals 44.27 foot-pounds; 1 foot-pound equals 0.0226 watt.

* Watts are units of power expressed per minute.
** Equivalents are based upon one liter of oxygen metabolizing carbohydrate. Energy equivalents would be slightly less on a mixed diet of carbohydrate, fat, and protein. For example, 1 liter of oxygen would equal only 4.82 kilocalories.

Approximate Caloric Expenditure Per Minute for Various Physical Activities

When using this appendix, keep these points in mind.

A. The figures are approximate and include the resting energy expenditure (REE). Thus, the total cost of the exercise includes not only the energy expended by the exercise itself, but also the amount you would have used anyway during the same period. Suppose you ran for 1 hour and the calculated energy cost was 800 Calories. During that same time at rest, your REE may have been 75 Calories, so the net cost of the exercise is 725 Calories.

B. The figures in the table are only for the time you are performing the activity. For example, in an hour of basketball, you may exercise strenuously only for 35 to 40 minutes, as you may take time-outs and may rest during foul shots. In general, record only the amount of time that you are actually exercising during the activity.

C. The energy cost, expressed in Calories per minute, will vary for different physical activities in a given individual depending on several factors. For example, the caloric cost of bicycling will vary depending on the type of bicycle, going uphill and downhill, and wind resistance. Walking with hand weights or ankle weights will increase energy output. Energy cost for swimming at a certain pace will depend on swimming efficiency, so the less efficient swimmer will expend more Calories. Thus, the values expressed here are approximations and may be increased or decreased depending upon various factors that influence energy cost for a specific physical activity.

D. Not all body weights could be listed, but you may approximate by using the closest weight listed.

E. There may be small differences between males and females, but not enough to make a significant difference in the total caloric value for most exercises.

425

Body weight

	Kilograms	45	48	50	52	55	57	59	61	64	66	68	70
	Pounds	100	105	110	115	120	125	130	135	140	145	150	155
Sedentary activities													
Lying quietly		1.0	1.0	1.1	1.1	1.2	1.3	1.3	1.4	1.4	1.5	1.5	1.5
Sitting and writing, card playing, etc.		1.2	1.3	1.4	1.5	1.5	1.6	1.7	1.7	1.8	1.8	1.9	2.0
Standing with light work, cleaning, etc.		2.7	2.9	3.0	3.1	3.3	3.4	3.5	3.7	3.8	3.9	4.1	4.2
Physical activities													
Archery		3.1	3.3	3.5	3.6	3.8	4.0	4.1	4.3	4.5	4.6	4.8	4.9
Badminton													
Recreational singles		3.6	3.8	4.0	4.2	4.4	4.6	4.7	4.9	5.1	5.3	5.4	5.6
Social doubles		2.7	2.9	3.0	3.1	3.3	3.4	3.5	3.7	3.8	3.9	4.1	4.2
Competitive		5.9	6.1	6.4	6.7	7.0	7.3	7.6	7.9	8.2	8.5	8.8	9.1
Baseball													
Player		3.1	3.3	3.4	3.6	3.8	4.0	4.1	4.3	4.4	4.5	4.7	4.8
Pitcher		3.9	4.1	4.3	4.5	4.7	4.9	5.1	5.3	5.5	5.7	5.9	6.0
Basketball													
Half court		3.0	3.1	3.3	3.5	3.6	3.8	3.9	4.1	4.2	4.4	4.5	4.7
Recreational		4.9	5.2	5.5	5.7	6.0	6.2	6.5	6.7	7.0	7.2	7.5	7.7
Vigorous competition		6.5	6.8	7.2	7.5	7.8	8.2	8.5	8.8	9.2	9.5	9.9	10.2
Bicycling, level (mph) (min/mile)													
5 12:00		1.9	2.0	2.1	2.2	2.3	2.4	2.5	2.6	2.7	2.8	2.9	3.0
10 6:00		4.2	4.4	4.6	4.8	5.1	5.3	5.5	5.7	5.9	6.1	6.4	6.6
15 4:00		7.3	7.6	8.0	8.4	8.7	9.1	9.5	9.8	10.0	10.5	10.9	11.3
20 3:00		10.7	11.2	11.7	12.3	12.8	13.3	13.9	14.4	14.9	15.5	16.0	16.5
Bowling		2.7	2.8	3.0	3.1	3.3	3.4	3.5	3.7	3.8	3.9	4.1	4.2
Calisthenics													
Light type		3.4	3.6	3.8	4.0	4.1	4.3	4.5	4.7	4.8	5.0	5.2	5.4
Timed vigorous		9.7	10.1	10.6	11.1	11.6	12.1	12.6	13.1	13.6	14.1	14.6	15.1
Canoeing (mph) (min/mile)													
2.5 24		1.9	2.0	2.1	2.2	2.3	2.4	2.5	2.6	2.7	2.8	2.9	3.0
4.0 15		4.4	4.6	4.9	5.1	5.3	5.5	5.8	6.0	6.2	6.4	6.7	6.9
5.0 12		5.7	6.0	6.3	6.6	6.9	7.2	7.5	7.8	8.1	8.4	8.7	9.0
Dancing													
Moderately (waltz)		3.1	3.3	3.5	3.6	3.8	4.0	4.1	4.3	4.5	4.6	4.8	4.9
Active (square, disco)		4.5	4.7	5.0	5.2	5.4	5.6	5.9	6.1	6.3	6.6	6.8	7.0
Aerobic (vigorously)		6.0	6.3	6.7	7.0	7.3	7.6	7.9	8.2	8.5	8.8	9.1	9.4

| 73 | 75 | 77 | 80 | 82 | 84 | 86 | 89 | 91 | 93 | 95 | 98 | 100 |
160	165	170	175	180	185	190	195	200	205	210	215	220
1.6	1.6	1.7	1.7	1.8	1.8	1.9	1.9	2.0	2.0	2.1	2.1	2.2
2.0	2.1	2.2	2.2	2.3	2.4	2.4	2.5	2.5	2.6	2.7	2.7	2.8
4.4	4.5	4.6	4.8	4.9	5.0	5.2	5.3	5.4	5.6	5.7	5.9	6.0
5.1	5.3	5.4	5.6	5.7	5.9	6.0	6.2	6.4	6.5	6.7	6.9	7.0
5.8	6.0	6.2	6.4	6.6	6.7	6.9	7.1	7.3	7.4	7.6	7.8	8.0
4.4	4.5	4.6	4.8	4.9	5.0	5.2	5.3	5.4	5.6	5.7	5.9	6.0
9.4	9.7	10.0	10.3	10.6	10.9	11.2	11.5	11.8	12.1	12.4	12.7	13.0
5.0	5.2	5.3	5.5	5.6	5.8	5.9	6.1	6.3	6.4	6.6	6.8	6.9
6.3	6.5	6.7	6.9	7.1	7.3	7.4	7.7	7.9	8.0	8.2	8.5	8.6
4.8	5.0	5.1	5.3	5.4	5.6	5.7	5.9	6.0	6.2	6.4	6.5	6.7
8.0	8.2	8.5	8.7	9.0	9.2	9.5	9.7	10.0	10.2	10.5	10.7	11.0
10.5	10.9	11.2	11.5	11.9	12.2	12.5	12.9	13.2	13.5	13.8	14.2	14.5
3.1	3.2	3.3	3.4	3.5	3.6	3.7	3.8	3.9	4.0	4.1	4.2	4.3
6.8	7.0	7.2	7.4	7.6	7.9	8.1	8.3	8.5	8.7	8.9	9.1	9.4
11.6	12.0	12.4	12.7	13.1	13.4	13.8	14.2	14.5	14.9	15.3	15.6	16.0
17.1	17.6	18.1	18.7	19.2	19.7	20.3	20.8	21.3	21.9	22.4	22.9	23.5
4.4	4.5	4.6	4.8	4.9	5.0	5.2	5.3	5.5	5.6	5.7	5.9	6.0
5.5	5.7	5.9	6.1	6.3	6.4	6.6	6.8	7.0	7.1	7.3	7.5	7.7
15.6	16.1	16.6	17.1	17.6	18.1	18.6	19.1	19.6	20.0	20.5	21.0	21.5
3.1	3.2	3.3	3.4	3.5	3.6	3.7	3.8	3.9	4.0	4.1	4.2	4.3
7.1	7.4	7.6	7.8	8.0	8.2	8.5	8.7	8.9	9.1	9.4	9.6	9.8
9.3	9.5	9.8	10.1	10.4	10.7	11.0	11.3	11.6	11.9	12.2	12.5	12.8
5.1	5.3	5.4	5.6	5.7	5.9	6.0	6.2	6.4	6.5	6.7	6.9	7.0
7.3	7.5	7.7	7.9	8.2	8.4	8.6	8.9	9.1	9.3	9.5	9.8	10.0
9.7	10.0	10.3	10.6	10.9	11.2	11.5	11.8	12.1	12.4	12.7	13.0	13.3

Body weight

Kilograms	45	48	50	52	55	57	59	61	64	66	68	70
Pounds	100	105	110	115	120	125	130	135	140	145	150	155
Fencing												
Moderately	3.3	3.5	3.6	3.8	4.0	4.1	4.3	4.5	4.6	4.8	5.0	5.2
Vigorously	6.6	7.0	7.3	7.7	8.0	8.3	8.7	9.0	9.4	9.7	10.0	10.4
Football												
Moderate	3.3	3.5	3.6	3.8	4.0	4.1	4.3	4.5	4.6	4.8	5.0	5.2
Touch, vigorous	5.5	5.8	6.1	6.4	6.6	6.9	7.2	7.5	7.8	8.0	8.3	8.6
Golf												
Twosome (carry clubs)	3.6	3.8	4.0	4.2	4.4	4.6	4.7	4.9	5.1	5.3	5.4	5.6
Foursome (carry clubs)	2.7	2.9	3.0	3.1	3.3	3.4	3.5	3.7	3.8	3.9	4.1	4.2
Power-cart	1.9	2.0	2.1	2.2	2.3	2.4	2.5	2.6	2.7	2.8	2.9	3.0
Handball												
Moderate	6.5	6.8	7.2	7.5	7.8	8.2	8.5	8.8	9.2	9.5	9.9	10.2
Competitive	7.7	8.0	8.4	8.8	9.2	9.6	10.0	10.4	10.8	11.1	11.5	11.9
Hiking, pack (3 mph)	4.5	4.7	5.0	5.2	5.4	5.6	5.9	6.1	6.3	6.6	6.8	7.0
Hockey, field	5.0	6.3	6.7	7.0	7.3	7.6	7.9	8.2	8.5	8.8	9.1	9.4
Hockey, ice	6.6	7.0	7.3	7.7	8.0	8.3	8.7	9.0	9.4	9.7	10.0	10.4
Horseback riding												
Walk	1.9	2.0	2.1	2.2	2.3	2.4	2.5	2.6	2.7	2.8	2.9	3.0
Sitting to trot	2.7	2.9	3.0	3.1	3.3	3.4	3.5	3.7	3.8	3.9	4.1	4.2
Posting to trot	4.2	4.4	4.6	4.8	5.1	5.3	5.5	5.7	5.9	6.1	6.4	6.6
Gallop	5.7	6.0	6.3	6.6	6.9	7.2	7.5	7.8	8.1	8.4	8.7	9.0
Horseshoes	2.5	2.6	2.8	2.9	3.0	3.1	3.3	3.4	3.5	3.7	3.8	3.9
Jogging (*see* Running)												
Judo	8.5	8.9	9.3	9.8	10.2	10.6	11.0	11.5	11.9	12.3	12.8	13.2
Karate	8.5	8.9	9.3	9.8	10.2	10.6	11.0	11.5	11.9	12.3	12.8	13.2
Mountain climbing	6.5	6.8	7.2	7.5	7.8	8.2	8.5	8.8	9.2	9.5	9.8	10.2
Paddle ball	5.7	6.0	6.3	6.6	6.9	7.2	7.5	7.8	8.1	8.4	8.7	9.0
Pool (billiards)	1.5	1.6	1.6	1.7	1.8	1.9	1.9	2.0	2.1	2.2	2.2	2.3
Racquetball	6.5	6.8	7.1	7.5	7.8	8.1	8.4	8.8	9.1	9.4	9.8	10.1
Roller skating (9 mph)	4.2	4.4	4.6	4.8	5.1	5.3	5.5	5.7	5.9	6.1	6.4	6.6
Running (steady state)												
(mph) (min/mile)												
5.0 12:00	6.0	6.3	6.6	7.0	7.3	7.6	7.9	8.2	8.5	8.8	9.1	9.4
5.5 10:55	6.7	7.0	7.3	7.7	8.0	8.4	8.7	9.0	9.4	9.7	10.0	10.4
6.0 10:00	7.2	7.6	8.0	8.4	8.7	9.1	9.5	9.8	10.2	10.6	10.9	11.3
7.0 8:35	8.5	8.9	9.3	9.8	10.2	10.6	11.0	11.5	11.9	12.3	12.8	13.2
8.0 7:30	9.7	10.2	10.7	11.2	11.6	12.1	12.6	13.1	13.6	14.1	14.6	15.1
9.0 6:40	10.8	11.3	11.9	12.4	12.9	13.5	14.0	14.6	15.1	15.7	16.2	16.8
10.0 6:00	12.1	12.7	13.3	13.9	14.5	15.1	15.7	16.4	17.0	17.6	18.2	18.8
11.0 5:28	13.3	14.0	14.6	15.3	16.0	16.7	17.3	18.0	18.7	19.4	20.0	20.7
12.0 5:00	14.5	15.2	16.0	16.7	17.4	18.2	18.9	19.7	20.4	21.1	21.9	22.6
Sailing, small boat	2.7	2.9	3.0	3.1	3.3	3.4	3.5	3.7	3.8	3.9	4.1	4.2
Skating, ice (9 mph)	4.2	4.4	4.6	4.8	5.1	5.2	5.5	5.7	5.9	6.1	6.4	6.6
Skating, in-line (13 mph)	9.5	10.0	10.5	10.9	11.5	12.0	12.4	12.8	13.4	13.9	14.3	14.7
Skiing, cross-country												
(mph) (min/mile)												
2.5 24:00	5.0	5.2	5.5	5.7	6.0	6.2	6.5	6.7	7.0	7.2	7.5	7.8
4.0 15:00	6.5	6.8	7.2	7.5	7.8	8.2	8.5	8.8	9.2	9.5	9.9	10.2
5.0 12:00	7.7	8.0	8.4	8.8	9.2	9.6	10.0	10.4	10.8	11.1	11.5	11.9

73	75	77	80	82	84	86	89	91	93	95	98	100
160	165	170	175	180	185	190	195	200	205	210	215	220
5.3	5.5	5.7	5.8	6.0	6.2	6.3	6.5	6.7	6.8	7.0	7.1	7.3
10.7	11.0	11.4	11.7	12.1	12.4	12.7	13.1	13.4	13.8	14.1	14.4	14.8
5.3	5.5	5.7	5.8	6.0	6.2	6.3	6.5	6.7	6.8	7.0	7.1	7.3
8.9	9.2	9.4	9.7	10.0	10.3	10.6	10.8	11.1	11.4	11.7	12.0	12.2
5.8	6.0	6.2	6.4	6.6	6.7	6.9	7.1	7.3	7.4	7.6	7.8	8.0
4.4	4.5	4.6	4.8	4.9	5.0	5.2	5.3	5.4	5.6	5.7	5.9	6.0
3.1	3.2	3.3	3.4	3.5	3.6	3.7	3.8	3.9	4.0	4.1	4.2	4.3
10.5	10.9	11.2	11.5	11.9	12.2	12.5	12.9	13.2	13.5	13.8	14.2	14.5
12.3	12.7	13.1	13.5	13.9	14.3	14.7	15.0	15.4	15.8	16.2	16.6	17.0
7.3	7.5	7.7	7.9	8.2	8.4	8.6	8.9	9.1	9.3	9.5	9.8	10.0
9.7	10.0	10.3	10.6	10.9	11.2	11.5	11.8	12.1	12.4	12.7	13.0	13.3
10.7	11.0	11.4	11.7	12.1	12.4	12.7	13.1	13.4	13.8	14.1	14.4	14.8
3.1	3.2	3.3	3.4	3.5	3.6	3.7	3.8	3.9	4.0	4.1	4.2	4.3
4.4	4.5	4.6	4.8	4.9	5.0	5.2	5.3	5.4	5.6	5.7	5.9	6.0
6.8	7.0	7.2	7.4	7.6	7.9	8.1	8.3	8.5	8.7	8.9	9.1	9.4
9.3	9.5	9.8	10.1	10.4	10.7	11.0	11.3	11.6	11.9	12.2	12.5	12.8
4.0	4.2	4.3	4.4	4.5	4.7	4.8	4.9	5.2	5.2	5.3	5.4	5.6
13.6	14.1	14.5	14.9	15.4	15.8	16.2	16.6	17.1	17.5	17.9	18.4	18.8
13.6	14.1	14.5	14.9	15.4	15.8	16.2	16.6	17.1	17.5	17.9	18.4	18.8
10.5	10.8	11.2	11.5	11.8	12.1	12.5	12.8	13.1	13.5	13.8	14.1	14.5
9.3	9.5	9.8	10.1	10.4	10.7	11.0	11.2	11.6	11.9	12.2	12.5	12.8
2.4	2.5	2.6	2.6	2.7	2.0	2.9	2.9	3.0	3.1	3.2	3.2	3.3
10.4	10.7	11.1	11.4	11.7	12.0	12.4	12.7	13.0	13.4	13.7	14.0	14.4
6.8	7.0	7.2	7.4	7.6	7.9	8.1	8.3	8.5	8.7	8.9	9.1	9.4
9.7	10.0	10.3	10.6	10.9	11.2	11.6	11.9	12.2	12.5	12.8	13.1	13.4
10.7	11.1	11.4	11.7	12.1	12.4	12.8	13.1	13.4	13.8	14.1	14.5	14.8
11.7	12.0	12.4	12.8	13.1	13.5	13.8	14.3	14.6	15.0	15.4	15.7	16.1
13.6	14.1	14.5	14.9	15.4	15.8	16.2	16.6	17.1	17.5	17.9	18.4	18.8
15.6	16.1	16.6	17.1	17.6	18.1	18.5	19.0	19.5	20.0	20.5	21.0	21.5
17.3	17.9	18.4	19.0	19.5	20.1	20.6	21.2	21.7	22.2	22.8	23.3	23.9
19.4	20.0	20.7	21.3	21.9	22.5	23.1	23.7	24.2	24.8	25.4	26.0	26.7
21.4	22.1	22.7	23.4	24.1	24.8	25.4	26.1	26.8	27.5	28.1	28.8	29.5
23.3	24.1	24.8	25.6	26.3	27.0	27.8	28.5	29.2	30.0	30.7	31.5	32.2
4.4	4.5	4.6	4.8	4.9	5.0	5.2	5.3	5.4	5.6	5.7	5.9	6.0
6.8	7.0	7.2	7.4	7.6	7.9	8.1	8.3	8.5	8.7	8.9	9.1	9.4
15.3	15.7	16.2	16.8	17.2	17.6	18.1	18.7	19.1	19.5	20.0	20.6	21.0
8.0	8.3	8.5	8.8	9.0	9.3	9.5	9.8	10.0	10.3	10.6	10.8	11.1
10.5	10.9	11.2	11.5	11.9	12.2	12.5	12.9	13.2	13.5	13.8	14.2	14.5
12.3	12.7	13.1	13.5	13.9	14.3	14.7	15.0	15.4	15.8	16.2	16.6	17.0

Body weight												
Kilograms	45	48	50	52	55	57	59	61	64	66	68	70
Pounds	100	105	110	115	120	125	130	135	140	145	150	155
Skiing, downhill	6.5	6.8	7.2	7.5	7.8	8.2	8.5	8.8	9.2	9.5	9.9	10.2
Soccer	5.9	6.2	6.6	6.9	7.2	7.5	7.8	8.1	8.4	8.7	9.0	9.3
Squash												
Normal	6.7	7.0	7.3	7.7	8.0	8.4	8.7	9.1	9.5	9.8	10.1	10.5
Competition	7.7	8.0	8.4	8.8	9.2	9.6	10.0	10.4	10.8	11.1	11.5	11.9
Swimming (yards/min)												
Backstroke												
25	2.5	2.6	2.8	2.9	3.0	3.1	3.3	3.4	3.5	3.7	3.8	3.9
30	3.5	3.7	3.9	4.1	4.2	4.4	4.6	4.8	4.9	5.1	5.3	5.5
35	4.5	4.7	5.0	5.2	5.4	5.6	5.9	6.1	6.3	6.6	6.8	7.0
40	5.5	5.8	6.1	6.4	6.6	6.9	7.2	7.5	7.8	8.0	8.3	8.6
Breaststroke												
20	3.1	3.3	3.5	3.6	3.8	4.0	4.1	4.3	4.5	4.6	4.8	4.9
30	4.7	5.0	5.2	5.4	5.7	5.9	6.2	6.4	6.7	6.9	7.1	7.4
40	6.3	6.7	7.0	7.3	7.6	8.0	8.3	8.6	8.9	9.3	9.6	9.9
Front crawl												
20	3.1	3.3	3.5	3.6	3.8	4.0	4.1	4.3	4.5	4.6	4.8	4.9
25	4.0	4.2	4.4	4.6	4.8	5.0	5.2	5.4	5.6	5.8	6.0	6.2
35	4.8	5.1	5.4	5.6	5.9	6.1	6.4	6.6	6.8	7.0	7.3	7.5
45	5.7	6.0	6.3	6.6	6.9	7.2	7.5	7.8	8.1	8.4	8.7	9.0
50	7.0	7.4	7.7	8.1	8.5	8.8	9.2	9.5	9.9	10.3	10.6	11.0
Table tennis	3.4	3.6	3.8	4.0	4.1	4.3	4.5	4.7	4.8	5.0	5.2	5.4
Tennis												
Singles, recreational	5.0	5.2	5.5	5.7	6.0	6.2	6.5	6.7	7.0	7.2	7.5	7.8
Doubles, recreational	3.4	3.6	3.8	4.0	4.1	4.3	4.5	4.7	4.8	5.0	5.2	5.4
Competition	6.4	6.7	7.1	7.4	7.7	8.1	8.4	8.7	9.1	9.4	9.8	10.1
Volleyball												
Moderate, recreational	2.9	3.0	3.2	3.3	3.5	3.6	3.8	3.9	4.1	4.2	4.4	4.5
Vigorous, competition	6.5	6.8	7.1	7.5	7.8	8.1	8.4	8.8	9.1	9.4	9.8	10.1
Walking												
(mph) (min/mile)												
1.0 60:00	1.5	1.6	1.7	1.8	1.8	1.9	2.0	2.1	2.2	2.2	2.3	2.4
2.0 30:00	2.1	2.2	2.3	2.4	2.5	2.6	2.8	2.9	3.0	3.1	3.2	3.3
2.3 26:00	2.3	2.4	2.5	2.7	2.8	2.9	3.0	3.1	3.2	3.4	3.5	3.6
3.0 20:00	2.7	2.9	3.0	3.1	3.3	3.4	3.5	3.7	3.8	3.9	4.1	4.2
3.2 18:45	3.1	3.3	3.4	3.6	3.8	4.0	4.1	4.3	4.4	4.5	4.7	4.8
3.5 17:10	3.3	3.5	3.7	3.9	4.0	4.2	4.4	4.6	4.7	4.9	5.1	5.3
4.0 15:00	4.2	4.4	4.6	4.8	5.1	5.3	5.5	5.7	5.9	6.1	6.4	6.6
4.5 13:20	4.7	5.0	5.2	5.4	5.7	5.9	6.2	6.4	6.7	6.9	7.1	7.4
5.0 12:00	5.4	5.7	6.0	6.3	6.5	6.8	7.1	7.4	7.7	7.9	8.2	8.4
5.4 11:10	6.2	6.6	6.9	7.2	7.5	7.9	8.2	8.5	8.8	9.2	9.5	9.8
5.8 10:20	7.7	8.0	8.4	8.8	9.2	9.6	10.0	10.4	10.8	11.1	11.5	11.9
Water skiing	5.0	5.2	5.5	5.7	6.0	6.2	6.5	6.7	7.0	7.2	7.5	7.8
Weight training	5.2	5.4	5.7	6.0	6.2	6.5	6.8	7.0	7.3	7.6	7.8	8.1
Wrestling	8.5	8.9	9.3	9.8	10.2	10.6	11.0	11.5	11.9	12.3	12.8	13.2

| 73 | 75 | 77 | 80 | 82 | 84 | 86 | 89 | 91 | 93 | 95 | 98 | 100 |
160	165	170	175	180	185	190	195	200	205	210	215	220
10.5	10.9	11.2	11.5	11.9	12.2	12.5	12.9	13.2	13.5	13.8	14.2	14.5
9.6	9.9	10.2	10.5	10.8	11.1	11.4	11.7	12.0	12.3	12.6	12.9	13.2
10.8	11.2	11.5	11.8	12.2	12.5	12.9	13.2	13.5	13.9	14.2	14.6	14.9
12.3	12.7	13.1	13.5	13.9	14.3	14.7	15.0	15.4	15.8	16.2	16.6	17.0
4.0	4.2	4.3	4.4	4.5	4.7	4.8	4.9	5.1	5.2	5.3	5.4	5.6
5.6	5.8	6.0	6.2	6.4	6.5	6.7	6.9	7.1	7.2	7.4	7.6	7.8
7.3	7.5	7.7	7.9	8.2	8.4	8.6	8.9	9.1	9.3	9.5	9.8	10.0
8.9	9.2	9.4	9.7	10.0	10.3	10.6	10.8	11.1	11.4	11.7	12.0	12.2
5.1	5.3	5.4	5.6	5.7	5.9	6.0	6.2	6.4	6.5	6.7	6.9	7.0
7.6	7.9	8.1	8.3	8.6	8.8	9.1	9.3	9.5	9.8	10.0	10.3	10.5
10.2	10.5	10.9	11.2	11.5	11.9	12.2	12.5	12.8	13.1	13.5	13.8	14.1
5.1	5.3	5.4	5.6	5.7	5.9	6.0	6.2	6.4	6.5	6.7	6.9	7.0
6.4	6.6	6.8	7.0	7.2	7.4	7.6	7.8	8.0	8.2	8.4	8.6	8.8
7.8	8.0	8.3	8.5	8.8	9.0	9.2	9.4	9.7	9.9	10.2	10.4	10.7
9.3	9.5	9.8	10.1	10.4	10.7	11.0	11.3	11.6	11.9	12.2	12.5	12.8
11.3	11.7	12.0	12.4	12.8	13.1	13.5	13.8	14.2	14.5	14.9	15.2	15.6
5.5	5.7	5.9	6.1	6.3	6.4	6.6	6.8	7.0	7.1	7.3	7.5	7.7
8.0	8.3	8.5	8.8	9.0	9.3	9.5	9.8	10.0	10.3	10.6	10.8	11.1
5.5	5.7	5.9	6.1	6.3	6.4	6.6	6.8	7.0	7.1	7.3	7.5	7.7
10.4	10.8	11.1	11.4	11.8	12.1	12.4	12.8	13.1	13.4	13.7	14.1	14.4
4.7	4.8	5.0	5.1	5.3	5.4	5.6	5.7	5.9	6.0	6.1	6.3	6.4
10.4	10.7	11.1	11.4	11.7	12.0	12.4	12.7	13.0	13.4	13.7	14.0	14.4
2.4	2.5	2.6	2.7	2.8	2.9	2.9	3.0	3.1	3.2	3.2	3.3	3.4
3.4	3.5	3.6	3.7	3.9	4.0	4.1	4.2	4.3	4.4	4.5	4.6	4.7
3.7	3.8	4.0	4.1	4.2	4.3	4.4	4.5	4.7	4.8	4.9	5.0	5.1
4.4	4.5	4.6	4.8	4.9	5.0	5.2	5.3	5.4	5.6	5.7	5.9	6.0
5.0	5.2	5.3	5.5	5.6	5.8	5.9	6.1	6.3	6.4	6.6	6.8	6.9
5.4	5.6	5.8	6.0	6.2	6.3	6.5	6.7	6.9	7.0	7.2	7.4	7.6
6.8	7.0	7.2	7.4	7.6	7.9	8.1	8.3	8.5	8.7	8.9	9.1	9.4
7.6	7.9	8.1	8.3	8.6	8.8	9.1	9.3	9.5	9.8	10.0	10.3	10.5
8.7	9.0	9.2	9.5	9.8	10.1	10.4	10.6	10.9	11.2	11.5	11.8	12.0
10.1	10.4	10.8	11.1	11.4	11.8	12.1	12.4	12.7	13.0	13.4	13.7	14.0
12.3	12.7	13.1	13.5	13.9	14.3	14.7	15.0	15.4	15.8	16.2	16.6	17.0
8.0	8.3	8.5	8.8	9.0	9.3	9.5	9.8	10.0	10.3	10.6	10.8	11.1
8.3	8.6	8.9	9.1	9.4	9.7	9.9	10.2	10.5	10.7	11.0	11.2	11.5
13.6	14.1	14.5	14.9	15.4	15.8	16.2	16.6	17.1	17.5	17.9	18.4	18.8

Self-Test on Drinking Habits and Alcoholism

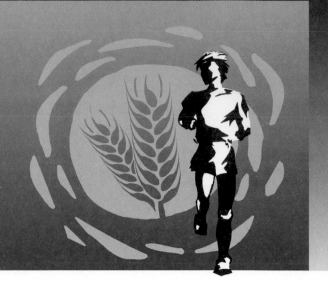

Here is a self-test to help you review the role alcohol plays in your life. These questions incorporate some of the common symptoms of alcoholism. This test is intended to help you determine if you or someone you know needs to find out more about alcoholism; it is not intended to be used to establish the diagnosis of alcoholism.

	Yes	No
1. Do you drink heavily when you are disappointed, under pressure or have had a quarrel with someone?	_____	_____
2. Have you ever been unable to remember part of the previous evening, even though your friends say you didn't pass out?	_____	_____
3. When drinking with other people, do you try to have a few extra drinks when others won't know about it?	_____	_____
4. Are you in more of a hurry to get your first drink of the day than you used to be?	_____	_____
5. Do you sometimes feel a little guilty about your drinking?	_____	_____
6. When you're sober, do you sometimes regret things you did or said while drinking?	_____	_____
7. Have you tried switching brands or drinks, or following different plans to control your drinking?	_____	_____
8. Have you sometimes failed to keep promises you made to yourself about controlling or cutting down on your drinking?	_____	_____
9. Have you ever had a DWI (driving while intoxicated) or DUI (driving under the influence of alcohol) violation, or any other legal problem related to your drinking?	_____	_____
10. Do you try to avoid family or close friends while you are drinking?	_____	_____

Any "yes" answer indicates you may be at greater risk for alcoholism. More than one "yes" answer may indicate the presence of an alcohol-related problem or alcoholism, and the need for consultation with an alcoholism professional. To find out more, contact the National Council on Alcoholism and Drug Dependence in your area.

Reprinted courtesy of the National Council on Alcoholism and Drug Dependence. For a brochure that contains these and other questions, contact the NCADD, 12 West 21st Street, New York, NY 10010.

Determination of Healthy Body Weight

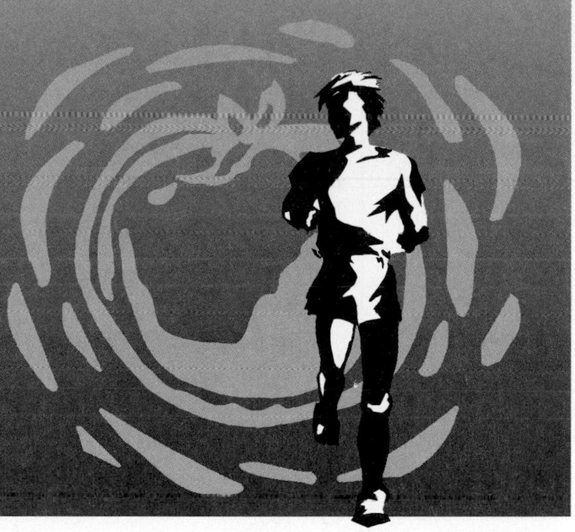

There are a number of different techniques utilized to determine a healthy body weight. The following three methods offer you an estimate of an appropriate body weight. Method A is based upon height-weight charts. Method B is based on the Body Mass Index (BMI). Method C is based upon body-fat percentage. Method D does not determine a desirable body weight but provides an assessment of desirable body-fat distribution.

Method A

1. Measure your height.

2. Measure your elbow width and determine your frame size from Table E.1.

    _____ Elbow width   _____ Frame size

3. Consult the Metropolitan height-weight tables to determine your desirable weight range. The midpoint is halfway into the range.

    _____ Height   _____ Frame size

    _____ Desirable weight range

    _____ Midpoint of range

4. Obtain your current weight (as close to nude weight as feasible).

    _____ Current body weight

5. Determination of desirable weight. You should attempt to reach the midpoint or lower end of the range.

    $\dfrac{\text{Current}}{\text{body weight}} - \dfrac{\text{Desirable}}{\text{weight}} = \dfrac{\text{Pounds of}}{\text{fat to lose}}$

    Your data:

    $\dfrac{\text{Current}}{\text{body weight}} - \dfrac{\text{Midpoint}}{\text{of range}} = \dfrac{\text{Pounds of}}{\text{fat to lose}}$

    _____ − _____ = _____

    $\dfrac{\text{Current}}{\text{body weight}} - \dfrac{\text{Low end}}{\text{of range}} = \dfrac{\text{Pounds of}}{\text{fat to lose}}$

    _____ − _____ = _____

Table E.1 Approximation of body frame size

Extend your arm and bend the forearm upward at a 90 degree angle. Keep fingers straight and turn the inside of your wrist toward your body. If you have a caliper, use it to measure the space between the two prominent bones on either side of your elbow. Without a caliper, place thumb and index finger of your other hand on these two bones. Measure the space between your fingers against a ruler or tape measure. For your height, compare it with figures in the right-hand column in the accompanying tables that list elbow measurements for medium-framed men and women. Measurements lower than those listed indicate that you have a small frame. Higher measurements indicate a large frame.

Height (ft/in.)*	Elbow breadth (in.)
Men	
5′1″–5′2″	2½″–2⅞″
5′3″–5′6″	2⅝″–2⅞″
5′7″–5′10″	2¾″–3″
5′11″–6′2″	2¾″–3⅛″
6′3″	2⅞″–3¼″
Women	
4′9″–5′2″	2¼″–2½″
5′3″–5′10″	2⅜″–2⅝″
5′11″	2½″–2¾″

*Height without shoes.
Used with permission of the Metropolitan Insurance Companies.

Table E.2 Desirable weights for females age 25 and over

Height (ft/in.)	(cm)	Small frame (lb)	(kg)	Medium frame (lb)	(kg)	Large frame (lb)	(kg)
5'10"	177.8	134–144	60.8–65.3	140–155	63.5–70.3	149–169	67.6–76.6
5'9"	175.3	130–140	59.0–63.5	136–151	61.7–68.5	145–164	65.8–74.4
5'8"	172.7	126–136	57.2–61.7	132–147	59.9–66.7	141–159	64.0–72.1
5'7"	170.2	122–131	55.3–59.4	128–143	58.1–64.9	137–154	62.1–69.9
5'6"	167.6	118–127	53.5–57.6	124–139	56.2–63.1	133–150	60.3–68.1
5'5"	165.1	114–123	51.7–55.8	120–135	54.4–61.2	129–146	58.5–66.2
5'4"	162.6	110–119	49.9–54.0	116–131	52.6–59.4	125–142	56.7–64.4
5'3"	160.0	107–115	48.5–52.2	112–126	50.8–57.2	121–138	54.9–62.6
5'2"	157.5	104–112	47.2–50.8	109–122	49.4–55.3	117–134	53.1–60.8
5'1"	154.9	101–109	45.8–49.4	106–118	48.1–53.5	114–130	51.7–59.0
5'0"	152.4	98–106	44.4–48.1	103–115	46.7–52.2	111–127	50.3–57.6
4'11"	149.8	95–103	43.1–46.7	100–112	45.4–50.8	108–124	49.0–56.2
4'10"	147.3	92–100	41.7–45.4	97–109	44.0–49.4	105–121	47.6–54.9
4'9"	144.7	90–97	40.8–44.0	94–106	42.6–48.1	102–118	46.3–53.5

For women between eighteen and twenty-five, subtract one pound for each year under 25. Height and weight measured without shoes or clothes.*

*If weighed with clothes, subtract approximate weight of clothes from recorded weight.
Used with permission of the Metropolitian Insurance Companies.

Table E.3 Desirable weights for males age 25 and over

Height (ft/in.)	(cm)	Small frame (lb)	(kg)	Medium frame (lb)	(kg)	Large frame (lb)	(kg)
6'3"	190.5	157–168	71.2–76.2	165–183	74.9–83.0	175–197	79.4–89.3
6'2"	188.0	153–164	69.4–74.4	160–178	72.6–80.8	171–192	77.6–87.1
6'1"	185.4	149–160	67.6–72.6	155–173	70.3–78.5	166–187	75.3–84.8
6'0"	182.9	145–155	65.8–70.3	151–168	68.5–76.2	161–182	73.0–82.6
5'11"	180.3	141–151	64.0–68.5	147–163	66.7–74.0	157–177	71.2–80.3
5'10"	177.8	137–147	62.1–66.7	143–158	64.9–71.7	152–172	69.0–78.0
5'9"	175.3	133–143	60.3–64.9	139–153	63.1–69.4	148–167	67.1–75.3
5'8"	172.7	129–138	58.5–62.6	135–149	61.2–67.6	144–163	65.3–74.0
5'7"	170.2	125–134	56.7–60.8	131–145	59.4–65.8	140–159	63.5–72.1
5'6"	167.6	121–130	54.9–59.0	127–140	57.6–63.5	135–154	61.2–69.9
5'5"	165.1	117–126	53.1–57.2	123–136	55.8–61.7	131–149	59.4–67.6
5'4"	162.6	114–122	51.7–55.3	120–132	54.4–59.9	128–145	58.1–65.8
5'3"	160.0	111–119	50.3–54.0	117–129	53.1–58.5	125–141	56.7–64.0
5'2"	157.5	108–116	49.0–52.6	114–126	51.7–57.2	122–137	55.3–62.1
5'1"	154.9	105–113	47.6–51.3	111–122	50.3–55.3	119–134	54.0–60.8

Height and weight measured without shoes or clothes.*

*If weighed with clothes, subtract approximate weight of clothes from recorded weight.
Used with permission of the Metropolitian Insurance Companies.

Method B

The BMI uses the metric system, so you need to determine your weight in kilograms and your height in meters. The formula is

$$\frac{\text{Body weight in kilograms}}{(\text{Height in meters})^2}$$

Dividing your body weight in pounds by 2.2 will give you your weight in kilograms. Multiplying your height in inches by 0.0254 will give you your height in meters.

$$\text{Your weight in kilograms} =$$

$$\frac{(\text{Your weight in pounds})}{2.2} = \underline{\hspace{1cm}}$$

$$\text{Your height in meters} =$$

$$(\text{Your height in inches}) \times 0.0254 = \underline{\hspace{1cm}}$$

$$\text{BMI} = \frac{\text{Body weight in kilograms}}{(\text{Height in meters})^2} = \underline{\hspace{1cm}}$$

Or you may use your weight in pounds and height in inches with the following formula:

$$\text{BMI} = \frac{\text{Body weight in pounds} \times 705}{\text{Height in inches}^2}$$

A BMI range of 20 to 25 is considered to be normal, but a suggested desirable range for females is 21.3 to 22.1 and for males is 21.9 to 22.4. BMI values above 27.8 for men and 27.3 for women have been associated with increased incidence rates for several health problems, including high blood pressure and diabetes. The American Dietetic Association, in their position statement on nutrition and physical fitness, notes that a BMI greater than 30 is classified as obese.

If you want to lower your body weight to a more desirable BMI, such as 22, use the following formula to determine what that weight should be; the weight is expressed in kilograms, so multiplying it by 2.2 will give you the desired weight in pounds.

$$\text{Kilograms body weight} =$$
$$\text{Desired BMI} \times (\text{Height in meters})^2$$

Here's a brief example for a woman who weighs 187 pounds and is 5′9″ tall; her BMI calculates to be 27.7, so her weight poses a health risk. If she wants to achieve a BMI of 23, she will need to reduce her weight to 155 pounds.

$$\text{Kilograms body weight} = 23 \times (1.753)^2 = 70.6$$

$$70.6 \text{ kg} \times 2.2 = 155 \text{ pounds}$$

To calculate your desirable body weight:

$$\text{Kilograms body weight} =$$

$$(\text{Your desired BMI}) \times (\text{Your height in meters})^2$$

$$\text{Kilograms body weight} = \underline{\hspace{1cm}} \times \underline{\hspace{1cm}}$$

$$\underline{\hspace{1cm}} \text{ kg} \times 2.2 = \underline{\hspace{1cm}} \text{ pounds}$$

Method C

For this method, you will need to know your body-fat percentage as determined by the procedure described in Table E.4 or another appropriate technique. You will also need to determine the body-fat percentage you desire to have. You may use Table 10.2 on page 323 as a guideline.

You will need to do the following calculations for the formula:

1. Determine your current lean body weight (LBW). Multiply your current body weight in pounds by your current percent body fat expressed as a decimal (20 percent would be .20) to obtain your pounds of body fat. Subtract your pounds of body fat from your current weight to give you your lean body weight (LBW).

2. Determine your desired body fat percentage and express it as a decimal.

$$\text{Desired body weight} = \frac{\text{LBM}}{1.00 - \text{Desired \% body fat}}$$

As an example, suppose we have a 200-pound male who is currently at 25 percent body fat but desires to get down to 20 percent as his first goal. Multiplying his current weight by his current percent body fat yields 50 pounds of body fat ($200 \times .25 = 50$); subtracting this from his current weight yields a LBM of 150 ($200 - 50$). If we plug his desired percent of 20 into the formula, he will need to reach a body weight of 187.5 to achieve this first goal.

$$\text{Desired body weight} = \frac{150}{1.00 - .20} = \frac{150}{.8} = 187.5$$

Your current body weight \underline{\hspace{1cm}}

Your current percent body fat \underline{\hspace{1cm}}

Your pounds of body fat \underline{\hspace{1cm}}

Your LBW \underline{\hspace{1cm}}

Your desired percent body fat \underline{\hspace{1cm}}

$$\text{Desired body weight} = \frac{\text{LBW}}{1.00 - ?} = \underline{\hspace{1cm}}$$

$$= \underline{\hspace{1cm}}$$

Table E.4 Generalized equations for predicting body fat

Measure the appropriate skinfolds for women (triceps, thigh, and suprailium sites) or men (chest, abdomen, and thigh sites) as illustrated in Figures E.1–E.4. You may use either the appropriate formula or the appropriate table on pages 439 and 440 to obtain the predicted body-fat percentage.

Women*	Men**
$BD = 1.0994921 - 0.0009929\ (X_1) + 0.0000023\ (X_1)^2 - 0.0001392\ (X_2)$	$BD = 1.10938 - 0.0008267\ (X_1) + 0.0000016\ (X_1)^2 - 0.0002574\ (X_2)$
BD = Body density	BD = Body density
X_1 = Sum of triceps, thigh, and suprailium skinfolds	X_1 = Sum of chest, abdomen and thigh skinfolds
X_2 = Age	X_2 = Age
	To calculate percent body fat, plug into Siri's equation
	$\left(\dfrac{4.95}{BD} - 4.5\right) \times 100$

*From Jackson, A., Pollock, M., and Ward, A. 1980. Generalized equations for predicting body density of women. *Medicine and Science in Sports and Exercise* 12:175–182.

**Jackson, A., and Pollock, M. 1978. Generalized equations for predicting body density of men. *British Journal of Nutrition* 40:497–504.

Method D

The waist:hip ratio (WHR) is a measure of regional fat distribution. Using a flexible (preferably metal) tape, measure the narrowest section of the bare waist as seen from the front while standing. Measure the hip girth at the largest circumference, which could be the hips, buttocks, or thighs, while standing. Wear tight clothing. Do not compress skin and fat with pressure from the tape. The measurement may be in either the English or metric system. The waist measurement alone may be used as a simple screening technique for abdominal obesity. Females with a waist of 39 inches or over, and men with a waist of 35 inches or over may be at increased risk.

Waist girth _____

Hip girth _____

Determine the ratio by dividing the waist girth by the hip girth.

$$\frac{\text{Waist girth}}{\text{Hip girth}} = \underline{\hspace{2cm}} = \underline{\hspace{2cm}}$$

Compare your results to the following rating scale for health risk.

Waist:hip ratio health risk rating scale

	Men	Women
Higher risk	>.95	>.85
Moderately high risk	.90–.95	.80–.85
Lower risk	<.90	<.80

Based on data from Van Itallie, T. B. Topography of body fat: Relationship to risk of cardiovascular and other diseases. In *Anthropometric standardization reference manual,* (pp. 143–149) ed. T. G. Lohman, A. F. Roche, and R. Martorell. Champaign, Ill: Human Kinetics. Copyright 1988 by T. G. Lohman, A. F. Roche, and R. Martorell. Reprinted by permission.

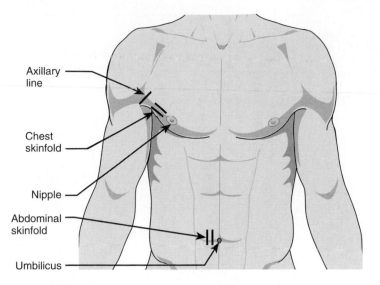

Axillary line

Chest skinfold

Nipple

Abdominal skinfold

Umbilicus

Figure E.1
The chest and abdomen skinfold. Chest —A diagonal fold is taken between the axillary fold and the nipple. Use a midway point for males, but only one-third the distance from the axilla for females. Abdomen—A vertical fold is taken about 2.5 centimeters (1 inch) to the side of the umbilicus.

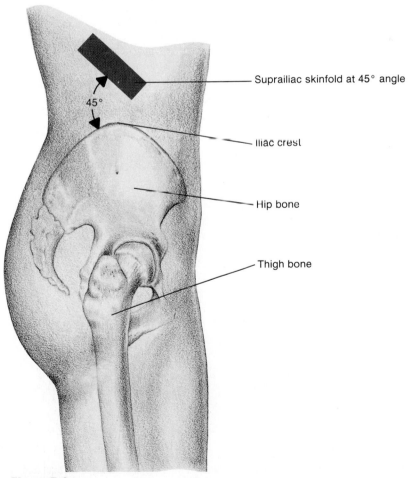

Suprailiac skinfold at 45° angle

45°

Iliac crest

Hip bone

Thigh bone

Figure E.2
The suprailiac skinfold. A diagonal fold is taken at about a 45-degree angle just above the crest of the ilium.

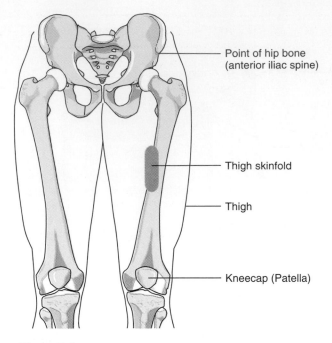

Figure E.3
The thigh skinfold. A vertical fold is taken on the front of the thigh midway between the anterior iliac spine and the patella.

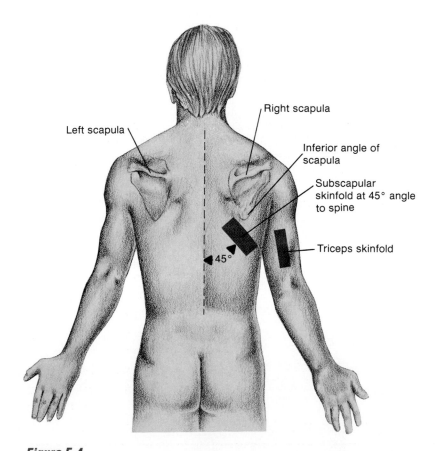

Figure E.4
The triceps and subscapular skinfolds. In the triceps skinfold, a vertical fold is taken over the triceps muscle one-half the distance from the acromion process to the olecranon process at the elbow. The subscapular skinfold is taken just below the lower angle of the scapula, at about a 45-degree angle to the spinal column.

Percent fat estimate for men: sum of chest, abdomen, and thigh skinfolds

Sum of skinfolds (mm)	Under 22	23–27	28–32	33–37	Age to last year 38–42	43–47	48–52	53–57	Over 57
8–10	1.3	1.8	2.3	2.9	3.4	3.9	4.5	5.0	5.5
11–13	2.2	2.8	3.3	3.9	4.4	4.9	5.5	6.0	6.5
14–16	3.2	3.8	4.3	4.8	5.4	5.9	6.4	7.0	7.5
17–19	4.2	4.7	5.3	5.8	6.3	6.9	7.4	8.0	8.5
20–22	5.1	5.7	6.2	6.8	7.3	7.9	8.4	8.9	9.5
23–25	6.1	6.6	7.2	7.7	8.3	8.8	9.4	9.9	10.5
26–28	7.0	7.6	8.1	8.7	9.2	9.8	10.3	10.9	11.4
29–31	8.0	8.5	9.1	9.6	10.2	10.7	11.3	11.8	12.4
32–34	8.9	9.4	10.0	10.5	11.1	11.6	12.2	12.8	13.3
35–37	9.8	10.4	10.9	11.5	12.0	12.6	13.1	13.7	14.3
38–40	10.7	11.3	11.8	12.4	12.9	13.5	14.1	14.6	15.2
41–43	11.6	12.2	12.7	13.3	13.8	14.4	15.0	15.5	16.1
44–46	12.5	13.1	13.6	14.2	14.7	15.3	15.9	16.4	17.0
47–49	13.4	13.9	14.5	15.1	15.6	16.2	16.8	17.3	17.9
50–52	14.3	14.8	15.4	15.9	16.5	17.1	17.6	18.2	18.8
53–55	15.1	15.7	16.2	16.8	17.4	17.9	18.5	19.1	19.7
56–58	16.0	16.5	17.1	17.7	18.2	18.8	19.4	20.0	20.5
59–61	16.9	17.4	17.9	18.5	19.1	19.7	20.2	20.8	21.4
62–64	17.6	18.2	18.8	19.4	19.9	20.5	21.1	21.7	22.2
65–67	18.5	19.0	19.6	20.2	20.8	21.3	21.9	22.5	23.1
68–70	19.3	19.9	20.4	21.0	21.6	22.2	22.7	23.3	23.9
71–73	20.1	20.7	21.2	21.8	22.4	23.0	23.6	24.1	24.7
74–76	20.9	21.5	22.0	22.6	23.2	23.8	24.4	25.0	25.5
77–79	21.7	22.2	22.8	23.4	24.0	24.6	25.2	25.8	26.3
80–82	22.4	23.0	23.6	24.2	24.8	25.4	25.9	26.5	27.1
83–85	23.2	23.8	24.4	25.0	25.5	26.1	26.7	27.3	27.9
86–88	24.0	24.5	25.1	25.7	26.3	26.9	27.5	28.1	28.7
89–91	24.7	25.3	25.9	26.5	27.1	27.6	28.2	28.8	29.4
92–94	25.4	26.0	26.6	27.2	27.8	28.4	29.0	29.6	30.2
95–97	26.1	26.7	27.3	27.9	28.5	29.1	29.7	30.3	30.9
98–100	26.9	27.4	28.0	28.6	29.2	29.8	30.4	31.0	31.6
101–103	27.5	28.1	28.7	29.3	29.9	30.5	31.1	31.7	32.3
104–106	28.2	28.8	29.4	30.0	30.6	31.2	31.8	32.4	33.0
107–109	28.9	29.5	30.1	30.7	31.3	31.9	32.5	33.1	33.7
110–112	29.6	30.2	30.8	31.4	32.0	32.6	33.2	33.8	34.4
113–115	30.2	30.8	31.4	32.0	32.6	33.2	33.8	34.5	35.1
116–118	30.9	31.5	32.1	32.7	33.3	33.9	34.5	35.1	35.7
119–121	31.5	32.1	32.7	33.3	33.9	34.5	35.1	35.7	36.4
122–124	32.1	32.7	33.3	33.9	34.5	35.1	35.8	36.4	37.0
125–127	32.7	33.3	33.9	34.5	35.1	35.8	36.4	37.0	37.6

From A. S. Jackson and M. L. Pollock, "Practical Assessment of Body Composition," May 1985, in *Physician and Sportsmedicine*. Reprinted with permission of McGraw-Hill, Inc.

Percent fat estimate for women: sum of triceps, suprailium, and thigh skinfolds

Sum of skinfolds (mm)	Under 22	23–27	28–32	33–37	38–42	43–47	48–52	53–57	Over 57
23–25	9.7	9.9	10.2	10.4	10.7	10.9	11.2	11.4	11.7
26–28	11.0	11.2	11.5	11.7	12.0	12.3	12.5	12.7	13.0
29–31	12.3	12.5	12.8	13.0	13.3	13.5	13.8	14.0	14.3
32–34	13.6	13.8	14.0	14.3	14.5	14.8	15.0	15.3	15.5
35–37	14.8	15.0	15.3	15.5	15.8	16.0	16.3	16.5	16.8
38–40	16.0	16.3	16.5	16.7	17.0	17.2	17.5	17.7	18.0
41–43	17.2	17.4	17.7	17.9	18.2	18.4	18.7	18.9	19.2
44–46	18.3	18.6	18.8	19.1	19.3	19.6	19.8	20.1	20.3
47–49	19.5	19.7	20.0	20.2	20.5	20.7	21.0	21.2	21.5
50–52	20.6	20.8	21.1	21.3	21.6	21.8	22.1	22.3	22.6
53–55	21.7	21.9	22.1	22.4	22.6	22.9	23.1	23.4	23.6
56–58	22.7	23.0	23.2	23.4	23.7	23.9	24.2	24.4	24.7
59–61	23.7	24.0	24.2	24.5	24.7	25.0	25.2	25.5	25.7
62–64	24.7	25.0	25.2	25.5	25.7	26.0	26.2	26.4	26.7
65–67	25.7	25.9	26.2	26.4	26.7	26.9	27.2	27.4	27.7
68–70	26.6	26.9	27.1	27.4	27.6	27.9	28.1	28.4	28.6
71–73	27.5	27.8	28.0	28.3	28.5	28.8	29.0	29.3	29.5
74–76	28.4	28.7	28.9	29.2	29.4	29.7	29.9	30.2	30.4
77–79	29.3	29.5	29.8	30.0	30.3	30.5	30.8	31.0	31.3
80–82	30.1	30.4	30.6	30.9	31.1	31.4	31.6	31.9	32.1
83–85	30.9	31.2	31.4	31.7	31.9	32.2	32.4	32.7	32.9
86–88	31.7	32.0	32.2	32.5	32.7	32.9	33.2	33.4	33.7
89–91	32.5	32.7	33.0	33.2	33.5	33.7	33.9	34.2	34.4
92–94	33.2	33.4	33.7	33.9	34.2	34.4	34.7	34.9	35.2
95–97	33.9	34.1	34.4	34.6	34.9	35.1	35.4	35.6	35.9
98–100	34.6	34.8	35.1	35.3	35.5	35.8	36.0	36.3	36.5
101–103	35.3	35.4	35.7	35.9	36.2	36.4	36.7	36.9	37.2
104–106	35.8	36.1	36.3	36.6	36.8	37.1	37.3	37.5	37.8
107–109	36.4	36.7	36.9	37.1	37.4	37.6	37.9	38.1	38.4
110–112	37.0	37.2	37.5	37.7	38.0	38.2	38.5	38.7	38.9
113–115	37.5	37.8	38.0	38.2	38.5	38.7	39.0	39.2	39.5
116–118	38.0	38.3	38.5	38.8	39.0	39.3	39.5	39.7	40.0
119–121	38.5	38.7	39.0	39.2	39.5	39.7	40.0	40.2	40.5
122–124	39.0	39.2	39.4	39.7	39.9	40.2	40.4	40.7	40.9
125–127	39.4	39.6	39.9	40.1	40.4	40.6	40.9	41.1	41.4
128–130	39.8	40.0	40.3	40.5	40.8	41.0	41.3	41.5	41.8

From A. S. Jackson and M. L. Pollock, "Practical Assessment of Body Composition," May 1985, in *Physician and Sportsmedicine*. Reprinted with permission of McGraw-Hill, Inc.

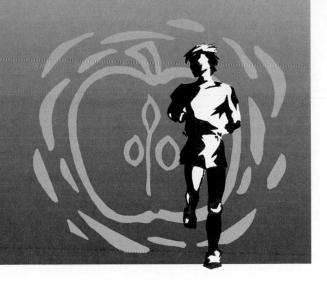

Exchange Lists for Meal Planning*

What are Exchange Lists?

Exchange lists are foods listed together because they are alike. Each serving of a food has about the same amount of carbohydrate, protein, fat, and Calories as the other foods on that list. That is why any food on a list can be "exchanged" or traded for any other food on the same list. For example, you can trade the slice of bread you might eat for breakfast for one-half cup of cooked cereal. Each of these foods equals one starch choice.

Exchange Lists

Foods are listed with their serving sizes, which are usually measured after cooking. When you begin, you should measure the size of each serving. This may help you learn to "eyeball" correct serving sizes.

The following chart shows the amount of nutrients in one serving from each list.

The exchange lists provide you with a lot of food choices (foods from the basic food groups, foods with added sugars, free foods, combination foods,

Groups/Lists	Carbohydrate (grams)	Protein (grams)	Fat (grams)	Calories
Carbohydrate group				
Starch	15	3	1 or less	80
Fruit	15	—	—	60
Milk				
Skim	12	8	0–3	90
Low-fat	12	8	5	120
Whole	12	8	8	150
Other carbohydrates	15	varies	varies	varies
Vegetables	5	2	—	25
Meat and meat substitutes group				
Very lean	—	7	0–1	35
Lean	—	7	3	55
Medium-fat	—	7	5	75
High-fat	—	7	8	100
Fat group	—	—	5	45

*The Exchange Lists are the basis of a meal planning system designed by a committee of the American Diabetes Association and the American Dietetic Association. While designed primarily for people with diabetes and others who must follow special diets, the Exchange Lists are based on principles of good nutrition that apply to everyone. © 1995 American Diabetes Association, Inc., American Dietetic Association.

and fast foods). This gives you variety in your meals. Several foods, such as dried beans and peas, bacon, and peanut butter, are on two lists. This gives you flexibility in putting your meals together. Whenever you choose new foods or vary your meal plan, monitor your blood glucose to see how these different foods affect your blood glucose level.

Most foods in the Carbohydrate group have about the same amount of carbohydrate per serving. You can exchange starch, fruit, or milk choices in your meal plan. Vegetables are in this group but contain only about 5 grams of carbohydrate.

A Word About Food Labels

Exchange information is based on foods found in grocery stores. However, food companies often change the ingredients in their products. That is why you need to check the Nutrition Facts panel of the food label.

The Nutrition Facts tell you the number of Calories and grams of carbohydrate, protein, and fat in one serving. Compare these numbers with the exchange information in this Appendix to see how many exchanges you will be eating. In this way, food labels can help you add foods to your meal plans.

Ask your dietitian to help you use food label information to plan your meals, or read pages 48–51 for more tips on how to use food labels.

Getting Started!

See your dietitian regularly when you are first learning how to use your meal plan and the exchange lists. Your meal plan can be adjusted to fit changes in your life-style, such as work, school, vacation, or travel. Regular nutrition counseling can help you make positive changes in your eating habits.

Careful eating habits will help you feel better and be healthier, too. Best wishes and good eating with *Exchange Lists for Meal Planning*.

Starch List

Cereals, grains, pasta, breads, crackers, snacks, starchy vegetables, and cooked dried beans, peas, and lentils are starches. In general, one starch is:

- 1/2 cup of cereal, grain, pasta, or starchy vegetable

- 1 ounce of a bread product, such as 1 slice of bread

- 3/4 to 1 ounce of most snack foods. (Some snack foods may also have added fat)

Nutrition tips

1. Most starch choices are good sources of B vitamins.

2. Foods made from whole grains are good sources of fiber.

3. Dried beans and peas are a good source of protein and fiber.

Selection tips

1. Choose starches made with little fat as often as you can.

2. Starchy vegetables prepared with fat count as one starch and one fat.

3. Bagels or muffins can be 2, 3, or 4 ounces in size, and can, therefore, count as 2, 3, or 4 starch choices. Check the size you eat.

4. Dried beans, peas, and lentils are also found on the Meat and Meat Substitutes list.

5. Regular potato chips and tortilla chips are found on the Other Carbohydrates list.

6. Most of the serving sizes are measured after cooking.

7. Always check Nutrition Facts on the food label.

One starch exchange equals
15 grams carbohydrate,
3 grams protein,
0–1 grams fat, and
80 Calories.

Bread

Bagel	1/2 (1 oz)
Bread, reduced-calorie	2 slices (1 1/2 oz)
Bread, white, wholewheat, pumpernickel, rye	1 slice (1 oz)
Bread sticks, crisp, 4 in. long × 1/2 in.	2 (2/3 oz)
English muffin	1/2
Hot dog or hamburger bun	1/2 (1 oz)
Pita, 6 in. across	1/2
Roll, plain, small	1 (1 oz)
Raisin bread, unfrosted	1 slice (1 oz)
Tortilla, corn, 6 in. across	1
Tortilla, flour, 7–8 in. across	1
Waffle, 4 1/2 in. square, reduced-fat	1

Cereals and grains

Bran cereals	1/2 cup
Bulgur	1/2 cup
Cereals	1/2 cup
Cereals, unsweetened, ready-to-eat	3/4 cup
Cornmeal (dry)	3 Tbsp
Couscous	1/3 cup
Flour (dry)	3 Tbsp
Granola, low-fat	1/4 cup
Grape-Nuts	1/4 cup
Grits	1/2 cup
Kasha	1/2 cup
Millet	1/4 cup
Muesli	1/4 cup
Oats	1/2 cup
Pasta	1/2 cup
Puffed cereal	1 1/2 cups

Rice milk . . . . 1/2 cup
Rice, white or brown . . . . 1/3 cup
Shredded Wheat . . . . 1/2 cup
Sugar-frosted cereal . . . . 1/2 cup
Wheat germ . . . . 3 Tbsp

Starchy vegetables

Baked beans . . . . 1/3 cup
Corn . . . . 1/2 cup
Corn on cob, medium . . . . 1 (5 oz)
Mixed vegetables with corn, peas,
   or pasta . . . . 1 cup
Peas, green . . . . 1/2 cup
Plantain . . . . 1/2 cup
Potato, baked or boiled . . . . 1 small (3 oz)
Potato, mashed . . . . 1/2 cup
Squash, winter (acorn, butternut) . . . . 1 cup
Yam, sweet potato, plain . . . . 1/2 cup

Crackers and snacks

Animal crackers 8
Graham crackers, 2 1/2 in. square 3
Matzoh . . . . 3/4 oz
Melba toast . . . . 4 slices
Oyster crackers 24
Popcorn (popped, no fat added
   or low-fat microwave) . . . . 3 cups
Pretzels . . . . 3/4 oz
Rice cakes, 4 in. across 2
Saltine-type crackers 6
Snack chips, fat-free (tortilla,
   potato) . . . . 15–20 (3/4 oz)
Whole-wheat crackers,
   no fat added . . . . 2–5 (3/4 oz)

Dried beans, peas, and lentils (Count as 1 starch exchange, plus 1 very lean meat exchange.)

Beans and peas (garbanzo, pinto,
   kidney, white, split, black-eyed) . . . . 1/2 cup
Lima beans . . . . 2/3 cup
Lentils . . . . 1/2 cup
Miso 🧂 . . . . 3 Tbsp

🧂 = 400 mg or more of sodium per serving.

Starchy foods prepared with fat (Count as 1 starch exchange, plus 1 fat exchange.)

Biscuit, 2 1/2 in. across 1
Chow mein noodles . . . . 1/2 cup
Corn bread, 2 in. cube . . . . 1 (2 oz)
Crackers, round butter type 6
Croutons . . . . 1 cup
French-fried potatoes . . . . 16–25 (3 oz)
Granola . . . . 1/4 cup
Muffin, small . . . . 1 (1 1/2 oz)
Pancake, 4 in. across 2
Popcorn, microwave . . . . 3 cups
Sandwich crackers, cheese or
   peanut butter filling 3
Stuffing, bread (prepared) . . . . 1/3 cup
Taco shell, 6 in. across 2
Waffle, 4 1/2 in. square 1
Whole-wheat crackers, fat added . . . . 4–6 (1 oz)

Some food you buy uncooked will weigh less after you cook it. Starches often swell in cooking so a small amount of uncooked starch will become a much larger amount of cooked food. The following table shows some of the changes.

Food (Starch group)	Uncooked	Cooked
Oatmeal	3 Tbsp	1/2 cup
Cream of Wheat	2 Tbsp	1/2 cup
Grits	3 Tbsp	1/2 cup
Rice	2 Tbsp	1/3 cup
Spaghetti	1/4 cup	1/2 cup
Noodles	1/3 cup	1/2 cup
Macaroni	1/4 cup	1/2 cup
Dried beans	1/4 cup	1/2 cup
Dried peas	1/4 cup	1/2 cup
Lentils	3 Tbsp	1/2 cup
Common measurements		
3 tsp = 1 Tbsp	4 ounces = 1/2 cup	
4 Tbsp = 1/4 cup	8 ounces = 1 cup	
5 1/3 Tbsp = 1/3 cup	1 cup = 1/2 pint	

Fruit list

Fresh, frozen, canned, and dried fruits and fruit juices are on this list. In general, one fruit exchange is:

- 1 small to medium fresh fruit
- 1/2 cup of canned or fresh fruit or fruit juice
- 1/4 cup of dried fruit.

Nutrition tips

1. Fresh, frozen, and dried fruits have about 2 grams of fiber per choice. Fruit juices contain very little fiber.

2. Citrus fruits, berries, and melons are good sources of vitamin C.

Selection tips

1. Count 1/2 cup cranberries or rhubarb sweetened with sugar substitutes as free foods.

2. Read the Nutrition Facts on the food label. If one serving has more than 15 grams of carbohydrate, you will need to adjust the size of the serving you eat or drink.

3. Portion sizes for canned fruits are for the fruit and a small amount of juice.

4. Whole fruit is more filling than fruit juice and may be a better choice.

5. Food labels for fruits may contain the words "no sugar added" or "unsweetened." This means that no sucrose (table sugar) has been added.

6. Generally, fruit canned in extra light syrup has the same amount of carbohydrate per serving as the "no sugar added" or the juice pack. All canned fruits on the fruit list are based on one of these three types of pack.

> One fruit exchange equals
> 15 grams carbohydrate and
> 60 Calories.
> The weight includes skin, core, seeds, and rind.

Fruit

Apple, unpeeled, small	1 (4 oz)
Applesauce, unsweetened	1/2 cup
Apples, dried	4 rings
Apricots, fresh	4 whole (5 1/2 oz)

Apricots, dried	8 halves
Apricots, canned	1/2 cup
Banana, small	1 (4 oz)
Blackberries	3/4 cup
Blueberries	3/4 cup
Cantaloupe, small	1/3 melon (11 oz) or 1 cup cubes
Cherries, sweet, fresh	12 (3 oz)
Cherries, sweet, canned	1/2 cup
Dates	3
Figs, fresh	1 1/2 large or 2 medium (3 1/2 oz)
Figs, dried	1 1/2
Fruit cocktail	1/2 cup
Grapefruit, large	1/2 (11 oz)
Grapefruit sections, canned	3/4 cup
Grapes, small	17 (3 oz)
Honeydew melon	1 slice (10 oz) or 1 cup cubes
Kiwi	1 (3 1/2 oz)
Mandarin oranges, canned	3/4 cup
Mango, small	1/2 fruit (5 1/2 oz) or 1/2 cup
Nectarine, small	1 (5 oz)
Orange, small	1 (6 1/2 oz)
Papaya	1/2 fruit (8 oz) or 1 cup cubes
Peach, medium, fresh	1 (6 oz)
Peaches, canned	1/2 cup
Pear, large, fresh	1/2 (4 oz)
Pears, canned	1/2 cup
Pineapple, fresh	3/4 cup
Pineapple, canned	1/2 cup
Plums, small	2 (5 oz)
Plums, canned	1/2 cup
Prunes, dried	3
Raisins	2 Tbsp
Raspberries	1 cup
Strawberries	1 1/4 cup whole berries
Tangerines, small	2 (8 oz)
Watermelon	1 slice (13 1/2 oz) or 1 1/4 cup cubes

Fruit juice

Apple juice/cider	1/2 cup
Cranberry juice cocktail	1/3 cup
Cranberry juice cocktail, reduced-calorie	1 cup
Fruit juice blends, 100% juice	1/3 cup
Grape juice	1/3 cup
Grapefruit juice	1/2 cup
Orange juice	1/2 cup
Pineapple juice	1/2 cup
Prune juice	1/3 cup

Milk List

Different types of milk and milk products are on this list. Cheeses are on the Meat list and cream and other dairy fats are on the Fat list. Based on the amount of fat they contain, milks are divided into skim/very low-fat milk, low-fat milk, and whole milk. One choice of these includes:

	Carbohydrate (grams)	Protein (grams)	Fat (grams)	Calories
Skim/very low-fat	12	8	0–3	90
Low-fat	12	8	5	120
Whole	12	8	8	150

Nutrition tips

1. Milk and yogurt are good sources of calcium and protein. Check the food label.

2. The higher the fat content of milk and yogurt, the greater the amount of saturated fat and cholesterol. Choose lower-fat varieties.

3. For those who are lactose intolerant, look for lactose-reduced or lactose-free varieties of milk.

Selection tips

1. One cup equals 8 fluid ounces or 1/2 pint.

2. Look for chocolate milk, frozen yogurt, and ice cream on the Other Carbohydrates list.

3. Nondairy creamers are on the Free Foods list.

4. Look for rice milk on the Starch list.

5. Look for soy milk on the Medium-fat Meat list.

One milk exchange equals
12 grams carbohydrate and
8 grams protein.

Skim and very low-fat milk (0–3 grams fat per serving)

Skim milk . . . . 1 cup
1/2% milk . . . . 1 cup
1% milk . . . . 1 cup
Nonfat or low-fat buttermilk . . . . 1 cup
Evaporated skim milk . . . . 1/2 cup
Nonfat dry milk . . . . 1/3 cup dry
Plain nonfat yogurt . . . . 3/4 cup
Nonfat or low-fat fruit-flavored
    yogurt sweetened with aspartame or
    with a nonnutritive sweetener . . . . 1 cup

Low-fat (5 grams fat per serving)

2% milk . . . . 1 cup
Plain low-fat yogurt . . . . 3/4 cup
Sweet acidophilus milk . . . . 1 cup

Whole milk (8 grams fat per serving)

Whole milk . . . . 1 cup
Evaporated whole milk . . . . 1/2 cup
Goat's milk . . . . 1 cup
Kefir . . . . 1 cup

Other Carbohydrates List

You can substitute food choices from this list for a starch, fruit, or milk choice on your meal plan. Some choices will also count as one or more fat choices.

Nutrition tips

1. These foods can be substituted in your meal plan, even though they contain added sugars or fat. However, they do not contain as many important vitamins and minerals as the choices on the Starch, Fruit, or Milk list.

2. When planning to include these foods in your meal, be sure to include foods from all the lists to eat a balanced meal.

Selection tips

1. Because many of these foods are concentrated sources of carbohydrate and fat, the portion sizes are often very small.

2. Always check Nutrition Facts on the food label. It will be your most accurate source of information.

3. Many fat-free or reduced-fat products made with fat replacers contain carbohydrate. When eaten in large amounts, they may need to be counted. Talk with your dietitian to determine how to count these in your meal plan.

4. Look for fat-free salad dressings in smaller amounts on the Free Foods list.

One exchange equals
15 grams carbohydrate, or
1 starch, or 1 fruit, or 1 milk.

Food	Serving size	Exchanges per serving
Angel food cake, unfrosted	1/12th cake	2 carbohydrates
Brownie, small, unfrosted	2 in. square	1 carbohydrate, 1 fat
Cake, unfrosted	2 in. square	1 carbohydrate, 1 fat
Cake, frosted	2 in. square	2 carbohydrates, 1 fat
Cookie, fat-free	2 small	1 carbohydrate
Cookie or sandwich cookie with creme filling	2 small	1 carbohydrate, 1 fat
Cupcake, frosted	1 small	2 carbohydrates, 1 fat
Cranberry sauce, jellied	1/4 cup	2 carbohydrates
Doughnut, plain cake	1 medium (1 1/2 oz)	1 1/2 carbohydrates, 2 fats
Doughnut, glazed	3 3/4 in. across (2 oz)	2 carbohydrates, 2 fats
Fruit juice bars, frozen, 100% juice	1 bar (3 oz)	1 carbohydrate
Fruit snacks, chewy (pureed fruit concentrate)	1 roll (3/4 oz)	1 carbohydrate
Fruit spreads, 100% fruit	1 Tbsp	1 carbohydrate
Gelatin, regular	1/2 cup	1 carbohydrate
Gingersnaps	3	1 carbohydrate
Granola bar	1 bar	1 carbohydrate, 1 fat
Granola bar, fat-free	1 bar	2 carbohydrates
Hummus	1/3 cup	1 carbohydrate, 1 fat
Ice cream	1/2 cup	1 carbohydrate, 2 fats
Ice cream, light	1/2 cup	1 carbohydrate, 1 fat
Ice cream, fat-free, no sugar added	1/2 cup	1 carbohydrate
Jam or jelly, regular	1 Tbsp	1 carbohydrate
Milk, chocolate, whole	1 cup	2 carbohydrates, 1 fat
Pie, fruit, 2 crusts	1/6 pie	3 carbohydrates, 2 fats
Pie, pumpkin or custard	1/8 pie	1 carbohydrate, 2 fats
Potato chips	12–18 (1 oz)	1 carbohydrate, 2 fats
Pudding, regular (made with low-fat milk)	1/2 cup	2 carbohydrates
Pudding, sugar-free (made with low-fat milk)	1/2 cup	1 carbohydrate
Salad dressing, fat free ▮	1/4 cup	1 carbohydrate
Sherbet, sorbet	1/2 cup	2 carbohydrates
Spaghetti or pasta sauce, canned ▮	1/2 cup	1 carbohydrate, 1 fat
Sweet roll or Danish	1 (2 1/2 oz)	2 1/2 carbohydrates, 2 fats

Food	Serving size	Exchanges per serving
Syrup, light	2 Tbsp	1 carbohydrate
Syrup, regular	1 Tbsp	1 carbohydrate
Syrup, regular	1/4 cup	4 carbohydrates
Tortilla chips	6–12 (1 oz)	1 carbohydrate, 2 fats
Yogurt, frozen, low-fat, fat-free	1/3 cup	1 carbohydrate, 0–1 fat
Yogurt, frozen, fat-free, no sugar added	1/2 cup	1 carbohydrate
Yogurt, low-fat with fruit	1 cup	3 carbohydrates, 0–1 fat
Vanilla wafers	5	1 carbohydrate, 1 fat

📍 = 400 mg or more sodium per exchange.

Vegetable List

Vegetables that contain small amounts of carbohydrates and Calories are on this list. Vegetables contain important nutrients. Try to eat at least 2 or 3 vegetable choices each day. In general, one vegetable exchange is:

- 1/2 cup of cooked vegetables or vegetable juice,

- 1 cup of raw vegetables.

If you eat 1 to 2 vegetable choices at a meal or snack, you do not have to count the calories or carbohydrates because they contain small amounts of these nutrients.

Nutrition tips

1. Fresh and frozen vegetables have less added salt than canned vegetables. Drain and rinse canned vegetables if you want to remove some salt.

2. Choose more dark green and dark yellow vegetables, such as spinach, broccoli, romaine, carrots, chilies, and peppers.

3. Broccoli, brussels sprouts, cauliflower, greens, peppers, spinach, and tomatoes are good sources of vitamin C.

4. Vegetables contain 1 to 4 grams of fiber per serving.

Selection tips

1. A 1-cup portion of broccoli is a portion about the size of a light bulb.

2. Tomato sauce is different from spaghetti sauce, which is on the Other Carbohydrates list.

3. Canned vegetables and juices are available without added salt.

4. If you eat more than 4 cups of raw vegetables or 2 cups of cooked vegetables at one meal, count them as 1 carbohydrate choice.

5. Starchy vegetables such as corn, peas, winter squash, and potatoes that contain larger amounts of Calories and carbohydrates are on the Starch list.

One vegetable exchange equals
5 grams carbohydrate,
2 grams protein,
0 grams fat, and
25 Calories.

Artichoke
Artichoke hearts
Asparagus
Beans (green, wax, Italian)
Bean sprouts
Beets
Broccoli
Brussels sprouts
Cabbage
Carrots
Cauliflower
Celery
Cucumber
Eggplant
Green onions or scallions
Greens (collard, kale, mustard, turnip)
Kohlrabi
Leeks
Mixed vegetables (without corn, peas, or pasta)
Mushrooms
Okra
Onions
Pea pods
Peppers (all varieties)
Radishes
Salad greens (endive, escarole, lettuce, romaine, spinach)
Sauerkraut 📍
Spinach
Summer squash
Tomato
Tomatoes, canned
Tomato sauce 📍
Tomato/vegetable juice 📍
Turnips
Water chestnuts
Watercress
Zucchini

📍 = 400 mg or more sodium per exchange.

Meat and Meat Substitutes List

Meat and meat substitutes that contain both protein and fat are on this list. In general, one meat exchange is:

- 1 oz meat, fish, poultry, or cheese,
- 1/2 cup dried beans.

Based on the amount of fat they contain, meats are divided into very lean, lean, medium-fat, and high-fat lists. This is done so you can see which ones contain the least amount of fat. One ounce (one exchange) of each of these includes:

	Carbohydrate (grams)	Protein (grams)	Fat (grams)	Calories
Very lean	0	7	0–1	35
Lean	0	7	3	55
Medium-fat	0	7	5	75
High-fat	0	7	8	100

Nutrition tips

1. Choose very lean and lean meat choices whenever possible. Items from the high-fat group are high in saturated fat, cholesterol, and Calories and can raise blood cholesterol levels.

2. Meats do not have any fiber.

3. Dried beans, peas, and lentils are good sources of fiber.

4. Some processed meats, seafood, and soy products may contain carbohydrate when consumed in large amounts. Check the Nutrition Facts on the label to see if the amount is close to 15 grams. If so, count it as a carbohydrate choice as well as a meat choice.

Selection tips

1. Weigh meat after cooking and removing bones and fat. Four ounces of raw meat is equal to 3 ounces of cooked meat. Some examples of meat portions are:

   - 1 ounce cheese = 1 meat choice and is about the size of a 1-inch cube
   - 2 ounces meat = 2 meat choices, such as 1 small chicken leg or thigh 1/2 cup cottage cheese or tuna
   - 3 ounces meat = 3 meat choices and is about the size of a deck of cards, such as 1 medium pork chop 1 small hamburger 1/2 of a whole chicken breast 1 unbreaded fish fillet

2. Limit your choices from the high-fat group to three times per week or less.

3. Most grocery stores stock Select and Choice grades of meat. Select grades of meat are the leanest meats. Choice grades contain a moderate amount of fat, and Prime cuts of meat have the highest amount of fat. Restaurants usually serve Prime cuts of meat.

5. "Hamburger" may contain added seasoning and fat, but ground beef does not.

6. Read labels to find products that are low in fat and cholesterol (5 grams or less of fat per serving).

7. Dried beans, peas, and lentils are also found on the Starch list.

8. Peanut butter, in smaller amounts, is also found on the Fats list.

9. Bacon, in smaller amounts, is also found on the Fats list.

Meal planning tips

1. Bake, roast, broil, grill, poach, steam, or boil these foods rather than frying.

2. Place meat on a rack so the fat will drain off during cooking.

3. Use a nonstick spray and a nonstick pan to brown or fry foods.

4. Trim off visible fat before or after cooking.

5. If you add flour, bread crumbs, coating mixes, fat, or marinades when cooking, ask your dietitian how to count it in your meal plan.

Very lean meat and substitutes list (One exchange equals 0 grams carbohydrate, 7 grams protein, 0–1 grams fat, and 35 Calories.)

One very lean meat exchange is equal to any one of the following items.

Poultry: Chicken or turkey (white meat, no skin), Cornish hen (no skin) . . . . 1 oz

Fish: Fresh or frozen cod, flounder, haddock, halibut, trout; tuna fresh or canned in water . . . . 1 oz

Shellfish: Clams, crab, lobster, scallops, shrimp, imitation shellfish . . . . 1 oz

Game: Duck or pheasant (no skin), venison, buffalo, ostrich . . . . 1 oz

Cheese with 1 gram or less fat per ounce:
Nonfat or low-fat cottage cheese . . . . 1/4 cup
Fat-free cheese . . . . 1 oz

Other: Processed sandwich meats with 1 gram or
less fat per ounce, such as deli thin, shaved meats,
chipped beef 🛆, turkey ham . . . . 1 oz
Egg whites 2
Egg substitutes, plain . . . . 1/4 cup
Hot dogs with 1 gram or less fat per ounce 🛆 1 oz
Kidney (high in cholesterol) . . . . 1 oz
Sausage with 1 gram or less fat per ounce . . . 1 oz

Count as one very lean meat and one starch
exchange.

Dried beans, peas, lentils (cooked) . . . . 1/2 cup

🛆 = 400 mg or more sodium per exchange.

Lean meat and substitutes list (One exchange equals 0 grams carbohydrate, 7 grams protein, 3 grams fat, and 55 Calories.)

One lean meat exchange is equal to any one of the following items.

Beef: USDA Select or Choice grades
of lean beef trimmed of fat, such as round,
sirloin, and flank steak; tenderloin;
roast (rib, chuck, rump); steak (T-bone,
porterhouse, cubed), ground round . . . . 1 oz
Pork: Lean pork, such as fresh ham; canned,
cured, or boiled ham; Canadian bacon 🛆;
tenderloin, center loin chop . . . . 1 oz
Lamb: Roast, chop, leg . . . . 1 oz
Veal: Lean chop, roast . . . . 1 oz
Poultry: Chicken, turkey (dark meat,
no skin), chicken white meat (with skin),
domestic duck or goose (well-drained
of fat, no skin) . . . . 1 oz
Fish:
Herring (uncreamed or smoked) . . . . 1 oz
Oysters . . . . 6 medium
Salmon (fresh or canned), catfish . . . . 1 oz
Sardines (canned) . . . . 2 medium
Tuna (canned in oil, drained) . . . . 1 oz
Game: Goose (no skin), rabbit . . . . 1 oz
Cheese:
4.5%-fat cottage cheese . . . . 1/4 cup
Grated Parmesan . . . . 2 Tbsp
Cheeses with 3 grams or less fat per ounce . . 1 oz
Other:
Hot dogs with 3 grams or less fat
per ounce . . . . 1 1/2 oz
Processed sandwich meat with 3 grams
or less fat per ounce, such as turkey
pastrami or kielbasa . . . . 1 oz
Liver, heart (high in cholesterol) . . . . 1 oz

Medium-fat meat and substitutes list (One exchange equals 0 grams carbohydrate, 7 grams protein, 5 grams fat, and 75 Calories.)

One medium-fat meat exchange is equal to any one of the
following items.

Beef: Most beef products fall into this category
(ground beef, meatloaf, corned beef,
short ribs, prime grades of meat trimmed
of fat, such as prime rib) . . . . 1 oz
Pork: Top loin, chop, Boston butt, cutlet . . . . . 1 oz
Lamb: Rib roast, ground . . . . 1 oz
Veal: Cutlet (ground or cubed, unbreaded) . . . 1 oz
Poultry: Chicken dark meat (with skin),
ground turkey or ground chicken,
fried chicken (with skin) . . . . 1 oz
Fish: Any fried fish product . . . . 1 oz
Cheese: With 5 grams or less fat per ounce
Feta . . . . 1 oz
Mozzarella . . . . 1 oz
Ricotta . . . . 1/4 cup (2 oz)
Other:
Egg (high in cholesterol, limit to 3 per week) . . 1
Sausage with 5 grams or less fat per ounce . . 1 oz
Soy milk . . . . 1 cup
Tempeh . . . . 1/4 cup
Tofu . . . . 4 oz or 1/2 cup

High-fat meat and substitutes list (One exchange equals 0 grams carbohydrate, 7 grams protein, 8 grams fat, and 100 Calories.)

Remember these items are high in saturated fat, cholesterol, and Calories and may raise blood cholesterol levels
if eaten on a regular basis. One high-fat meat exchange
is equal to any one of the following items.

Pork: Spareribs, ground pork, pork sausage . . . 1 oz
Cheese: All regular cheeses, such as American 🛆,
cheddar, Monterey Jack, Swiss . . . . 1 oz
Other: Processed sandwich meats with
8 grams or less fat per ounce, such as
bologna, pimento loaf, salami . . . . 1 oz
Sausage, such as bratwurst, Italian,
knockwurst, Polish, smoked 🛆 . . . . 1 oz
Hot dog (turkey or chicken) 🛆 1 (10/lb)
Bacon . . . . 3 slices (20 slices/lb)

Count as one high-fat meat plus one fat exchange.

Hot dog (beef, pork, or combination) 🛆 . . 1 (10/lb)
Peanut butter (contains unsaturated fat) . . . 2 Tbsp

🛆 = 400 mg or more sodium per exchange.

Fat List

Fats are divided into three groups, based on the main type of fat they contain: monounsaturated, polyunsaturated, and saturated. Small amounts of monounsaturated and polyunsaturated fats in the foods we eat are linked with good health benefits. Saturated fats are linked with heart disease and cancer. In general, one fat exchange is:

- 1 teaspoon of regular margarine or vegetable oil,

- 1 tablespoon of regular salad dressings.

Nutrition tips

1. All fats are high in Calories. Limit serving sizes for good nutrition and health.

2. Nuts and seeds contain small amounts of fiber, protein, and magnesium.

3. If blood pressure is a concern, choose fats in the unsalted form to help lower sodium intake, such as unsalted peanuts.

Selection tips

1. Check the Nutrition Facts on food labels for serving sizes. One fat exchange is based on a serving size containing 5 grams of fat.

2. When selecting regular margarine, choose those with liquid vegetable oil as the first ingredient. Soft margarines are not as saturated as stick margarines. Soft margarines are healthier choices. Avoid those listing hydrogenated or partially hydrogenated fat as the first ingredient.

3. When selecting low-fat margarines, look for liquid vegetable oil as the second ingredient. Water is usually the first ingredient.

4. When used in smaller amounts, bacon and peanut butter are counted as fat choices. When used in larger amounts, they are counted as high-fat meat choices.

5. Fat-free salad dressings are on the Other Carbohydrates list and the Free Foods list.

6. See the Free Foods list for nondairy coffee creamers, whipped topping, and fat-free products, such as margarines, salad dressings, mayonnaise, sour cream, cream cheese, and nonstick cooking spray.

Monounsaturated fats list (One fat exchange equals 5 grams fat and 45 Calories.)

Avocado, medium	1/8 (1 oz)
Oil (canola, olive, peanut)	1 tsp
Olives: ripe (black)	8 large
green, stuffed 🧂	10 large
Nuts	
almonds, cashews	6 nuts
mixed (50% peanuts)	6 nuts
peanuts	10 nuts
pecans	4 halves
Peanut butter, smooth or crunchy	2 tsp
Sesame seeds	1 Tbsp
Tahini paste	2 tsp

Polyunsaturated fats list (One fat exchange equals 5 grams fat and 45 Calories.)

Margarine: stick, tub, or squeeze	1 tsp
lower-fat (30% to 50% vegetable oil)	1 Tbsp
Mayonnaise: regular	1 tsp
reduced-fat	1 Tbsp
Nuts, walnuts, English	4 halves
Oil (corn, safflower, soybean)	1 tsp
Salad dressing: regular 🧂	1 Tbsp
reduced-fat	2 Tbsp
Miracle Whip Salad Dressing®: regular	2 tsp
reduced-fat	1 Tbsp
Seeds: pumpkin, sunflower	1 Tbsp

🧂 = 400 mg or more sodium per exchange.

Saturated fats list* (One fat exchange equals 5 grams of fat and 45 Calories.)

Bacon, cooked	1 slice (20 slices/lb)
Bacon, grease	1 tsp
Butter: stick	1 tsp
whipped	2 tsp
reduced-fat	1 Tbsp
Chitterlings, boiled	2 Tbsp (1/2 oz)
Coconut, sweetened, shredded	2 Tbsp
Cream, half and half	2 Tbsp
Cream cheese: regular	1 Tbsp (1/2 oz)
reduced-fat	2 Tbsp (1 oz)
Fatback or salt pork, see below†	
Shortening or lard	1 tsp
Sour cream: regular	2 Tbsp
reduced-fat	3 Tbsp

*Saturated fats can raise blood cholesterol levels.
†Use a piece 1 in. × 1 in. × 1/4 in. if you plan to eat the fatback cooked with vegetables. Use a piece 2 in. × 1 in. × 1/2 in. when eating only the vegetables with the fatback removed.

Free Foods List

A *free food* is any food or drink that contains less than 20 Calories or less than 5 grams of carbohydrate per serving. Foods with a serving size listed should be limited to three servings per day. Be sure to spread them out throughout the day. If you eat all three servings at one time, it could affect your blood glucose level. Foods listed without a serving size can be eaten as often as you like.

Fat-free or reduced-fat foods

Cream cheese, fat-free . . . . 1 Tbsp
Creamers, nondairy, liquid . . . . 1 Tbsp
Creamers, nondairy, powdered . . . . 2 tsp
Mayonnaise, fat-free . . . . 1 Tbsp
Mayonnaise, reduced-fat . . . . 1 tsp
Margarine, fat-free . . . . 4 Tbsp
Margarine, reduced-fat . . . . 1 tsp
Miracle Whip®, nonfat . . . . 1 Tbsp
Miracle Whip®, reduced-fat . . . . 1 tsp
Nonstick cooking spray
Salad dressing, fat-free . . . . 1 Tbsp
Salad dressing, fat-free, Italian . . . . 2 Tbsp
Salsa . . . . 1/4 cup
Sour cream, fat-free, reduced-fat . . . . 1 Tbsp
Whipped topping, regular or light . . . . 2 Tbsp

Sugar-free or low-sugar foods

Candy, hard, sugar-free . . . . 1 candy
Gelatin dessert, sugar-free
Gelatin, unflavored
Gum, sugar-free
Jam or jelly, low-sugar or light . . . . 2 tsp
Sugar substitutes†
Syrup, sugar-free . . . . 2 Tbsp

†Sugar substitutes, alternatives, or replacements that are approved by the Food and Drug Administration (FDA) are safe to use. Common brand names include:
Equal® (aspartame)
Sprinkle Sweet® (saccharin)
Sweet One® (acesulfame K)
Sweet-10® (saccharin)
Sugar Twin® (saccharin)
Sweet 'n Low® (saccharin)

Drinks

Bouillon, broth, consommé 🥄
Bouillon or broth, low-sodium
Carbonated or mineral water
Cocoa powder, unsweetened . . . . 1 Tbsp
Coffee
Club soda
Diet soft drinks, sugar-free
Drink mixes, sugar-free
Tea
Tonic water, sugar-free

Condiments

Catsup . . . . 1 Tbsp
Horseradish
Lemon juice
Lime juice
Mustard
Pickles, dill 🥄 . . . . 1 1/2 large
Soy sauce, regular or light 🥄
Taco sauce . . . . 1 Tbsp
Vinegar

Seasonings

Be careful with seasonings that contain sodium or are salts, such as garlic or celery salt, and lemon pepper.

Flavoring extracts
Garlic
Herbs, fresh or dried
Pimento
Spices
Tabasco® or hot pepper sauce
Wine, used in cooking
Worcestershire sauce

🥄 = 400 mg or more of sodium per choice.

Combination Foods List

Many of the foods we eat are mixed together in various combinations. These combination foods do not fit into any one exchange list. Often it is hard to tell what is in a casserole dish or prepared food item. This is a list of exchanges for some typical combination foods. This list will help you fit these foods into your meal plan. Ask your dietitian for information about any other combination foods you would like to eat.

Food entrees

Food entrees	Serving size	Exchanges per serving
Tuna noodle casserole, lasagna, spaghetti with meatballs, chili with beans, macaroni and cheese ♣	1 cup (8 oz)	2 carbohydrates, 2 medium-fat meats
Chow mein (without noodles or rice)	2 cups (16 oz)	1 carbohydrate, 2 lean meats
Pizza, cheese, thin crust ♣	1/4 of 10 in. (5 oz)	2 carbohydrates, 2 medium-fat meats, 1 fat
Pizza, meat topping, thin crust ♣	1/4 of 10 in. (5 oz)	2 carbohydrates, 2 medium-fat meats, 2 fats
Pot pie ♣	1 (7 oz)	2 carbohydrates, 1 medium-fat meat, 4 fats

Frozen entrees

Frozen entrees	Serving size	Exchanges per serving
Salisbury steak with gravy, mashed potato ♣	1 (11 oz)	2 carbohydrates, 3 medium-fat meats, 3–4 fats
Turkey with gravy, mashed potato, dressing ♣	1 (11 oz)	2 carbohydrates, 2 medium-fat meats, 2 fats
Entree with less than 300 calories ♣	1 (8 oz)	2 carbohydrates, 3 lean meats

Soups

Soups	Serving size	Exchanges per serving
Bean ♣	1 cup	1 carbohydrate, 1 very lean meat
Cream (made with water) ♣	1 cup (8 oz)	1 carbohydrate, 1 fat
Split pea (made with water) ♣	1/2 cup (4 oz)	1 carbohydrate
Tomato (made with water) ♣	1 cup (8 oz)	1 carbohydrate
Vegetable beef, chicken noodle, or other broth-type ♣	1 cup (8 oz)	1 carbohydrate

♣ = 400 mg or more sodium per exchange.

Fast Foods*

Food	Serving size	Exchanges per serving
Burritos with beef ♣	2	4 carbohydrates, 2 medium-fat meats, 2 fats
Chicken nuggets ♣	6	1 carbohydrate, 2 medium-fat meats, 1 fat
Chicken breast and wing, breaded and fried ♣	1 each	1 carbohydrate, 4 medium-fat meats, 2 fats
Fish sandwich/tartar sauce ♣	1	3 carbohydrates, 1 medium-fat meat, 3 fats
French fries, thin	20–25	2 carbohydrates, 2 fats
Hamburger, regular	1	2 carbohydrates, 2 medium-fat meats
Hamburger, large ♣	1	2 carbohydrates, 3 medium-fat meats, 1 fat
Hot dog with a bun ♣	1	1 carbohydrate, 1 high-fat meat, 1 fat
Individual pan pizza ♣	1	5 carbohydrates, 3 medium-fat meats, 3 fats
Soft-serve cone	1 medium	2 carbohydrates, 1 fat
Submarine sandwich ♣	1 sub (6 in.)	3 carbohydrates, 1 vegetable, 2 medium-fat meats, 1 fat
Taco, hard shell ♣	1 (6 oz)	2 carbohydrates, 2 medium-fat meats, 2 fats
Taco, soft shell ♣	1 (3 oz)	1 carbohydrate, 1 medium-fat meat, 1 fat

♣ = 400 mg or more of sodium per serving.

*Ask at your fast-food restaurant for nutrition information about your favorite fast foods.

Calories, Percent Fat, and Cholesterol in Selected Fast-Food Restaurant Products*

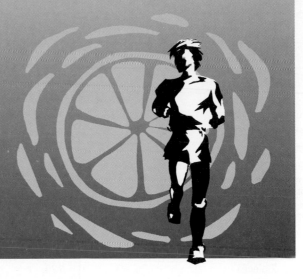

	Calories	% Fat Calories	Cholesterol (milligrams)
Arby's			
Regular roast beef	383	43	43
Beef'n Cheddar	508	47	52
Chicken breast fillet	445	45	45
Potato cakes	204	48	0
Turkey sub	486	35	51
Garden salad	117	40	12
Burger King			
Dutch apple pie	300	46	0
Double cheeseburger	600	53	135
Double Whopper with cheese	960	59	195
Onion rings	310	42	0
Vanilla milk shake (medium)	300	17	20
Croissan'wich with sausage/egg/cheese	600	68	260
Salad dressing, Thousand Island	140	79	15
Salad dressing, reduced Calorie Italian	15	33	0
Hardee's			
Ham biscuit	400	45	15
Hamburger, regular	270	37	35
Mesquite bacon cheeseburger	370	43	45
Big country breakfast (sausage)	1,000	59	570
Garden salad	220	55	40
Chicken fillet	480	33	35
Fisherman's fillet	560	43	65
Fried chicken, breast	370	35	75

	Calories	% Fat Calories	Cholesterol (milligrams)
KFC			
BBQ baked beans	190	13	5
Coleslaw	180	44	5
Mashed potatoes with gravy	120	42	1
Side breast (original recipe)	400	55	135
Side breast (extra tasty crispy)	470	53	80
Chicken sandwich	497	40	52
Long John Silver's			
Batter-dipped fish sandwich	320	37	30
Popcorn shrimp	280	46	85
Fish with batter, 1 piece	170	59	30
Hush puppies, 2 pieces	120	33	0
McDonald's			
Hamburger	255	31	35
Arch Deluxe	550	51	90
Big Mac	560	50	85
Grilled chicken deluxe	440	41	60
Chicken McNuggets (6 pieces)	290	52	60
French fries (large)	450	44	0
Hotcakes with margarine and syrup	580	26	15
Egg McMuffin	290	38	235
Breakfast burrito	320	56	195
Sausage biscuit	430	60	35
Low-fat apple bran muffin	300	10	0
Grilled chicken salad deluxe	120	8	45
Pizza Hut			
Thin 'N Crispy cheese, 2 medium slices	420	38	40
Pan, cheese, 2 medium slices	600	40	50
Thin 'N Crispy, Meat Lover's, 2 medium slices	620	48	70
Stuffed Crust, Meat Lover's, 2 medium slices	1,000	42	120
Personal pan pizza, supreme (whole pizza)	710	39	60

	Calories	% Fat Calories	Cholesterol (milligrams)
Subway			
Subway Club	300	18	37
Turkey breast	276	13	20
Tuna (regular mayo)	522	57	31
Veggie Delite	223	12	0
Taco Bell			
Bean burrito	391	28	5
Beef burrito	432	39	57
Taco, beef	180	55	32
Soft taco, beef	223	45	32
Soft taco, chicken	223	40	58
Nachos Supreme	364	44	17
Taco salad	838	58	79
Wendy's			
Plain single hamburger	360	39	65
Grilled chicken sandwich	310	22	65
Plain potato, baked	310	0	0
Potato with broccoli and cheese	470	25	5
Chicken nuggets (6 pieces)	280	64	50

* All fast-food restaurants have pamphlets describing the nutrient content of all foods they serve, in many cases including whole sandwiches and meals, but also individual components such as bread, meat, vegetables, condiments, etc. Fast-food offerings change often, so use these free publications to assess the quality of their products. Just ask for a copy at the counter.

A Cardiac Risk Index

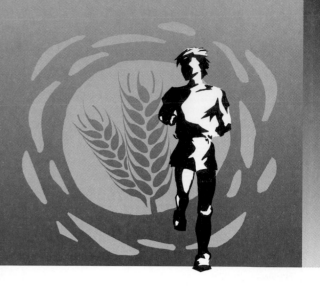

To score your cardiac risk index, total the point values from the small boxes as they relate to you for each of the eight factors listed.

1. *Age*	10 to 20 1	21 to 30 2	31 to 40 3	41 to 50 4	51 to 60 6	61 to 70 and over 8
2. *Heredity*	No known history of heart disease 1	1 relative with cardiovascular disease over 60 2	2 relatives with cardiovascular disease over 60 3	1 relative with cardiovascular disease under 60 4	2 relatives with cardiovascular disease under 60 6	3 relatives with cardiovascular disease under 60 8
3. *Weight*	More than 5 lbs. below standard weight 0	Standard weight 1	5–20 lbs. overweight 2	21–35 lbs. overweight 3	36–50 lbs. overweight 5	51–65 lbs. overweight 7
4. *Tobacco smoking*	Nonuser 0	Cigar and/or pipe 1	10 cigarettes or less a day 2	20 cigarettes a day 3	30 cigarettes a day 5	40 cigarettes a day or more 8
5. *Exercise*	Intensive occupational and recreational exertion 1	Moderate occupational and recreational exertion 2	Sedentary work and intense recreational exertion 3	Sedentary occupational and moderate recreational exertion 5	Sedentary work and light recreational exertion 6	Complete lack of all exercise 8
6. *Cholesterol or % fat in diet*	Cholesterol below 180 mg. Diet contains no animal or solid fats 1	Cholesterol 181–205 mg. Diet contains 10% animal or solid fats 2	Cholesterol 206–230 mg. Diet contains 20% animal or solid fats 3	Cholesterol 231–255 mg. Diet contains 30% animal or solid fats 4	Cholesterol 256–280 mg. Diet contains 40% animal or solid fats 5	Cholesterol 281–330 mg. Diet contains 50% animal or solid fats 7
7. *Blood pressure*	100 upper reading 1	120 upper reading 2	140 upper reading 3	160 upper reading 4	180 upper reading 6	200 or over upper reading 8
8. *Sex*	Female 1	Female over 45 2	Male 3	Bald Male 4	Bald short male 6	Bald short stocky male 7

Total score: _____

Cardiovascular disease risk index scoring table

Group I 6 to 11 = very low risk		*Group IV* 26 to 32 = high risk
Group II 12 to 17 = low risk		*Group V* 33 to 42 = dangerous risk
Group III 18 to 25 = average risk		*Group VI* 42 to 60 = extremely dangerous risk

Reprinted with permission of Dr. John Boyer, San Diego State University, San Diego, California.

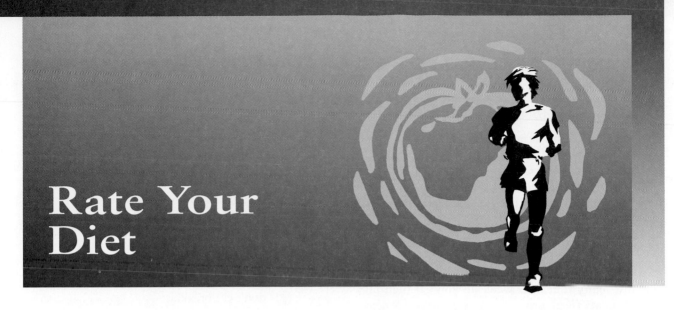

Rate Your Diet

These 39 questions will give you a rough sketch of your typical eating habits. The (+) or (−) number for each answer instantly pats you on the back for good eating habits or alerts you to problems you didn't even know you had. The quiz focuses on fat, saturated fat, cholesterol, sodium, sugar, fiber, and fruits and vegetables, It doesn't attempt to cover everything in your diet. Also, it doesn't try to measure precisely how much of the key nutrients you eat.

Instructions

Next to each answer is a number with a + or − sign in front of it. **Circle the number that corresponds to the answer you choose.** That's your score for the question. If two or more answers apply, circle each one. Then average them to get your score for the question.

How to average. In answering question 19, for example, if your sandwich-eating is equally divided among tuna salad (−2), roast beef (+1), and turkey breast (+3), add the three scores (which gives you +2) and then divide by three. That gives you a score of +2/3 for the question. Round it to +1.

Pay attention to serving sizes, which we give when needed. For example, a serving of vegetables is 1/2 cup. If you usually eat one cup of vegatables at a time, count it as two servings.

The Quiz
Fruits, vegetables, grains & beans

1. **How many servings of fruit or 100% fruit juice do you eat per day?** (*OMIT fruit snacks like Fruit Roll-Ups and fruit-on-the-bottom yogurt. One serving = one piece or 1/2 cup of fruit or 6 oz. of fruit juice.*)
   (a) 0 . . . . −3   (d) 2 . . . . +1
   (b) less than 1 . . . −2   (e) 3 . . . . +2
   (c) 1 0   (f) 4 or more . . . +3

2. **How many servings of non-fried vegetables do you eat per day?** (*One serving = 1/2 cup. INCLUDE potatoes.*)
   (a) 0 0   (d) 2 . . . . +1
   (b) less than 1 . . . −2   (e) 3 . . . . +2
   (c) 1 0   (f) 4 or more . . . +3

3. **How many servings of vitamin-rich vegetables do you eat per week?** (*One serving = 1/2 cup. ONLY count broccoli, Brussels sprouts, carrots, collards, kale, red pepper, spinach, sweet potatoes, or winter squash.*)
   (a) 0 . . . . −3   (c) 4 to 6 . . . . . . +2
   (b) 1 to 3 . . . . . . +1   (d) 7 or more . . . +3

4. **How many servings of leafy green vegetables do you eat per week?** (*One serving =1/2 cup cooked or 1 cup raw. ONLY count collards, kale, mustard greens, romaine lettuce, spinach, or Swiss chard.*)
   (a) 0 . . . . −3   (d) 3 to 4 . . . . . . +2
   (b) less than 1 . . . −2   (e) 5 or more . . . +3
   (c) 1 to 2 . . . . . . +1

5. **How many times per week does your lunch or dinner contain grains, vegetables, or beans, but little or no meat, poultry, fish, eggs, or cheese?**
   (a) 0 . . . . −1   (c) 3 to 4 . . . . . . +2
   (b) 1 to 2 . . . . . . +1   (d) 5 or more . . . +3

6. **How many times per week do you eat beans, split peas, or lentils?** (*OMIT green beans.*)
   (a) 0 . . . . −3   (d) 2 . . . . +1
   (b) less than 1 . . . −1   (e) 3 . . . . +2
   (c) 1 0   (f) 4 or more . . . +3

7. **How many servings of grains do you eat per day?** (*One serving =1 slice of bread, 1 oz. of crackers, 1 large pancake, 1 cup pasta or cold cereal, or 1/2 cup granola, cooked cereal, rice, or bulgur. OMIT heavily sweetened cold cereals.*)
   (a) 0 . . . . −3   (d) 5 to 7 . . . . . . +2
   (b) 1 to 2 0   (e) 8 or more . . . +3
   (c) 3 to 4 . . . . . . +1

8. **What type of bread, rolls, etc., do you eat?**
   (a) 100% whole wheat as the only flour . . . . +3
   (b) whole wheat flour as the 1st or 2nd flour . . . +2
   (c) rye, pumpernickel, or oatmeal . . . . +1
   (d) white, French, or Italian 0

9. **What kind of breakfast cereal do you eat?**
   (a) whole-grain (like oatmeal or Wheaties) . . . . +3
   (b) low-fiber (like Cream of Wheat or
       Corn Flakes) 0
   (c) sugary low-fiber (like Frosted Flakes)
       or low-fat granola . . . . −1
   (d) regular granola . . . . −2

Meat, poultry & seafood

10. **How many times per week do you eat high-fat red meats** (*hamburgers, pork chops, ribs, hot dogs, pot roast, sausage, bologna, steaks other than round steak, etc.*)**?**
    (a) 0 . . . . +3   (d) 2 . . . . −2
    (b) less than 1 . . . . . +2   (e) 3 . . . . −3
    (c) 1 . . . . −1   (f) 4 or more . . . . . . −4

11. **How many times per week do you eat lean red meats** (*hot dogs, or luncheon meats with no more than 2 grams of fat per serving, round steak, or pork tenderloin*)**?**
    (a) 0 . . . . +3   (d) 2–3 . . . . −1
    (b) less than 1 . . . . . +1   (e) 4–5 . . . . −2
    (c) 1 0   (f) 6 or more . . . . . . −3

12. **After cooking, how large is the serving of red meat you eat?** (*To convert from raw to cooked, reduce by 25 percent. For example, 4 oz. of raw meat shrinks to 3 oz. after cooking. There are 16 oz. in a pound.*)
    (a) 6 oz. or more . . . −3   (c) 3 oz. or less 0
    (b) 4 to 5 oz. . . . . −2   (d) don't eat
                                          red meat . . . . +3

13. **If you eat red meat, do you trim the visible fat when you cook or eat it?**
    (a) yes . . . . +1   (b) no . . . . −3

14. **What kind of ground meat or poultry do you eat?**
    (a) regular ground beef . . . . −4
    (b) ground beef that's 11% to 25% fat . . . . −3
    (c) ground chicken or 10% fat ground beef . . . . . −2
    (d) ground turkey . . . . −1
    (e) ground turkey breast . . . . +3
    (f) don't eat ground meat or poultry . . . . +3

15. **What chicken parts do you eat?**
    (a) breast . . . . +3   (d) wing . . . . −2
    (b) drumstick . . . . . . +1   (e) don't eat poultry +3
    (c) thigh . . . . −1

16. **If you eat poultry, do you remove the skin before eating?**
    (a) yes . . . . +2   (b) no . . . . −3

17. **If you eat seafood, how many times per week?**
    (*OMIT deep-fried foods, tuna packed in oil, and mayonnaise-laden tuna salad—low-fat mayo is okay.*)
    (a) less than 1 0   (c) 2 . . . . +2
    (b) 1 . . . . +1   (d) 3 or more . . . . . . +3

Mixed foods

18. **What is your most typical breakfast?** (*SUBTRACT an extra 3 points if you also eat sausage.*)
    (a) biscuit sandwich or croissant sandwich . . . . . −4
    (b) croissant, danish, or doughnut . . . . −3
    (c) eggs . . . . −3
    (d) pancakes, French toast, or waffles . . . . −1
    (e) cereal, toast, or bagel (no cream cheese) . . . +3
    (f) low-fat yogurt or low-fat cottage cheese . . . . +3
    (g) don't eat breakfast 0

19. **What sandwich fillings do you eat?**
    (a) regular luncheon meat, cheese, or egg salad . −3
    (b) tuna or chicken salad or ham . . . . −2
    (c) peanut butter 0
    (d) roast beef . . . . +1
    (e) low-fat luncheon meat . . . . +1
    (f) tuna or chicken salad made
        with fat-free mayo . . . . +3
    (g) turkey breast or hummus . . . . +3

20. **What do you order on your pizza?** (*Subtract 1 point if you order extra cheese, cheese-filled crust, or more than one meat topping.*)
    (a) no cheese with at least one vegetable
        topping . . . . +3
    (b) cheese with at least one vegetable
        topping . . . . −1
    (c) cheese . . . . −2
    (d) cheese with one meat topping . . . . −3
    (e) don't eat pizza . . . . +3

21. **What do you put on your pasta?** (*ADD one point if you also add sautéed vegetables.*)
    (a) tomato sauce or red clam sauce . . . . +3
    (b) meat sauce or meat balls . . . . −1
    (c) pesto or another oily sauce . . . . −3
    (d) Alfredo or another creamy sauce . . . . −4

22. **How many times per week do you eat deep-fried foods** (*fish, chicken, french fries, potato chips, etc.*)**?**
    (a) 0 . . . . +3   (d) 3 . . . . −2
    (b) 1 0   (e) 4 or more . . . . . . −3
    (c) 2 . . . . −1

23. **At a salad bar, what do you choose?**
    (a) nothing, lemon, or vinegar . . . . +3
    (b) fat-free dressing . . . . +2
    (c) low- or reduced-Calorie dressing . . . . +1
    (d) oil and vinegar . . . . −1
    (e) regular dressing . . . . −2
    (f) cole slaw, pasta salad, or potato salad . . . . . . −2
    (g) cheese or eggs . . . . −3

24. **How many times per week do you eat canned or dried soups or frozen dinners?** (*OMIT lower-sodium, low-fat ones.*)
    (a) 0 . . . . +3   (d) 3 to 4 . . . . –2
    (b) 1 0   (e) 5 or more . . . . . . –3
    (c) 2 . . . . –1

25. **How many servings of low-fat calcium-rich food do you eat per day?** (*One serving = 2/3 cup low-fat or nonfat milk or yogurt, 1 oz. low-fat cheese, 1 1/2 oz. sardines, 3 1/2 oz. canned salmon with bones, 1 oz. tofu made with calcium sulfate, 1 cup collards or kale, or 200 mg of a calcium supplement.*)
    (a) 0 . . . . –3   (d) 2 . . . . +2
    (b) less than 1 . . . . . –1   (e) 3 or more . . . . . . +3
    (c) 1 . . . . +1

26. **How many times per week do you eat cheese?** (*INCLUDE pizza, cheeseburgers, lasagna, tacos or nachos with cheese, etc. OMIT foods made with low-fat cheese.*)
    (a) 0 . . . . +3   (d) 3 . . . . –2
    (b) 1 . . . . +1   (e) 4 or more . . . . . . –3
    (c) 2 . . . . –1

27. **How many egg yolks do you eat per week?** (*ADD 1 yolk for every slice of quiche you eat.*)
    (a) 0 . . . . +3   (d) 3 . . . . –1
    (b) 1 . . . . +1   (e) 4 . . . . –2
    (c) 2 0   (f) 5 or more . . . . . . –3

Fats & oils

28. **What do you put on your bread, toast, bagel, or English muffin?**
    (a) stick butter or cream cheese . . . . –4
    (b) stick margarine or whipped butter . . . . –3
    (c) regular tub margarine . . . . –2
    (d) light tub margarine or whipped light butter . . . . –1
    (e) jam, fat-free margarine, or fat-free cream cheese 0
    (f) nothing . . . . +3

29. **What do you spread on your sandwiches?**
    (a) mayonnaise . . . . –2
    (b) light mayonnaise . . . . –1
    (c) catsup, mustard, or fat-free mayonnaise . . . . +1
    (d) nothing . . . . +2

30. **With what do you make tuna salad, pasta salad, chicken salad, etc?**
    (a) mayonnaise . . . . –2   (d) low-fat yogurt . . +2
    (b) light mayonnaise –1
    (c) fat-free
        mayonnaise   0

31. **What do you use to sauté vegetables or other foods?** (*Vegetable oil includes safflower, corn, sunflower, and soybean.*)
    (a) butter or lard . . . –3   (d) olive or
    (b) margarine . . . . . . –2   canola oil . . . . . . +1
    (c) vegetable oil or   (e) broth . . . . +2
        light margarine . –1   (f) cooking spray . . . +3

Beverages

32. **What do you drink on a typical day?**
    (a) water or club soda . . . . +3
    (b) caffeine-free coffee or tea 0
    (c) diet soda . . . . –1
    (d) coffee or tea (up to 4 a day) . . . . –1
    (e) regular soda (up to 2 a day) . . . . –2
    (f) regular soda (3 or more a day) . . . . –3
    (g) coffee or tea (5 or more a day) . . . . –3

33. **What kind of "fruit" beverage do you drink?**
    (a) orange, grapefruit, prune or
        pineapple juice . . . . +3
    (b) apple, grape, or pear juice . . . . +1
    (c) cranberry juice blend or cocktail 0
    (d) fruit "drink," "ade," or "punch" . . . . –3

34. **What kind of milk do you drink?**
    (a) whole . . . . –3   (c) 1% low-fat . . . . . +2
    (b) 2% fat . . . . –1   (d) skim . . . . +3

Desserts & snacks

35. **What do you eat as a snack?**
    (a) fruits or   (e) nuts or granola
        vegetables . . . . . +3   bar . . . . –2
    (b) low-fat yogurt . . +2   (f) candy bar or
    (c) low-fat crackers . +1   pastry . . . . –3
    (d) cookies or fried
        chips . . . . –2

36. **Which of the following "salty" snacks do you eat?**
    (a) potato chips, corn chips, or popcorn . . . . –3
    (b) tortilla chips . . . . –2
    (c) salted pretzels or light microwave popcorn . . –1
    (d) unsalted pretzels . . . . +2
    (e) baked tortilla or potato chips or homemade
        air-popped popcorn . . . . +3
    (f) don't eat salty snacks . . . . +3

37. **What kind of cookies do you eat?**
    (a) fat-free cookies . . . . +2
    (b) graham crackers or reduced-fat cookies . . . . . +1
    (c) oatmeal cookies . . . . –1
    (d) sandwich cookies (like Oreos) . . . . –2
    (e) chocolate coated, chocolate chip,
        or peanut butter . . . . –3
    (f) don't eat cookies . . . . +3

38. **What kind of cake or pastry do you eat?**
    - (a) cheesecake . . . . −4
    - (b) pie or doughnuts. . . . . −3
    - (c) cake with frosting. . . . . −2
    - (d) cake without frosting . . . . −1
    - (e) muffins 0
    - (f) angelfood, fat-free cake, or fat-free pastry . . . +1
    - (g) don't eat cakes or pastries . . . . +3

39. **What kind of frozen dessert do you eat?**
    (SUBTRACT 1 point for each of the following toppings: hot fudge, nuts or chocolate candy bars or pieces.)
    - (a) gourmet ice cream . . . . −4
    - (b) regular ice cream . . . . −3
    - (c) frozen yogurt or light ice cream . . . . −1
    - (d) sorbet, sherbet, or ices . . . . −1
    - (e) non-fat frozen yogurt or fat-free ice cream . . +1
    - (f) don't eat frozen desserts. . . . . +3

Scoring your diet

Add up your score for each question.

Score

0 or below	**Oops!**	We don't staple *Nutrition Action* shut, you know.
1 to 29	**Hmmm.**	Don't be discouraged. This eating business is tough.
30 to 59	**Yesss!**	Congratulations. You can invite us over to eat any day.
60 or above	**C-o-o-o-l.**	Our photographer should be at your door any second.

American College of Sports Medicine Position Stand: The Recommended Quantity and Quality of Exercise for Developing and Maintaining Cardiorespiratory and Muscular Fitness in Healthy Adults

This Position Stand replaces the 1978 ACSM position paper, "The Recommended Quantity and Quality of Exercise for Developing and Maintaining Fitness in Healthy Adults."

Increasing numbers of persons are becoming involved in endurance training and other forms of physical activity, and, thus, the need for guidelines for exercise prescription is apparent. Based on the existing evidence concerning exercise prescription for healthy adults and the need for guidelines, the American College of Sports Medicine (ACSM) makes the following recommendations for the quantity and quality of training for developing and maintaining cardiorespiratory fitness, body composition, and muscular strength and endurance in the healthy adult:

1. Frequency of training: 3–5 d $\cdot$ wk^{-1}.

2. Intensity of training: 60–90% of maximum heart rate (HR$_{max}$), or 50–85% of maximum oxygen uptake (VO$_{2max}$) or HR$_{max}$ reserve.[1]

3. Duration of training: 20–60 min of continuous aerobic activity. Duration is dependent on the intensity of the activity; thus, lower intensity activity should be conducted over a longer period of time. Because of the importance of "total fitness" and the fact that it is more readily attained in longer duration programs, and because of the potential hazards and compliance problems associated with high

intensity activity, lower to moderate intensity activity of longer duration is recommended for the nonathletic adult.

4. Mode of activity: any activity that uses large muscle groups, can be maintained continuously, and is rhythmical and aerobic in nature, e.g., walking-hiking, running-jogging, cycling-bicycling, cross-country skiing, dancing, rope skipping, rowing, stair climbing, swimming, skating, and various endurance game activities.

5. Resistance training: Strength training of a moderate intensity, sufficient to develop and maintain fat-free weight (FFW), should be an integral part of an adult fitness program. One set of 8–12 repetitions of eight to ten exercises that condition the major muscle groups at least 2 d$\cdot$wk^{-1} is the recommended minimum.

Rationale and Research Background
Introduction

The questions "How much exercise is enough," and "What type of exercise is best for developing and maintaining fitness?" are frequently asked. It is recognized that the term "physical fitness" is composed of a variety of characteristics included in the broad categories of cardiovascular-respiratory fitness, body composition, muscular strength and endurance, and flexibility. In this context fitness is defined as the ability to perform moderate to vigorous levels of physical activity without undue fatigue and the capability of maintaining such ability throughout life (167). It is also recognized that the adaptive response to training is complex and includes peripheral, central, structural, and functional factors

---

[1] Maximum heart rate reserve is calculated from the difference between resting and maximum heart rate. To estimate training intensity, a percentage of this value is added to the resting heart rate and is expressed as a percentage of HR$_{max}$ reserve (85).

(5,172). Although many such variables and their adaptive response to training have been documented, the lack of sufficient in-depth and comparative data relative to frequency, intensity, and duration of training makes them inadequate to use as comparative models. Thus, in respect to the above questions, fitness is limited mainly to changes in VO_{2max}, muscular strength and endurance, and body composition, which includes total body mass, fat weight (FW), and FFW. Further, the rationale and research background used for this position stand will be divided into programs for cardiorespiratory fitness and weight control and programs for muscular strength and endurance.

Fitness versus Health Benefits of Exercise

Since the original position statement was published in 1978, an important distinction has been made between physical activity as it relates to health versus fitness. It has been pointed out that the quantity and quality of exercise needed to attain health-related benefits may differ from what is recommended for fitness benefits. It is now clear that lower levels of physical activity than recommended by this position statement may reduce the risk for certain chronic degenerative diseases and yet may not be of sufficient quantity or quality to improve VO_{2max} (71,72, 98,167). ACSM recognizes the potential health benefits of regular exercise performed more frequently and for a longer duration, but at lower intensities than prescribed in this position statement (13A,71,100,120,160). ACSM will address the issue concerning the proper amount of physical activity necessary to derive health benefits in another statement.

Need for Standardization of Procedures and Reporting Results

Despite an abundance of information available concerning the training of the human organism, the lack of standardization of testing protocols and procedures, of methodology in relation to training procedures and experimental design, and of a preciseness in the documentation and reporting of the quantity and quality of training prescribed make interpretation difficult (123,133,139, 164,167). Interpretation and comparison of results are also dependent on the initial level of fitness (42,43,58, 114,148,151,156), length of time of the training experiment (17,45,125,128,139,145,150), and specificity of the testing and training (5,43,130,139,145A,172). For example, data from training studies using subjects with varied levels of VO_{2max}, total body mass, and FW have found changes to occur in relation to their initial values (14,33,109,112,113,148,151); i.e., the lower the initial VO_{2max} the larger the percentage of improvement found, and the higher the FW the greater the reduction. Also, data evaluating trainability with age, comparison of the different magnitudes and quantities of effort, and comparison of the trainability of men and women may have been influenced by the initial fitness levels.

In view of the fact that improvement in the fitness variables discussed in this position statement continues over many months of training (27,86,139,145,150), it is reasonable to believe that short-term studies conducted over a few weeks have certain limitations. Middle-aged sedentary and older participants may take several weeks to adapt to the initial rigors of training, and thus need a longer adaptation period to get the full benefit from a program. For example, Seals et al. (150) exercise trained 60–69-yr-olds for 12 months. Their subjects showed a 12% improvement in VO_{2max} after 6 months of moderate intensity walking training. A further 18% increase in VO_{2max} occurred during the next 6 months of training when jogging was introduced. How long a training experiment should be conducted is difficult to determine, but 15–20 wk may be a good minimum standard. Although it is difficult to control exercise training experiments for more than 1 yr, there is a need to study this effect. As stated earlier, lower doses of exercise may improve VO_{2max} and control or maintain body composition, but at a slower rate.

Although most of the information concerning training described in this position statement has been conducted on men, the available evidence indicates that women tend to adapt to endurance training in the same manner as men (19,38,46,47,49,62,65,68,90,92,122,166).

Exercise Prescription for Cardiorespiratory Fitness and Weight Control

Exercise prescription is based upon the frequency, intensity, and duration of training, the mode of activity (aerobic in nature, e.g., listed under No. 4 above), and the initial level of fitness. In evaluating these factors, the following observations have been derived from studies conducted for up to 6–12 months with endurance training programs.

Improvement in VO_{2max} is directly related to frequency (3,6,50,75–77,125,126,152,154,164), intensity (3,6,26,29,58,61,75–77,80,85,93,118,152,164) and duration (3,29,60,61,70,75–77,101,109,118,152,162,164,168) of training. Depending upon the quantity and quality of training, improvement in VO_{2max} ranges from 5 to 30% (8,29,30,48,59,61,65,67,69,75–77,82,84,96,99,101,102, 111,115,119,123,127,139,141,143,149,150,152,153,158, 164,168,173). These studies show that a minimum increase in VO_{2max} of 15% is generally attained in programs that meet the above stated guidelines. Although changes in VO_{2max} greater than 30% have been shown, they are usually associated with large total body mass and FW loss, in cardiac patients, or in persons with a very low initial level of fitness. Also, as a result of leg fatigue or a lack of motivation, persons with low initial fitness may have spuriously low initial VO_{2max} values. Klissouras (94A) and Bouchard (16A) have shown that human variation in the trainability of VO_{2max} is important and related to current phenotype level. That is, there is a genetically determined pretraining status of the trait and capacity to adapt to physical training. Thus, physiological results should be interpreted with respect to both genetic variation and the quality and quantity of training performed.

Intensity-Duration   Intensity and duration of training are interrelated, with total amount of work accomplished being an important factor in improvement in fitness (12,20,27,48,90,92,123,127,128,136,149,151,164). Although more comprehensive inquiry is necessary, present evidence suggests that, when exercise is performed above the minimum intensity threshold, the total amount of work accomplished is an important factor in fitness development (19,27,126,127,149,151) and maintenance (134). That is, improvement will be similar for activities performed at a lower intensity-longer duration compared to higher intensity-shorter duration if the total energy costs of the activities are equal. Higher intensity exercise is associated with greater cardiovascular risk (156A), orthopedic injury (124,139) and lower compliance to training than lower intensity exercise (36,105,124,146). Therefore, programs emphasizing low to moderate intensity training with longer duration are recommended for most adults.

The minimal training intensity threshold for improvement in VO_{2max} is approximately 60% of the HR_{max} (50% of VO_{2max} or HR_{max} reserve) (80,85). The 50% of HR_{max} reserve represents a heart rate of approximately 130–135 beats $\cdot$ min^{-1} for young persons. As a result of the age-related change in maximum heart rate, the absolute heart rate to achieve this threshold is inversely related to age and can be as low as 105–115 beats $\cdot$ min^{-1} for older persons (35,65,150). Patients who are taking beta-adrenergic blocking drugs may have significantly lower heart rate values (171). Initial level of fitness is another important consideration in prescribing exercise (26,90,104,148,151). The person with a low fitness level can achieve a significant training effect with a sustained training heart rate as low as 40–50% of HR_{max} reserve, while persons with higher fitness levels require a higher training stimulus (35,58,152,164).

Classification of Exercise Intensity   The classification of exercise intensity and its standardization for exercise prescription based on a 20–60 min training session has been confusing, misinterpreted, and often taken out of context. The most quoted exercise classification system is based on the energy expenditure ($kcal \cdot min^{-1} \cdot kg^{-1}$) of industrial tasks (40,89). The original data for this classification system were published by Christensen (24) in 1953 and were based on the energy expenditure of working in the steel mill for an 8-h day. The classification of industrial and leisure-time tasks by using absolute values of energy expenditure have been valuable for use in the occupational and nutritional setting. Although this classification system has broad application in medicine and, in particu-

lar, making recommendations for weight control and job placement, it has little or no meaning for preventive and rehabilitation exercise training programs. To extrapolate absolute values of energy expenditure for completing an industrial task based on an 8-h work day to 20–60 min regimens of exercise training does not make sense. For example, walking and jogging/running can be accomplished at a wide range of speeds; thus, the relative intensity becomes important under these conditions. Because the endurance training regimens recommended by ACSM for nonathletic adults are geared for 60 min or less of physical activity, the system of classification of exercise training intensity shown in Table 1 is recommended (139). The use of a realistic time period for training and an individual's relative exercise intensity makes this system amenable to young, middle-aged, and elderly participants, as well as patients with a limited exercise capacity (3,137,139).

Table 1 also describes the relationship between relative intensity based on percent HR_{max}, percentage of HR_{max} reserve or percentage of VO_{2max}, and the rating of perceived exertion (RPE) (15,16,137). The use of heart rate as an estimate of intensity of training is the common standard (3,139).

The use of RPE has become a valid tool in the monitoring of intensity in exercise training programs (11,37,137,139). It is generally considered an adjunct to heart rate in monitoring relative exercise intensity, but once the relationship between heart rate and RPE is known, RPE can be used in place of heart rate (23,139). This would not be the case in certain patient populations where a more precise knowledge of heart rate may be critical to the safety of the program.

Table 1 **Classification of intensity of exercise based on 20–60 min of endurance training**

Relative intensity (%)			
HR_{max}*	VO_{2max}* or HR_{max} reserve	Rating of Perceived Exertion	Classification of Intensity
< 35%	< 30%	< 10	Very light
35–59%	30–49%	10–11	Light
60–79%	50–74%	12–13	Moderate (somewhat hard)
80–89%	75–84%	14–16	Heavy
≥ 90%	≥ 85%	> 16	Very heavy

Source: From M. L. Pollock and J. H. Wilmore, *Exercise in Health and Disease: Evaluation and Prescription for Prevention and Rehabilitation*, 2d ed. Copyright © 1990 W. B. Saunders, Philadelphia, PA. Reprinted by permission.

* HR_{max} = maximum heart rate; VO_{2max} = maximum oxygen uptake

Frequency The amount of improvement in VO_{2max} tends to plateau when frequency of training is increased above 3 d·wk^{-1} (50,123,139). The value of the added improvement found with training more than 5 d·wk^{-1} is small to not apparent in regard to improvement in VO_{2max} (75–77,106,123). Training of less than 2 d·wk^{-1} does not generally show a meaningful change in VO_{2max} (29,50,118,123,152,164).

Mode If frequency, intensity, and duration of training are similar (total kcal expenditure), the training adaptations appear to be independent of the mode of aerobic activity (101A,118,130). Therefore, a variety of endurance activities, e.g., those listed above, may be used to derive the same training effect.

Endurance activities that require running and jumping are considered high impact types of activity and generally cause significantly more debilitating injuries to beginning as well as long-term exercisers than do low impact and non-weight bearing type activities (13,93,117, 124,127,135,140,142). This is particularly evident in the elderly (139). Beginning joggers have increased foot, leg, and knee injuries when training is performed more than 3 d·wk^{-1} and longer than 30 min duration per exercise session (135). High intensity interval training (run-walk) compared to continuous jogging training was also associated with a higher incidence of injury (124,136). Thus, caution should be taken when recommending the type of activity and exercise prescription for the beginning exerciser. Orthopedic injuries as related to overuse increase linearly in runners/joggers when performing these activities (13,140). Thus, there is a need for more inquiry into the effect that different types of activities and the quantity and quality of training has on injuries over short-term and long-term participation.

An activity such as weight training should not be considered as a means of training for developing VO_{2max}, but it has significant value for increasing muscular strength and endurance and FFW (32,54,107,110,165). Studies evaluating circuit weight training (weight training conducted almost continuously with moderate weights, using 10–15 repetitions per exercise session with 15–30 s rest between bouts of activity) show an average improvement in VO_{2max} of 6% (1,51–54,83,94,108,170). Thus, circuit weight training is not recommended as the only activity used in exercise programs for developing VO_{2max}.

Age Age in itself does not appear to be a deterrent to endurance training. Although some earlier studies showed a lower training effect with middle-aged or elderly participants (9,34,79,157,168), more recent studies show the relative changes in VO_{2max} to be similar to younger age groups (7,8,65,132,150,161,163). Although more investigation is necessary concerning the rate of improvement in VO_{2max} with training at various ages, at present it appears that elderly participants need longer periods of time to adapt (34,132,150). Earlier studies showing moderate to no improvement in VO_{2max} were conducted over a short time span (9), or exercise was conducted at a moderate to low intensity (34), thus making the interpretation of the results difficult.

Although VO_{2max} decreases with age and total body mass and FW increase with age, evidence suggests that this trend can be altered with endurance training (22,27,86–88,139). A 9% reduction in VO_{2max} per decade for sedentary adults after age 25 has been shown (31,73), but for active individuals the reduction may be less than 5% per decade (21,31,39,73). Ten or more yr follow-up studies where participants continued training at a similar level showed maintenance of cardiorespiratory fitness (4,87,88,138). A cross-sectional study of older competitive runners showed progressively lower values in VO_{2max} from the fourth to seventh decades of life, but also showed less training in the older groups (129). More recent 10-yr follow-up data on these same athletes (50–82 yr of age) showed VO_{2max} to be unchanged when training quantity and quality remained unchanged (138). Thus, lifestyle plays a significant role in the maintenance of fitness. More inquiry into the relationship of long-term training (quantity and quality), for both competitors and noncompetitors, and physiological function with increasing age is necessary before more definitive statements can be made.

Maintenance of Training Effect In order to maintain the training effect, exercise must be continued on a regular basis (18,25,28,47,97,111,144,147). A significant reduction in cardiorespiratory fitness occurs after 2 wk of detraining (25,144), with participants returning to near pretraining levels of fitness after 10 wk (47) to 8 months of detraining (97). A loss of 50% of their initial improvement in VO_{2max} has been shown after 4–12 wk of detraining (47,91,144). Those individuals who have undergone years of continuous training maintain some benefits for longer periods of detraining than subjects from short-term training studies (25). While stopping training shows dramatic reductions in VO_{2max}, reduced training shows modest to no reductions for periods of 5–15 wk (18, 75–77,144). Hickson et al., in a series of experiments where frequency (75), duration (76), or intensity (77) of training were manipulated, found that, if intensity of training remained unchanged, VO_{2max} was maintained for up to 15 wk when frequency and duration of training were reduced by as much as 2/3. When frequency and duration of training remained constant and intensity of training was reduced by 1/3 or 2/3, VO_{2max} was significantly reduced. Similar findings were found in regards to reduced strength training exercise. When strength training exercise was reduced from 3 or 2 d·wk^{-1} to at least 1 d·wk^{-1}, strength was maintained for 12 wk of reduced training (62). Thus, it appears that missing an exercise session periodically or reducing training for up to 15 wk will not adversely affect VO_{2max} or muscular strength and endurance as long as training intensity is maintained.

Even though many new studies have given added insight into the proper amount of exercise, investigation is necessary to evaluate the rate of increase and decrease of fitness when varying training loads and reduction in training in relation to level of fitness, age, and length of time in training. Also, more information is needed to better identify the minimal level of exercise necessary to maintain fitness.

Weight Control and Body Composition Although there is variability in human response to body composition change with exercise, total body mass and FW are generally reduced with endurance training programs (133,139,171A), while FFW remains constant (123,133,139,169) or increases slightly (116,174). For example, Wilmore (171A) reported the results of 32 studies that met the criteria for developing cardiorespiratory fitness that are outlined in this position stand and found an average loss in total body mass of 1.5 kg and percent fat of 2.2%. Weight loss programs using dietary manipulation that result in a more dramatic decrease in total body mass show reductions in both FW and FFW (2,78,174). When these programs are conducted in conjunction with exercise training, FFW loss is more modest than in programs using diet alone (78,121). Programs that are conducted at least 3 d·wk^{-1} (123,125,126,128,169), of at least 20 min duration (109,123,169), and of sufficient intensity to expend approximately 300 kcal per exercise session (75 kg person)[2] are suggested as a threshold level for total body mass and FW loss (27,64,77,123,133,139). An expenditure of 200 kcal per session has also been shown to be useful in weight reduction if the exercise frequency is at least 4 d·wk^{-1} (155). If the primary purpose of the training program is for weight loss, then regimens of greater frequency and duration of training and low to moderate intensity are recommended (2,139). Programs with less participation generally show little or no change in body composition (44,57,93,123,133,159,162,169). Significant increases in VO$_{2max}$ have been shown with 10–15 min of high intensity training (6,79,109,118,123,152,153); thus, if total body mass and FW reduction are not considerations, then shorter duration, higher intensity programs may be recommended for healthy individuals at low risk for cardiovascular disease and orthopedic injury.

Exercise Prescription for Muscular Strength and Endurance

The addition of resistance/strength training to the position statement results from the need for a well-rounded program that exercises all the major muscle groups of the body. Thus, the inclusion of resistance training in adult fitness programs should be effective in the development and maintenance of FFW. The effect of exercise training is specific to the area of the body being trained (5,43,145A,172). For example, training the legs will have little or no effect on the arms, shoulders, and trunk muscles. A 10-yr follow-up of master runners who continued their training regimen, but did no upper body exercise, showed maintenance of VO$_{2max}$ and a 2-kg reduction of FFW (138). Their leg circumference remained unchanged, but arm circumference was significantly lower. These data indicate a loss of muscle mass in the untrained areas. Three of the athletes who practiced weight training exercise for the upper body and trunk muscles maintained their FFW. A comprehensive review by Sale (145A) carefully documents available information on specificity of training.

Specificity of training was further addressed by Graves et al. (63). Using the bilateral knee extension exercise, they trained four groups: group A, first $\frac{1}{2}$ of the range of motion; group B, second $\frac{1}{2}$ of the range of motion; group AB, full range of motion; and a control group that did not train. The results clearly showed that the training result was specific to the range of motion trained, with group AB getting the best full range effect. Thus, resistance training should be performed through a full range of motion for maximum benefit (63,95).

Muscular strength and endurance are developed by the overload principle, i.e., by increasing more than normal the resistance to movement or frequency and duration of activity (32,41,43,74,145). Muscular strength is best developed by using heavy weights (that require maximum or nearly maximum tension development) with few repetitions, and muscular endurance is best developed by using lighter weights with a greater number of repetitions (10,41,43,145). To some extent, both muscular strength and endurance are developed under each condition, but each system favors a more specific type of development (43,145). Thus, to elicit improvement in both muscular strength and endurance, most experts recommend 8–12 repetitions per bout of exercise.

Any magnitude of overload will result in strength development, but higher intensity effort at as near maximal effort will give a significantly greater effect (43,74,101B,103,145,172). The intensity of resistance training can be manipulated by varying the weight load, repetitions, rest interval between exercises, and number of sets completed (43). Caution is advised for training that emphasizes lengthening (eccentric) contractions, compared to shortening (concentric) or isometric contractions, as the potential for skeletal muscle soreness and injury is accentuated (3A,84A).

Muscular strength and endurance can be developed by means of static (isometric) or dynamic (isotonic or isokinetic) exercises. Although each type of training has its favorable and weak points, for healthy adults, dynamic resistance exercises are recommended. Resistance training for the average participant should be rhythmical,

---

[2] Haskell and Haskell et al. (71,72) have suggested the use of 4 kcal·kg^{-1} of body weight of energy expenditure per day for a minimum standard for use in exercise programs.

performed at a moderate to slow speed, move through a full range of motion, and not impede normal forced breathing. Heavy resistance exercise can cause a dramatic acute increase in both systolic and diastolic blood pressure (100A,101C).

The expected improvement in strength from resistance training is difficult to assess because increases in strength are affected by the participants' initial level of strength and their potential for improvement (43,66,74,114,172). For example, Mueller and Rohmert (114) found increases in strength ranging from 2 to 9% per week depending on initial strength levels. Although the literature reflects a wide range of improvement in strength with resistance training programs, the average improvement for sedentary young and middle-aged men and women for up to 6 months of training is 25–30%. Fleck and Kraemer (43), in a review of 13 studies representing various forms of isotonic training, showed an average improvement in bench press strength of 23.3% when subjects were tested on the equipment with which they were trained and 16.5% when tested on special isotonic or isokinetic ergometers (six studies). Fleck and Kraemer (43) also reported an average increase in leg strength of 26.6% when subjects were tested with the equipment that they trained on (six studies) and 21.2% when tested with special isotonic or isokinetic ergometers (five studies). Results of improvement in strength resulting from isometric training have been of the same magnitude as found with isotonic training (17,43,62,63).

In light of the information reported above, the following guidelines for resistance training are recommended for the average healthy adult. A minimum of 8–10 exercises involving the major muscle groups should be performed a minimum of two times per week. A minimum of one set of 8–12 repetitions to near fatigue should be completed. These minimal standards for resistance training are based on two factors. First, the time it takes to complete a comprehensive, well-rounded exercise program is important. Programs lasting more than 60 min per session are associated with higher dropout rates (124). Second, although greater frequencies of training (17,43,56) and additional sets or combinations of sets and repetitions elicit larger strength gains (10,32,43,74, 145,172), the magnitude of difference is usually small. For example, Braith et al. (17) compared training 2 d·wk^{-1} with 3 d·wk^{-1} for 18 wk. The subjects performed one set of 7–10 repetitions to fatigue. The 2 d·wk^{-1} group showed a 21% increase in strength compared to 28% in the 3 d·wk^{-1} group. In other words, 75% of what could be attainted in a 3 d·wk^{-1} program was attained in 2 d·wk^{-1}. Also, the 21% improvement in strength found by the 2 d·wk^{-1} regimen is 70–80% of the improvement reported by other programs using additional frequencies of training and combinations of sets and repetitions (43). Graves et al. (62,63), Gettman et al. (55), Hurley et al. (83) and Braith et al. (17) found that programs using one set to fatigue showed a greater than 25% increase in strength. Although resistance training equipment may provide a better graduated and quantitative stimulus for overload than traditional calisthenic exercises, calisthenics and other resistance types of exercise can still be effective in improving and maintaining strength.

Summary

The combination of frequency, intensity, and duration of chronic exercise has been found to be effective for producing a training effect. The interaction of these factors provides the overload stimulus. In general, the lower the stimulus the lower the training effect, and the greater the stimulus the greater the effect. As a result of specificity of training and the need for maintaining muscular strength and endurance, and flexibility of the major muscle groups, a well-rounded training program including resistance training and flexibility exercises is recommended. Although age in itself is not a limiting factor to exercise training, a more gradual approach in applying the prescription at older ages seems prudent. It has also been shown that endurance training of fewer than 2 d·wk^{-1}, at less than 50% of maximum oxygen uptake and for less than 10 min·d^{-1}, is inadequate for developing and maintaining fitness for healthy adults.

In the interpretation of this position statement, it must be recognized that the recommendations should be used in the context of participants' needs, goals, and initial abilities. In this regard, a sliding scale as to the amount of time allotted and intensity of effort should be carefully gauged for both the cardiorespiratory and muscular strength and endurance components of the program. An appropriate warm-up and cool-down, which would include flexibility exercises, is also recommended. The important factor is to design a program for the individual to provide the proper amount of physical activity to attain maximal benefit at the lowest risk. Emphasis should be placed on factors that result in permanent lifestyle change and encourage a lifetime of physical activity.

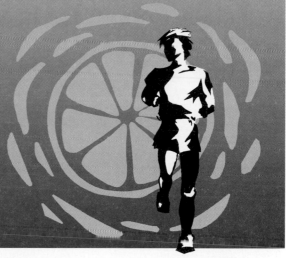

Energy Pathways of Carbohydrate, Fat, and Protein

6C → two 3C molecules

Figure K.1 In glycolysis, 1 glucose molecule is converted into 2 pyruvic acid molecules in nine separate steps. In addition to 2 pyruvic acids, these products include 2 molecules of NADH and 4 molecules of ATP. Since 2 molecules were used at the beginning of glycolysis, however, the net gain is 2 ATP per glucose molecule. When oxygen supply is inadequate, pyruvic acid may be converted into lactic acid (step 10), permitting the regeneration of NAD to enable energy production via glycolysis to continue.

Glucose ($C_6H_{12}O_6$)

ATP ①
ADP

Glucose 6–phosphate

②

Fructose 6–phosphate

ATP ③
ADP

Fructose 1,6–diphosphate

Dihydroxy-acetone phosphate

④

3–Phosphoglyceraldehyde   3–Phosphoglyceraldehyde

P_i P_i
NAD ⑤   NAD ⑤
2H   2H
NADH   NADH

1,3–Diphosphoglyceric acid   1,3–Diphosphoglyceric acid

ADP ⑥   ADP ⑥
ATP   ATP

3–Phosphoglyceric acid   3–Phosphoglyceric acid

⑦   ⑦

2–Phosphoglyceric acid   2–Phosphoglyceric acid

⑧   ⑧

Phosphoenolpyruvic acid   Phosphoenolpyruvic acid

ADP ⑨   ⑨ ADP
ATP   ATP

NAD   NAD
NADH + H⁺   NADH + H⁺

Lactic Acid ($C_3H_6O_3$) ⑩ Pyruvic acid ($C_3H_4O_3$)   Pyruvic acid ($C_3H_4O_3$) ⑩ Lactic Acid ($C_3H_6O_3$)

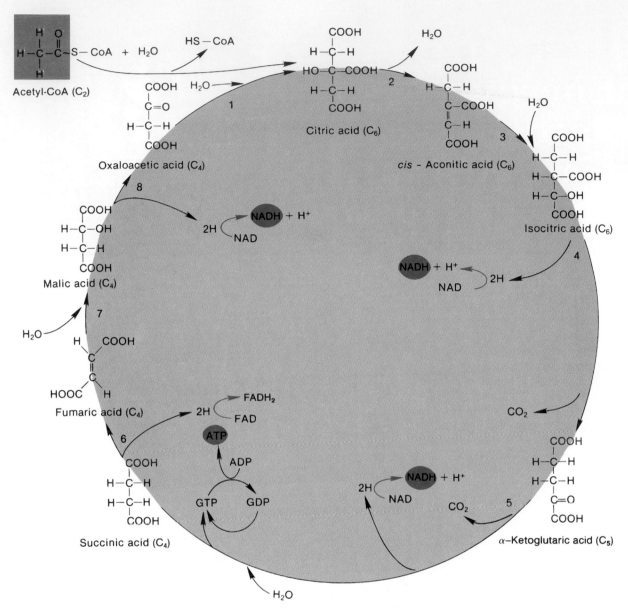

Figure K.2 The Krebs cycle. Acetyl CoA combines with oxaloacetic acid to form citric acid. At various stages of the Krebs cycle, hydrogen ions and electrons are removed by NAD (nicotinamide adenine dinucleotide) and FAD (flavin adenine dinucleotide) for passage through the electron transport system and the generation of ATP. Only small amounts of high energy phosphates (guanosine triphosphate, GTP) are generated directly in the Krebs cycle.

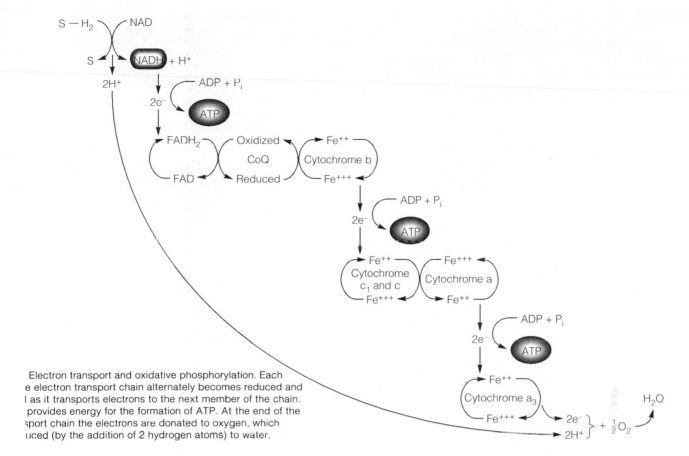

Electron transport and oxidative phosphorylation. Each
e electron transport chain alternately becomes reduced and
l as it transports electrons to the next member of the chain.
provides energy for the formation of ATP. At the end of the
sport chain the electrons are donated to oxygen, which
uced (by the addition of 2 hydrogen atoms) to water.

Figure K.3 Electron transport and oxidative phosphorylation. Each element in the electron transport chain alternately becomes reduced and then oxidized as it transports electrons to the next member of the chain. This process provides energy for the

formation of ATP. At the end of the electron transport chain the electrons are donated to oxygen, which becomes reduced (by the addition of 2 hydrogen atoms) to water.

Figure K.4 Energy pathways for fatty acids. Triglycerides in the adipose tissue may be catabolized by hormone-sensitive lipase, with the fatty acids being released to the plasma and binding with albumin; the glycerol component is transported to the liver for metabolism. A receptor at the muscle cell transports the fatty acid into the muscle cell where it is converted into fatty acyl CoA by an enzyme (fatty acyl CoA synthetase). The fatty acyl CoA is then transported into the mitochondria with carnitine as a carrier. The fatty acyl CoA, which is a combination of acetyl CoA units, then undergoes beta-oxidation, a process that splits off the acetyl CoA units for entrance into the Krebs cycle.

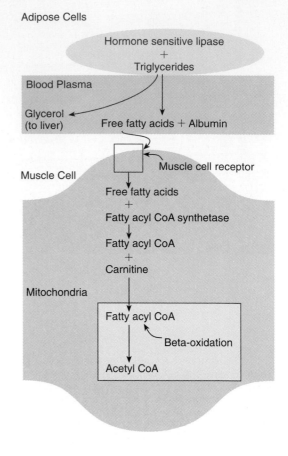

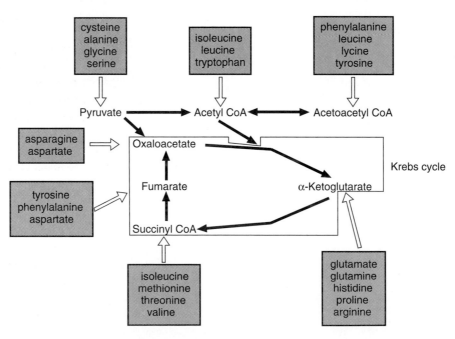

Figure K.5 Metabolic fates of various amino acids. Various amino acids, after deamination, may enter into energy pathways at different sites.

American College of Sports Medicine Position Stand: Exercise and Fluid Replacement

Summary

American College of Sports Medicine. Position Stand on Exercise and Fluid Replacement. *Med. Sci. Sports Exerc.*, Vol. 28, No. 1, pp. i–vii, 1996. It is the position of the American College of Sports Medicine that adequate fluid replacement helps maintain hydration and, therefore, promotes the health, safety, and optimal physical performance of individuals participating in regular physical activity. This position statement is based on a comprehensive review and interpretation of scientific literature concerning the influence of fluid replacement on exercise performance and the risk of thermal injury associated with dehydration and hyperthermia. Based on available evidence, the American College of Sports Medicine makes the following general recommendations on the amount and composition of fluid that should be ingested in preparation for, during, and after exercise or athletic competition:

1) It is recommended that individuals consume a nutritionally balanced diet and drink adequate fluids during the 24-h period before an event, especially during the period that includes the meal prior to exercise, to promote proper hydration before exercise or competition.

2) It is recommended that individuals drink about 500 ml (about 17 ounces) of fluid about 2 h before exercise to promote adequate hydration and allow time for excretion of excess ingested water.

This pronouncement was written for the American College of Sports Medicine by: Victor A. Convertino, Ph.D., FACSM (Chair); Lawrence E. Armstrong, Ph.D., FACSM; Edward F. Coyle, Ph.D., FACSM; Gary W. Mack, Ph.D., Michael N. Sawka, Ph.D., FACSM; Leo C. Senay, Jr., Ph.D., FACSM, and W. Michael Sherman, Ph.D., FACSM. Used by permission of the American College of Sports Medicine.

3) *During* exercise, athletes should start drinking early and at regular intervals in an attempt to consume fluids at a rate sufficient to replace all the water lost through sweating (i.e., body weight loss), or consume the maximal amount that can be tolerated.

4) It is recommended that ingested fluids be cooler than ambient temperature [between 15° and 22°C (59° and 72°F)] and flavored to enhance palatability and promote fluid replacement. Fluids should be readily available and served in containers that allow adequate volumes to be ingested with ease and with minimal interruption of exercise.

5) Addition of proper amounts of carbohydrates and/or electrolytes to a fluid replacement solution is recommended for exercise events of duration greater than 1 h since it does not significantly impair water delivery to the body and may enhance performance. During exercise lasting less than 1 h, there is little evidence of physiological or physical performance differences between consuming a carbohydrate-electrolyte drink and plain water.

6) During intense exercise lasting longer than 1 h, it is recommended that carbohydrates be ingested at a rate of 30–60 g $\cdot$ h^{-1} to maintain oxidation of carbohydrates and delay fatigue. This rate of carbohydrate intake can be achieved without compromising fluid delivery by drinking 600–1200 ml $\cdot$ h^{-1} of solutions containing 4%–8% carbohydrates (g $\cdot$ 100 ml^{-1}). The carbohydrates can be sugars (glucose or sucrose) or starch (e.g., maltodextrin).

7) Inclusion of sodium (0.5–0.7 g $\cdot$ l^{-1} of water) in the rehydration solution ingested during exercise lasting longer than 1 h is recommended since it may be advantageous in enhancing palatability, promoting fluid retention, and possibly preventing hyponatremia in certain individuals who

drink excessive quantities of fluid. There is little physiological basis for the presence of sodium in an oral rehydration solution for enhancing intestinal water absorption as long as sodium is sufficiently available from the previous meal.

Introduction

Disturbances in body water and electrolyte balance can adversely affect cellular as well as systemic function, subsequently reducing the ability of humans to tolerate prolonged exercise. Water lost during exercise-induced sweating can lead to dehydration of both intracellular and extracellular fluid compartments of the body. Even a small amount of dehydration (1% body weight) can increase cardiovascular strain as indicated by a disproportionate elevation of heart rate during exercise, and limit the ability of the body to transfer heat from contracting muscles to the skin surface where heat can be dissipated to the environment. Therefore, consequences of body water deficits can increase the probability for impairing exercise performance and developing heat injury.

The specific aim of this position statement is to provide appropriate guidelines for fluid replacement that will help avoid or minimize the debilitating effects of water and electrolyte deficits on physiological function and exercise performance. These guidelines will also address the rationale for inclusion of carbohydrates and electrolytes in fluid replacement drinks.

Hydration Before Exercise

Fluid replacement following exercise represents hydration prior to the next exercise bout. Any fluid deficit prior to exercise can potentially compromise thermoregulation during the next exercise session if adequate fluid replacement is not employed. Water loss from the body due to sweating is a function of the total thermal load that is related to the combined effects of exercise intensity and ambient conditions (temperature, humidity, wind speed) (62,87). In humans, sweating can exceed 30 g • min^{-1} (1.8 kg • h^{-1}) (2,31). Water lost with sweating is derived from all fluid compartments of the body, including the blood (hypovolemia) (72), thus causing an increase in the concentration of electrolytes in the body fluids (hypertonicity) (85). People who begin exercise when hypohydrated with concomitant hypovolemia and hypertonicity display impaired ability to dissipate body heat during subsequent exercise (26,28,61,85,86). They demonstrate a faster rise in body core temperature and greater cardiovascular strain (28,34,82,83). Exercise performance of both short duration and high power output, as well as prolonged moderate intensity endurance activities, can be impaired when individuals begin exercise with the burden of a previously incurred fluid deficit (1,83), an effect that is exaggerated when activity is performed in a hot environment (81).

During exercise, humans typically drink insufficient volumes of fluid to offset sweat losses. This observation has been referred to as "voluntary dehydration" (33,77). Following a fluid volume deficit created by exercise, individuals ingest more fluid and retain a higher percentage of ingested fluid when electrolyte deficits are also replaced (71). In fact, complete restoration of a fluid volume deficit cannot occur without electrolyte replacement (primarily sodium) in food or beverage (39,89). Electrolytes, primarily sodium chloride, and to a lesser extent potassium, are lost in sweat during exercise. The concentration of Na$^+$ in sweat averages ~50 mmol • l^{-1} but can vary widely (20–100 mmol • l^{-1}) depending on the state of heat acclimation, diet, and hydration (6). Despite knowing the typical electrolyte concentration of sweat, determination of a typical amount of total electrolyte loss during thermal or exercise stress is difficult because the amount and composition of sweat varies with exercise intensity and environmental conditions. The normal range of daily U.S. intake of sodium chloride (NaCl) is 4.6 to 12.8 g (~80–220 mmol) and potassium (K$^+$) is 2–4 g (50–100 mmol) (63). Exercise bouts that produce electrolyte losses in the range of normal daily dietary intake are easily replenished within 24 h following exercise and full rehydration is expected if adequate fluids are provided. When meals are consumed, adequate amounts of electrolytes are present so that the composition of the drink becomes unimportant. However, it is important that fluids be available during meal consumption since most persons rehydrate primarily during and after meals. In the absence of meals, more complete rehydration can be accomplished with fluids containing sodium than with plain water (32,55,71).

To avoid or delay the detrimental effects of dehydration during exercise, individuals appear to benefit from fluid ingested prior to competition. For instance, water ingested 60 min before exercise will enhance thermoregulation and lower heart rate during exercise (34,56). However, urine volume will increase as much as 4 times that measured without preexercise fluid intake. Pragmatically, ingestion of 400–600 ml of water 2 h before exercise should allow renal mechanisms sufficient time to regulate total body fluid volume and osmolality at optimal preexercise levels and help delay or avoid detrimental effects of dehydration during exercise.

Fluid Replacement During Exercise

Without adequate fluid replacement during prolonged exercise, rectal temperature and heart rate will become more elevated compared with a well-hydrated condition (13,19,29,54). The most serious effect of dehydration resulting from the failure ___ replace fluids during exercise is impaired heat diss___ which can ___ body core temperature to dan___ h level___ ___). Exercise-induced deh___ body fluids and impairs skin blood flow (26,53,54,65), and has been associated with reduced sweat rate (26,85), thus limiting evaporative heat loss, which accounts for more than 80% of heat loss in a hot-dry environment. Dehydration (i.e, 3% body weight loss) can also elicit significant reduction in cardiac output during exercise since a reduction in stroke volume can be greater than the increase in heart rate (53,80). Since a net result of electrolyte and water imbalance associated with failure to adequately replace fluids during exercise is an increased rate of heat storage, dehydration induced by exercise presents a potential for the development of heat-related disorders (24), including potentially life-threatening heat stroke (88,92). It is therefore reasonable to surmise that fluid replacement that offsets dehydration and excessive elevation in body heat during exercise may be instrumental in reducing the risk of thermal injury (37).

To minimize the potential for thermal injury, it is advocated that water losses due to sweating during exercise be replaced at a rate equal to the sweat rate (5,19,66,73). Inadequate water intake can lead to premature exhaustion. During exercise, humans do not typically drink as much water as they sweat and, at best, voluntary drinking only replaces about two-thirds of the body water lost as sweat (36). It is common for individuals to dehydrate by 2%–6% of their body weight during exercise in the heat despite the availability of adequate amounts of fluid (33,35,66,73). In many athletic events, the volume and frequency of fluid consumption may be limited by the rules of competition (e.g., number of rest periods or time outs) or their availability (e.g., spacing of aid stations along a race course). While large volumes of ingested fluids ($\geq 1 \, l \cdot h^{-1}$) are tolerated by exercising individuals in laboratory studies, field observations indicate that most participants drink sparingly during competition. For example, it is not uncommon for elite runners to ingest less than 200 ml of fluid during distance events in a cool environment lasting more than 2 h (13,66). Actual rates of fluid ingestion are seldom more than 500 ml $\cdot$ h^{-1} (66,68) and most athletes allow themselves to become dehydrated by 2–3 kg of body weight in sports such as running, cycling, and the triathlon. It is clear that perception of thirst, an imperfect index of the magnitude of fluid deficit, cannot be used to provide complete restoration of water lost by sweating. As such, individuals participating in prolonged intense exercise must rely on strategies such as monitoring body weight loss and ingesting volumes of fluid during exercise at a rate equal to that lost from sweating, i.e., body weight reduction, to ensure complete fluid replacement. This can be accomplished by ingesting beverages that enhance drinking at a rate of one pint of fluid per pound of body weight reduction. While gastrointestinal discomfort has been reported by individuals who have attempted to drink at rates equal to their sweat rates, especially in excess of 1 l $\cdot$ h^{-1} (10,13,52,57,66), this response appears to be individual and there is no clear association

between the volume of ingested fluid and symptoms of gastrointestinal distress. Further, failure to maintain hydration during exercise by drinking appropriate amounts of fluid may contribute to gastrointestinal symptoms (64,76). Therefore, individuals should be encouraged to consume the maximal amount of fluids during exercise that can be tolerated without gastrointestinal discomfort up to a rate equal to that lost from sweating.

Enhancing palatability of an ingested fluid is one way of improving the match between fluid intake and sweat output. Water palatability is influenced by several factors including temperature and flavoring (25,36). While most individuals prefer cool water, the preferred water temperature is influenced by cultural and learned behaviors. The most pleasurable water temperature during recovery from exercise was 5°C (78), although when water was ingested in large quantities, a temperature of ~15°–21°C was preferred (9,36). Experiments have also demonstrated that voluntary fluid intake is enhanced if the fluid is flavored (25,36) and/or sweetened (27). It is therefore reasonable to expect that the effect of flavoring and water temperature should increase fluid consumption during exercise, although there is insufficient evidence to support this hypothesis. In general, fluid replacement beverages that are sweetened (artificially or with sugars), flavored, and cooled to between 15° and 21°C should stimulate fluid intake (9,25,36,78).

The rate at which fluid and electrolyte balance will be restored is also determined by the rate at which ingested fluid empties from the stomach and is absorbed from the intestine into the blood. The rate at which fluid leaves the stomach is dependent on a complex interaction of several factors, such as volume, temperature, and composition of the ingested fluid, and exercise intensity. The most important factor influencing gastric emptying is the fluid volume in the stomach (52,68,75). However, the rate of gastric emptying of fluid is slowed proportionately with increasing glucose concentration above 8% (15,38). When gastric fluid volume is maintained at 600 ml or more, most individuals can still empty more than 1000 ml $\cdot$ h^{-1} when the fluids contain a 4%–8% carbohydrate concentration (19,68). Therefore, to promote gastric emptying, especially with the presence of 4%–8% carbohydrate in the fluid, it is advantageous to maintain the largest volume of fluid that can be tolerated in the stomach during exercise (e.g., 400–600 ml). Mild to moderate exercise appears to have little or no effect on gastric emptying while heavy exercise at intensities greater than 80% of maximal capacity may slow gastric emptying (12,15). Laboratory and field studies suggest that during prolonged exercise, frequent (every 15–20 min) consumption of moderate (150 ml) to large (350 ml) volumes of fluid is possible. Despite the apparent advantage of high gastric fluid volume for promoting gastric emptying, there should be some caution associated with maintaining high gastric fluid volume. People differ in their gastric emptying rates as well as their tolerance to gastric volumes, and it has not been determined if the ability to tolerate high gastric volumes can be improved by drinking during training. It is also unclear whether complaints of gastrointestinal symptoms by athletes during competition are a function of an unfamiliarity of exercising with a full stomach or because of delays in gastric emptying (57). It is therefore recommended that individuals learn their tolerance limits for maintaining a high gastric fluid volume for various exercise intensities and durations.

Once ingested fluid moves into the intestine, water moves out of the intestine into the blood. Intestinal absorptive capacity is generally adequate to cope with even the most extreme demands (30); and at intensities of exercise that can be sustained for more than 30 min, there appears to be little effect of exercise on intestinal function (84). In fact, dehydration consequent to failure to replace fluids lost during exercise reduces the rate of gastric emptying (64,76), supporting the rationale for early and continued drinking throughout exercise.

Electrolyte and Carbohydrate Replacement During Exercise

There is little physiological basis for the presence of sodium in an oral rehydration solution for enhancing intestinal water absorption as long as sodium is sufficiently available in the gut from the previous meal or in the pancreatic secretions (84). Inclusion of sodium (<50 mmol $\cdot$ l^{-1}) in fluid replacement drinks during exercise has not shown consistent improvements in retention of ingested fluid in the vascular compartment (20,23,44,45). A primary rationale for electrolyte supplementation with fluid replacement drinks is, therefore, to replace electrolytes lost from sweating during exercise greater than 4–5 h in duration (3). Normal plasma sodium concentration is 140 mmol $\cdot$ l^{-1}, making sweat ($\sim$50 mmol $\cdot$ l^{-1}) hypotonic relative to plasma. At a sweat rate of 1.5 l $\cdot$ h^{-1}, a total sodium deficit of 75 mmol $\cdot$ h^{-1} could occur during exercise. Drinking water can lower elevated plasma electrolyte concentrations back toward normal and restore sweating (85,86), but complete restoration of the extracellular fluid compartment cannot be sustained without replacement of lost sodium (39,70,89). In most cases, this can be accomplished by normal dietary intake (63). If sodium enhances palatability, then its presence in a replacement solution may be justified because drinking can be maximized by improving taste qualities of the ingested fluid (9,25).

The addition of carbohydrates to a fluid replacement solution can enhance intestinal absorption of water (30,84). However, a primary role of ingesting carbohydrates in a fluid replacement beverage is to maintain blood glucose concentration and enhance carbohydrate oxidation during exercise that lasts longer than 1 h, especially when muscle glycogen is low (11,14,17,18,50,60). As a result, fatigue can be delayed by carbohydrate ingestion during exercise of duration longer than 1 h which normally causes fatigue without carbohydrate ingestion (11). To maintain blood glucose levels during continuous moderate-to-high intensity exercise, carbohydrates should be ingested throughout exercise at a rate of 30–60 g $\cdot$ h^{-1}. These amounts of carbohydrates can be obtained while also replacing relatively large amounts of fluid if the concentration of carbohydrates is kept below 10% (g $\cdot$ 100 ml^{-1} of fluid). For example, if the desired volume of ingestion is 600–1200 ml $\cdot$ h^{-1}, then the carbohydrate requirements can be met by drinking fluids with concentrations in the range of 4%–8% (19). With this procedure, both fluid and carbohydrate requirements can be met simultaneously during prolonged exercise. Solutions containing carbohydrate concentrations >10% will cause a net movement of fluid into the intestinal lumen because of their high osmolality, when such solutions are ingested during exercise. This can result in an effective loss of water from the vascular compartment and can exacerbate the effects of dehydration (43).

Few investigators have examined the benefits of adding carbohydrates to water during exercise events lasting less than 1 h. Although preliminary data suggest a potential benefit for performance (4,7,48), the mechanism is unclear. It would be premature to recommend drinking something other than water during exercise lasting less than 1 h. Generally, the inclusion of glucose, sucrose, and other complex carbohydrates in fluid replacement solutions have equal effectiveness in increasing exogenous carbohydrate oxidation, delaying fatigue, and improving performance (11,16,79,90). However, fructose should not be the predominant carbohydrate because it is converted slowly to blood glucose—not readily oxidized (41,42)—which does not improve performance (8). Furthermore, fructose may cause gastrointestinal distress (59).

Fluid Replacement and Exercise Performance

Although the impact of fluid deficits on cardiovascular function and thermoregulation is evident, the extent to which exercise performance is altered by fluid replacement remains unclear. Although some data indicate that drinking improves the ability to perform short duration athletic events (1 h) in moderate climates (7), other data suggest that this may not be the case (40). It is likely that the effect of fluid replacement on performance may be most noticeable during exercise of duration greater than 1 h and/or at extreme ambient environments.

The addition of a small amount of sodium to rehydration fluids has little impact on time to exhaustion during mild prolonged (>4 h) exercise in the heat (73), ability to complete 6 h of moderate exercise (5), or capacity to perform during simulated time trials (20,74). A sodium deficit, in combination with ingestion and retention of a large volume of fluid with little or no electrolytes, has led to low plasma sodium levels in a very few marathon or ultra-marathon athletes (3,67). Hyponatremia (blood sodium concentration between 117 and 128 mmol $\cdot$ l^{-1}) has been observed in ultra endurance athletes at the end of competition and is associated with disorientation, confusion, and in most cases, grand mal seizures (67,69). One major rationale for inclusion of sodium in rehydration drinks is to avoid hyponatremia. To prevent development of this rare condition during prolonged (>4 h) exercise, electrolytes should be present in the fluid or food during and after exercise.

Maintenance of blood glucose concentrations is necessary for optimal exercise performance. To maintain blood glucose concentration during fatiguing exercise greater than 1 h (above 65% VO$_{2max}$), carbohydrate ingestion is necessary (11,49). Late in prolonged exercise, ingested carbohydrates become the main source of carbohydrate energy and can delay the onset of fatigue (17,19,21, 22,51,58). Data from field studies designed to test these concepts during athletic competition have not always demonstrated delayed onset of fatigue (46,47,91), but the inability to control critical factors (such as environmental conditions, state of training, drinking volumes) make confirmation difficult. Inclusion of carbohydrates in a rehydration solution becomes more important for optimal performance as the duration of intense exercise exceeds 1 h.

Conclusion

The primary objective for replacing body fluid loss during exercise is to maintain normal hydration. One should consume adequate fluids during the 24-h period before an event and drink about 500 ml (about 17 ounces) of fluid about 2 h before exercise to promote adequate hydration and allow time for excretion of excess ingested water. To minimize risk of thermal injury and impairment of exercise performance during exercise, fluid replacement should attempt to equal fluid loss. At equal exercise intensity, the requirement for fluid replacement becomes greater with increased sweating during environmental thermal stress. During exercise lasting longer than 1 h, a) carbohydrates should be added to the fluid replacement solution to maintain blood glucose concentration and delay the onset of fatigue, and b) electrolytes (primarily NaCl) should be added to the fluid replacement solution to enhance palatability and reduce the probability for development of hyponatremia. During exercise, fluid and carbohydrate requirements can be met simultaneously by ingesting 600–1200 ml $\cdot$ h^{-1} of solutions containing 4%–8% carbohydrate. During exercise greater than 1 h, approximately 0.5–0.7 g of sodium per liter of water would be appropriate to replace that lost from sweating.

Acknowledgment

This pronouncement was reviewed for the American College of Sports Medicine by members-at-large, the Pronouncement Committee, and by: David L. Costill, Ph.D., FACSM, John E. Greenleaf, Ph.D., FACSM, Scott J. Montain, Ph.D., and Timothy D. Noakes, M.D., FACSM.

References

1. Armstrong, L. E., D. L. Costill, and W. J. Fink. Influence of diuretic-induced dehydration on competitive running performance. *Med. Sci. Sports Exerc.* 17:456–461, 1985.
2. Armstrong, L. E., R. W. Hubbard, B. H. Jones, and J. J. Daniels. Preparing Alberto Salazar for the heat of the 1984 Olympic marathon. *Physician Sportsmed.* 14:73–81, 1986.
3. Armstrong, L. E., W. C. Curtis, R. W. Hubbard, R. P. Francesconi, R. Moore, and E. W. Askew. Symptomatic hyponatremia during prolonged exercise in heat. *Med. Sci. Sports Exerc.* 25:543–549, 1993.
4. Ball, T. C., S. Headley, and P. Vanderburgh. Carbohydrate-electrolyte replacement improves sprint capacity following 50 minutes of high-intensity cycling. *Med. Sci. Sports Exerc.* 26:S196, 1994 (abstract).
5. Barr, S. I., D. L. Costill, and W. J. Fink. Fluid replacement during prolonged exercise: effects of water, saline, or no fluid. *Med. Sci. Sports Exerc.* 23:811–817, 1991.
6. Bean, W. B. and L. W. Eichna. Performance in relationship to environmental temperature. Reactions of normal young men to simulated desert environment. *Fed. Proc.* 2:144–158, 1943.
7. Below, P. R. and E. F. Coyle. Fluid and carbohydrate ingestion individually benefit intense exercise lasting one hour. *Med. Sci. Sports Exerc.* 27:200–210, 1995.
8. Bjorkman, O., K. Sahlin, L. Hagenfeldt, and J. Wahren. Influence of glucose and fructose ingestion on the capacity for long-term exercise. *Clin. Physiol.* 4:483–494, 1984.
9. Boulze, D., P. Montastruc, and M. Cabanac. Water intake, pleasure and water temperature in humans. *Physiol. Behav.* 30:97–102, 1983.
10. Brouns, F., W. H. M. Saris, and N. J. Rehrer. Abdominal complaints and gastrointestinal function during long-lasting exercise. *Int. J. Sports Med.* 8:175–189, 1987.
11. Coggan, A. R. and E. F. Coyle. Carbohydrate ingestion during prolonged exercise: effects on metabolism and performance. *Exerc. Sport Sci. Rev.* 19.1–40, 1991.
12. Costill, D. L. Gastric emptying of fluids during exercise. In: *Perspectives in Exercise Science and Sports Medicine, Vol. 3, Fluid Homeostasis During Exercise*, C. V. Gisolfi and D. R. Lamb (Eds.). Carmel, IN: Benchmark Press, Inc., 1990, pp. 97–128.
13. Costill, D. L., W. F. Krammer, and A. Fisher. Fluid ingestion during distance running. *Arch. Environ. Health* 21:520–525, 1970.
14. Costill, D. L. and M. Hargreaves. Carbohydrate nutrition and fatigue. *Sports Med.* 13:86–92, 1992.
15. Costill, D. L. and B. Saltin. Factors limiting gastric emptying during rest and exercise. *J. Appl. Physiol.* 37:679–683, 1974.
16. Coyle, E. F. Timing and method of increased carbohydrate intake to cope with heavy training, competition and recovery. *J. Sports Sci.* 9:29–52, 1991.
17. Coyle, E. F., A. R. Coggan, M. K. Hemmert, and J. L. Ivy. Muscle glycogen utilization during prolonged strenuous exercise when fed carbohydrate. *J. Appl. Physiol.* 61:165–172, 1986.
18. Coyle, E. F., J. M. Hagberg, B. F. Hurley, W. H. Martin, A. A. Ehsani, and J. O. Holloszy. Carbohydrate feeding during prolonged strenuous exercise can delay fatigue. *J. Appl. Physiol.* 55:230–235, 1983.
19. Coyle, E. F. and S. J. Montain. Benefits of fluid replacement with carbohydrate during exercise. *Med. Sci. Sports Exerc.* 24 (Suppl. 9):S234–S330, 1992.

20. Criswell, D., K. Renshler, S. K. Powers, R. Tulley, M. Cicale, and K. Wheeler. Fluid replacement beverages and maintenance of plasma volume during exercise: role of aldosterone and vasopressin. *Eur. J. Appl. Physiol.* 65:445–451, 1992.

21. Davis, J. M., W. A. Burgess, C. A. Slentz, W. P. Bartoli, and R. R. Pate. Effects of ingesting 6% and 12% glucose/electrolyte beverages during prolonged intermittent cycling in the heat. *Eur. J. Appl. Physiol.* 57:563–569, 1988.

22. Davis, J. M., D. R. Lamb, R. R. Pate, C. A. Slentz, W. A. Burgess, and W. P. Bartoll. Carbohydrate-electrolyte drinks: effects on endurance cycling in heat. *Am. J. Clin. Nutr.* 48:1023–1030, 1988.

23. Deuster, P. A., A. Singh, A. Hofmann, F. M. Moses, and G. C. Chrousos. Hormonal responses to ingesting water or a carbohydrate beverage during a 2 h run. *Med. Sci. Sports Exerc.* 24:72–79, 1992.

24. Eichna, L. W., W. B. Bean, W. F. Ashe, and N. Nelson. Performance in relation to environmental temperature. Reactions of normal young men to hot, humid (simulated jungle) environment. *Bull. Johns Hopkins Hosp.* 76:25–58, 1945.

25. Engell, D. and E. Hirsch. Environmental and sensory modulation of fluid intake in humans. In: *Thirst: Physiological and Psychological Aspects.* D. J. Ramsay and D. A. Booth (Eds.). Berlin: Springer-Verlag, 1990, pp. 382–402.

26. Fortney, S. M. Effect of hyperosmolality on control of blood flow and sweating. *J. Appl. Physiol.* 57:1688–1695, 1984.

27. Fortney, S. M., E. R. Nadel, C. B. Wenger, and J. R. Bove. Effect of acute alterations of blood volume on circulatory performance in humans. *J. Appl. Physiol.* 50:292–298, 1981.

28. Fortney, S. M., E. R. Nadel, C. B. Wenger, and J. R. Bove. Effect of blood volume on sweating rate and body fluids in exercising humans. *J. Appl. Physiol.* 51:1594–1600, 1981.

29. Gilsolfi, C. V. and J. R. Copping. Thermal effects of prolonged treadmill exercise in the heat. *Med. Sci. Sports* 6:108–113, 1974.

30. Gisolfi, C. V., R. W. Summers, and H. P. Schedl. Intestinal absorption of fluids during a rest and exercise. In: *Perspectives in Exercise Science and Sports Medicine, Vol. 3, Fluid Homeostasis During Exercise.* C. V. Gisolfi and D. L. Lamb (Eds.). Carmel, IN: Benchmark Press, Inc., 1990, pp. 129–180.

31. Gisolfi, C. V., K. J. Spranger, R. W. Summers, H. P. Schedl, and T. L. Bleiler. Effects of cycle exercise on intestinal absorption in humans. *J. Appl. Physiol.* 71:2518–2527, 1991.

32. Gonzalez-Alonso, J., C. L. Heapes, and E. F. Coyle. Rehydration after exercise with common beverages and water. *Int. J. Sports Med.* 13:399–406, 1992.

33. Greenleaf, J. E. and F. Sargent II. Voluntary dehydration in man. *J. Appl. Physiol.* 20:719–724, 1965.

34. Greenleaf, J. E. and B. L. Castle. Exercise temperature regulation in man during hypohydration and hyperhydration. *J. Appl. Physiol.* 30:847–853, 1971.

35. Greenleaf, J. E., P. J. Brock, L. C. Keil, and J. T. Morse. Drinking and water balance during exercise and heat acclimation. *J. Appl. Physiol.* 54:414–419, 1983.

36. Hubbard, R. W., O. Maller, M. N. Sawka, R. N. Francesconi, L. Drolet, and A. J. Young. Voluntary dehydration and alliesthesia for water. *J. Appl. Physiol.* 57:868–875, 1984.

37. Hubbard, R. W. and L. E. Armstrong. The heat illness: biochemical, ultrastructural, and fluid-electrolyte considerations. In: *Human Performance Physiology and Environmental Medicine at Terrestrial Extremes.* K. B. Pandolf, M. N. Sawka, and R. R. Gonzales (Eds.). Indianapolis: Benchmark Press, Inc., 1988, pp. 305–360.

38. Hunt, J. N. and M. T. Knox. Regulation of gastric emptying. In: *Handbook of Physiology.* Vol. IV. Washington, DC: American Physiological Society, 1969, pp. 1917–1935.

39. Lassiter, W. E. Regulation of sodium chloride distribution within the extracellular space. In: *The Regulation of Sodium and Chloride Balance.* D. W. Seldin and G. Giebisch (Eds.). New York: Raven Press, Inc., 1990, pp. 23–58.

40. Levine, L., M. S. Rose, R. P. Francesconi, P. D. Neufer, and M. N. Sawka. Fluid replacement during sustained activity in the heat: Nutrient solution vs. water. *Aviat. Space Environ. Med.* 62:559–564, 1991.

41. Massicotte, D., F. Perronnet, C. Allah, C. Hillaire-Marcel, M. Ledoux, and G. Brisson. Metabolic response to [13C]glucose and [13C]fructose ingestion during exercise. *J. Appl. Physiol.* 61:1180–1184, 1986.

42. Massicotte, D., F. Perronnet, G. Brisson, K. Bakkouch, and C. Hillaire-Marcel. Oxidation of glucose polymer during exercise: comparison of glucose and fructose. *J. Appl. Physiol.* 66:179–183, 1989.

43. Maughan, R. J. Thermoregulation and fluid balance in marathon competition at low ambient temperature. *Int. J. Sports Med.* 6:25–19, 1985.

44. Maughan, R. J., C. E. Fenn, M. Gleeson, and J. B. Leiper. Metabolic and circulatory responses to the ingestion of glucose polymers and glucose-electrolyte solutions during exercise in man. *Eur. J. Appl. Physiol.* 56:356–362, 1987.

45. Maughan, R. J., C. E. Fenn, M. Gleeson, and J. B. Leiper. Effects of fluid, electrolyte, and substrate ingestion on endurance capacity. *Eur. J. Appl. Physiol.* 58:481–486, 1989.

46. Millard-Stafford, M., P. B. Sparling, L. B. Rosskopf, B. T. Hinson, and L. J. Dicarlo. Carbohydrate-electrolyte replacement during a simulated triathlon in the heat. *Med. Sci. Sports Exerc.* 22:621–628, 1990.

47. Millard-Stafford, M., P. B. Sparling, L. B. Rosskopf, and L. J. Dicarlo. Carbohydrate-electrolyte replacement improves distance running performance in the heat. *Med. Sci. Sports Exerc.* 24:934–940, 1992.

48. Millard-Stafford, M., L. B. Rosskopf, T. K. Snow, and B. T. Hinson. Pre-exercise carbohydrate-electrolyte ingestion improves one-hour running performance in the heat. *Med. Sci. Sports Exerc.* 26:S196, 1994 (abstract).

49. Mitchell, J. B., D. L. Costill, J. A. Houmard, M. G. Flynn, W. J. Fink, and J. D. Beltz. Effects of carbohydrate ingestion on gastric emptying and exercise performance. *Med. Sci. Sports Exerc.* 20:110–115, 1988.

50. Mitchell, J. B., D. L. Costill, J. A. Houmard, W. J. Fink, D. D. Pascoe, and D. R. Pearson. Influence of carbohydrate dosage on exercise performance and glycogen metabolism. *J. Appl. Physiol.* 67:1843–1849, 1989.

51. Mitchell, J. B., D. L. Costill, J. A. Houmard, W. J. Fink, R. A. Robergs, and J. A. Davis. Gastric emptying: influence of prolonged exercise and carbohydrate concentration. *Med. Sci. Sports Exerc.* 21:269–274, 1989.

52. Mitchell, J. B. and K. W. Voss. The influence of volume of fluid ingested on gastric emptying and fluid balance during prolonged exercise. *Med. Sci. Sports Exerc.* 23:314–319, 1991.

53. Montain, S. J. and E. F. Coyle. Fluid ingestion during exercise increases skin blood flow independent of increases in blood volume. *J. Appl. Physiol.* 73:903–910, 1992.

54. Montain, S. J. and E. F. Coyle. The influence of graded dehydration on hyperthermia and cardiovascular drift during exercise. *J. Appl. Physiol.* 73:1340–1350, 1992.

55. Morimoto, T., K. Mike, H. Nose, S. Yamada, K. Kirakawa, and C. Matsubara. Changes in body fluid and its composition during heavy sweating and effect of fluid and electrolyte replacement. *Jpn. J. Biometeorol.* 18:31–39, 1981.

56. Moroff, S. V. and D. B. Bass. Effects of overhydration on man's physiological responses to work in the heat. *J. Appl. Physiol.* 20:267–270, 1965.

57. Moses, F. M. The effect of exercise on the gastrointestinal tract. *Sports Med.* 9:159–172, 1990.

58. Murray, R., D. E. Eddy, T. W. Murray, J. G. Seifert, G. L. Paul, and G. A. Halaby. The effect of fluid and carbohydrate feeding during intermittent cycling exercise. *Med. Sci. Sports Exerc.* 19:597–604, 1987.

59. Murray, R., G. L. Paul, J. G. Seifert, D. E. Eddy, and G. A. Halaby. The effects of glucose, fructose, and sucrose ingestion during exercise. *Med. Sci. Sports Exerc.* 21:275–282, 1989.

60. Murray, R., G. L. Paul, J. G. Siefert, and D. E. Eddy. Responses to varying rates of carbohydrate ingestion during exercise. *Med. Sci. Sports Exerc.* 23:713–718, 1991.

61. Nadel, E. R., S. M. Fortney, and C. B. Wenger. Effect of hydration state on circulatory and thermal regulations. *J. Appl. Physiol.* 49:715–721, 1980.

62. Nadel, E. R., C. B. Wenger, M. F. Roberts, J. A. J. Stolwijk, and E. Cafarelli. Physiological defenses against hyperthermia of exercise. *Ann. N. Y. Acad. Sci.* 301:98–110, 1977.

63. National Research Council. *Recommended Dietary Allowances,* 10th Ed. Washington, DC: National Academy Press, 1989, pp. 250–255.

64. Neufer, P. D., A. J. Young, and M. N. Sawka. Gastric emptying during exercise: effects of heat stress and hypohydration. *Eur. J. Appl. Physiol.* 58:433–439, 1989.

65. Nishiyasu, T., X. Shi, G. W. Mack, and E. R. Nadel. Effect of hypovolemia on forearm vascular resistance control during exercise in the heat. *J. Appl. Physiol.* 71:1382–1386, 1991.

66. Noakes, T. D. Fluid replacement during exercise. *Exerc. Sports Sci. Rev.* 21:297–330, 1993.

67. Noakes, T. D., R. J. Norma, R. H. Buck, J. Godlonton, K. Stevenson, and D. Pittaway. The incidence of hyponatremia during prolonged ultraendurance exercise. *Med. Sci. Sports Exerc.* 22:165–170, 1990.

68. Noakes, T. D., N. J. Rehrer, and R. J. Maughan. The importance of volume in regulating gastric emptying. *Med. Sci. Sports Exerc.* 23:307–313, 1991.

69. Noakes, T. D., N. Goodwin, B. L. Rayner, T. Branken, and R. K. N. Taylor. Water intoxication: a possible complication during endurance exercise. *Med. Sci. Sports Exerc.* 17:370–375, 1985.

70. Nose, H., M. Morita, T. Yawata, and T. Morimoto. Recovery of blood volume and osmolality after thermal dehydration in rats. *Am. J. Physiol.* 251:R492–R498, 1986.

71. Nose, H., G. W. Mack, X. Shi, and E. R. Nadel. Role of osmolality and plasma volume during rehydration in humans. *J. Appl. Physiol.* 65:325–331, 1988.

72. Nose, H., G. W. Mack, X. Shi, and E. R. Nadel. Shift in body fluid compartments after dehydration in humans. *J. Appl. Physiol.* 65:318–324, 1988.

73. Pitts, G. C., R. E. Johnson, and F. C. Consolazio. Work in the heat as affected by intake of water, salt, and glucose. *Am. J. Physiol.* 142:253–259, 1944.

74. Powers, S. K., J. Lawler, S. Dodd, R. Tulley, G. Landry, and K. Wheeler. Fluid replacement drinks during high intensity exercise: effects on minimizing exercise-induced disturbances in homeostasis. *Eur. J. Appl. Physiol.* 60:54–60, 1990.

75. Rehrer, N. J. The maintenance of fluid balance during exercise. *Int. J. Sports Med.* 15:122–125, 1994.

76. Rehrer, N. J., E.J. Beckers, F. Brouns, F. Ten Hoor, and W. H. M. Saris. Effects of dehydration on gastric emptying and gastrointestinal distress while running. *Med. Sci. Sports Exerc.* 22:790–795, 1990.

77. Rothstein, A., E. F. Adolph, and J. H. Wills. Voluntary dehydration. In: *Physiology of Man In the Desert,* E. F. Adolph (Ed.). New York: Interscience, 1947, pp. 254–270.

78. Sandick, B. L., D. B. Engell, and O. Maller. Perception of water temperature and effects for humans after exercise. *Physiol. Behav.* 32:851–855, 1984.

79. Saris, W. H. M., B. H. Goodpaster, A. E. Jeukendrup, F. Brouns, D. Halliday, and A. J. M. Wagenmakers. Exogenous carbohydrate oxidation from different carbohydrate sources during exercise. *J. Appl. Physiol.* 75:2168–2172, 1993.

80. Sawka, M. N., R. G. Knowlton, and J. B. Critz. Thermal and circulatory responses to repeated bouts of prolonged running. *Med. Sci. Sports* 11:177–180, 1979.

81. Sawka, M. N., R. P. Francesconi, A. J. Young, and K. B. Pandolf. Influence of hydration level and body fluids on exercise performance in the heat. *J.A.M.A.* 252:1165–1169, 1984.

82. Sawka, M. N., A. J. Young, R. P. Francesconi, S. R. Muza, and K. B. Pandolf. Thermoregulatory and blood responses during exercise at graded hypohydration levels. *J. Appl. Physiol.* 59:1394–1401, 1985.

83. Sawka, M. N. and K. B. Pandolf. Effects of body water loss on physiological function and exercise performance. In: *Perspectives in Exercise Science and Sports Medicine. Vol. 3. Fluid Homeostasis during Exercise.* C. V. Gilsolfi and D. R. Lamb (Eds.). Carmel, IN: Benchmark Press, Inc., 1990, pp. 1–38.

84. Schedl, H. P., R. J. Maughan, and C. V. Gisolfi. Intestinal absorption during rest and exercise: implications for formulating an oral rehydration solution (ORS). *Med. Sci. Sports Exerc.* 26:267–280, 1994.

85. Senay, L. C., Jr. Relationship of evaporative rates to serum [Na+], [K+], and osmolarity in acute heat stress. *J. Appl. Physiol.* 25:149–152, 1968.

86. Senay, L. C., Jr. Temperature regulation and hypohydration: a singular view. *J. Appl. Physiol.* 47:1–7, 1979.

87. Shapiro, Y., K. B. Pandolf, and R. F. Goldman. Predicting sweat loss response to exercise, environment, and clothing. *Eur. J. Appl. Physiol.* 48:83–96, 1982.

88. Sutton, J. R. Clinical Implications of Fluid Imbalance. In: *Perspectives in Exercise Science and Sports Medicine, Vol. 3. Fluid Homeostasis During Exercise.* C. V. Gisolfi and D. R. Lamb (Eds.). Carmel, IN: Benchmark Press, Inc., 1990, pp. 425–455.

89. Takamata, A., G. W. Mack, C. M. Gillen, and E. R. Nadel. Sodium appetite, thirst, and body fluid regulation in humans during rehydration without sodium replacement. *Am. J. Physiol. (Regulatory Integrative Comp. Physiol.)* 266:R1493–R1502, 1994.

90. Wagenmakers, J. M., F. Brouns, W. H. M. Saris, and D. Halliday. Oxidation rates of orally ingested carbohydrate during prolonged exercise in men. *J. Appl. Physiol.* 75:2774–2780, 1993.

91. Wells, C. L., T. A. Schrader, J. R. Stern, and G. S. Krahenbuhl. Physiological responses to a 20-mile run under three fluid replacement treatments. *Med. Sci. Sports Exerc.* 17:364–369, 1985.

92. Wyndham, C. H. Heat stroke and hyperthermia in marathon runners. *Am. N. Y. Acad. Sci.* 301:128–138, 1977.

Healthy People 2000: Objectives for Physical Activity and Nutrition*

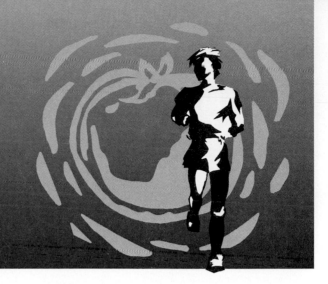

Unstructured Physical Activity

1. Increase to at least 30 percent the proportion of people aged 6 and older who engage regularly, preferably daily, in light to moderate physical activity for at least 30 minutes per day

2. Reduce to no more than 15 percent the proportion of people aged 6 and older who engage in no leisure-time physical activity

Structured Physical Activity

1. Increase to at least 20 percent the proportion of people aged 18 and older and to at least 75 percent the proportion of children and adolescents aged 6 through 17 who engage in vigorous physical activity that promotes the development and maintenance of cardiorespiratory fitness three or more days per week for 20 or more minutes per occasion

2. Increase to at least 40 percent the proportion of people aged 6 and older who regularly perform physical activities that enhance and maintain muscular strength, muscular endurance, and flexibility

3. Increase to at least 50 percent the proportion of overweight people aged 12 and over who have adopted sound dietary practices combined with regular physical activity to attain an appropriate body weight

*Selected objectives for unstructured physical activity, structured physical activity, and nutrition. For full information, see the full report, U.S. Department of Health and Human Services Public Health Service. *Healthy People 2000: National Health Promotion and Disease Prevention Objectives.* Washington, DC: U.S. Government Printing Office, 1991.

Nutrition

1. Reduce dietary fat intake to an average of 30 percent of Calories or less and average saturated-fat intake to less than 10 percent of Calories

2. Increase complex-carbohydrate and fiber-containing foods in the diets to five or more daily servings for vegetables (including legumes) and fruits, and to six or more daily servings for grain products

3. Increase to at least 50 percent the proportion of overweight people aged 12 and older who have adopted sound dietary practices combined with regular physical activity to attain an appropriate body weight

4. Increase calcium intake so that at least 50 percent of youth aged 12 through 24 and 50 percent of pregnant and lactating women consume three or more servings daily of foods rich in calcium, and at least 50 percent of people aged 25 and older consume two or more servings daily

5. Decrease salt and sodium intake so that at least 65 percent of home-meal preparers prepare foods without adding salt, at least 80 percent of people avoid using salt at the table, and at least 40 percent of adults regularly purchase foods modified or lower in sodium

6. Reduce iron deficiency to less than 3 percent among children and among women in childbearing age

7. Increase to at least 85 percent the proportion of people aged 18 and older who use food labels to make nutritious food selections

Internet Sources of Reliable Information on Nutrition as Related to Health, Exercise and Sports

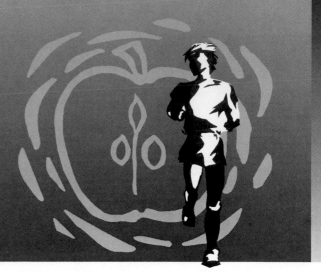

The Internet is an enormous worldwide network of interconnected computers. Internet sites are primarily commercial, educational, government and military institutions that contain vast repositories of information. The World Wide Web (WWW), often simply called the Web, is a collection of computer files, a specific location on the Internet. Each Web site is identified with an address known as uniform resource locator (URL) which may be accessed by use of Hyper Text Transfer Protocol (http). A Web address appears like http://www.anysite.com. Some Internet sites do not use the www. You may connect to a Web site on the Internet with your home computer, provided you have a phone line, a modem, an Internet provider (such as America Online), and a browser (such as Netscape Navigator). Most colleges and universities provide students resources for access to the Internet, and most libraries offer training programs for students to become familiar with using the Internet to obtain information.

A search engine is a program that permits you to locate specific Web sites on the Internet. Several popular search engines include Alta Vista (http://altavista.digital.com), Infoseek (http://guide.infoseek.com), WebCrawler (http://webcrawler.com), and Yahoo (http://www.yahoo.com). Two medicine specific search engines are Achoo (http://www.achoo.com) and Health AtoZ (http://Healthatoz.com).

Unfortunately, you can not always rely on the information you see on the WWW. One must be cautious when using the Internet to obtain health-related information. The Federal Trade Commission (FTC) has indicated that numerous WWW sites contain promotions for various products and services claiming to help cure, treat or prevent a wide variety of health problems. Unfortunately, most of these claims, particularly for dietary supplements,

are fraudulent. You may obtain a free brochure entitled *Fraudulent Health Claims: Don't Be Fooled* by contacting the FTC via their Web site listed below.

Numerous Web sites provide information on nutrition and exercise as they are related to health and fitness. An excellent starting point is the Tufts University Nutrition Navigator; its Web site address is http://www.navigator.tufts.edu. The Nutrition Navigator provides a rating guide to other nutrition Web sites, evaluating the reliability of the information they provide. You may also access these other Web sites directly from Nutrition Navigator.

The following Web sites (many included in the Nutrition Navigator) are considered to be sources of reliable information. The Web site should provide you with the address and phone numbers of the organization, if needed. Many of these national organizations also have regional affiliates that you may find in your local phone book or by contacting local health agencies or hospitals. The Web sites listed were current at the time of publication of this book, but may have changed. Your library should be able to provide you with current Web site addresses for other relevant sources of nutrition information.

American Anorexia/Bulimia Association (AABA)
http://members.aol.com/AmAnBu

American Cancer Society
http://www.cancer.org

American Dietetic Association (ADA)
Sports and Cardiovascular Nutritionists (SCAN)
http://www.catright.org

American Heart Association
http://www.amhrt.org

American Institute of Nutrition
http://www.nutrition.org

American Medical Association
http://www.ama-assn.org

Centers for Disease Control and Prevention (CDC)
http://www.cdc.gov

Consumer Information Center
http://www.pueblo.gsa.gov/food.htm

Department of Health and Human Services
http://www.os.dhhs.gov

Department of Health and Human Services
Healthfinder
http://www.healthfinder.gov

Dietitians of Canada (Formerly Canadian Dietetic
Association)
http://www.dietitians.ca

Federal Trade Commission
http://www.ftc.gov

Food and Drug Administration
Office of Consumer Affairs
Center for Food Safety and Applied Nutrition
http://www.fda.gov

GatorAde Sports Science Institute
http://www.gssiweb.com

International Food Information Council (IFIC)
http://ificinfo.health.org

National Clearinghouse for Alcohol and Drug
Information
http://www.health.org

National Council against Health Fraud
http://www.ncahf.org
http://www.quackwatch.com

National Institutes of Health
http://www.nih.gov/health/consumer/conicd.htm

National Osteoporosis Foundation
http://www.nof.org

President's Council on Physical Fitness and Sports
http://os.dhhs.gov/

United States Department of Agriculture
Food and Nutrition Information Center
National Agriculture Library
http://www.nal.usda.gov/fnic/

Shape Up America
http://www.shapeup.org

United States Olympic Committee
http://www.olympic-usa.org

USA Today Health: Diet
http://www.usatoday.com/life/health/diet/
lhdie000.htm

If you are interested in doing scientific literature searches, the following sites provide access to Medline, the computerized literature retrieval system of the National Library of Medicine.

Medscape
http://www.medscape.com

National Library of Medicine
http://www.nlm.nih.gov

The following USDA Web site provides data on the nutrient composition of most foods. Included in the analysis of each food is the water content (g), energy (Calories and kilojoules), protein (g), total fat (g), carbohydrate (g), total dietary fiber (g), ash (g), minerals (Ca, Fe, Mg, P, K, Na, Zn, Cu, Mn), vitamins (C, thiamin, riboflavin, niacin, pantothenic acid, B-6, folate, B-12, A, E), eight saturated fatty acids, four monounsaturated fatty acids, seven polyunsaturated fatty acids, cholesterol, phytosterols, and eighteen amino acids.

http://www.nal.usda.gov/fnic/cgi-bin/nut_search.pl

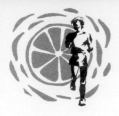

Glossary

AAS *See* anabolic/androgenic steroids.

acclimatization The ability of the body to undergo physiological adaptations so that the stress of a given environment, such as high environmental temperature, is less severe.

acetaldehyde An intermediate breakdown product of alcohol.

acetic acid A naturally occurring saturated fatty acid; a precursor for the Krebs cycle when converted into acetyl CoA.

acetyl CoA The major fuel for the oxidative processes in the body, being derived from the breakdown of glucose and fatty acids.

acid-base balance A relative balance of acid and base products in the body so that an optimal pH is maintained in the tissues, particularly the blood.

acidosis A disturbance of the normal acid-base balance in which excess acids accumulate in the body. Lactic acid production during exercise may lead to acidosis.

acute exercise bout A single bout of exercise that will produce various physiological reactions dependent upon the nature of the exercise; a single workout.

additives Substances added to food to improve flavor, color, texture, stability, or for similar purposes.

adenosine triphosphate *See* ATP.

ADH The antidiuretic hormone secreted by the pituitary gland; its major action is to conserve body water by decreasing urine formation.

adrenaline A hormone secreted by the adrenal medulla; it is a stimulant and prepares the body for "fight or flight."

aerobic Relating to energy processes that occur in the presence of oxygen.

aerobic glycolysis Oxidative processes in the cell that liberate energy in the metabolism of the carbohydrate glycogen.

aerobic lipolysis Oxidative processes in the cell that liberate energy in the metabolism of fats.

aerobic walking Rapid walking designed to elevate the heart rate so that a training effect will occur; more strenuous than ordinary leisure walking.

alanine A nonessential amino acid.

alcohol A colorless liquid with depressant effects; ethyl alcohol or ethanol is the alcohol designed for human consumption.

alcohol dehydrogenase An enzyme in the liver that initiates the breakdown of alcohol to acetaldehyde.

alcoholism A rather undefined term used to describe individuals who abuse the effect of alcohol; an addiction or habituation that may result in physical and/or psychological withdrawal effects.

aldosterone The main electrolyte-regulating hormone secreted by the adrenal cortex; primarily controls sodium and potassium balance.

allithiamine A derivative of thiamine.

alpha-ketoacid Specific acids associated with different amino acids and released upon deamination or transamination; for example, the breakdown of glutamate yields alpha-ketoglutarate.

alpha-linolenic acid An omega-3 fatty acid considered to be an essential nutrient.

alpha-tocopherol The most biologically active alcohol in vitamin E.

alpha-tocopherol equivalent The amount of other forms of tocopherol to equal the vitamin E activity of one milligram of alpha-tocopherol.

amenorrhea Absence or cessation of menstruation.

amino acids The chief structural material of protein, consisting of an amino group (NH_2) and an acid group (COOH) plus other components.

amino group The nitrogen-containing component of amino acids (NH_2).

aminostatic theory A theory suggesting that hunger is controlled by the presence or absence of amino acids in the blood acting upon a receptor in the hypothalamus.

ammonia A metabolic by-product of the oxidation of glutamine; it may be transformed into urea for excretion from the body.

amylopectin A branched-chain starch.

amylose A straight-chain starch that is more resistant to digestion compared to amylopectin.

anabolic/androgenic steroids Drugs designed to mimic the actions of testosterone to build muscle tissue (anabolism) while minimizing the androgenic effects (masculinization).

anabolism Constructive metabolism, the process whereby simple body compounds are formed into more complex ones.

anaerobic Relating to energy processes that occur in the absence of oxygen.

anaerobic glycolysis Metabolic processes in the cell that liberate energy in the metabolism of the carbohydrate glycogen without the involvement of oxidation.

anaerobic threshold The intensity of exercise at which the individual begins to increase the proportion of energy derived from anaerobic means, principally the lactic acid system. *Also see* steady-state threshold and OBLA.

android-type obesity Male-type obesity in which the body fat accumulates in the abdominal area and is a more significant risk factor for chronic disease than is gynoid-type obesity.

anemia In general, subnormal levels of circulating RBCs and hemoglobin; there are many different types of anemia.

angina The pain experienced under the breastbone or in other areas of the upper body when the heart is deprived of oxygen.

anhidrotic heat exhaustion Heat exhaustion associated with diminished secretion or absence of sweat.

anion A negatively charged ion, or electrolyte.

anorexia athletica A form of anorexia nervosa observed in athletes involved in sports in which low percentages of body fat may enhance performance, such as gymnastics and ballet.

anorexia nervosa A serious nervous condition, particularly among teenage girls and young women, marked by a loss of appetite and leading to various degrees of emaciation.

anthropometry Use of body girths and diameters to evaluate body composition.

antibodies Protein substances developed in the body in reaction to the presence of a foreign substance, called an antigen; natural antibodies are also present in the blood. They are protective in nature.

antidiuretic hormone *See* ADH.

antioxidant A compound that may protect other compounds from the effects of oxygen. The antioxidant itself interferes with oxidative processes.

antipromoters Compounds that block the actions of promoters, agents associated with the development of certain diseases, such as cancer.

apolipoprotein A class of special proteins associated with the formation of lipoproteins. A variety of apolipoproteins have been identified and are involved in the specific functions of the different lipoproteins.

appetite A pleasant desire for food for the purpose of enjoyment that is developed through previous experience; believed to be controlled in humans by an appetite center, or appestat, in the hypothalamus.

arginine An essential amino acid.

arteriosclerosis Hardening of the arteries; *also see* atherosclerosis.

ascorbic acid   Vitamin C.

aspartame   An artificial sweetener made from amino acids.

aspartates   Salts of aspartic acid, an amino acid.

atherosclerosis   A specific form of arteriosclerosis characterized by the formation of plaque on the inner layers of the arterial wall.

athletic amenorrhea   The cessation of menstruation in athletes, believed to be caused by factors associated with participation in strenuous physical activity.

ATP   Adenosine triphosphate, a high-energy phosphate compound found in the body; one of the major forms of energy available for immediate use in the body.

ATPase   The enzyme involved in the splitting of ATP and the release of energy.

ATP-PC system   The energy system for fast, powerful muscle contractions; uses ATP as the immediate energy source, the spent ATP being quickly regenerated by breakdown of the PC. ATP and PC are high-energy phosphates in the muscle cell.

basal metabolic rate   *See* BMR.

Basic Four Food Groups   Grouping of foods into four categories that can be used as a means to educate individuals on how to obtain essential nutrients. The four groups are meat, milk, bread-cereal, and fruit-vegetable.

BCAA   Branched-chain amino acids (leucine, isoleucine, and valine). Three essential amino acids that help form muscle tissue.

bee pollen   A nutritional product containing minute amounts of protein and some vitamins that has been advertised to be possibly ergogenic for some athletes.

behavior modification   Relative to weight-control methods, behavioral patterns, or the way one acts, may be modified to help achieve weight loss.

beriberi   A deficiency disease attributed to lack of thiamin (vitamin B_1) in the diet.

beta-carotene   A precursor for vitamin A found in plants.

beta glucan   Gummy form of water-soluble fiber useful in reducing serum cholesterol; oats are a good source.

beta-oxidation   Process in the cells whereby 2-carbon units of acetic acid are removed from long-chain fatty acids for conversion to acetyl CoA and oxidation via the Krebs cycle.

bile   A fluid secreted by the liver into the intestine that aids in the breakdown process of fats.

bile salts   Active salts found in bile; cholesterol is part of their structure.

binge-purge syndrome   An eating behavior characterized by excessive hunger leading to gorging, followed by guilt and purging by vomiting. *Also see* bulimia nervosa.

bioavailability   In relation to nutrients in food, the amount that may be absorbed into the body.

bioelectrical impedance analysis (BIA)   A method to calculate percentage of body fat by measuring electrical resistance due to the water content of the body.

biotin   A component of the B complex.

bisphosphonates   Drugs used to inhibit bone resorption, but not mineralization, to help prevent bone loss and increase bone mineral density; Fosamax is one brand.

blood alcohol content (BAC)   The concentration of alcohol in the blood, usually expressed as milligram percent.

blood alcohol level   *See* blood alcohol content.

blood glucose   Blood sugar; the means by which carbohydrate is carried in the blood; normal range is 70–120 mg/ml.

blood pressure   The pressure of the blood in the blood vessels; usually used to refer to arterial blood pressure. *Also see* systolic blood pressure and diastolic blood pressure.

BMI   *See* Body Mass Index.

BMR   The basal metabolic rate; measurement of energy expenditure in the body under resting, postabsorptive conditions, indicative of the energy needed to maintain life under these basal conditions.

body image   The image or impression the individual has of his or her body. A poor body image may lead to personality problems.

Body Mass Index (BMI)   An index calculated by a ratio of height to weight, used as a measure of obesity.

body plethysmography   A body composition technique using a special chamber to measure air displacement; similar to water displacement theory associated with underwater weighing.

branched-chain amino acids   *See* BCAA.

bread exchange   One bread exchange in the Food Exchange System contains 15 grams of carbohydrate, 3 grams of protein, and 80 Calories.

brown fat   A special form of adipose tissue that is designed to produce heat; small amounts are found in humans in the area of vital organs such as the heart and lungs.

bulimia nervosa   An eating disorder involving a loss of control over the impulse to binge; the binge-purge syndrome.

bulk-up method   A method of weight training designed to increase muscle mass; uses high resistance and moderate volume with many different muscle groups.

CAD   Coronary artery disease; atherosclerosis in the coronary arteries.

caffeine   A stimulant drug found in many food products such as coffee, tea, and cola drinks; stimulates the central nervous system.

calciferol   A synthetic vitamin D.

calcium   A silver-white metallic element essential to human nutrition.

caloric concept of weight control   The concept that Calories are the basis of weight control. Excess Calories will add body weight while caloric deficiencies will contribute to weight loss.

caloric deficit   A negative caloric balance whereby more Calories are expended than consumed; a weight loss will occur.

Calorie   A Calorie is a measure of heat energy. A small calorie represents the amount of heat needed to raise one gram of water one degree Celsius. A large Calorie (kilocalorie, KC, or C) is 1,000 small calories.

calorimeter   A device used to measure the caloric value of a given food, or heat production of animals or humans.

carbohydrates   A group of compounds containing carbon, hydrogen, and oxygen. Glucose, glycogen, sugar, starches, fiber, cellulose, and the various saccharides are all carbohydrates.

carbohydrate loading   A dietary method used by endurance-type athletes to help increase the carbohydrate (glycogen) levels in their muscles and liver.

carcinogenicity   The potential of a substance to cause cancer.

carnitine   A chemical that facilitates the transfer of fatty acids into the mitochondria for subsequent oxidation.

catabolism   Destructive metabolism whereby complex chemical compounds in the body are degraded to simpler ones.

catalase   An enzyme that helps neutralize free radicals.

cation   A positively charged ion or electrolyte.

cellulite   A name given to the lumpy fat that often appears in the thigh and hip region of women. Cellulite is simply normal fat in small compartments formed by connective tissue, but may contain other compounds that bind water.

cellulose   The fibrous carbohydrate that provides the structural backbone for plants; plant fiber.

Celsius   A thermometer scale that has a freezing point of 0° and a boiling point of 100°; also known as the centigrade scale.

cerebrospinal fluid (CSF)   The fluid found in the brain and spinal cord.

CHD   Coronary heart disease; a degenerative disease of the heart caused primarily by arteriosclerosis or atherosclerosis of the coronary vessels of the heart.

chloride   A compound of chlorine present in a salt form carrying a negative charge; Cl⁻, an anion.

cholecalciferol   The product of irradiation of 7-dehydrocholesterol found in the skin. *Also see* vitamin D_3.

cholesterol   A fat-like pearly substance, an alcohol, found in all animal fat and oils; a main constituent of some body tissues and body compounds.

choline   A substance associated with the B complex that is widely distributed in both plant and animal tissues; involved in carbohydrate, fat, and protein metabolism.

chromium   A whitish metal essential to human nutrition; it is involved in carbohydrate metabolism via its role with insulin.

chronic-training effect   Physiological changes in the body, brought on by repeated bouts of exercise, that will help make the body more efficient during exercise.

chylomicron   A particle of emulsified fat found in the blood following the digestion and assimilation of fat.

circuit aerobics   A combination of aerobic and weight-training exercises designed to elicit the specific benefits of each type of exercise.

circuit training   A method of training in which exercises are arranged in a circuit or sequence. May be designed with weight training to help convey an aerobic training effect.

cirrhosis   A degenerative disease of the liver, one cause being excessive consumption of alcohol.

cis   The chemical structure of unsaturated fatty acids in which the hydrogen ions are on the same side of the double bond.

clinical obesity   Obesity determined by a clinical procedure.

Clostridium   A bacteria commonly involved in food poisoning.

cobalamin   The cobalt-containing complex common to all members of the vitamin B_{12} group; often used to designate cyanocobalamin.

cobalt   A gray, hard metal that is a component of vitamin B_{12}.

coenzyme   An activator of an enzyme; many vitamins are coenzymes.

coenzyme Q10   *See* CoQ10.

colon   The large intestine.

complementary proteins   Combining plant foods such as rice and beans so that essential amino acids deficient in one of the foods are provided by the other in order to obtain a balanced intake of essential amino acids.

complete protein   A protein that contains all nine essential amino acids in the proper proportions. Animal protein is complete protein.

complex carbohydrates   A term used to describe foods high in starch, such as bread, cereals, fruits, and vegetables as contrasted to simple carbohydrates such as table sugar.

concentric method   A method of weight training in which the muscle shortens.

conduction   In relation to body temperature, the transfer of heat from one substance to another by direct contact.

convection   In relation to body temperature, the transfer of heat by way of currents in either air or water.

copper   A reddish metallic element essential to human nutrition; it functions with iron in the formation of hemoglobin and the cytochromes.

CoQ10   A coenzyme involved in the electron transport system in the mitochondria.

core temperature   The temperature of the deep tissues of the body, usually measured orally or rectally; *also see* shell temperature.

coronary artery disease   *See* CAD.

coronary heart disease   *See* CHD.

coronary occlusion   Closure of coronary arteries that may precipitate a heart attack; occlusion may be partial or complete closure.

coronary risk factors   Behaviors (smoking) or body properties (cholesterol levels) that may predispose an individual to coronary heart disease.

coronary thrombosis   Occlusion (closure) of coronary arteries, usually by a blood clot.

cortisol   A hormone secreted by the adrenal cortex with gluconeogenic potential, helping to convert amino acids to glucose.

creatine   A nitrogen-containing compound found in the muscles, usually complexed with phosphate to form phosphocreatine.

cruciferous vegetables   Vegetables in the cabbage family, such as broccoli, cauliflower, kale, and all cabbages.

cyanocobalamin   Vitamin B_{12}.

cysteine   A breakdown product of cystine. It is also a sulfur-containing amino acid.

cystine   A sulfur-containing amino acid.

cytochromes   Any one of a class of pigment compounds that play an important role in cellular oxidative processes.

Daily Reference Values (DRVs)   The DRVs are recommended daily intakes for the macronutrients (carbohydrate, fat, and protein) as well as cholesterol, sodium, and potassium. On a food label, the DRV is based on a 2,000 Calorie diet.

Daily Value (DV)   A term used in food labeling; the DV is based on a daily energy intake of 2,000 Calories and for the food labeled, presents the percentage of the RDI and the DRV recommended for healthy Americans. *See* RDI and DRV.

deamination   Removal of an amine group, or nitrogen, from an amino acid.

dehydration   A reduction of the body water to below the normal level of hydration; water output exceeds water intake.

dehydroepiandrosterone (DHEA)   A natural steroid hormone produced endogenously by the adrenal gland. May be marketed as a nutritional sports ergogenic as derived from herbal precursors.

depressant   Drugs or agents that will depress or lower the level of bodily functions, particularly central nervous system functioning.

DEXA   *See* dual energy X-ray absorptiometry.

DHA   Docasahexanoic acid, an omega-3 fatty acid found in fatty fish.

DHAP   Dihydroxyacetone and pyruvate, the combination of two by-products of glycolysis.

DHEA   *See* dehydroepiandrosterone.

diabetes mellitus   A disorder of carbohydrate metabolism due to disturbances in production or utilization of insulin; results in high blood glucose levels and loss of sugar in the urine.

diarrhea   Frequent passage of a watery fecal discharge due to a gastrointestinal disturbance.

diastolic blood pressure   The blood pressure in the arteries when the heart is at rest between beats.

dietary fiber   Fiber in plant foods that cannot be hydrolyzed by the digestive enzymes.

dietary-induced thermogenesis (DIT)   The increase in the basal metabolic rate following the ingestion of a meal. Heat production is increased.

dietary supplement   A food product, added to the total diet, that contains either vitamins, minerals, herbs, botanicals, amino acids, metabolites, constituents, extracts, or combinations of these ingredients.

Dietary Supplement Health and Education Act   Act passed by the United States Congress defining a dietary supplement (*see* dietary supplement); legislation to control advertising and marketing.

2,3–diphosphoglyceride   A by-product of carbohydrate metabolism in the red blood cell; helps the hemoglobin unload oxygen to the tissues.

disaccharides   Any one of a class of sugars that yield two monosaccharides on hydrolysis; sucrose is the most common.

dispensable amino acids   *See* nonessential amino acids.

DIT   *See* dietary-induced thermogenesis.

diuretics   A class of agents that stimulate the formation of urine; used as a means to reduce body fluids.

diverticulosis   Weak spots in the wall of the large intestine that may bulge out like a weak spot in a tire inner tube. May become infected leading to diverticulitis.

DNA   Deoxyribonucleic acid; a complex protein found in chromosomes that is the carrier of genetic information and the basis of heredity.

docasahexanoic acid   *See* DHA.

doping   Official term used by the International Olympic Committee to depict the use of drugs in sports in attempts to enhance performance.

doubly-labeled water technique   A technique using labeled water to study energy metabolism.

DRV   *See* Daily Reference Values.

DSHEA   *See* Dietary Supplement Health and Education Act.

dual energy X-ray absorptiometry   A computerized X-ray technique at two energy levels to image body fat, lean tissues, and bone mineral content.

dumping syndrome   Movement of fluid from the blood to the intestines by osmosis. May occur when a concentrated sugar solution is consumed in large quantities, causing symptoms such as weakness and gastrointestinal distress.

duration concept   One of the major concepts of aerobic exercise; duration refers to the amount of time spent exercising during each session.

DV   *See* Daily Value.

DXA   *See* dual energy X-ray absorptiometry.

eating disorder   A psychological disorder centering on the avoidance, excessive consumption, or purging of food, such as anorexia nervosa and bulimia nervosa.

eccentric method   A weight-training method in which the muscle undergoes a lengthening contraction.

eicosanoids   Derivatives of fatty acid oxidation in the body, including prostaglandins, thromboxanes, and leukotrienes.

eicosapentaenoic acid   *See* EPA.

electrolyte   A substance that, when in a solution, conducts an electric current.

electrolyte solution   A solution that contains ions and can conduct electricity; often the ions of salts such as sodium and chloride are called electrolytes; *also see* ions.

electron transfer system A highly structured array of chemical compounds in the cell that transport electrons and harness energy for later use.

element Relative to chemistry, a substance that cannot be subdivided into substances different from itself; many elements are essential to human life.

EMR Exercise metabolic rate; an increased metabolic rate due to the need for increased energy production; during exercise, the REE may be increased more than twenty-fold.

endocrine system The body system consisting of glands that secrete hormones, which have a wide variety of effects throughout the body.

energy The ability to do work; energy exists in various forms, notably mechanical, heat, and chemical in the human body.

English system A measurement system based upon the foot, pound, quart, and other nonmetric units; *also see* metric system.

enzyme A complex protein in the body that serves as a catalyst, facilitating reactions between various substances without being changed itself.

EPA Eicosapentaenoic acid, an omega-3 fatty acid found in fatty fish.

ephedrine A stimulant with somewhat weaker effects than amphetamine; found in some commercial dietary supplements.

epidemiological research A study of certain populations to determine the relationship of various risk factors to epidemic diseases or health problems.

epinephrine A hormone secreted by the adrenal medulla that stimulates numerous body processes to enhance energy production, particularly during intense exercise.

epithelial cells The layer of cells that covers the outside and inside surfaces of the body, including the skin and the lining of the gastrointestinal system.

ergogenic aids Work-enhancing agents that are used in attempts to increase athletic or physical performance capacity.

ergogenic effect The physiological or psychological effect that an ergogenic substance is designed to produce.

ergolytic effect An agent or substance that may lead to decreases in work productivity or physical performance. *See also* ergogenic effect.

Escherichia A bacteria commonly involved in food poisoning.

essential amino acids Those amino acids that must be obtained in the diet and cannot be synthesized in the body. Also known as indispensable amino acids.

essential fat Fat in the body that is an essential part of the tissues, such as cell membrane structure, nerve coverings, and the brain; *also see* storage fat.

essential fatty acid Those unsaturated fatty acids that may not be synthesized in the body and must be obtained in the diet, e.g., linoleic fatty acid.

essential nutrients Those nutrients found to be essential to human life and optimal functioning.

ester Compound formed from the combination of an organic acid and an alcohol.

Estimated Safe and Adequate Daily Dietary Intakes (ESADDI) Part of the RDA. Daily allowances for selected nutrients that are based upon available scientific evidence to be safe and adequate to meet human needs.

ethanol Alcohol; ethyl alcohol.

ethyl alcohol Alcohol; ethanol.

evaporation The conversion of a liquid to a vapor, which consumes energy; evaporation of sweat cools the body by using body heat as the energy source.

exercise A form of structured physical activity generally designed to enhance physical fitness; exercise usually refers to strenuous physical activity.

exercise frequency In an aerobic exercise program, the number of times per week that an individual exercises.

exercise intensity The tempo, speed, or resistance of an exercise. Intensity can be increased by working faster, doing more work in a given amount of time.

exercise metabolic rate *See* EMR.

exercise sequence *See* principle of exercise sequence.

exercise stimulus The means whereby one elicits a physiological response; running, for example, can be the stimulus to increase the heart rate and other physiological functions.

exertional heat stroke Heat stroke that is precipitated by exercise in a warm or hot environment.

experimental research Study that manipulates an independent variable (cause) to observe the outcome on a dependent variable (effect).

extracellular water Body water that is located outside the cells; often subdivided into the intravascular water and the intercellular, or interstitial, water.

faddism Relative to nutrition, the use of dietary fads based upon theoretical principles that may or may not be valid; usually used in a negative sense, as in quackery.

fasting Starvation; abstinence from eating that may be partial or complete.

fast-twitch fibers Muscle fibers characterized by high contractile speed

fat exchange A fat exchange in the Food Exchange System contains 5 grams of fat and 45 Calories.

fat-free mass The remaining mass of the human body following the extraction of all fat.

fat substitutes Various substances used as substitutes for fats in food products; two popular brands are Simplesse and Olestra.

fatigue A generalized or specific feeling of tiredness that may have a multitude of causes; may be mental or physical.

fat loading A term to describe practices used to maximize the use of fats as an energy source during exercise, particularly a low-carbohydrate, high-fat diet.

fat patterning The deposition of fat in specific areas of the human body, such as the stomach, thighs, or hips. Genetics plays an important role in fat patterning.

fats Triglycerides; a combination, or ester, of three fatty acids and glycerol.

fatty acids Any one of a number of aliphatic acids containing only carbon, oxygen, and hydrogen; they may be saturated or unsaturated.

FDA *See* Food and Drug Administration.

female athlete triad The triad of disordered eating, amenorrhea, and osteoporosis sometimes seen in female athletes involved in sports where excess body weight may be detrimental to performance.

female-type obesity *See* gynoid-type obesity.

ferritin The form in which iron is stored in the tissues.

fetal alcohol effects (FAE) Symptoms noted in children born to women who consumed alcohol during pregnancy; not as severe as fetal alcohol syndrome.

fetal alcohol syndrome (FAS) The cluster of physical and mental symptoms seen in the child of a mother who consumes excessive alcohol during pregnancy.

FFA Free fatty acids, formed by the hydrolysis of triglycerides.

fiber In general, the indigestible carbohydrate in plants that forms the structural network; *also see* cellulose.

First Law of Thermodynamics The law that energy cannot be created nor destroyed; energy can be converted from one form to another.

flatulence Gas or air in the gastrointestinal tract, particularly the intestines.

fluoride A salt of hydrofluoric acid; a compound of fluorine that may be helpful in the prevention of tooth decay.

folacin Collective term for various forms of folic acid.

folate Salt of folic acid; form found in foods.

folic acid A water-soluble vitamin that appears to be essential in preventing certain types of anemia.

food additives *See* additives.

food allergy An adverse immune response to an otherwise harmless food. *Also see* food hypersensitivity.

food cultism Treating a particular food as if it possesses special properties, such as prevention or treatment of disease or improvement of athletic performance, usually without scientific justification.

Food and Drug Administration Federal agency tasked with the responsibilities to monitor safety of foods and drugs sold in the United States.

Food Exchange System The system developed by the American Dietetic Association and other health groups that categorizes foods by content of carbohydrate, fat, protein, and Calories. Used as a basis for diet planning.

Food Guide Pyramid A food group approach to healthful nutrition, containing five food groups: breads, cereal, rice, and pasta; fruits; vegetables; meat, poultry, fish, dry beans, eggs, and nuts; milk, yogurt, and cheese; and fats, oils, sweets (not an official food group).

food hypersensitivity Some individuals may develop clinical symptoms, such as migraine headaches, gastrointestinal distress, or hives and itching when certain foods are eaten.

food intolerance A general term for any adverse reaction to a food or food component not involving the immune system; an example is lactose intolerance.

food poisoning Foodborne illness caused by bacteria such as Salmonella, Escherichia, Staphylococcus, and Clostridium.

foot-pound   A unit of work whereby the weight of 1 pound is moved through a distance of 1 foot.

Fosamax   A commercial bisphosphonate product.

free fatty acids   *See* FFA.

free radicals   An atom or compound in which there is an unpaired electron. Thought to cause cellular damage.

fructose   A monosaccharide known as levulose or fruit sugar; found in all sweet fruits.

fruit exchange   One fruit exchange in the Food Exchange System contains 15 grams of carbohydrate and 60 Calories.

fruitarian   A type of vegetarian who subsides solely on fruits, fruit products, and nuts.

fTRP:BCAA ratio   The ratio of free tryptophan to branched-chain amino acids; a high ratio is theorized to elicit fatigue in prolonged endurance events.

galactose   A monosaccharide formed when lactose is hydrolyzed into glucose and galactose.

gastric emptying   The rate at which substances, particularly fluids, empty from the stomach; high gastric emptying rates are advisable for sports drinks.

generally recognized as safe   *See* GRAS.

ginseng   A general term for a variety of natural chemical plant extracts derived from the family Araliaceae; extract contains ginsenosides and other chemicals that may influence human physiology.

glucagon   A hormone secreted by the pancreas; basically it exerts actions just the opposite of insulin, i.e., it responds to hypoglycemia and helps to increase blood sugar levels.

glucarate   A compound found in cruciferous vegetables that is thought to block the actions of cancer-causing agents.

glucogenic amino acids   Amino acids that may undergo deamination and be converted into glucose through the process of gluconeogenesis.

gluconeogenesis   The formation of carbohydrates from molecules that are not themselves carbohydrate, such as amino acids and the glycerol from fat.

glucose   A monosaccharide; a thick, sweet, syrupy liquid.

glucose-alanine cycle   The cycle in which alanine is released from the muscle and is converted to glucose in the liver.

glucose-electrolyte solutions   Solutions designed to replace sweat losses; contain varying proportions of water, glucose, sodium, potassium, chloride, and other electrolytes.

glucose polymer   A combination of several glucose molecules into a more complex carbohydrate.

glucose polymer solutions   Fluid replacement beverages containing primarily water and glucose polymers.

glucostatic theory   The theory that hunger and satiety are controlled by the glucose level in the blood; the receptors that respond to the blood glucose level are in the hypothalamus.

glutathione peroxidase   An enzyme that helps neutralize free radicals.

glycemic index   An index expressing the effects of various foods on the rate and amount of increase in blood glucose levels.

glycerate   A commercial product containing glycerol; marketed to athletes.

glycerin   *See* glycerol.

glycerol   Glycerin, a clear syrupy liquid; an alcohol that combines with fatty acids to form triglycerides.

glycogen   A polysaccharide that is the chief storage form of carbohydrate in animals; it is stored primarily in the liver and muscles.

glycogen-sparing effect   The theory that certain dietary techniques, such as the use of caffeine, may facilitate the oxidation of fatty acids for energy and thus spare the utilization of glycogen.

glycolysis   The degradation of sugars into smaller compounds; the main quantitative anaerobic energy process in the muscle tissue.

gout   The deposit of uric acid by-products in and about the joints contributing to inflammation and pain; usually occurs in the knee or foot.

gram calorie   A small calorie; *see* Calorie.

GRAS   Generally recognized as safe; a classification for food additives indicating that they most likely are not harmful for human consumption.

gums   A form of water-soluble dietary fiber found in plants.

gynoid-type obesity   Female-type obesity; body fat is deposited primarily about the hips and thighs. *Also see* android-type obesity.

HDL   High-density lipoprotein; a protein-lipid complex in the blood that facilitates the transport of triglycerides, cholesterol, and phospholipids. *Also see* HDL cholesterol.

HDL cholesterol   High-density lipoprotein cholesterol; one mechanism whereby cholesterol is transported in the blood. High HDL levels are somewhat protective against CHD.

health-related fitness   Those components of physical fitness whose improvement have health benefits, such as cardiovascular fitness, body composition, flexibility, and muscular strength and endurance.

Healthy North American Diet   A diet plan based upon healthful eating principles that is designed to help prevent or treat common chronic diseases in the United States, Canada and Mexico, particularly cardiovascular disease and cancer.

heat-balance equation   Heat balance is dependent upon the interrelationships of metabolic heat production and loss or gain of heat by radiation, convection, conduction, and evaporation.

heat cramps   Painful muscular cramps or tetany following prolonged exercise in the heat without water or salt replacement.

heat exhaustion   Weakness or dizziness from overexertion in a hot environment.

heat index   The apparent temperature determined by combining air temperature and relative humidity.

heat stroke   Elevated body temperature of 105.8° F or greater caused by exposure to excessive heat gains or production and diminished heat loss.

heat syncope   Fainting caused by excessive heat exposure.

hematuria   Blood or red blood cells in the urine.

heme iron   The iron in the diet associated with hemoglobin in animal meats.

hemicellulose   A form of dietary fiber found in plants. Differs from cellulose in that it may be hydrolyzed by dilute acids outside of the body. Not hydrolyzed in the body.

hemochromatosis   Presence of excessive iron in the body resulting in an enlarged liver and bronze pigmentation of the skin.

hemoglobin   The protein-iron pigment in the red blood cells that transports oxygen.

hemolysis   A rupturing of red blood cells with a release of hemoglobin into the plasma.

hepatitis   An inflammatory condition of the liver.

HGH   *See* human growth hormone.

hidden fat   In foods, the fat that is not readily apparent, such as the high fat content of cheese.

high blood pressure   *See* hypertension.

high-density lipoprotein   *See* HDL.

high-fructose corn syrup   A common high-Calorie sweetener used as a food additive; derived from the partial hydrolysis of corn starch.

histidine   An essential amino acid.

HMB   Beta-hydroxy-beta-methylbutyrate, a metabolic by-product of the amino acid leucine, alleged to retard the breakdown of muscle protein during strenuous exercise.

homeostasis   A term used to describe a condition of normalcy in the internal body environment.

hormone   A chemical substance produced by specific body cells, secreted into the blood and then acting on specific target tissues.

hormone sensitive lipase   An enzyme that catalyzes triglycerides into free fatty acids and glycerol.

HR max   The normal maximal heart rate of an individual during exercise.

HR reserve   The mathematical difference, or reserve, between the resting HR and maximal HR. A percentage of this reserve may be added to the resting HR to determine exercise intensity.

HSL   *See* hormone sensitive lipase.

human growth hormone (HGH)   A hormone released by the pituitary gland that regulates growth; also involved in fatty acid metabolism.

hunger   A basic physiological desire to eat that is normally caused by a lack of food; may be accompanied by stomach contractions.

hunger center   A collection of nerve cells in the hypothalamus that is involved in the control of feeding reflexes.

hydrodensitometry   Another term for the underwater weighing technique.

hydrogenated fats   Fats to which hydrogen has been added, usually causing them to be saturated.

hydrolysis   A mechanism for splitting substances into smaller compounds by the addition of water; enzyme action.

hypercholesteremia   Elevated blood cholesterol levels.

hyperglycemia   Elevated blood glucose levels.

hyperhydration   The practice of increasing the body-water stores by fluid consumption prior to an athletic event; a state of increased water content in the body.

hyperkalemia   An increased concentration of potassium in the blood.

hyperlipidemia   Elevated blood lipid levels.

hyperplasia   The formation of new body cells.

hypertension   A condition with various causes whereby the blood pressure is higher than normal.

hyperthermia   Unusually high body temperature; fever.

hypertonic   Relative to osmotic pressure, a solution that has a greater concentration of solute or salts, hence higher osmotic pressure, in comparison to another solution.

hypertriglyceridemia   Elevated blood levels of triglycerides.

hypertrophy   Excessive growth of a cell or organ; in pathology, an abnormal growth.

hypervitaminosis   A pathological condition due to an excessive vitamin intake, particularly the fat-soluble vitamins A and D.

hypoglycemia   A low blood sugar level.

hypohydration   Dehydration; a state of decreased water content in the body.

hypokalemia   A decreased concentration of potassium in the blood.

hyponatremia   A decreased concentration of sodium in the blood.

hypothalamus   A part of the brain involved in the control of involuntary activity in the body; contains many centers for neural control such as temperature, hunger, appetite and thirst.

hypothermia   Unusually low body temperature.

hypotonic   Having an osmotic pressure lower than that of the solution to which it is compared.

incomplete protein   Protein food that does not possess the proper amount of essential amino acids; characteristic of plant foods in general.

Index of Nutritional Quality   *See* INQ.

indicator nutrients   These eight nutrients, if provided in adequate supply through a varied diet, should provide adequate amounts of the other essential nutrients. The eight are protein, vitamin A, thiamin, riboflavin, niacin, vitamin C, calcium, and iron.

indispensable amino acids   *See* essential amino acids.

indoles   Phytochemicals believed to help prevent various diseases.

infrared interactance   Use of infrared technology to estimate body composition.

initial fitness level   The physical fitness level of an individual prior to the onset of a physical conditioning program.

in-line skating   An exercise-skating technique with specially-designed shoes for use on sidewalks and similar surfaces.

inosine   A nucleoside of the purine family that serves as a base for the formation of a variety of compounds in the body; theorized to be ergogenic.

inositol   A member of the B complex, although its role in human nutrition has not been established; not classified as a vitamin.

INQ   Index of Nutritional Quality; a mathematical means of determining the quality of any given food relative to its content of a specific nutrient.

insensible perspiration   Perspiration on the skin not detectable by ordinary senses.

insoluble dietary fiber   Dietary fiber that is not soluble in water, such as cellulose. *Also see* soluble dietary fiber.

insulin   A hormone secreted by the pancreas involved in carbohydrate metabolism.

insulin response   Blood insulin levels rise following the ingestion of sugar and the resultant hyperglycemia; the insulin causes the sugar to be taken up by the muscles and fat cells, possibly creating a reactive hypoglycemia.

intercellular water   Body water found between the cells; also known as interstitial water.

intermittent high-intensity exercise   Short-term bouts of high-intensity exercise interspersed with short periods of recovery.

International Unit   *See* IU.

International Unit System   *See* SI.

interstitial water   *See* intercellular water.

interval training   A method of physical training in which periods of activity are interspersed with periods of rest.

intestinal absorption   The rate at which substances, particularly fluids and carbohydrate, are absorbed into the body; a fast rate of intestinal absorption is a desirable characteristic of sports drinks.

intracellular water   Body water that is found within the cells.

intravascular water   Body water found in the vascular system, or blood vessels.

involuntary dehydration   Unintentional loss of body fluids during exercise under warm or hot environmental conditions.

iodine   A nonmetallic element that is necessary for the proper development and functioning of the thyroid gland.

ions   Particles with an electrical charge; anions are negative and cations are positive.

iron   A metallic element essential for the development of several chemical compounds in the body, notably hemoglobin.

iron-deficiency anemia   Anemia caused by an inadequate intake or absorption of iron, resulting in impaired hemoglobin formation.

iron deficiency without anemia   A condition in which the hemoglobin levels are normal but several indices of iron status in the body are below normal levels.

ischemia   Lack of blood supply.

isoflavones   Phytochemicals believed to help prevent various diseases.

isoleucine   An essential amino acid.

isokinetic   Literally meaning "same speed"; in weight training an isokinetic machine is used to control the speed of muscle contraction.

isometric   Literally meaning "same length"; in weight training the resistance is set so that the muscle will not shorten.

isotonic   Literally meaning "equal tension or pressure"; in weight training the resistance is set so there is supposed to be equal tension in the muscle through a range of motion, but this is rarely achieved owing to movement of body parts. Isotonic also means equal osmotic pressures between two solutions.

IU   International Unit; a method of expressing the quantity of some substance, such as vitamins, which is an internationally developed and accepted standard.

jogging   A term used to designate slow running; although the distinction between running and jogging is relative to the individual involved, a common value used for jogging is a 9-minute mile or slower.

joule   A measure of work in the metric system; a newton of force applied through a distance of one meter.

KC   Kilocalorie or Kcal; *see* Calorie.

ketogenesis   The formation of ketones in the body from other substances, such as fats and proteins.

ketogenic amino acids   Amino acids that may be deaminated, converted into ketones and eventually into fat.

ketones   An organic compound containing a carbonyl group; ketone acids in the body, such as acetone, are the end products of fat metabolism.

ketosis   The accumulation of excess ketones in the blood; since ketones are acids, acidosis occurs.

key-nutrient concept   The concept that if certain key nutrients are adequately supplied by the diet, the other essential nutrients will also be present in adequate amounts. *Also see* indicator nutrients.

KGM   Kilogram-meter; a measure of work in the metric system whereby 1 kilogram of weight is moved through a distance of 1 meter; however, the joule is the recommended unit to express work.

kidney stones   Compounds in the pelvis of the kidney formed from various salts such as carbonates, oxalates, and phosphates.

kilocalorie   A large Calorie; *see* Calorie.

kilogram   A unit of mass in the metric system; in ordinary terms, 1 kilogram is the equivalent of 2.2 pounds.

kilogram-meter *See* KGM.

kilojoule One thousand joules; one kilojoule (kJ) is approximately 0.25 kilocalorie.

Krebs cycle The main oxidative reaction sequence in the body that generates ATP; also known as the citric acid or tricarboxylic acid cycle.

lactic acid The anaerobic end product of glycolysis; it has been implicated as a causative factor in the etiology of fatigue.

lactic acid system The energy system that produces ATP anaerobically by the breakdown of glycogen to lactic acid; used primarily in events of maximal effort for one to two minutes.

lactose A white crystalline disaccharide that yields glucose and galactose upon hydrolysis; also known as milk sugar.

lactose intolerance Gastrointestinal disturbances due to an intolerance to lactose in milk; caused by deficiency of lactase, an enzyme that digests lactose.

lactovegetarian A vegetarian who includes milk products in the diet as a form of high-quality protein.

LDL Low-density lipoprotein; a protein-lipid complex in the blood that facilitates the transport of triglycerides, cholesterol, and phospholipids. *Also see* LDL cholesterol.

LDL cholesterol Low-density lipoprotein cholesterol; a mechanism whereby cholesterol is transported in the blood. High blood levels are associated with increased incidence of CHD.

lean body mass The body weight minus the body fat, composed primarily of muscle, bone, and other nonfat tissue.

lecithin A fatty substance of a class known as phospholipids; said to have the therapeutic properties of phosphorous.

legume The fruit or pod of vegetables including soybeans, kidney beans, lima beans, garden peas, black-eyed peas, and lentils; high in protein.

leptin Regulatory hormone produced by fat cells; when released into the circulation, it influences the hypothalamus to control appetite.

leucine An essential amino acid.

leukotrienes Eicosanoids that possess hormone-like activity in numerous cells in the body.

levulose Fructose.

lignin A noncarbohydrate form of dietary fiber.

limiting amino acid An amino acid deficient in a specific plant food, making it an incomplete protein; methionine is a limiting amino acid in legumes while lysine is deficient in grain products.

linoleic acid An essential fatty acid.

lipase An enzyme that catabolizes fats into fatty acids and glycerol.

lipids A class of fats or fat-like substances characterized by their insolubility in water and solubility in fat solvents; triglycerides, fatty acids, phospholipids, and cholesterol are important lipids in the body.

lipoic acid A coenzyme that functions in oxidative decarboxylation, or removal of carbon dioxide from a compound.

lipoprotein A combination of lipid and protein possessing the general properties of proteins. Practically all the lipids of the plasma are present in this form.

lipoprotein (a) Serum lipid factor very similar to the LDL, being in the upper LDL density range and containing apolipoprotein (a); high levels are associated with increased risk for CHD.

lipoprotein lipase An enzyme involved in the metabolism of lipoproteins.

lipostatic theory The theory that hunger and satiety are controlled by the lipid level in the blood.

liquid meals Food in a liquid form designed to provide a balanced intake of essential nutrients.

liquid-protein diets Protein in a liquid form; a common form consists of protein predigested into simple amino acids.

liver glycogen The major storage form of carbohydrate in the liver.

long-chain fatty acids (LCFA) Fatty acids containing chains with 12 or more carbons.

long-haul concept Relative to weight control, the idea that weight loss via exercise should be gradual, and one should not expect to lose large amounts of weight in a short time.

L-tryptophan One form of tryptophan. L is for levo (left), or the direction in which polarized light is rotated when various organic compounds are analyzed.

lysine An essential amino acid.

macrominerals Those minerals essential to human nutrition with an RDA in excess of 100 mg/day: calcium, magnesium, phosphorous, sodium, potassium, chloride.

macronutrients Dietary nutrients needed by the body in daily amounts greater than a few grams, such as carbohydrate, fat, protein, and water.

magnesium A white metallic mineral element essential in human nutrition.

magnetic resonance imaging Magnetic-field and radio-frequency waves used to image body tissues; useful for imaging visceral fat.

Ma Huang A Chinese plant extract theorized to be ergogenic; contains ephedrine, a stimulant.

major minerals *See* macrominerals.

male-type obesity *See* android-type obesity.

malnutrition Poor nutrition that may be due to inadequate amounts of essential nutrients. Too many Calories leading to obesity is also a form of malnutrition. *Also see* subclinical malnutrition.

maltodextrin A glucose polymer that exerts lesser osmotic effects compared with glucose; used in a variety of sports drinks as the source of carbohydrate.

maltose A white crystalline disaccharide that yields two molecules of glucose upon hydrolysis.

manganese A metallic element essential in human nutrition.

maximal heart rate *See* HR max.

maximal heart rate reserve The difference between the maximal HR and resting HR. A percentage of this reserve, usually 60–90 percent, is added to the resting HR to get the target HR for aerobics training programs.

maximal oxygen uptake *See* VO$_2$ max.

MCTs Medium-chain triglycerides. Triglycerides containing fatty acids with carbon chain lengths of 6–12 carbons.

meat exchange One very lean meat exchange in the Food Exchange System contains 0–1 gram of fat, 7 grams of protein, and 35 Calories; a lean meat exchange contains 3 grams of fat, 7 grams of protein and 55 Calories; a medium-fat meat exchange has an additional 2 grams of fat and totals 75 Calories; a high-fat exchange has 5 additional grams of fat and totals 100 Calories.

Mediterranean Food Guide Pyramid A food group approach to healthful nutrition that includes basic food groups, but also lists olive oil and wine as components of the diet; *see* Food Guide Pyramid.

medium-chain fatty acids (MCFA) Fatty acids containing chains with 6–12 carbons.

medium-chain triglycerides *See* MCTs.

megadose An excessive amount of a substance in comparison to a normal dose of RDA; usually used to refer to vitamins.

menoquinone The animal form of vitamin K.

meta-analysis A statistical technique to summarize the findings of numerous studies in an attempt to provide a quantitatively based conclusion.

metabolic aftereffects of exercise The theory that the aftereffects of exercise will cause the metabolic rate to be elevated for a time, thus expending Calories and contributing to weight loss.

metabolic rate The energy expended to maintain all physical and chemical changes occurring in the body.

metabolic syndrome The syndrome of symptoms often seen with android-type obesity, particularly hyperinsulinemia, hypertriglyceridemia, and hypertension.

metabolic water The water that is a by-product of the oxidation of carbohydrate, fat, and protein in the body.

metabolism The sum total of all physical and chemical processes occurring in the body.

metalloenzyme An enzyme that needs a mineral component, such as zinc, in order to function effectively.

methionine An essential amino acid.

metric system A method of measurement based upon units of ten.

METS A measurement unit of energy expenditure; one MET equals approximately 3.5 ml O$_2$/kg body weight/minute.

microgram   One millionth of a gram (μg).

micronutrients   Dietary nutrients needed by the body in daily amounts less than a few grams, such as vitamins and minerals.

milk exchange   One skim milk exchange in the Food Exchange System contains 12 grams of carbohydrate, 8 grams of protein, a trace of fat, and 90 Calories. A low-fat exchange contains 120 Calories whereas whole milk has 150 Calories.

milligram   One thousandth of a gram.

millimole   One thousandth of a mole.

mineral   An inorganic element occurring in nature.

mitochondria   Structures within the cells that serve as the location for the aerobic production of ATP.

mole   One mole is the gram molecular weight of a compound, which is the quantity of a substance that equals its molecular weight.

molybdenum   A hard, heavy, silvery-white metallic element.

monosaccharides   Simple sugars (glucose, fructose, and galactose) that cannot be broken down by hydrolysis.

monounsaturated fatty acids   Fatty acids that have a single double bond.

morbid obesity   Severe obesity in which the incidence of life-threatening diseases is increased significantly.

MPF factor   Muscle protein factor; an unknown property of meat, fish, and poultry that facilitates the absorption of nonheme iron found in plant foods.

MRI   *See* magnetic resonance imaging.

muscle glycogen   The form in which carbohydrate is stored in the muscle.

muscle hypertrophy   An increase in the size of the muscle.

myocardial infarction   Death of heart tissue following cessation of blood flow; may be caused by coronary occlusion.

myoglobin   An iron-containing compound, similar to hemoglobin, found in the muscle tissues; it binds oxygen in the muscle cells.

narcotic   Any agent that produces insensibility to pain.

National Weight Control Registry   A data base of individuals who have lost 30 pounds of weight or more and have kept it off for a year.

Nautilus   A brand of exercise equipment designed for strength-training programs; uses a principle to help provide optimal resistance throughout the full range of motion.

negative caloric balance   A condition whereby the caloric output exceeds the caloric intake, thus contributing to a weight loss.

negative nitrogen balance   A condition in which dietary protein is insufficient to meet the nitrogen needs of the body. More nitrogen is excreted than is retained in the body.

net protein utilization   *See* NPU.

neural tube defects   Birth defects involving incomplete formation of the neural tube in the spinal column of newborn children; may lead to paralysis; may be prevented by adequate folate intake.

neuropeptide Y   Neuropeptide produced in the hypothalamus; a potent appetite stimulant.

neutron activation analysis   A sophisticated, noninvasive method of analyzing body structure and function.

newton   A unit of force that will accelerate 1 kilogram of mass 1 meter per second per second.

niacin   Nicotinamide; nicotinic acid; part of the B complex and an important part of several coenzymes involved in aerobic energy processes in the cells.

niacin equivalent   A unit of measure of niacin activity in a food related to both the amount of niacin present and that obtainable from tryptophan; about 60 mg tryptophan can be converted to 1 mg niacin.

nickel   A silvery-white metallic element.

nicotinamide   An amide of nicotinic acid; niacin.

nicotinic acid   Niacin.

nitrogen   A colorless, tasteless, odorless gas comprising about 80 percent of the atmospheric gas; an essential component of protein that is formed in plants during their developmental process.

nitrogen balance   A dietary state in which the input and output of nitrogen is balanced so that the body neither gains nor loses protein tissue.

nonessential amino acids   Amino acids that may be formed in the body and thus need not be obtained in the diet; also known as dispensable amino acids. *See* essential amino acids.

nonessential nutrient   A nutrient that may be formed in the body from excess amounts of other nutrients.

nonheme iron   Iron that is found in plant foods; *see* heme iron.

nonprotein nitrogen   Nitrogen in the body and foods that is associated with nonprotein compounds.

normohydration   The state of normal hydration, or normal body-water levels, as compared with hypohydration and hyperhydration.

NPU   Net protein utilization; a technique used to assess protein quality.

NPY   *See* neuropeptide Y.

NTD   *See* neural tube defects.

nutraceutical   A nutrient that may function as a pharmaceutical when taken in certain quantities.

nutrient   Substances found in food that provide energy, promote growth and repair of tissues, and regulate metabolism.

nutrient density   A concept related to the degree of concentration of nutrients in a given food; *also see* the related concept INQ.

nutrition   The study of foods and nutrients and their effect on health, growth, and development of the individual.

nutritional labeling   A listing of selected key nutrients and Calories on the label of commercially prepared food products.

obesity   An excessive accumulation of body fat; usually reserved for those individuals who are 20–30 percent or more above the average weight for their size.

OBLA   Onset of blood lactic acid. The intensity level of exercise at which the blood lactate begins to accumulate rapidly.

octacosanol   A solid white alcohol found in wheat germ oil.

Olestra   A commercially produced substitute for dietary fat.

omega-3 fatty acids   Polyunsaturated fatty acids that have a double bond between the third and fourth carbon from the terminal, or omega, carbon. EPA and DHA found in fish oils are theorized to prevent coronary heart disease.

onset of blood lactic acid   *See* OBLA.

oral contraceptives   Birth control pills used to prevent conception.

oral rehydration therapy   Fluids balanced in nutrients that help restore normal hydration levels in the body and prevent excessive dehydration.

organic foods   Foods that are stated to be grown without the use of man-made chemicals such as pesticides and artificial fertilizers.

ORT   *See* oral rehydration therapy.

osmolality   Osmotic concentration determined by the ionic concentration of the dissolved substance per unit of solvent.

osmoreceptors   Receptors in the body that react to changes in the osmotic pressure of the blood.

osmotic pressure   A pressure that produces a diffusion between solutions that have different concentrations.

osteomalacia   A disease characterized by softening of the bones, leading to brittleness and increased deformity; caused by a deficiency of vitamin D.

osteoporosis   Increased porosity or softening of the bone.

overload principle   *See* principle of overload.

overtraining syndrome   Symptoms associated with excessive training, such as tiredness, sleeplessness, and elevated heart rate.

overweight   Body weight greater than that which is considered normal; *also see* obesity.

ovolactovegetarian   A vegetarian who also consumes eggs and milk products as a source of high-quality animal protein.

ovovegetarian   A vegetarian who includes eggs in the diet to help obtain adequate amounts of protein.

oxalates   Salts of oxalic acid, which are found in green leafy vegetables such as spinach and beet greens.

oxidized LDL   An oxidized form of low-density lipoprotein that has increased atherogenic potential.

oxygen consumption   The total amount of oxygen utilized in the body for the production of energy; it is directly related to the metabolic rate.

oxygen system   The energy system that produces ATP via the oxidation of various foodstuffs, primarily fats and carbohydrates.

PABA   Para-aminobenzoic acid; although not a vitamin, often grouped with the B complex.

pangamic acid   A term often associated with "vitamin B$_{15}$," the essentiality of which has not been established; often contains calcium gluconate and dimethylglycine.

pantothenic acid   A vitamin of the B complex.

para-aminobenzoic acid   *See* PABA.

partially hydrogenated fats   Polyunsaturated fats that are not fully saturated with hydrogen through a hydrogenation process; *also see* trans fatty acids.

PC   Phosphocreatine; a high-energy phosphate compound found in the body cells; part of the ATP-PC energy system.

peak bone mass   The concept of maximizing the amount of bone mineral content during the formative years of childhood and young adulthood.

pectin   A form of soluble dietary fiber found in some fruits.

pellagra   A deficiency disease caused by inadequate amounts of niacin in the diet.

pentose   A simple sugar containing five carbons instead of six as in glucose.

peptides   Small compounds formed by the union of two or more amino acids; known also as dipeptides, tripeptides, etc., depending upon the number of amino acids combined.

perceptual-motor activities   Physical activities characterized by the perception of a given stimulus and culminating in an appropriate motor, or movement, response.

peripheral vascular disease   Atherosclerosis or blockage of the peripheral arteries.

pernicious anemia   A severe progressive form of anemia that may be fatal if not treated with vitamin B$_{12}$. Usually caused by inability to absorb B$_{12}$, not a dietary deficiency of B$_{12}$.

pescovegetarian   A vegetarian who eats fish, but not poultry.

pesticides   Poisons used to destroy pests of various types, including plants and animals.

pH   The abbreviation used to express the level of acidity of a solution; a low pH represents high acidity.

phenylalanine   An essential amino acid.

phenylketonuria (PKU)   Congenital lack of an enzyme to metabolize phenylalanine, an essential amino acid. May lead to mental retardation if not detected early in life.

phosphagens   Compounds such as ATP and phosphocreatine that serve as a source of high energy in the body cells.

phosphates   Salts of phosphoric acid, purported to possess ergogenic qualities.

phosphocreatine   *See* PC.

phospholipids   Lipids containing phosphorus that in hydrolysis yield fatty acids, glycerol, and a nitrogenous compound. Lecithin is an example.

phosphorus   A nonmetallic element essential to human nutrition.

phosphorus:calcium ratio   The ratio of calcium to phosphorus intake in the diet; the normal ratio is 1:1.

photon absorptiometry   An analytical, noninvasive technique designed to assess bone density.

phylloquinone   Vitamin K; essential in the blood clotting process.

physical activity   Any activity that involves human movement; in relation to health and physical fitness, physical activity is often classified as structured and unstructured.

physical conditioning   Methods used to increase the efficiency or capacity of a given body system so as to improve physical or athletic performance.

physical fitness   A set of abilities individuals possess to perform specific types of physical activity. *Also see* health-related fitness and sports-related fitness.

phytates   Salts of phytic acids; produced in the body during the digestion of certain grain products; can combine with some minerals such as iron and possibly decrease their absorption.

phytochemicals   Chemical substances, other than nutrients, found in plants that are theorized to possess medicinal properties to help prevent various diseases.

phytoestrogens   Phytochemicals that may compete with natural endogenous estrogens; believed to help prevent certain forms of cancer associated with excess estrogen activity in the body.

picolinate   A natural derivative of tryptophan; commercially it is bound to chromium as a means to enhance chromium absorption.

PKU   *See* phenylketonuria.

plaque   The material that forms in the inner layer of the artery and contributes to atherosclerosis. It contains cholesterol, lipids, and other debris.

platelet aggregability   Function of platelets to promote clumping together of red blood cells.

PMS   Premenstrual syndrome. A condition associated with a wide variety of symptoms during the time prior to menses.

polypeptides   A combination of a number of simple amino acids; *also see* peptide.

polysaccharide   A carbohydrate that upon hydrolysis will yield more than ten monosaccharides.

polyunsaturated fatty acids   Fats that contain two or more double bonds and thus are open to hydrogenation.

POMS   Profile of mood states. An inventory to evaluate mood states such as anger, vigor, etc.

positive caloric balance   A condition whereby caloric intake exceeds caloric output; the resultant effect is a weight gain.

Positive Health Life-style   A life-style characterized by health behaviors designed to promote health and longevity by helping to prevent many of the chronic diseases afflicting modern society.

postabsorptive state   The period after a meal has been absorbed from the gastrointestinal tract; in BMR tests it is usually a period of approximately 12 hours.

potassium   A metallic element essential in human nutrition; it is the principal cation present in the intracellular fluids.

power   Work divided by time; the ability to produce work in a given period of time.

power-endurance continuum   In relation to strength training, the concept that power or strength is developed by high resistance and few repetitions, whereas endurance is developed by low resistance and many repetitions.

PRE   Progressive resistive exercise.

pre-event nutrition   Dietary intake prior to athletic competition; may refer to a 2- to 3-day period prior to an event or the immediate pre-event meal.

premenstrual syndrome   *See* PMS.

Pritikin program   A dietary program developed by Nathan Pritikin, which severely restricts the intake of certain foods like fats and cholesterol and greatly increases the consumption of complex carbohydrates.

profile of mood states   *See* POMS.

principle of exercise sequence   Relative to a weight-training workout, the lifting sequence is designed so that different muscle groups are utilized sequentially so as to be fresh for each exercise.

principle of overload   The major concept of physical training whereby one imposes a stress greater than that normally imposed upon a particular body system.

principle of progressive resistance exercise (PRE)   A training technique, primarily with weights, whereby resistance is increased as the individual develops increased strength levels.

principle of recuperation   A principle of physical conditioning whereby adequate rest periods are taken for recuperation to occur so that exercise may be continued.

principle of specificity of training   The principle that physical training should be designed to mimic the specific athletic event in which one competes. Specific human energy systems and neuromuscular skills should be stressed.

proline   A nonessential amino acid.

promoters   Substances or agents necessary to support or promote the development of a disease once it is initiated.

proof   Relative to alcohol content, proof is twice the percentage of alcohol in a solution; 80-proof whiskey is 40 percent alcohol.

prostaglandins   Eicosanoids that possess hormone-like activity in numerous cells in the body.

proteases   Enzymes that catalyze proteins.

protein   Any one of a group of complex organic compounds containing nitrogen; formed from various combinations of amino acids.

protein-Calorie insufficiency   A major health problem in certain parts of the world where the population suffers from inadequate intake of protein and total Calories.

protein complementarity   The practice among vegetarians of eating foods together from two or more different food groups, usually legumes, nuts, or beans with grain products, in order to ensure a balanced intake of essential amino acids.

protein-sparing effect An adequate intake of energy Calories, as from carbohydrate, will decrease somewhat the rate of protein catabolism in the body and hence spare protein. This is the basis of the protein-sparing modified fast, or diet.

proteinuria The presence of proteins in the urine.

provitamin A Carotene, a substance in the diet from which the body may form vitamin A.

psyllium A plant product that contains both water-soluble and insoluble dietary fiber.

purines The end products of nucleoprotein metabolism, which may be formed in the body; they are nonprotein nitrogen compounds that are eventually degraded to uric acid.

PVD See peripheral vascular disease.

pyridoxal A component of the vitamin B group.

pyridoxamine A part of the vitamin B group; an analog of pyridoxine.

pyridoxine A component of the vitamin B complex, vitamin B_6.

pyruvate The end product of glycolysis. Under aerobic conditions it may be converted into acetyl CoA, whereas under anaerobic conditions it is converted into lactic acid.

quackery Misrepresentation of the facts to deceive the consumer.

quality Calories Calories in foods that are accompanied by substantial amounts of nutrients. Skim milk contains quality Calories as it provides considerable amounts of protein, calcium, and other nutrients, while cola drinks provide similar Calories but no nutrients.

radiation Electromagnetic waves given off by an object; the body radiates heat to a cool environment.

rating of perceived exertion See RPE.

RDA Recommended Dietary Allowances; the levels of intake of essential nutrients considered to be adequate to meet the known nutritional needs of practically all healthy persons.

RDI See Reference Daily Intakes.

RE Retinol equivalent; a measure of vitamin A activity in food as measured by preformed vitamin A or carotene, provitamin A; 1 RE equals 5 IU.

reactive hypoglycemia A decrease in blood glucose caused by an excessive insulin response to hyperglycemia associated with a substantial intake of high-glycemic-index foods.

Recommended Dietary Allowances See RDA.

recommended dietary goals Dietary goals for Americans that have been established by a U.S. Senate subcommittee on nutrition; goals stress dietary reduction of fat, cholesterol, salt, and sugar, and increase of complex carbohydrates.

recuperation principle See principle of recuperation.

REE See resting energy expenditure.

Reference Daily Intakes (RDIs) The RDI is used in food labeling as the recommended daily intake for protein and selected vitamins and minerals. It replaces the old U.S. RDA (United States Recommended Daily Allowance).

regional fat distribution Deposition of fat in different regions of the body. See also android- and gynoid-type obesity.

relative humidity The percentage of moisture in the air compared to the amount of moisture needed to cause saturation, which is taken as 100.

relative-weight method A method of determining obesity by comparing the weight of an individual to standardized height and weight tables.

repetition maximum (RM) In weight training, the amount of weight that can be lifted for a specific number of repetitions.

repetitions In relation to weight training or interval training, the number of times that an exercise is done.

resting energy expenditure (REE) The energy required to drive all physiological processes while in a state of rest.

resting metabolic rate See RMR.

retinol Vitamin A.

retinol equivalent See RE.

riboflavin Vitamin B_2, a member of the B complex.

ribose A five-carbon sugar found in several body compounds, such as riboflavin.

risk factor Associated factors that increase the risk for a given disease, for example, cigarette smoking and lung cancer.

RMR Resting metabolic rate; also see BMR and REE.

RNA Ribonucleic acid; nuclear material involved in the formation of proteins in cells.

RPE Rating of perceived exertion; a subjective rating, on a numerical scale, used to express the perceived difficulty of a given work task.

running Although the distinction between running and jogging is relative to the individual involved, a common value used for running is 7 mph or faster.

saccharide A series of carbohydrates ranging from simple sugars (monosaccharides) to complex carbohydrates (polysaccharides).

saccharine An artificial sweetener made from coal tar.

SAD Seasonal affective disorder. Symptoms associated with various seasons of the year, e.g., depression in winter months.

Salmonella A bacteria commonly involved in food poisoning.

salt-depletion heat exhaustion Weakness caused by excessive loss of electrolytes due to excessive sweating.

satiety center A group of nerve cells in the hypothalamus that responds to certain stimuli in the blood and provides a sensation of satiety.

saturated fatty acids Fats that have all chemical bonds filled.

SCFA See short-chain fatty acids.

scurvy A deficiency caused by a lack of vitamin C in the diet; symptoms include weakness, bleeding gums, and anemia.

SDA Specific dynamic action; often used to represent the increased energy cost observed during the metabolism of protein in the body. Also see dietary-induced thermogenesis and TEF.

Seasonal affective disorder See SAD.

secondary amenorrhea Cessation of menstruation after the onset of puberty; primary amenorrhea is the lack of menstruation prior to menarche.

selenium A nonmetallic element resembling sulfur; an essential nutrient.

semivegetarian An individual who refrains from eating red meat but includes white meat such as fish and chicken in a diet stressing vegetarian concepts.

serotonin A neurotransmitter in the brain; may induce a sense of relaxation and drowsiness, possibly associated with fatigue; may also depress the appetite.

serum lipid level The concentration of lipids in the blood serum.

set-point theory The weight-control theory that postulates that each individual has an established normal body weight. Any deviation from this set point will lead to changes in body metabolism to return the individual to the normal weight.

sets In weight training, a certain number of repetitions constitutes a set; for example, a lifter may do three sets of six repetitions per set.

settling-point theory Theory that the body weight set point may be increased or decreased through interactions of genetics and the environment; an environment rich in high-fat foods may lead to a higher set point so that the body settles in at a higher weight and fat content.

shell temperature The temperature of the skin; also see core temperature.

short-chain fatty acids (SCFA) Fatty acids with chains containing less than six carbons.

SI Le Systeme International d'Unite, or the International System of Units; a system of measurement based upon the metric system.

silicon A nonmetallic element.

simple carbohydrates Usually used to refer to table sugar, or sucrose, a disaccharide; may refer also to other disaccharides and the monosaccharides.

Simplesse A commercially produced fat substitute derived from protein.

skinfold technique A technique used to compute an individual's percentage of body fat; various skinfolds are measured and a regression formula is used to compute the body fat.

sling psychrometer A device that incorporates both a dry-bulb and wet-bulb thermometer, thus providing a heat-stress index incorporating both temperature and relative humidity.

slow-twitch fibers Red muscle fibers that have a slow contraction speed; designed for aerobic-type activity.

Smilax A commercial plant extract theorized to produce anabolic effects.

sodium A soft metallic element; combines with chloride to form salt; the major extracellular cation in the human body.

sodium bicarbonate $NaHCO_3$; a sodium salt of carbonic acid that serves as a buffer of acids in the blood, often referred to as the alkaline reserve.

soluble dietary fiber Dietary fibers in plants such as gums and pectins that are soluble in water.

specific dynamic action *See* SDA.

specific heat The amount of energy or heat needed to raise the temperature of a unit of mass, such as 1 kilogram of body tissue, 1 degree Celsius.

specificity of training *See* principle of specificity of training.

sport nutrition The application of nutritional principles to sport with the intent of maximizing performance.

sports anemia A temporary condition of low hemoglobin levels often observed in athletes during the early stages of training.

sports bars Commercial food products targeted to athletes and physically active individuals containing various concentrations of carbohydrate, fat and protein; some products contain other nutrients, such as antioxidants.

sports drinks Popular term for various glucose-electrolyte fluid replacement drinks.

sports gels Commercial food products targeted to athletes; consist primarily of carbohydrate in a gel form.

sports-related fitness Components of physical fitness that, when improved, have implications for enhanced sport performance, such as agility and power.

spot reducing The theory that exercising a specific body part, such as the thighs, will facilitate the loss of body fat from that spot.

standard error of measurement or estimate A measure of variability about the mean. Sixty-eight percent of the population is within one standard error above and below the mean, while about 95 percent is within two standard errors.

standardized exercise An exercise task that conforms to a specific standardized protocol.

standards of identity A list of ingredients that are specified for a particular food product, such as mayonnaise; food manufacturers need not label ingredients if the product conforms to such specifications.

Staphylococcus A bacteria commonly involved in food poisoning.

steady state A level of metabolism, usually during exercise, when the oxygen consumption satisfies the energy expenditure and the individual is performing in an aerobic state.

steady-state threshold The intensity level of exercise at which the production of energy appears to shift rapidly to anaerobic mechanisms, such as when a rapid rise in blood lactic acid exists. The oxygen system will still supply a major portion of the energy, but the lactic acid system begins to contribute an increasing share.

sterols Substances similar to fats because of their solubility characteristics; the most commonly known sterol is cholesterol.

stimulus period In exercise programs, the time period over which the stimulus is applied, such as a HR of 150 for 15 minutes.

storage fat Fat that accumulates and is stored in the adipose tissue; *also see* essential fat.

strength-endurance continuum In relation to strength training, the concept that power or strength is developed by high resistance and few repetitions and that endurance is developed by low resistance and many repetitions.

structured physical activity A planned program of physical activities usually designed to enhance physical fitness; structured physical activity is often referred to as exercise.

subclinical malnutrition A nutrient-deficiency state in which no clinical signs of the nutrient deficiency are observable, but other nonspecific symptoms such as fatigue may be present.

subcutaneous fat The body fat found immediately under the skin; evaluated by skinfold calipers.

sucrose Table sugar, a disaccharide; yields glucose and fructose upon hydrolysis.

sulfur A pale yellow nonmetallic element essential in human nutrition; component of the sulfur-containing amino acids.

sumo wrestling A form of wrestling in Japan.

superoxide dismutase An enzyme in body cells that helps neutralize free radicals.

systolic blood pressure The blood pressure in the arteries when the heart is contracting and pumping blood.

target heart rate range In an aerobic exercise program, the heart-rate level that will provide the stimulus for a beneficial training effect.

TDEE *See* total daily energy expenditure.

TEE *See* thermic effect of exercise.

TEF *See* thermic effect of food.

testosterone The male sex hormone responsible for male secondary sex characteristics at puberty; it has anabolic and androgenic effects.

thermic effect of exercise (TEE) Increased muscular contraction produces additional heat.

thermic effect of food (TEF) The increased body heat production associated with the digestion, assimilation, and metabolism of energy nutrients in a meal just consumed.

thermogenesis The production of heat; metabolic processes in the body generate heat constantly.

thiamin Vitamin B_1.

threonine An essential amino acid.

threshold stimulus The minimal level of exercise intensity needed to stimulate gains in physical fitness.

thromboxanes Eicosanoids that possess hormone-like activity in numerous cells in the body.

thyroxine A hormone secreted by the thyroid gland that is involved in the control of the metabolic rate.

tin A white metallic element.

tocopherol Generic name for an alcohol that has the activity of vitamin E.

tonicity Tension or pressure as related to fluids; fluids with high osmolality exhibit hypertonicity while fluids with low osmolality exhibit hypotonicity.

total body electrical impedance A sophisticated method of measuring the resistance provided by water in the body as a means to predict body composition.

total body fat The sum total of the body's storage fat and essential fat stores.

total daily energy expenditure The total amount of energy expended during the day, including REE, TEF, and TEE.

trabecular bone The spongy bone structure found inside the bone, as contrasted with the more compact bone on the outside.

trace minerals Those minerals essential to human nutrition that have an RDA less than 100 mg.

trans fatty acids Unsaturated fatty acids in which the hydrogen ions are on opposite sides of the double bond.

triglycerides One of the many fats formed by the union of glycerol and fatty acids.

triose A simple sugar having three carbon atoms.

tryptophan An essential amino acid.

Type I muscle fiber The slow-twitch red fiber that provides energy primarily by the oxygen system.

Type IIa muscle fiber The fast-twitch red fiber that provides energy by both the oxygen system and the lactic acid system.

Type IIb muscle fiber The fast-twitch white fiber that provides energy primarily by the lactic acid system.

tyrosine A nonessential amino acid.

ubiquinone *See* CoQ_{10}.

UCP *See* uncoupling protein.

uncoupling protein A protein believed to stimulate thermogenesis in fat tissues; uncouples thermogenesis with the production of ATP, so no ATP is generated in this process.

underwater weighing A technique for measuring the percentage of body fat in humans.

United States Recommended Daily Allowances *See* U.S. RDA.

Universal Gym A brand name for exercise equipment, particularly weights for strength development.

unsaturated fatty acids Fatty acids that contain double or triple bonds and hence can add hydrogen atoms.

unstructured physical activity Many of the normal, daily physical activities that are generally not planned as exercise, such as walking to work, climbing stairs, gardening, domestic activities, and games and other childhood pursuits.

urea The chief nitrogenous constituent of urine and the final product of the decomposition of proteins in the body.

uric acid A crystalline end product of purine metabolism; commonly involved in gout and the formation of kidney stones.

U.S. RDA   The United States Recommended Daily Allowances; the RDA figures used on labels, representing the percentage of the RDA for a given nutrient contained in a serving of the food. The U.S. RDA are now known as the Reference Daily Intake (RDI).

valine   An essential amino acid.

Valsalva phenomenon   A condition in which a forceful exhalation is attempted against a closed epiglottis and no air escapes; such a straining may cause the person to faint.

vanadium   A light gray metallic element.

vanadyl sulfate   A salt form of vanadium; marketed for its anabolic potential.

vascular water   The body water contained in the blood vessels; a part of the extracellular water.

vasodilation   An increase in the size of the blood vessels, usually referring to the arterial system.

vegan   Vegetarian who eats no animal products.

vegetable exchange   One vegetable exchange in the Food Exchange System contains 5 grams of carbohydrate, 2 grams of protein and 25 Calories.

vegetarian   One whose food is of vegetable or plant origin; *also see* lactovegetarian, ovovegetarian, ovolactovegetarian, pescovegetarian, semivegetarian, and vegan.

very-low-Calorie diet (VLCD)   A diet containing less than 800 Calories per day.

very low-density lipoprotein   *See* VLDL.

visceral fat   The deep fat found in the abdominal area; needs special measuring techniques, such as MRI.

vitamin, natural   Often referred to as a vitamin derived from natural sources; i.e., food in nature; contrast with vitamin, synthetic.

vitamin, synthetic   An artificial vitamin commercially produced from the separate components of the vitamin.

vitamin A   Retinol, an unsaturated aliphatic alcohol; fat soluble.

vitamin B_1   Thiamin; the antineuritic vitamin.

vitamin B_2   Riboflavin.

vitamin B_6   Pyridoxine and related compounds.

vitamin B_{12}   Cyanocobalamin.

vitamin B_{15}   Not a vitamin but marketed as one; usual composition is calcium gluconate and dimethylglycine (DMG).

vitamin C   Ascorbic acid; the antiscorbutic vitamin.

vitamin D   Any one of related sterols that have antirachitic properties; fat soluble.

vitamin D_3   The prohormone form of vitamin D, also known as cholecalciferol, formed in the skin by irradiation from the sun. Released into the blood and eventually converted by the kidney to the hormone form of vitamin D.

vitamin deficiency   Subnormal body-vitamin levels due to inadequate intake or absorption; specific disorders are linked with deficiencies of specific vitamins.

vitamin E   Alpha-tocopherol, one of three tocopherols; fat soluble.

vitamin K   The antihemorrhagic, or clotting vitamin; fat soluble.

vitamins   A general term for a number of substances deemed essential for the normal metabolic functioning of the body.

VLDL   Very low-density lipoproteins; a protein-lipid complex in the blood that transports triglycerides, cholesterol, and phospholipids; has a very low density. *Also see* HDL cholesterol and LDL cholesterol.

voluntary dehydration   Intentional loss of body fluids in attempts to reduce body mass for sports competition; techniques include exercise, sauna, and diuretics.

VO_2 max   Maximal oxygen uptake; measured during exercise, the maximal amount of oxygen consumed reflects the body's ability to utilize oxygen as an energy source; equals the cardiac output times the arteriovenous oxygen difference.

waist:hip ratio   The mathematical ratio of the waist girth to the hip girth, usually taken as the smallest waist measurement and the largest hip measurement; may be referred to as gut:butt ratio.

warm-down   A phase after an exercise session during which the individual gradually tapers the level of activity—for example, by jogging slowly after a fast run.

warm-up   Low-level exercises used to increase the muscle temperature and/or stretch the muscles prior to a strenuous exercise bout.

water   A tasteless, colorless, odorless fluid essential to life, composed of two parts hydrogen and one part oxygen (H_2O).

water-depletion heat exhaustion   Weakness caused by excessive loss of body fluids such as through exercise-induced dehydration in a hot or warm environment.

water intoxication   Consumption of excessive amounts of water leading to dilution of body electrolytes. *See also* hyponatremia.

watt   A unit of power in the SI; one watt equals about 6 kilogram-meters per minute.

WBGT Index   Wet-bulb globe thermometer index; a heat-stress index based upon four factors measured by the wet-bulb globe thermometer.

weight cycling   Repetitive loss and regain of body weight; often called yo-yo dieting.

wet-bulb globe thermometer   A device that takes into account the various factors determining heat stress: air temperature, air movement, radiation heat, and humidity.

wheat germ oil   Oil extracted from the embryo of wheat, high in linoleic fatty acid, vitamin E, and octacosanol.

work   Effort expended to accomplish something; in terms of physics, force times distance.

xerophthalmia   Dryness of the conjunctiva and cornea of the eye, which may lead to blindness if untreated; caused by a deficiency of vitamin A.

xylitol   A sugar alcohol that may be obtained from fruits.

yohimbine   A plant extract theorized to stimulate testosterone production and elicit anabolic effects.

zinc   A blue-white crystalline metallic element essential to human nutrition.

zone diet   A high-protein diet plan; the 40-30-30 plan consisting of 40 percent Calories from carbohydrate, and 30 percent each from protein and fat.

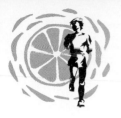

Index